MENTAL HEALTH

A Person-centred Approach
Third edition

T0201278

Australia and Aotearoa New Zealand are nations with diverse communities, and their mental health workers are required to use person-centred approaches to connect with, support and care for people from different backgrounds. *Mental Health: A Person-centred Approach* equips students with the tools they need to provide exceptional, person-focused care when supporting improvement in the mental health of diverse communities.

This third edition has been updated and restructured to provide a logical and comprehensive guide to mental health practice. It includes new chapters on trauma-informed care, different mental health conditions and diagnoses, suicide and self-harm, and the mental health of people with intellectual or developmental disabilities. Significant updates have been made to the chapters on the social and emotional well-being of First Nations and mental health assessment.

Taking a narrative approach, the text interweaves personal stories from consumers, carers and workers with lived experience. Each chapter highlights 'Translation to practice', to help students understand how they might apply theoretical concepts in their day-to-day practice; 'Interprofessional perspectives' to reflect the realities of client contexts and interactions with health and social services; and reflection and end-of-chapter questions and activities to test students' understanding of key theories.

Written by experts in the field, *Mental Health: A Person-centred Approach* remains an essential resource for mental health students.

Nicholas Procter is a professor in the UniSA Clinical and Health Sciences and Inaugural Chair of Mental Health Nursing at the University of South Australia.

Rhonda L. Wilson is a professor of nursing in the School of Nursing and Midwifery, University of Newcastle, Australia and a professor of nursing in the School of Nursing at Massey University, Aotearoa New Zealand. Proudly Wiradjuri, Rhonda now lives and works respectfully on Darkingjung Country.

Helen P. Hamer is an independent consultant with many years of experience in mental health nursing. She holds honorary lecturer positions in the University of Auckland and Yale University.

Denise McGarry is a lecturer in mental health nursing in the School of Nursing, College of Health and Medicine at the University of Tasmania.

Mark Loughhead is the inaugural lecturer of lived experience in mental health within the Nursing and Midwifery Program at the University of South Australia.

Cambridge University Press acknowledges the Australian Aboriginal and Torres Strait Islander peoples of this nation. We acknowledge the traditional custodians of the lands on which our company is located and where we conduct our business. We pay our respects to ancestors and Elders, past and present. Cambridge University Press is committed to honouring Australian Aboriginal and Torres Strait Islander peoples' unique cultural and spiritual relationships to the land, waters and seas, and their rich contribution to society.

Cambridge University Press acknowledges the Māori people as *tangata whenua* of Aotearoa New Zealand. We pay our respects to the First Nation Elders of New Zealand, past, present and emerging.

MENTAL HEALTH
A Person-centred Approach
THIRD EDITION

Edited by
Nicholas Procter
Rhonda L. Wilson
Helen P. Hamer
Denise McGarry
Mark Loughhead

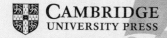
CAMBRIDGE
UNIVERSITY PRESS

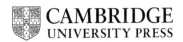

Shaftesbury Road, Cambridge CB2 8EA, United Kingdom

One Liberty Plaza, 20th Floor, New York, NY 10006, USA

477 Williamstown Road, Port Melbourne, VIC 3207, Australia

314–321, 3rd Floor, Plot 3, Splendor Forum, Jasola District Centre, New Delhi – 110025, India

103 Penang Road, #05–06/07, Visioncrest Commercial, Singapore 238467

Cambridge University Press is part of Cambridge University Press & Assessment, a department of the University of Cambridge.

We share the University's mission to contribute to society through the pursuit of education, learning and research at the highest international levels of excellence.

www.cambridge.org
Information on this title: www.cambridge.org/highereducation/isbn/9781108984621

First published 2014
Second edition 2017
Third edition 2022 (version 2, June 2023)

Cover designed by Anne-Marie Reeves
Typeset by Integra Software Services Pvt. Ltd
Printed in Singapore by Markono Print Media Pte Ltd, March 2023

A catalogue record for this publication is available from the British Library.

A catalogue record for this book is available from the National Library of Australia.

ISBN 978-1-108-98462-1 Paperback

Additional resources for this publication are available at www.cambridge.org/highereducation/isbn/9781108984621/resources

Foreword: Carer

In 2013, I was waiting to turn right at the traffic lights when I suddenly became aware of a young man standing at the pedestrian crossing on the opposite side of the road. I looked again at the handsome face. The blonde hair, cut in a style I remember so well. The man was wearing blue jeans and a denim jacket. My heart skipped a beat. The resemblance. Once again, the universe had found a way to bring him back to me for a few moments. My son, Nicholas. My son who, in November 2000, had died in the psychiatric ward of a public hospital in Adelaide. He was 26 years old.

I'd visited Nicholas in hospital shortly before he died. We went for a walk in the grounds of the hospital that day, and I noticed one of the other patients, an elderly woman, was following us. We sat down on a bench and the woman came and stood close by. After a while Nicholas got up and walked over to the woman. He put his hand on her arm very gently and in a quiet voice I heard him say, 'My mother and I are having some time together, would you mind very much moving further away?' The woman nodded and without speaking moved away a little. We started to talk but we were interrupted again; this time the woman had started to sing. Looking over at Nicholas she sang to him. The words of the song were: 'A certain smile, a certain face can lead an unsuspecting heart on a merry chase.' It was an unlikely serenade but he listened attentively to her until she finished singing, then he turned back to me, and we continued our conversation.

At that moment I knew that despite the illness, his essential kindness hadn't left him. That, despite the illness, the essence of Nicholas had not changed. I knew, too, that he'd let her know she mattered. Was valued. He did it by listening to her story. A story that she had sung to him with the words of an old love song.

In this book you will meet courageous people who live with mental illness, and also the people who love and care for them. You will come to know their experiences through reading their stories. It has taken trust for them to share their stories; a trust in you, that as you read them it will be with an open as well as an inquiring mind.

Are stories important? My children, when they were little, seemed to think so. 'Tell me a story,' was a favourite way for them to push back the night, to delay the lights being put out, or to chase away a bad dream with a happy-ever-after ending.

As a young wife and mother of newly born twins and a little one-year-old daughter, Sarah, one of my favourite times was when an invitation would come from my kindly neighbour, Vivian, to 'put the kettle on'. I'd bundle the children into the big old pram and set off to her house across the road.

Sarah had been born with a major heart abnormality and was often in need of urgent medical attention. I was often anxious in those days, and the chance to talk it over with my neighbour, to 'tell her my story' was a great release. 'Tell me about it,' Vivian would say and, sitting in the sunny family room, drinking cups of tea, I'd tell her about the worries of the day.

Often, it concerned me not being able to coax Sarah to eat or even drink very much. The medication prescribed to help regulate her little heart also had the unfortunate side-effect of being an appetite suppressant.

'Is her colour too pale? Do her little fingers look blue to you?' I'd want to know. Sometimes, all I needed was reassurance that all was well. At other times we would decide that maybe it was best to call in the local doctor to have a look at Sarah. But always it was that listening ear – as well as wise counsel that my friend gave me – that was important to me.

The founders of Alcoholics Anonymous believed stories were important. The remarkable program of recovery from addiction devised by them includes the regular attendance of members at meetings, where they are encouraged to tell their stories and to listen to the stories of others. Along with the 12 steps or suggestions, it is in the listening and in the telling of stories that Bill Wilson and Dr Bob believed a transformation could occur.

'Is it real or is it pretend?' my children would ask me sometimes as I'd start the bedtime story. The day that Nicholas, now an adult arrived at my apartment and, looking wildly around, produced a notepad and pen and wrote 'Don't talk. We are being monitored by agents … ' I knew that the pretend story he was writing was very real to him. I tried to reassure him that he was safe, but the words I wrote on the notepad that he gave me didn't help him. I knew he was very ill, that something was terribly wrong. Eventually, I phoned a friend and together we managed to get Nicholas into my car and drove to the hospital. He was admitted immediately. A few hours later I was told that he'd been transferred to a psychiatric ward and that the diagnosis was drug-induced psychosis.

Nicholas was 22 years old when this first admission occurred. He'd been studying at university and had an ambition to become a writer. But after this time his life changed; there were more hospital admissions and he was diagnosed with mental illness and drug dependency – comorbidity.

Over the following four years there were some periods of relative well-being. Nicholas spent a number of times at a Buddhist retreat in New South Wales and learned the practice of meditation. He travelled to India and Nepal. He fell in love and told me that one day they would have an amazing child together. He tried to get back to studying again.

But drugs came back into his life, and this time the anti-psychotic medication he'd been prescribed was not effective. Nicholas rang to tell me that he'd decided to go into hospital as a voluntary patient, to be introduced to a drug his doctor advised might help him. 'Clonazepam does have risks of major side-effects and would need to be carefully monitored', I was advised by his doctor. 'It's worth a try, Mum', he told me as I drove with him to the hospital. He was admitted and commenced the process of coming off one anti-psychotic medication and being introduced to another.

Sometime later, Nicholas rang me from the hospital. 'I've decided to quit drugs, Mum, and I'm going to start a methadone treatment tomorrow.' He went on to explain that it was all arranged. The hospital would organise a taxi to take him to the nearby clinic, and then after he'd been given the methadone a taxi would be called to return him back to the hospital. He'd decided to turn his life around. A new medication for the mental illness and a new treatment to come off heroin. He rang me the night before he died and we talked about the new treatments. We ended the call as we always did: 'I love you, Mum', he told me. 'And I love you too, Nicholas … '

Three days after starting the methadone treatment combination with Clonazepam Nicholas was found dead on the floor near his hospital bed. The autopsy result was death due to mixed drug toxicity. A coroner's report two years later resulted in a verdict of 'accidental death by drug toxicity', with strong recommendations for changes to procedures by hospital administrations in relation to treatment of drug withdrawal when combined with certain anti-psychotic drugs.

A week after Nicholas died, I received a call from the hospital's social worker, who offered to deliver his possessions that were left at the hospital. They were given to me in a green plastic bin-liner. His doona with a large blood stain. Although I'd read in the autopsy report of the internal haemorrhage he'd had moments before he died, I had not understood that reality until I saw the blood-stained doona.

I looked at the rest of his possessions the hospital had returned to me. His Doc Martens. Blue jeans. A denim jacket. A t-shirt with 'Champion' written across the front. A portable chess set. A transistor radio. A writing pad and biro. The book he'd been reading, with a piece of paper folded as a bookmark, Gore Vidal's *Judgement of Paris*. There was also a black wallet I'd given him a few years earlier. Neatly tucked into one of the folds was a receipt. It was dated two days before he died. It was a receipt for a layby; a $5 deposit on a black leather jacket at St Vincent de Paul's Opportunity Shop. The shop was near the clinic where Nicholas had gone to receive the methadone treatment.

In those last days he'd been creating a new life for himself –

A new medication to take away the psychosis
A way out of dependency on drugs
And a new-to-him black leather jacket to wear.
He'd been creating a happy-ever-after ending to his story.

To all the students reading this book, I wish you every success with your studies. It's my belief that mental illness is one of the great challenges of our time. To find a cure for schizophrenia. A medication without major side-effects. To care for people with mental illness in times of crisis with insight and compassion … these are my hopes for you.

Margaret O'Donnell

Foreword: Consumer

The best nurse I ever had walked beside me and never got in my way. She would appear unobtrusively by my side and gently encourage me to get off my bed and go for walks with her. She hardly said a thing to me, but I could feel her calmness and acceptance through all the static of my distress. Other nurses got in my way; they tore off my blankets, threatened me, berated me for being inappropriate or for not facing the world, or gave me strange looks when I expressed my pain.

In their training and professional development, nurses learn many things – much of it is irrelevant to the experience of the person using the service. I do not remember any of the nurses I encountered for their professional skills. But I do remember them for their human qualities. Above all, I remember the nurses who were kind and compassionate.

Compassion is hard to teach and impossible to enforce, but it is the single most important attribute any mental health professional needs to develop. Compassion means being able to stand in the shoes of the other and be with the person in her or his distress. It allows the helper to stand on the ledge between deflecting the other person's pain and losing herself or himself in it. Compassion takes a strong sense of self, patience and an acceptance of difference.

Unfortunately, compassion cannot thrive in services that control people and pathologise their experience. A recovery based, trauma-informed service promotes people's autonomy, respects their subjectivity and does not tolerate iatrogenic harm; this is the best setting for compassion to grow. Wherever we work in the mental health system we have a responsibility to foster compassion, not only in our one-to-one relationships with the people who use the service and our colleagues, but also in creating a service environment that encourages empowering and respectful relationships at all levels. A person-centred service is meaningless without compassion.

Mental Health: A Person-centred Approach is a recovery-based text for undergraduate nurses in Australia and New Zealand. This book is a compass for your journey to becoming a mental health nurse whose compassion service users will remember.

Mary O'Hagan

Contents

3 Māori mental health   44

Kerri Butler and Jacquie Kidd

4 The social and emotional well-being of First Nations Australians   61

Katrina D. Ward and Rhonda L. Wilson

9   Use of psychotropic medicines in mental health care   173

Mark Loughhead, Simon Bell, Davi Macedo and Nicholas Procter

16   Intellectual and developmental disability   360
Henrietta Trip, Margaret Hughes, Reece Adams and Isaac Tait

17   Mental health of children and young people   379
Rhonda L. Wilson and Serena Riley

About the authors

Editors

Nicholas Procter PhD MBA GradDip Adult Ed BA CertAdvClinNsg RN. Nicholas is the University of South Australia's Inaugural Chair of Mental Health Nursing and director of the Mental Health and Suicide Prevention Research and Education Group, located within UniSA Clinical and Health Sciences.

Rhonda L. Wilson RN BNSc NM(Hons) PhD. Rhonda is a professor of nursing in the School of Nursing and Midwifery, University of Newcastle, Australia and a professor of nursing in the School of Nursing, Massey University, Aotearoa New Zealand. She is proudly Wiradjuri, raised on Anaiwan land, and lives and works respectfully on Darkingjung Country. Rhonda is an internationally regarded mental health nursing academic with collaborations throughout Australia, Aotearoa New Zealand, Scandinavia, Europe, the United Kingdom and the United States. She has wide-ranging experience in clinical mental health nursing in rural and regional Australia, and in teaching nursing and mental health curricula to undergraduate and postgraduate students. Her main research interests are in mental health, digital health and the social and emotional well-being of First Nations, and to design and support innovative digital health interventions suitable for the promotion of mental health, well-being and recovery among diverse and hard-to-reach populations throughout the world.

Helen P. Hamer is an independent consultant with many years of experience in mental health nursing, and a Fellow at Te Ao Māramatanga: New Zealand College of Mental Health Nurses. Helen's research focuses on citizenship, social justice and social inclusion for people with mental health problems. Helen is recognised internationally as a leader in the development of consumers as co-researchers and academics, and the facilitation of recovery-focused and trauma-informed practice. Helen holds honorary lecturer positions at the University of Auckland, School of Nursing and Yale University's Programme for Recovery and Community Health, Department of Psychiatry.

Denise McGarry PhD. Denise is a credentialled mental health nurse and a Fellow of the Australian College of Mental Health Nurses. She teaches at the University of Tasmania, in the School of Nursing, College of Health and Medicine, as a lecturer in mental health nursing. In this capacity she enjoys working with undergraduate and postgraduate students.

Mark Loughhead is the inaugural lecturer of lived experience in mental health within the Nursing and Midwifery Program at the University of South Australia. His work aims to promote lived-experience perspectives relating to personal recovery and person-centred care, and the redesign of mental health supports and systems with lived-experience leadership and co-production. Mark is a lived-experience leader within his university's Mental Health Suicide Prevention Research and Education Group. There, he guides research and education relating to the lived-experience workforce and the recovery-orientated practice skills of lived-experience and clinical workforces. His background includes 25 years in community mental health education, consumer advocacy and tertiary education.

Contributors

Reece Adams has a background in occupational therapy and has worked in the field of intellectual and developmental disabilities for the past 17 years. Reece is the Head of the Centre for Developmental Disability Health, Victoria, within Monash Health in Victoria, Australia. He is also a member of the International Association for the Scientific Study of Intellectual and Developmental Disabilities (IASSIDD) and the IASSIDD Health Special Interest Research Committee, as well as an Associate Member of the Australian Association for Developmental Disability Medicine.

Amy Baker PhD BHSc(Hons)(OccTh) BAppSc(OccTh). Amy is a lecturer in the Occupational Therapy Program at the University of South Australia. She has undertaken research and projects in a range of areas including autism, palliative care, loss, grief and human flourishing in the context of mental illness. Amy's research and teaching focus on mental health and suicide prevention, including the psychosocial effects of community gardens and healing environments, and the effects of severe mental illness on work. She also has strong interests in engaging people from culturally and linguistically diverse backgrounds in this field, and in research approaches that are qualitative and participatory in nature.

Kirsty Baker is a lecturer in mental health nursing at the University of South Australia. She teaches within the Bachelor of Nursing and Graduate Diploma of Mental Health Nursing courses. She has a special interest in psychosis and consumer preference of care. She continues to work as a clinical mental health nurse in the emergency department setting, where she provides mental health assessment and supportive nursing care for consumers and their families in times of crisis.

Jane Barrington is a mental health nurse with a particular interest in curriculum development in mental health nursing education. She has a background in working with service users who have experienced significant trauma and mental distress subsequent to interpersonal abuse. Jane is interested in social justice and social change as strategies for reducing mental distress in Aotearoa New Zealand.

Simon Bell is a professor and the Director of the Centre for Medicine Use and Safety at Monash University and an adjunct professor of geriatric pharmacotherapy in the Faculty of Health Sciences at the University of Eastern Finland. His research interests primarily relate to the use of medicines among older people, particularly psychotropic and analgesic medicines.

Kerri Butler is *tangata whai ite ora* and has worked in the field of mental health in various roles, including lived-experience leadership roles. She is from the Ngapuhi *iwi* in the Hokianga and has Ngati Porou affiliations with the east coast of Aotearoa New Zealand.

Andrea E. Donaldson is a senior lecturer in the School of Health at Massey University, Manawatu campus, in Aotearoa New Zealand, where she teaches in mental health and addictions programs for undergraduate and postgraduate nursing students. She has been a registered nurse for 20 years and has worked in a variety of practice areas, such as cardiothoracic and vascular health, high-dependency unit, cardiology, surgery, emergency, adult mental health and forensic mental health. Andrea is also a qualified biochemist and has a PhD in forensic science. She is of Ngati Manipoto descent in the Waikato region of Aotearoa New Zealand. Andrea's research interests are in nursing education, mental health and forensic science, where she is investigating non-fatal strangulation and its mental health consequences.

Monika Ferguson PhD. Monika is a research fellow in mental health and suicide prevention at UniSA's Clinical and Health Sciences faculty. She obtained her PhD in psychology at the same university and has completed postgraduate studies in suicide prevention studies at Griffith University. Her program of research is funded by Suicide Prevention Australia and focuses on educational interventions to reduce suicide and improve support for people following a suicide attempt. Monika teaches in mental health programs for undergraduate and postgraduate students and is actively involved in curriculum design.

Lisa Hodge PhD. Lisa is a research fellow in the Institute for Health and Sport, and Deputy Leader of the Active Living and Public Health Group at Victoria University. Her research focuses on the link between eating disorders and trauma, in particular, and mental health more broadly, as well as arts-based research methods. Lisa's recent book is entitled *Eating Disorders and Child Sexual Abuse* (2021).

Margaret Hughes is a senior nursing lecturer in Aotearoa New Zealand with an interest in disability nursing and its inclusion nursing education programs. Margaret's focus is on how the families of people living with a disability are included, welcomed and valued in the health system.

Mary Anne Kenny BJuris LLB LLM. Mary Anne is an associate professor of law at Murdoch University. She researches and publishes in the areas of refugee law and human rights. Mary Anne is the former Chair of the Law Reform Commission of Western Australia. She has been a legal practitioner for over 25 years.

Jacquie Kidd PhD MN RN. Jacquie is a mental health nurse of Māori (Ngāpuhi) descent. She is an associate professor at Auckland University of Technology in Aotearoa New Zealand and has a research focus on co-designing solutions to health inequity with Māori communities.

Debra Lampshire is an expert by experience and a professional teaching fellow at the University of Auckland in Aotearoa New Zealand, and has an extensive background as a mental health educator. She is employed by Auckland District Health Board as a project manager for the psychological interventions for an enduring mental illness project. In this unique and innovative position, Debra works in the clinical setting, leading the development of psychological strategies for positive symptoms of psychosis, and she is the first non-clinician to do so. She is Aotearoa New Zealand chairperson of the International Society for Psychological and Social Interventions for Psychoses (ISPS) and a member of its international executive committee. Debra has received both the 'Making a Difference' award and the Supreme award from Attitude ACC for her leadership in mental health in New Zealand and internationally.

Davi Macedo PhD. Davi is a research associate in the UniSA Mental Health and Suicide Prevention Research and Education Group. His research work focuses on risk and protective factors for the mental health and well-being of vulnerable populations. He obtained his PhD at the University of Adelaide, looking at the effects of racism on Aboriginal children's social and emotional well-being. He is investigating principles for adapting trauma-informed practice and person-centred approaches when responding to people in mental distress – including self-harm and suicidal crisis – during the COVID-19 pandemic. Davi also practices as a psychologist, working with young people and families with complex needs.

Kerry Mawson is a registered nurse with qualifications in mental health, drug and alcohol counselling and higher education. Kerry has worked in a variety of clinical areas including drug and alcohol services, adult mental health and adolescent services. She has held a teaching position at the Australian Catholic University for 13 years while maintaining her clinical practice in various roles at a major teaching hospital. She is a clinical supervisor and panel member for the Nursing and Midwifery Council, regularly speaks at training days and conferences and has a publication history. Kerry works as an educational consultant for Mental Health Drug and Alcohol Services at a local health district in Sydney, New South Wales.

Kate Rhodes RN BPsych BHSc(Hons)PhD. Kate is an experienced mental health clinician and academic, active in the development, delivery and evaluation of mental health programs within UniSA's Clinical and Health Sciences. Kate has worked clinically as a registered nurse for over 30 years in general medical, developmental disability, predominantly in mental health. She has extensive experience across a range of mental health settings including crisis intervention in suicide prevention, emergency mental health assessment, and mental health and suicide prevention education. After completing a first-class honours degree in psychology in 2011, Kate graduated with a PhD in the School of Medicine at Flinders University, South Australia in 2017. Throughout her career Kate has demonstrated extensive understanding of community engagement in mixed-methods research and evaluation, report writing and high-level reviews of evidence.

Serena Riley RN BN (UNE) GCPaedNurs GCNeoNurs. Serena is a registered nurse. After completing a Bachelor of Nursing at the University of New England, Armidale in New South Wales, Serena completed two graduate certificate courses, in paediatrics and neonatal special care. Her position as a senior clinical nurse within the paediatric unit, alongside her personal history of recovery from a mental illness, has given Serena unique perspective and understanding when caring for patients with mental health issues. Serena has also undertaken humanitarian work in India, South Africa, Uganda, Egypt and Greece, where she observed some of the unique challenges faced by people across the globe. Serena works within the Queensland health sector, specialising in the treatment of people recovering from eating disorders.

Bernadette Solomon is a senior lecturer in mental health and addictions at Massey University, Auckland in Aotearoa New Zealand. She has been a registered and psychiatric nurse for over 30 years. Bernadette has extensive experience as a mental health nurse academic and educator, and her specialty practice is in forensic mental health nursing. Bernadette's research has focused on mental health recovery and explored the experience and meaning of recovery-oriented practice for nurses working in acute in-patient mental health services. She is particularly passionate about the empowering potential of embedding recovery-oriented practice into mental health services and nurse education. Her other research interests are in nursing education, mental health and forensic mental health, where she is investigating non-fatal strangulation and its mental health consequences.

Anne Storey is a nurse practitioner in the Royal Prince Alfred Parent and Baby Unit Mental Health Service, Sydney Local Health Service in New South Wales.

Isaac Tait is a consumer of health services who lives with several disabilities in Aotearoa New Zealand. Isaac is also a successful artist and a member of a mixed-abilities drama group providing social commentary on living and working with a disability.

Sue Thomson is a registered psychiatric and comprehensive nurse. Over the past 42 years Sue has worked in mental health services, primarily with older adults as a nurse specialist, community mental health nurse, charge nurse, facility manager and as the Northern Regional Dementia Behavioural Support and Advisory Coordinator for all of Auckland and Northland in Aotearoa New Zealand. Sue took on the role of General Manager Mental Health and Aged Care for a large non-government organisation in 2019, managing multiple services for all ages, including a dementia unit and a private hospital seeking to provide an activities-based approach to a population with significant behavioural symptoms of dementia. In dementia services, Sue's specialist areas continue to include those with early onset dementia, management of the behavioural and psychological symptoms of dementia, and dementia in people with pre-existing functional disorders.

Henrietta Trip RN DipNS BN MHealSc(Nurs)(Dist) PhD(Otago). Henrietta is a senior lecturer and academic lead in the Master of Health Sciences program, at the Centre for Postgraduate Nursing Studies, University of Otago, Christchurch, in Aotearoa New Zealand. Her teaching focuses primarily on healthcare access and equity for populations considered vulnerable, and on developing knowledge and capacity for nursing to work alongside these populations. Henrietta's research is specifically linked to long-term conditions, self-efficacy, supported decision-making and management practices for people with learning, intellectual or developmental disability, with a particular interest in the effects and responsiveness of social models of disability.

Katrina D. Ward RN MBA MMHN BN DipCouns DipSEWB. Katrina is a descendant of the Ngiyampaa people whose country is located in the Central North West of New South Wales. Katrina has lived and worked in the health sector for most of her life and is passionate about promoting and improving the physical and emotional well-being of Aboriginal people. She has a wealth of clinical mental health knowledge and experience, particularly in the areas of social and emotional well-being, suicide intervention, grief and loss, and substance abuse. Katrina is the Chief Operations Manager at Walgett and Brewarrina Aboriginal Medical Services. As an Aboriginal person working in a senior role within the Aboriginal Community Controlled Health Organisation (ACCHO) sector, Katrina is keen to assist in nurturing young Aboriginal people to follow their hopes and dreams, and to believe that anything is achievable. Through sharing her personal achievements, Katrina strives to raise hope and inspiration for individuals in recognising that self-determination and having a positive attitude can assist in achieving their dreams. She supports education as a means to becoming empowered and increasing general knowledge as a pathway to achieving personal goals and successes throughout life's journey.

Personal narrative contributors

Breeana Alder is the Nursing Unit Manager of the Transplant Unit at Royal Prince Alfred Hospital, Sydney, New South Wales. Breeana previously worked as the clinical nurse educator in the same unit.

Seung An has been working as a pharmacist for over 10 years, in various specialty areas in hospitals as well as community pharmacies. She has been specialising in mental health pharmacy as a clozapine coordinator since 2019, at the Professor Marie Bashir Centre (PMBC) in Camperdown, New South Wales. Seung is the secretary of the Medication Reference Committee Meeting at PMBC and has been ensuring medication safety and quality use of medicines. She enjoys staff education, including for pharmacy students, pharmacists and medical and nursing staff.

Michael Barton PhD MEd (Counselling and Guidance) BEd. Michael is Director of Teaching and Learning at a New South Wales independent school.

Edwina Casey RN. Edwina completed her nursing degree at the University of New England, in New South Wales, in 2012. At that time, she found her mental health placement an eye-opening clinical experience. Not only did she discover mental health as a completely different aspect of nursing, but also a demanding yet a rewarding area of nursing to be a part of – one that many nurses and other health professionals underestimate. Edwina is undertaking her new graduate year in Hobart, Tasmania, in a cardiothoracic ward. She encourages nursing students to make the most of their mental health unit and clinical placement, and to rise to the challenge of promoting a greater awareness of mental health in rural and remote areas in Australia.

Rachael Casey has 16 years of experience as a nurse in various areas, including renal and liver transplant, gastroenterology and drug health, during which she has been a clinical nurse educator and nursing unit manager in these units. Rachael has undertaken postgraduate study, including a Graduate Certificate in Renal Nursing, Masters of Clinical Nursing, Masters of Healthcare Leadership, and Masters of Health Management. Rachael has been nominated and has received awards for Excellence in Education, Excellence in Management and Excellence in Clinical Leadership.

Phil Escott has been working with Sydney Local Health District, New South Wales as a senior peer support worker for over 20 years. He is passionate about engaging with consumers in clinical settings to provide hope, offer kindness and empathy, and to enable personal recovery. Phil is an example of someone who has recovered from mental health challenges and uses his lived experience to empower other consumers in their own journeys to recovery. Phil also gives presentations, runs groups and collaborates in research, and provides mentoring for new peer workers.

Michael Evans is a security manager for Royal Prince Alfred Hospital, Sydney in New South Wales. He has been a leader in the progression of security in hospitals for staff, patients and visitors for many years.

Shane Fenwick MTheol GradDipTheol BAPsych. Shane has 10 years' experience in working and volunteering in the not-for-profit sector. He has worked with at-risk young people, refugees, people living with psychosocial disability, and in faith-based community development. Having had his own lived experiences, Shane is passionate about improving outcomes for those living with mental health issues and illness. He is currently undertaking the Master of Occupational Therapy at the University of Sydney, with plans to work as a mental health clinician.

Matthew Halpin is an established, lived-experience and mental health leader with diverse experience across peer workforce development, lived-experience leadership, research, and state and national reform. Matt is an assistant director at the National Mental Health Commission, where he has worked across national policy and reform, including national disaster mental health support and stigma-reduction strategies.

Alison Hansen is a mental health nurse and lecturer at Monash University in Victoria, with a background in forensic mental health nursing, specifically working with women in this setting. She is undertaking in a Doctor of Philosophy (Nursing) to explore the use and experiences of seclusion by women in forensic mental health settings. Alison has taught in and coordinated pre-registration programs, and has taught in post-registration nursing programs, with her main teaching focus being on mental health and law and ethics for nurses. Alison's teaching passion is in supporting students to think critically about their practice and to challenge ideas and promote mental health in order to break down barriers and support inclusion within a supportive learning environment. She has a strong interest in reducing stigma, supporting recovery-oriented mental health practice, and reducing, and where possible, eliminating the use of restrictive interventions.

James Robert Hindman MBA MBusMan BN. James has worked in a variety of roles in emergency, acute and community mental health care in regional and rural New South Wales. He is passionate about improving services through service design, profession development and reflective practices.

Jemima Isbester is a survivor of childhood trauma, mental health issues, addiction, domestic violence, homelessness and suicidality. She is passionate about structures of support that hold space for meaning-making, such as intentional peer support, open dialogue, 'Mad studies', hearing voices and alternatives to suicide, and the integration of peer work into clinical mental health services. Her pronouns are she and her.

Tara McAndrew is a registered paramedic and lecturer at the University of Tasmania, with over 20 years' experience in the field. Tara is passionate about education in mental health and understands the unique role paramedics play in caring for people in the community. Tara has established a mental health education program for student paramedics that is highly regarded among industry professionals.

Paul McNamara RGN RPN BN MMHN Cert IMH CMHN FACMHN. Paul is a mental health nurse working Cairns. He has established an extensive professional social media portfolio using the homophone 'meta4RN' (read as either 'metaphor RN' or 'meta for RN'). For more information about Paul visit his website at meta4RN.com and/or follow him via @meta4RN on Twitter, Facebook, YouTube or Instagram.

Rosalie Menadue has worked as a mental health nurse with in-patients at The Rozelle Hospital and Concord Centre for Mental Health, and as a community case manager and clinician in the Acute Care Service in the Sydney Local Health District in New South Wales. She is a clinical nurse specialist at Buduwa, a Step Up, Step Down PARC model facility located in Burwood, Sydney. She has also been an active branch official (as president, secretary and/or delegate) in the New South Wales Nurses and Midwives' Association.

Leigh Murray is a family advisor for mental health services in Auckland District Health Board and the Chair for Family Connections (National Education Alliance for Borderline Personality Disorder) in Aotearoa New Zealand.

Bonnee Nash has been working as a peer support worker for two years and is passionate about breaking down stigmas around addiction and mental health. She advocates giving a voice to the voiceless and role modelling that there is hope for recovery and living a life with quality and purpose. Bonnee loves hiking, photography and helping people to help themselves, through highlighting their own strengths and capacity to grow, evolve and change.

Kathryn Sweegers has 10 years' experience in non-government mental health support working in a variety of roles, including carer support, early intervention mental health support for children and young people, and management of national psychosocial support programs for individuals living with severe and persistent mental health issues.

Emily Walker is a registered nurse working as a clinical nurse consultant at Royal Prince Alfred Hospital Sydney, New South Wales. She works in the emergency department, general and mental health hospital setting, with people who may experience substance use issues.

Geraldine White works as a mental health nurse practitioner in Consultation Liaison Psychiatry at Canterbury Hospital, which includes working as the clinical lead for the Sydney Local Health District Transitional Nurse Practitioner Team. Geraldine commenced undergraduate nursing studies in 1987, and completed a master's degree in 1992. Her career has spanned in-patient nursing, community nursing, crisis team nursing, consultation liaison nursing and psychotherapy. Geraldine has worked in private practice and has contracted to non-government organisations. She converted her nursing degree to a nurse practitioner qualification and registration in 2007.

Acknowledgements

The authors are extremely grateful to Emily Baxter, Lucy Russell and other staff at Cambridge University Press for their thoughtful guidance and support, and to Renée Otmar for her editing excellence. We also gratefully acknowledge the lived and living experience of consumers and carers, for their wisdom and guidance, and the contributions of practitioners who have openly discussed and shared their stories and experiences.

The editors and Cambridge University Press would like to thank the following for permission to reproduce material in this book.

Figure 4.1: generated on Wordclouds.com. **Figure 7.1**: from Van Orden, K. A., Witte, T. K., Cukrowicz, K. C., Braithwaite, S. R., Selby, E. A. & Joiner, T. E., Jr. (2010). The interpersonal theory of suicide. *Psychological Review*, *117*(2): 575–600. © 2010 by American Psychological Association. Reproduced with permission. **Figure 8.1**: © Australian Institute of Health and Welfare. Licenced under Creative Commons BY 3.0 licence, https://creativecommons.org/licenses/by/3.0/au/. **Figure 8.2**: © Ministry of Health. Licenced under Creative Commons BY 4.0 licence, https://creativecommons.org/licenses/by/4.0/. **Figure 12.1**: © Yee Mon Oo 2021. Reproduced with permission. **Figure 13.1**: © King's Fund. Reproduced with permission. **Figures 13.2–13.4** and **13.6**: © Commonwealth of Australia 2011. Reproduced with permission. **Figure 13.5**: © Mitchell Institute at Victoria University, Melbourne. Reproduced with permission. **Figure 15.1**: © Domestic Abuse Intervention Project, 2017. Reproduced with permission. **Figure 15.2**: © The Royal College of Psychiatrists 2006 from Read, J., Hammersley, P. & Rudegeair, T. (2007). Why, when and how to ask about childhood abuse. *Advances in Psychiatric Treatment*, *13*(2): 101–10. Reproduced with permission. **Figures 17.1** and **17.2**: © Elinor Irvine. Reproduced with permission. **Figure 19.1**: © Commonwealth of Australia. Licenced under Creative Commons Attribution 4.0 International (CC BY 4.0), https://creativecommons.org/licenses/by/4.0/.

Table 13.1: © International Diabetes Federation 2006. Reproduced with permission. **Table 13.2**: © Commonwealth of Australia 2011. Reproduced with permission.

Extract from The Uluru Statement of the Heart: © Commonwealth of Australia 2017. Licenced under Creative Commons Attribution 4.0 International licence, https://creativecommons.org/licenses/by/4.0/legalcode.

Every effort has been made to trace and acknowledge copyright. The publisher apologises for any accidental infringement and welcomes information that would redress this situation.

Introduction to mental health and mental illness

Human connectedness and the collaborative consumer narrative

Nicholas Procter, Amy Baker, Kirsty Baker, Lisa Hodge,
Davi Macedo and Monika Ferguson

1

LEARNING OBJECTIVES

At the completion of this chapter, you should be able to:

1 Describe the nature and scope of a narrative approach in mental health practice.
2 Explain key concepts of trauma-informed practice and what it means in the context of person-centred care, and meaningful engagement between practitioners and consumers, carers and family members.
3 Explain key concepts such as mental health and mental illness; identify and discuss the determinants of mental health such as social, cultural, biological, environmental, employment/work and societal determinants; and discuss stigma and beliefs about mental illness and its effect on help-seeking.
4 Contextualise mental health nursing as a specialist field in which support is built in collaboration; and discuss enablers and barriers to meaningful engagement between practitioners and consumers, carers and family members.
5 Discuss collaborative practice in mental health care in the context of recovery; and discuss consumer participation, human rights, vulnerability and practical aspects of human connectedness as a means of engaging with people and communities at risk.

Introduction

This chapter reflects a coming together of key issues and themes embedded in everyday work with **consumers** and **carers**. In recent times, the definition of a carer has expanded to include immediate family and friends, and also to include extended family members such as grandparents and cousins. In transcultural and other contexts, it is important to use humanistic language, in line with a recovery approach; for example, the terms 'support person/people' and 'support networks' may be preferable to the term 'carer' in mental health practice and mental health nursing. This approach provides a foundation for human connectedness and sets the consumer narrative as central to mental health practice and to mental health nursing, specifically.

consumer – a person who uses or has used a mental health service, or who has a lived experience of a mental illness

carer – a person who provides assistance, care and support for someone who has a mental illness

PERSONAL NARRATIVE

Michael's story

My name is Michael. I'm 24 years old and single. I was recently taken to the emergency department of my local hospital, by ambulance. Apparently, my mother was concerned because she could not rouse me. I've been told that upon arrival the level of alcohol detected from my breath was pretty high, and I'd also taken some Valium tablets. Once the alcohol level in my system was reduced, I was referred to the hospital's mental health team for assessment. I spoke to a nurse, Melissa, and explained that, although I am aware of the risk of using alcohol with other drugs, I had no intention of trying to hurt myself.

I used to be a sociable, funny guy at school, with loads of friends. When I was 21, I was assaulted during a night out with friends in the city. Since then, everything seems to have been off – completely changed. I've noticed a change in my personality and behaviour. I often feel irritable and tearful, lacking energy and motivation. I feel down most days, and I've given up on finding work after I lost my job last year. I also have nightmares, so I use alcohol to get to sleep. For the past three years, I have been drinking around eight beers a night and up to 16 beers on weekend nights. To help me get to sleep, I take two to three Valium tablets most nights, and I also occasionally smoke cannabis. I know that this isn't helping but I don't know what else to do.

I talked to Melissa about how I often feel isolated from others and hopeless about my situation. At times, I've even thought of ending it all. These kinds of thoughts tend to be worse when I've been drinking and can't sleep. I explained to Melissa that I also have trouble being in crowds. I live in shared accommodation, and I visit the local supermarket for groceries once per fortnight. My brother visits me weekly; he tries to encourage me to get out of the house but I find this too stressful. I would really like to get back to being the person I used to be. I'd like to find a job and be able to catch up with my friends again, but I feel so overwhelmed and don't know how to get better.

REFLECTIVE QUESTIONS

- What are some of the signs of concern about Michael's mental health and well-being?
- Do you think some people might be at higher risk to experience mental health difficulties after adverse life events?

A narrative approach to mental health

The story of Michael – and many others within this book – is central to both the narrative and person-centred approach taken in each chapter. A person-centred approach is concerned with human connectedness: the capacity for feelings to be received and understood, and lives to be revealed. A narrative approach illuminates the needs of the person with a mental health condition, their family, carers and **practitioner** through an interactive process of dialogue and information exchange. At a deeper level, narrative is a means of storytelling.

Given the complex and dynamic nature of working with people experiencing mental illness, interprofessional cooperation is not only required but essential. In this book we refer to different professional categories: nurses, mental health nurses, practitioners, medical practitioners and health workers, to illustrate the range of interprofessional roles and contexts in which care takes place. Reference to one category is not meant to exclude additional health and human services workers whose intervention can potentially benefit people receiving care.

Storytelling is a profoundly human capacity. Both the teller and listener work together – in interaction – to build meaning. The listener experiences the reality of being the narrator and actively contributes to the storytelling. A narrative is thus constructed in cooperation, based in shared experience and knowledge (Michel & Valach, 2011). Such activity is central to the practice of mental health nursing. This is because the discourse itself involves stories that together become a joint action.

The alternative to a narrative approach is application of a structured or mechanistic style of engagement and interaction. Rather than creating a forum for the sharing of various perspectives and possibilities, this approach is largely monologic. In an interview situation (for example) the interviewee is asked a list of questions. Learning is by a predetermined 'case study' that is defined by a distinctive feature, disease or condition. There is an absence of knowing the person, who they are and what they stand for and, in some instances, the person is lost completely. In this situation, a person's life is subjected to being impersonally processed, with little opportunity to contribute a perspective on what actually lies behind their situation, life difficulty or aspiration to live a healthy and socially engaged life.

A narrative approach in the context of this book has special meaning. By combining the best evidence in mental health with the opportunity to know and understand the human connections that can and should be made in mental health care, this book adopts an all-encompassing approach to engaging with, responding to and supporting people with mental illness. It signals a change in the nature and context of learning by promoting alternative points of view and lived experience in mental health. Each chapter encompasses relevant information pitched at a level suited to an undergraduate student while simultaneously making sense of the consumer's and/or carer's voice and experience. The consumers, carers and practitioners who have contributed to this book have changed their names to protect their anonymity. Each has had a direct experience in recovering from mental illness, using mental health services or providing mental health support. This form of writing is valuable for both student and academic readers, as it draws from key evidence in the field as well as our relationship to it. The desired outcome of narrative thinking is for the chapters and adjunctive learning materials to reveal a new story through conversational partnership between the student and the text. Dominant themes are examined, discussed and, where necessary, challenged. If the student can empathically put themselves in the place of the person

practitioner – a professional in health or human services working with people who have lived experiences of mental distress, and their carers and family members

with a mental illness, then it will be possible to move beyond current thinking toward new and fresh thinking. This task can be made more productive through reflective questions and thinking about opportunities for translation to practice.

How can we start thinking about a narrative approach to mental health care?

A narrative approach to mental health care invites the person, practitioners and carers to cooperate in building an understanding of what care means for the person in a given context and situation. To consider how these approaches might look like in practice, reflect on the following questions:

- What questions would you ask a person about their experiences of mental health conditions? What do you think would be important to know?
- Based on your own experiences in health or mental health services, what would you like a nurse, mental health nurse or other practitioner to know about the way you are feeling about your current condition?
- What are some of the challenges for practitioners and other health workers in adopting a narrative approach to mental health care? Why do you think this happens?

Trauma-informed practice

A narrative approach to understanding mental health is closely aligned with the idea of trauma-informed practice. Put succinctly, trauma-informed practice means that services and professionals (including managers and supervisors) engage with consumers and carers in a trauma-informed manner. This assumes that many people seeking a service could potentially have experienced significant trauma at some point in their lives. It does this to help prevent an escalation of distress and deterioration in behavioural, emotional, physical and psychological well-being. Health and human services are guided by the goal of achieving optimal health and well-being for the consumer, underpinned by best practices regarding safety, agency, connection, belonging, meaning, identity, justice, dignity and value. Professional groups work from the premise of universal understanding, whereby the workers assume that all people accessing a service have experienced some form of trauma. In this context, trauma is defined as 'the personal experience of interpersonal violence including sexual abuse, physical abuse, severe neglect, loss and/or the witnessing of violence, terrorism and/or disasters' (National Association of State Mental Health Program Directors Centre for Trauma Informed Care (NCTIC), 2015). Such events are usually repetitive, intentional, prolonged and severe, which means that the effect of trauma can be pervasive and complex.

Universal understanding of trauma as a potential feature in the life of a person with a mental health condition arises from the highly influential Adverse Childhood Experiences (ACE) study (Felitti et al., 1998). The ACE study involved a comprehensive survey of more than 13 000 participants to identify adverse experiences of psychological, physical or sexual abuse; violence against mother; or living with household members who were substance abusers, mentally ill or suicidal, or ever imprisoned. The study reported that people often experience more than one category of ACEs. Multiple ACEs were linked to the presence of multiple risk factors for poor health outcomes later in life. Noticeably longer exposure to ACEs increased the likelihood of risk factors for several of the major causes of death in adulthood (Felitti et al., 1998; Felitti, 2002).

With such significant evidence, the underlying assumption within trauma-informed care is a universal precaution to 'do no harm' (Muskett, 2014), and with the purpose of preventing, ameliorating and not exacerbating the negative effects of trauma. Taking into account the work of Elliot and colleagues (2005) and the National Centre for Trauma Informed Care (NCTIC; 2015), a trauma-informed practitioner, program, organisation or system is one that:

- realises the widespread effect of trauma on the development and coping strategies of the individual, and potential paths to recovery
- recognises signs and experiences of trauma in consumers, families, staff and others involved in the system
- strives for therapeutic relationships that develop safety and trust in the individual (that is, non-traumatising, comforting relationships)
- demonstrates respect for the individual's need for safety, respect and acceptance
- emphasises the person's strengths by focusing on adaptations rather than symptoms; resilience rather than a reliance on pathology alone
- works towards maximising the individual's choice and control over their recovery
- responds by fully integrating knowledge about and implications of trauma into policies, procedures and practices
- actively seeks to resist re-traumatisation.

Defining mental health and mental illness

Mental health

Mental health is an overall state of well-being and functioning. It is closely related to the ability to cope with and bounce back from adversity, solve problems in everyday life, manage when things are difficult and cope with everyday stressors. Mental health is made possible by a supportive social, friendship and family environment, work–life balance, physical health and, in many instances, reduced stress and trauma.

A survey by the Australian Institute of Family Studies over 12 years (2001–12) of more than 27 000 people aged between 15 and 90 years enquired into participants' satisfaction with common life events. The study revealed that, overall, Australians were content with their lives (Qu, de Vaus & AIFS, 2015). Participants were asked to give a score on a scale of zero to 10 (maximum score) to indicate their happiness and contentment across their life events. The average score across domains was seven. Similarly, a mean score of 7.4 was observed in a nationally representative sample in 2017 (Park, Joshanloo & Scheifinger, 2019). This suggests that, overall, Australians have been happy and content with their lives in the recent past. However, several million people are living with a mental illness.

The most recent data on prevalence estimates of mental illness, based on a diagnostic tool, is from the 2007 National Survey of Mental Health and Wellbeing. The study estimated that, of the 16 million Australians aged 16–85 years in 2007, almost half (45 per cent, or 7.3 million) would experience a mental condition at some point in their lives (Australian

Bureau of Statistics (ABS), 2007). This percentage would now correspond to 8.7 million people (Australian Institute of Health and Welfare (AIHW), 2019). Each year, an estimated one in five (approximately 3.9 million in 2017) Australians present with a mental disorder (ABS, 2007; AIHW, 2019). It is also estimated that in 2019–20, 4.4 million patients (approximately 17 per cent of the Australian population) received a mental-health related prescription, and in 2018–19, $10.6 billion was spent on mental-health related services (AIHW, 2021a). Another indicator of the effects of mental health conditions is the burden of disease. This is a measure of the estimated effects of different health conditions in terms of years of life lost or years of life lived with disability/impaired functioning. In 2018, Australians suffered a greater burden of living with illness (52%) than from premature death (48%). Anxiety (6.4 per 1000) and depression (5.8 per 1000) conditions were the second cause of non-fatal burden, behind coronary heart disease and lung cancer (AIHW, 2021b). This means these are the second-largest conditions that prevent people from living meaningful, fruitful and productive lives.

Mental illness

Mental illness is a clinically diagnosable condition that significantly interferes with an individual's cognitive, emotional and/or social abilities (Department of Health, 2009). The diagnosis of mental illness is generally made according to the classification systems of the *Diagnostic and Statistical Manual of Mental Disorders* (DSM) (American Psychiatric Association (APA), 2013) or the International Classification of Diseases (ICD) (World Health Organization (WHO), 2013a; Department of Health, 2009). Mental illness affects people of all ages, nationalities and socio-economic backgrounds, and affects the lives of many people in our communities, as well as their families and friends. The experience of mental illness is common, with the most recent national data from diagnostic tools indicating that 45 per cent of the population (aged 16 years and older) in Australia and 40 per cent in Aotearoa New Zealand have experienced a mental illness at some point in their lives (ABS, 2007; Oakley Browne, Well & Scott, 2006). Moreover, approximately one in five adults in Australia and Aotearoa New Zealand experience a mental illness each year (ABS, 2007; Oakley Browne et al., 2006).

According to the most recent diagnostic information, in both Australia and Aotearoa New Zealand, mental illness is more commonly experienced by young people. The prevalence of mental illness is typically highest in people aged between 16 and 24 years. This includes the experience of anxiety and depression, conditions associated with substance misuse and longer-term conditions such as anxiety, chronic and recurrent depression and schizophrenia. Comorbidity (the experience of more than one condition or disease simultaneously by an individual) is quite high. For example, of those individuals in Aotearoa New Zealand who experience an illness over 12 months, 37 per cent experience more than one (Oakley Browne et al., 2006). The most likely co-occurrence is of anxiety and mood conditions (Oakley Browne et al., 2006). In both countries, women are more likely to experience mental illness than men, and this is largely accounted for by the higher incidence of anxiety conditions among women (ABS, 2007, 2018; Ministry of Health, 2015). Despite the relatively high prevalence of mental illness among adults in Australia and Aotearoa New Zealand, between 61 and 65 per cent of people with a 12-month or longer mental health condition do not receive treatment for their mental illness (ABS, 2007; Oakley Browne et al., 2006). In Australia, however, an increase in treatment rates has been observed, with a rise from about 36 per cent in 2007 to approximately 46 per cent in 2009–10 (ABS 2007; Whiteford et al., 2014).

Rates of mental illness among Aboriginal and Torres Strait Islander peoples are currently undetermined. However, the 2012–13 Australian Aboriginal and Torres Strait Islander Health Survey (AIHW, 2015) indicates that Indigenous people are 2.7 times more likely than non-Indigenous Australians to report either high or very high levels of psychological distress, which indicates a higher probability of mental illness. Similarly, the 12-month prevalence of mental illness among Māori and Pacific Islander peoples is 29.5 per cent and 24.4 per cent, respectively (compared to 21 per cent for the broader Aotearoa New Zealand population; Oakley Browne et al., 2006); this also indicates a higher incidence of mental illness among individuals in these populations.

Contemporary approaches

As is sometimes seen in the popular media, cinema and TV, people with a mental illness are typically portrayed as only having an illness; one that is best managed away from the community and subject to closed institutional care and, in some instances, inhumane treatment. While it is important to communicate factors associated with diagnostic categories, nowadays the practice of mental health care in Australia and Aotearoa New Zealand places a strong emphasis on human rights, personhood, advocacy, care in the least restrictive environment, early intervention and safety for people with a mental illness.

Let's take the story of Michael and relate it to events in South Australia as an example of a contemporary approach. On 1 July 2010, a new Mental Health Act took effect in South Australia, the *Mental Health Act 2009* (SA), with the broad purposes of protecting the rights and liberties of people with mental illness; ensuring that their dignity and liberty are retained as far as may be consistent with their protection; protecting the public; and the proper delivery of services. The Act also aims to ensure the accessibility and delivery of specialist treatment, care, rehabilitation and support services for people with mental illness, and the creation of appropriate and effective processes for engagement between consumers and service providers, including transportation and orders for community treatment, detention and treatment. For a person like Michael, the Act means that staff must engage with him in a meaningful and collaborative way in the design of a care plan to enable Michael's full recovery with dignity (Mendoza et al., 2013). Michael must also be supported through provision of appropriate transportation, should it be required under the Act for him to receive compulsory in-patient treatment.

Social determinants of mental health

The social determinants of health are the circumstances in which people are born, grow up, live and work, and the systems that are in place to support them to deal with illness (Commission on Social Determinants of Health, 2008). These circumstances are all shaped by wider societal factors, and by the social and economic conditions in which people live. Mental health promotion is therefore not only the responsibility of the healthcare sector, but also of many other sectors such as housing, education and employment (World Health Organization (WHO) and Calouste Gulbenkian Foundation, 2014).

According to Keleher and Armstrong (2005), the social determinants of mental health can be categorised into four areas (see Table 1.1).

Table 1.1 The four social determinants of mental health

Social determinant	Description
Individual	A person's ability to manage their feelings, thoughts and life in general, their emotional resilience and ability to deal with stress. Adequate rest, sleep and proper nutrition also contribute to an overall sense of well-being and ability to cope.
Community	A person's social supports, social connectedness, having a good sense of belonging and an opportunity to actively participate in their community. For some people with strong cultural and social affiliations, understanding and responding to a mental health condition is largely guided and derived from self-identity through community affiliation and cultural belonging.
Organisation	Factors such as safe housing, employment options and educational opportunities, access to good transport and a political system that enhances mental health. This also includes mentally healthy workplace practices known to support people in mental distress.
Whole society	Social structures that exist in education, employment and justice to address inequities and promote access and support to people who are vulnerable.

Source: Adapted from Keleher and Armstrong (2005).

Keleher and Armstrong (2005) suggested that mental health promotion can enhance supportive social conditions and create positive environments for the good mental health and well-being of populations, communities and individuals. Mental health promotion requires action to influence determinants of mental health and to address inequity through the implementation of effective, multi-level interventions across a wide number of sectors, policies, programs, settings and environments (Keleher & Armstrong, 2005, p. 13).

The mental health practitioner acts as an advocate for people with mental illness in accessing services in housing, education and employment, with the aim of developing beneficial outcomes in a way that enables the consumer to retain as much control as possible over how it is carried out.

TRANSLATION TO PRACTICE

Understanding the social determinants of mental health can help us guide our practice

Nabil is a 36-year old man with a Syrian background who presents for consultation due to physical and mental health concerns. He reports having lost 5 kilograms in the past two weeks, along with his appetite, and being sleep deprived for two nights. Nabil is on unpaid leave and is concerned about maintaining his job as his ability to concentrate is affected. He has recently divorced, which contributes to his feelings of isolation (his main source of support was his former wife's family). Nabil discloses that he had lived in a refugee camp for three years and recently nightmares and flashbacks about this experience have become more frequent. Nabil reports feeling like he has no control of what is happening around him. He also discloses having diabetes and not being able to properly monitor his diet or medication.

Consider what factors at the individual, community, organisation and societal levels could have contributed to Nabil's mental health difficulties. What kind of support at each level could improve Nabil's sense of well-being? Consider the specific intervention and services in your response.

The practitioner understands how stigma might prevent consumers from taking up opportunities to engage with available resources. The expectation of consumer advocacy is thus individual empowerment. The mental health practitioner stands alongside the consumer, to strengthen their voice and to enhance their resilience (Department of Health, 2013).

Mental illness and life expectancy

Mental illness can have a significant effect on life expectancy. A systematic review and meta-analysis of 148 English-language studies reported that people with a mental illness had a mortality rate 2.22 times higher than the general population, with an estimated 8 million worldwide deaths per year being attributable to mental illness (Walker, McGee & Druss, 2015). The review found a median reduction in life expectancy of 10.1 years for people with a diagnosis of mental illness, with a greater risk for mortality among those diagnosed with psychoses, mood disorders and anxiety. An Australian survey of people living with psychotic illness (n = 1825) (of whom just under 50 per cent had a diagnosis of schizophrenia) reported that, in the previous month, 33 per cent of participants did not have breakfast on any day of the week (Morgan et al., 2011). In the same survey, 41.5 per cent ate only one serving or less of vegetables a day, and 7.1 per cent did not eat any vegetables at all (Morgan et al., 2011).

Since nutrition is inextricably linked to physical health, it is not surprising that the major cause of death in people with a diagnosed mental illness is not suicide, as many believe, but cardiovascular diseases. While mental health practitioners are well-practised in assessing risk of self-harm, they are less familiar with assessing risk of cardiovascular disease. Given that people with a serious mental illness are more likely to be inactive, obese and smoke, compared to the general population, it can be seen that the incidence of metabolic syndrome is more common in this population group (Parish, 2011). It must be noted that, in addition to the effects of second-generation anti-psychotic medications, inactivity, overweight and obesity are also the results of psychotropic medication. In this circumstance, poor physical health is associated with the combined elements of the mental health condition as well treatment by psychotropic medication (Correll, Detraux, De Lepeleire & De Hert, 2015).

The largest proportion of deaths due to non-communicable disease in people diagnosed with a mental illness is closely associated with metabolic syndrome, namely cardiovascular diseases (48 per cent), followed by cancers, chronic respiratory diseases and diabetes, which alone is directly responsible for 3.5 per cent of deaths. Behavioural risk factors, including tobacco use, harmful use of alcohol, physical inactivity and an unhealthy diet, are estimated to be responsible for about 80 per cent of coronary heart disease and cerebrovascular disease. Behavioural risk factors for metabolic syndrome are associated with four key metabolic changes: hypertension, obesity, hyperglycaemia and hyperlipidaemia (WHO, 2012). A large-scale, systematic review and meta-analysis reported that approximately one in three patients diagnosed with schizophrenia present with a metabolic syndrome (Mitchell et al., 2013).

The combined and cumulative nature of diet, lifestyle and treatment factors have substantial effects on both quality of life and life expectancy. A systematic review covering studies from 25 countries concluded that people with schizophrenia have a standardised mortality ratio for all-cause mortality of 2.58, or 2.5 times the risk of dying (Saha, Chant & McGrath, 2007). Also important is the knowledge that the physical health care needs of people with a mental illness are often neglected by health care workers, due to stigma. Often, physical complaints are disregarded by practitioners who label the consumer as anxious or somatically focused. Given the vast amount of evidence that people with a mental illness are more likely to suffer poor cardio-metabolic health (Correll et al., 2015), practitioners need to listen carefully to the needs of consumers and act to reduce the incidence of cardiovascular disease.

Mental health practitioners and nurses work at the intersection of mental and physical health, and they have a vital role to play in improving standards of physical care. Mental health workers have an important role in monitoring how medications affect consumers and their physical health needs. Psychotropic and other forms of medication can cause, or at least contribute towards, adverse physical health effects, including premature disability and death. There is tremendous scope to improve the quality of physical care for people with a severe mental illness through direct care practices, such as including questions about health symptoms in standard health assessments, sharing information between medical practitioners and specialists, and offering advice on diet, exercise and sleeping habits, when necessary (Happell et al., 2011).

At the same time, many people with mental health conditions are not formally engaged with mainstream mental health services in an integrated and sustainable way (Mendoza et al., 2013). Collaborative practice in mental health must be inclusive of this group and may occur through other health contacts such as primary care and community health services. Health promotion activities, illness prevention and early intervention are all ways in which the mental health practitioner, together with the multidisciplinary team, can provide the best care to people with a mental illness who are at risk of developing life-threatening conditions (Happell et al., 2011).

Mental illness and substance misuse

Among people diagnosed with mental illness, there is an emerging picture worldwide suggesting that illicit substance involvement is on the rise (WHO, 2013b). Boredom among young people and increased exposure to substances such as cannabis, amphetamines and methamphetamines are believed to have contributed to the breakdown of traditional, community-based groups (such as clubs and societies), which foster belonging and encourage peer support and community involvement (Procter, 2008). Referred to as 'comorbidity' or 'dual diagnosis', the co-occurrence of a mental health condition and a substance misuse condition is both complex and widespread. It is well established that drug and alcohol misuse is commonly experienced by people with a mental health condition. According to the Australian National Mental Health and Wellbeing Survey (ABS, 2007) 63 per cent of Australians who reported that they had misused drugs nearly every day within the previous 12 months had also experienced a mental health condition in the same time period. More recently, in 2016, people who reported drinking at risky levels were 1.2–1.3 times as likely to self-report having received a mental health diagnoses or mental health-related treatment. The same risk was 2.5 times higher among those who reported smoking daily. Mental health conditions or very high levels of psychological distress are especially common among people who engage in illicit drug use. People who use methamphetamines, for example, are three times as likely to self-disclose a mental health diagnosis when compared to the non-illicit drug using population (AIHW, 2017).

Comorbid mental health and alcohol and other drug conditions are more likely to be experienced by young people with a background involving trauma, including being a refugee, when compared to their Australian-born peers. Studies have shown that significant barriers to service engagement and service provision exist for young people from refugee backgrounds with one condition, and Posselt and colleagues (2014) reported that the risk may increase for those experiencing comorbidity, as they not only face disrupted or fragmented cultural affiliations and 'cultural and linguistic barriers, but are also often required to effectively navigate two different service sectors' (p. 19).

Mental illness and homelessness

The prevalence of mental illness among homeless people in Australia is equally as significant, with research suggesting that rates of mental illness in homeless people are four to five times higher than in the general population (Schizophrenia Fellowship of NSW Inc., 2008). More specifically, of the 241 000 people aged 10 years and over who received support from specialist homelessness agencies in 2017, one in three (over 81 000) reported a current mental health condition (AIHW, 2019). These background factors are often closely associated with a lack of supportive accommodation options for people with mental health conditions, the transfer of people with unstable mental health conditions to community settings, the episodic nature of mental illness and uncontrolled use of, and access to, illicit stimulants (Schizophrenia Fellowship of NSW Inc., 2008).

Mental illness and violence/aggression

A recent review of the literature examining crime and violence in people with schizophrenia, with and without comorbid substance-use conditions, concluded that although most people with the condition do not engage in criminal behaviour, schizophrenia is associated with increased risk of violent offending, independent of substance misuse status. Besides offending, people with schizophrenia receive police intervention due to participating in family violence more often than those without the condition (Short et al., 2013). Having a diagnosis of schizophrenia is claimed to be a particularly strong risk factor for violence in females, yet this finding is not conclusive. This situation is made more difficult when we take into account two intersecting and interrelated issues. First is the notion that people with severe mental illness experience significantly more problems in interpersonal relationships, and family members may often be the targets of violent behaviour (Short et al., 2013). Second is the considerable and continuing stigma and prejudice associated with mental illness in the wider community (Pescosolido, 2013).

Mental illness and risk

Some people are more vulnerable and at higher risk of developing a mental illness than others. The factors that may contribute to a person's risk include trauma and abuse, social isolation, homelessness, socio-economic disadvantage, physical or intellectual disability and genetic predisposition. Harmful use of alcohol and other drugs can significantly increase the occurrence of mental illness. We also know that people from Aboriginal, Torres Strait Islander and Māori communities are more vulnerable to developing a mental illness secondary to intergenerational trauma suffered during European settlement and colonisation (Council of Australian Governments (COAG), 2012; Stewart-Harawira, 2005). Some people with mental illness experience disadvantage such as lowered educational achievement, lack of social connectedness, poverty, poor physical health and reduced life expectancy. These disadvantages may influence whether someone with a mental health condition is able to access the help needed. Practitioners are responsible for being aware of these risk factors and how they affect the lives of people with mental illness.

The first signs of mental illness may emerge in childhood, adolescence or early adulthood. Young people at risk of developing a mental illness may be those who have been bullied at school, are children of parents with a mental illness or children linked with the criminal justice system, or refugees, or children brought up in traumatic circumstances. These children or young people at risk may already be linked to services that offer counselling, or may be part of a youth group. It is therefore important for the wider community, across cultures and across the lifespan, to be able to identify and respond to people in mental distress in order to offer support early and reduce the risk of the person's situation becoming worse and more distressing (COAG, 2012).

Mental illness and stigma

stigma – a form of prejudice that involves inaccurate and hurtful representations of people due to belonging to a social group; in the case of people with mental illness, those representations are dehumanising and might include being violent, manipulative, comical or incompetent

Stigma and discrimination are factors that can prevent a person from seeking help for their troubles and concerns. In general, the public – including some health professionals – perceives people who experience mental illness as difficult, dangerous and unpredictable, and those with chronic mental health conditions such as schizophrenia are the most feared (Mental Health Council of Australia (MHCA), 2011). This perception can result in perpetual discrimination, othering and stigma (Corrigan, Rafacz & Rusch, 2011). Stigma can be defined as a spoiled identity that discredits a person in society who possesses an attribute that makes them different from others and perceived as less desirable; a person who is considered bad, sinister, dangerous or weak (Goffman, 1963). These negative attributes are devalued in a particular social context, and are endorsed by a set of prejudicial attitudes and discriminatory behaviours (Corrigan, 2004; Corrigan et al., 2011). Stigma exists in the behaviour and responses of others, and in institutional decision-making (e.g. decision-making about insurance cover or travel and employment opportunities). It is often also internalised by the stigmatised persons themselves, affecting their sense of self, their self-esteem and perceived capacities (Corrigan et al., 2011).

Stigma can also be manifested at an implicit level due to strongly associated ideas between concepts – in this case mental health and mental illness – and the meaning and interpretation we learn about them from social messages. For example, a derogatory stereotype identified in the general public is that people with an experience of mental illness have limited abilities for independence and have weak characters (Link et al., 1999). Since health practitioners might have been exposed to similar socialisation processes, the same stereotypes are often also held about people with mental illness, potentially influencing the quality of care delivered to consumers and carers.

On one side of the spectrum, health professionals can be perceived as being insensitive and having low expectations of people with mental illness, but also as benevolent and paternalistic, on the other (Lamont & Dickens, 2019; Wahl & Aroesty-Cohen, 2010). Implicit stigma has been linked to mental health professionals' tendency to over-diagnose (Peris, Teachman & Nosek, 2008). Especially relevant to this discussion are findings that perceptions of people with mental illness experiences include that they are dangerous and that implicit stigma is associated with lower recovery attitudes. Practitioners with stereotypical ideas were less likely to endorse a process of change based on promotion of hope, empowerment and resilience (Stull et al., 2017).

Mental health practitioners need to challenge the problem of stigma, which can be deeply embedded in people's experience of the labels of mental illness, and can lead to their competence being questioned. Implicitly held beliefs can manifest subconsciously and therefore practitioners must be aware of their own implicit biases and how these can influence their practice. They need to support efforts to prevent mental ill health and promote health, wellness and resilience. Practitioners need to support the rights of people with mental illness and enable them to participate in meaningful ways in society. Community awareness through mental health promotion can reduce discrimination and increase opportunities for prevention and early intervention (Commonwealth of Australia, 2009).

Beliefs about mental illness

Another important part of the understanding and experience of working with people who have a mental illness is consideration of the beliefs about what causes or contributes to the onset of mental illness. Different potential reasons or causes for mental illness that have been suggested range from life events such as the loss of significant relationships to genetic factors, substance misuse and factors such as witchcraft or spiritual possession (Choudhry et al., 2016; Larkings & Brown, 2018; Stefanovics et al., 2016). Explanations for the origins of mental illness are often clustered into broader categories, such as biological, psychological or social factors (Choudhry et al., 2016). Other classifications for causal factors include factors that are considered internal or external, or controllable or uncontrollable by the person (Elliott, Maitoza & Schwinger, 2011). It is thought that beliefs about the origins of mental illness are affected by factors including a person's sex or gender identity, cultural background or belief system (Choudhry et al., 2016; Stefanovics et al., 2016; Von Lersner et al., 2019).

Within the biomedical model of psychiatry, mental illness is largely attributed to malfunctioning in the brain. However, people who have lived with mental illness propose a much wider range of possible reasons (Elliott et al., 2011). Increasingly, the field of trauma experience is being identified by consumers as an approach that offers different, non-pathological ways of describing distress, experience and attempted coping behaviours (Muskett, 2014). This approach, along with other alternative views and languages to describe them can be found among consumers with significant experience of formal mental health care. Many consumers develop alternative explanations for their experiences and are often critical of the psychiatric language of disorder and illness. Consumers may seek views and responses from helpers who accept alternative views and are not based on 'fear of risk' responses or 'being fixed' (Our Consumer Place, 2010).

Sandy Jeffs is an Australian writer who has been diagnosed with schizophrenia; in her writing she has pondered the possibilities of what may have been the basis for, or contributed to, the onset of mental illness in her situation:

> How does one explain the experience of falling into madness, one's mind fracturing? Somewhere in there festers my fraught relationships with my parents, the early experience of sexual assault, a confused attraction to Catholicism, and contradictory feelings of self-loathing and self-aggrandisement … My childhood was awful. I have wondered many times whether its crushing weight was what tipped my fragile mind over the edge. Or was my madness simply a biochemical imbalance that would have developed anyway? (Jeffs, 2009, p. 18)

The process of considering these possibilities was an important one for Jeffs, who noted that 'through the process of uncovering and reconstructing my life in sequence and through reflection,

I can make sense of it' (Jeffs, 2009, p. 18). Making sense of mental illness is a process that often involves moving between – or abandoning – various beliefs and making it a period marked by both movement and uncertainty (Kaite et al., 2015). The explanations people attribute to mental illnesses are important for a range of reasons. Beliefs about the causes of mental illness may influence people's preferences and expectations for treatment and engagement (Choudhry et al., 2016), and therefore also carry important consequences for recovery.

Mental health care focuses on consumer recovery as a principle for care delivery that embodies the concepts of consumer self-determination, resilience and self-management in determining nursing interventions. Contemporary care should also promote access to peer support workers and groups. Peer support creates opportunity for the consumer to explore diverse aspects of their experience, and to learn about the self and others, in practical and meaningful ways outside of the clinical context. This may include access to peer-based models, such as the Hearing Voices groups (Longden, Read & Dillon, 2018) or Alternatives to Suicide (Western Massachusetts Recovery Learning Community, 2020). Promoting hope and therapeutic optimism in people with a mental illness is an essential ingredient of person-centred care that all practitioners need to practise. The aim is to develop the person's self-confidence and to promote belief in their own capacity to recover, reach goals and transcend boundaries (Edward et al., 2011).

Mental health nursing

Mental health nursing is primarily concerned with responding to people with mental illness and supporting them with a recovery framework. Mental health nursing practice is grounded in the needs of consumers and deployed to the person's support and carer network, where this exists. This book seeks to demonstrate this practice using a range of techniques. In developing each chapter, the authors draw on input from people with lived experience of mental illnesses, their families, carers and practitioners at various levels to help illuminate key issues.

The approach in this book is consistent with what many believe to be fundamental to mental health nursing. The Australian College of Mental Health Nurses (ACMHN; 2015) states that 'mental health nursing is a unique interpersonal process, which promotes and maintains behaviours that contribute to human flourishing for individuals and communities'.

Mental health nursing can be therapeutic in itself, as it is centred in developing an honest and trusting relationship of care. The concepts of caring and compassion are implicated in mental health nursing practice, where the goal is to support people experiencing difficulties in their social, emotional and physical functioning. In addition, mental health nursing is centred on empowering people to become active and – whenever possible – autonomous in making self-care related choices and voicing their own needs. The practice of care expands from the person to their peers and carers, in a comprehensive approach to promoting mental health care (ACMHN, 2015).

The mental health nurse is a non-judgemental, ethically aware professional who responds to the needs of the consumer in a flexible and open manner. The practitioner works alongside people with a mental illness to empower, advocate and support individuals and their families to find ways of coping with the difficulties they face. The practitioner helps the person to discover and ascribe individual meaning to their experiences and to explore opportunities for recovery and personal growth.

PERSONAL NARRATIVE

Alex: Michael's nurse

Working as a clinical mental health nurse in the city's major emergency department, I received a referral from an emergency department's medical officer for a young man named Michael. Michael had been brought in by ambulance after his mother found him at home, unable to be roused. Michael had consumed alcohol and taken an overdose of 40 mg diazepam. On arrival, his breath alcohol reading indicated an estimated 0.32 blood alcohol content (BAC). Michael was referred to me once his BAC had reduced to 0.05.

I approached Michael in a relatively low-key manner and explained who I was. He agreed to talk to me about how he had been feeling and why he took an overdose of medication the previous night.

Michael said he had been feeling down 'for ages' and has been using more and more alcohol and marijuana to help him cope. Using his description of the situation, I considered Michael's experiences to be symptoms of trauma and distress, which developed over the previous three years.

I needed to explore Michael's mental state prior to this time, so I asked him about his childhood and his experience of school. Michael said he had been a sociable, popular guy at school who enjoyed spending time with friends. Michael said this all changed after he was assaulted in the city when he was 21 years old.

At this point it was important to assess Michael's risk, so I asked him why he had taken 40 mg of diazepam. He said he was intoxicated and wanted to get some uninterrupted sleep, and so took more than the prescribed dose of diazepam. I asked Michael whether he believed this would end his life, which he denied. He appeared to be shocked by the question. He said that he had not thought it would harm him and, although he sometimes does have fleeting thoughts of ending his life, he would never intentionally try to hurt himself. He said he felt upset that his mother had found him in this state. Michael explained that he wanted help to improve his situation, as he had not spoken to anyone about this before. I repeated back to Michael all that he had told me and asked whether I had missed anything. I thanked Michael for opening up to me and telling me his story. I reassured Michael that his situation could be helped and that his symptoms were treatable with the right support.

I discussed my assessment with the consultant psychiatrist, who agreed to refer Michael to the community mental health team and link him with a cognitive behavioural therapy specialist and psychiatrist who might consider commencement of an anti-depressant. I would also provide Michael with information for community drug and alcohol services to support him in psychosocial activities and other supports to help reduce his alcohol, marijuana and benzodiazepine use. A letter would be sent to Michael's general practitioner (GP) with the mental health assessment and a suggested plan for follow-up.

REFLECTIVE QUESTIONS

- How might you engage someone like Michael in conversation so that he feels valued and respected?
- What sorts of behaviours would show Michael that you are engaged in his story and would help him to feel respected and valued?
- What qualities or characteristics, such as compassion, do you think are important to engage effectively with someone like Michael?

Mental health nursing as a specialist field

Mental health nursing is a specialist field of nursing that focuses on meeting the mental health needs of the consumer, in partnership with family, significant others and the community, in any setting. It is a specialised, interpersonal process embodying the concept of caring, which is designed to be therapeutic by:

1 supporting and advocating for consumers to optimise their health status in a manner that is congruent with their explanatory model and life situation;
2 encouraging consumers to take an active role in decisions about their health care;
3 genuinely involving family, significant others and communities in the care and support of consumers; and
4 being proactive in the care and support of consumers, in support of citizenship and human rights.

Some of the predominant clinical roles of the mental health practitioner are to work collaboratively to assess consumers' mental health needs and provide therapeutic support where possible. The mental health practitioner works from a body of knowledge as well as from an experimental basis for which feelings can be received and lives revealed. 'Evidence-based health care is the conscientious use of current best evidence in making decisions about the care of individual patients or the delivery of health services' (Cochrane, 2014). These combined elements of the consumer narrative and evidence-based care help to ensure that the consumer is provided with the highest possible standard of care, based upon present and future needs.

The importance of trust in mental health nursing

As in most relationships, it is widely acknowledged that trust is a core component of clinical engagement between mental health consumers and practitioners (Gardner, McCutcheon & Fedoruk, 2010; Hellwig, 1993; Junghan et al., 2007; Killaspy et al., 2009; Kirsh & Tate, 2006; Vecchi, Van Hasselt & Romano, 2005). It is also recognised that trust is something that takes time to establish (Addis & Gamble, 2004). There is increasing literature highlighting that mistrust is often a key reason people disengage from mental health services (Priebe et al., 2005; Watts & Priebe, 2002). Trust is a fundamental requirement for effective and contemporary mental health service delivery. Thus, in the mental health context – one that may be characterised by significant human interaction to establish therapeutic relationships – it is important to understand the nature, scope and consequences surrounding how trust is facilitated. From this perspective, we can begin to understand how this contributes to consumer engagement, both in the immediate instance and in the future.

Mental health nurses working with people who are experiencing mental distress may encounter difficult and sometimes complex negotiations and decisions. Such decisions may have to be made at a time when the person is distressed, angry or confused, and when the causes of their behaviour are unclear. Being empathetic to consumers' experiences is considered an important means by which to demonstrate 'genuine care'. Without genuine care to facilitate and communicate empathy, the ability to engage in the future may be hindered.

REFLECTIVE QUESTION

Think of situations in which you have felt distressed and/or anxious. Aside from the details of the situation you were in, write down three things that helped you to reduce the feelings you had at that time.

Recovery

Recovery is the active process of people with mental illness moving toward achieving well-being and a satisfying life, despite the presence of mental illness. The meaning of this term is in contrast to other understandings of the term 'recovery', such as a return to a previous level of functioning. Recovery is generally not viewed by people with a mental illness to be a return to a previous state, since their experiences of living with mental illness, including factors such as treatment, hospitalisation and stigma, have likely changed their lives irrevocably (Davidson, 2003). Thus, recovery has been characterised as a journey that is 'deeply personal' (Anthony, 1993), individual (Jeffs, 2009) or unique (Deegan, 1996). Recovery is often a transformative process (Jeffs, 2009) of accepting the presence of mental illness and in redefining the self as more than a mental illness (Deegan, 1996).

A person seeking to be in recovery assumes responsibility for their own mental health, in partnership with family, carers and mental health practitioners. As such, recovery from mental illness does not occur in isolation, but with assistance from key others. Recovery is facilitated by the deeply human responses of others (Anthony, 1993). This means valuing and respecting the lived experience of people with mental illness, their family members and carers.

The importance of hope, resilience and reconnection is paramount. Therapeutic optimism on the part of the practitioner is an important factor in this regard, and is defined as a 'practitioner's self-reported, specific expectancies regarding client outcomes in a clinical setting' (Byrne & Sullivan, 2006, p. 11). Optimism is made therapeutic as it facilitates the processing of negative information, gives rise to thorough and flexible ways to be supportive and promotes the development of coping and problem-solving skills.

Working collaboratively with consumers, helping and supporting their reconnection with a social life and meaningful activities, in particular social activities outside of the mental health environment, such as gaining employment or volunteering in the wider community, are important to being in recovery. Having roles and routines provide a sense of purpose and goals around which everyday life can be structured. Recovery is not a linear process. It continues to occur even when symptoms recur. Therapeutic optimism can help to facilitate resilience and enhance coping skills to manage life's challenges.

REFLECTIVE QUESTIONS

- What do you consider to be the key enablers in helping people to achieve optimal recovery?
- What factors or conditions do you think would create challenges to being in recovery?
- How might the idea of therapeutic optimism be developed and deployed in Michael's situation?

Collaborative practice in mental health nursing

Collaborative practice involves taking time and setting the context for a personable relationship with a consumer and their family. This approach is marked by genuine empathy for the person and belief in the benefits of meaningful engagement. For Alex, spending time with Michael requires much more than taking a predefined nursing or medical history. In taking the opportunity to meet with Michael, there is also an opportunity to talk about ways to help him feel connected and safe in his new environment. In preparing to discuss his admission, Alex enquires about Michael's understanding of his current situation. This means exploring any concerns he may have and the practical steps that can be taken to work together, with dignity and respect, and in partnership with others, to help address these concerns.

Collaborative practice with carers and family members

Collaborative practice also involves working with family members and carers. Mental health carers provide unpaid care and support to family members or friends who have a mental illness. Carers may range from children through to older adults, and may be from any cultural background. Carers are central to the care and support of people with a mental illness and are the major providers of care in the community (Carers Australia, 2012). The role of caring for someone with a mental illness is not always understood by others, as the tasks undertaken may be quite different to what is generally understood as a 'caring' role (Carers Australia, 2012). For example, tasks associated with caring for someone with a physical disability, such as assistance with bathing or cooking, may not be undertaken to support a person with a mental illness. Instead, the role of caring in this context may include tasks such as providing emotional or social support, helping the person to organise their daily schedule or dealing with emergencies.

Many people do not identify themselves as carers, as it is often assumed that carers receive payment for care. Stigma may be another reason for not identifying as a carer of a person with a mental illness. This may be especially pronounced in cultures that view mental illness as having serious, widespread effects on the families of people who have a mental illness; for example, if mental illness is viewed as something that will bring a curse upon family or community members. Therefore, the estimated number of carers for people with mental illness is likely to be largely underestimated. Furthermore, some consumers may not view a family member or friend who provides them with care and support as a carer. These issues summarise some of the challenges in being a carer for someone with a mental illness.

Carers are a valuable, yet under-utilised source of information about the well-being of a person with mental illness. Carers quite often know the person with a mental illness very well and for a long time. As such, they may have information that can be useful in supporting the person in their recovery. However, due to the many challenges related to being a carer of a person with a mental illness, carers may not seek or receive sufficient support. It is important to ask carers about their own support systems, such as family or friends, and whether they require additional help or support, such as counselling or being connected with carer support groups.

PERSONAL NARRATIVE

Zoe's story

My name is Zoe. I'm a 32-year-old engineer, and I'm married with two young children. I am also the carer of David, my older brother. David is 36 years old and has lived with a bipolar condition for the past 15 years. When David was 21 years old, our father died following a gun accident. David was particularly close to our father, often describing him as his best friend. Our parents had divorced prior to our father's passing, and David has had little contact with our mother since they separated.

At the time of our father's death, David was in his final year of study to become a lawyer. David became deeply depressed, refusing to eat or talk. He was hospitalised for three months, where he was given electroconvulsive treatment (ECT). Upon returning home, David found it difficult to continue his studies or socialise. He would spend most of his time watching TV and sleeping, a situation that continued for some years. I would usually visit David every second day, and I would try to encourage him to go for a walk, help me with the shopping, or join in social activities. David's old friends would also ask to visit but he declined. To try and maintain some of his friendships, I helped David to set up a Facebook account, but unfortunately he rarely used it.

One day, I noticed David behaving differently – he was very chatty and upbeat, talking about going to a party he had been invited to through Facebook. I thought this behaviour was odd and out of character, but I was relieved that he no longer seemed so down. The next time I visited, David seemed to be a completely different person. He had invited all of the neighbours over and was hosting a martini evening. When he ushered me into the house, I was made to feel like royalty. David was speaking at such a rate that I could barely make sense of what he was saying. He was certainly the 'life of the party', but I couldn't help feeling that I and the other guests were a captive audience. I was concerned about David's behaviour, so I decided to stay until the party finished. The last guests left at 4.00 a.m. By 7.00 a.m., David was still wide awake, singing, cleaning and wearing strange clothes. By midnight the following day, David had still not slept and had become agitated with me and his neighbours, who had asked him to turn the music down. I began to feel increasingly threatened, so I called the police. David repeated that 'the devil would be here to intervene soon'. Instead, the police visited and, shortly afterwards David was taken to the psychiatric hospital.

REFLECTIVE QUESTIONS

- What do you think Zoe might have been feeling or experiencing before and after David was taken to hospital?
- Once David becomes well again, how might he feel about the situation, including Zoe's involvement that led to him being taken to hospital?
- In the long term, what kinds of supports or resources might Zoe need access to for her to be able to provide good care and support for David?

INTERPROFESSIONAL PERSPECTIVES

The importance of making meaningful connections with consumers and carers in mental health cannot be overstated. The same can also be said with regard to interprofessional connections. One of the outcomes of mainstreaming mental health services into the community is that nurses working in general health and hospital settings have increased contact with people experiencing mental health issues and mental illness. For this reason, interprofessional care is an increasingly important aspect of clinical practice.

As nurses, we are not expected to take sole clinical or administrative responsibility when responding to a person with mental illness. At the very least, we should have fundamental skills to be able to engage therapeutically and to undertake a screening mental state assessment, carefully documenting our findings and talking with colleagues about appropriate support, referral pathways, immediate care and treatment.

It is at this point that we should be aware of our clinical networks, professional strengths and limitations – of what catches our eye, our ear (all of our senses, really) – and be willing to seek the assistance and support of colleagues for appropriate advice and specialist referral. Clinical supervision – where we engage with more experienced peers in discussing cases and seeking for advice – can be useful to guarantee people will receive the best available care and reduce any concerns we might have about our skills.

The initial contact with a person with mental illness is particularly important, but often it occurs in less-than-ideal circumstances, such as in a busy and noisy emergency room, the unfamiliar surroundings of a person's home, or on the telephone. In some instances, particularly when working with people from diverse cultural and linguistic backgrounds, it may be difficult to speak with the person in private, and confidentiality can be a concern.

It is important to remember that even when people are distressed and facing extreme life circumstances, they may have recently perceived rejection or other negative situations. As such, a considerable degree of expertise and patience may be required to establish therapeutic rapport. This can be an effective pathway to establishing safety and dignity for all concerned and can be achieved by indicating that we wish to try and understand what is happening to the person, and that a certain amount of time has been set aside in order to do so. This approach can help to create a context for human connectedness so that feelings are able to be explored and lives revealed. Such actions are important in their own right and are also known to favourably help reduce the likelihood of additional distress and suffering.

Source: Adapted from Procter (2008).

SUMMARY

This chapter has presented stories and information, supplemented by activities designed to deepen your understanding of:

- The *narrative approach* as a means of storytelling, which is central to mental health practice. It creates a dialogue, enables new ways of thinking and new perspectives, and maintains personhood for the consumer.

- The *determinants of mental health and mental illness,* which are interrelated across social, personal, occupational and cultural aspects of our lives. Knowing the importance of these determinants helps practitioners understand how and why mental health can be promoted and ill health prevented. While lived experience of mental health and illness is critical in advancing fresh understandings of person-centred care, equally important is the relationship of the consumer and their family with accompanying evidence and national survey data.
- The requirement for *contemporary mental health care and practical support* for people with a mental health condition to incorporate notions of person-centred practice that has value and meaning for the consumer. Engaging with individuals and communities at risk involves much more than simply knowing what needs to be done; it incorporates practices marked by supporting human rights and promoting recovery with dignity.
- *Trauma-informed practitioners or services* such as those that work from the fundamental principles of trauma awareness. That is, working to provide comfort and to avoid re-traumatisation, while simultaneously empowering consumers in meaningful decision-making, safety, trustworthiness, choice and collaboration. A trauma-informed practitioner works within the context of a universal understanding and belief that symptoms and experiences related to trauma are coping strategies developed to manage traumatic experiences. Helping and supporting consumers, family members and carers to develop strengths and skills is an important guide to best practice.
- *First-person accounts of lived experience in mental health* from the perspective of consumers, carers and practitioners. As discussion, reflection and analysis unfolds, encouraging readers to reflect on their practice, they are also preparing for the future. This is an important attribute of both professional practice and trauma-informed practice, in particular, across a range of health care disciplines and clinical settings.

CRITICAL THINKING/LEARNING ACTIVITIES

1 Consider Michael's story and his experiences. What interventions or services might he need to help him build resilience, to enable his recovery with dignity?
2 What does the term 'recovery' mean in the field of mental health? How does this differ from its meaning in other areas of health?
3 What are some of the key roles undertaken by a carer of a person with a mental illness?
4 What are the four key metabolic changes people with mental illness are at risk of developing? How can the risk of these changes be minimised?
5 How can stigma affect the lived experience of a person with a mental illness and their family or carers?

LEARNING EXTENSION

The following is a list of terms used to refer to people with a mental illness.

Consumer	Service user	Mentally retarded
Lunatic	Mentally ill	Crazy
Survivor	Client	Mad
Mental health problem	Eccentric	Patient

Write a paragraph answering the following questions:

- How would you feel if these terms were applied to you and/or your family?
- Would any of them be more or less acceptable to you? Explain your answer.

FURTHER READING

O'Hagan, M. (2013). Straight Answers to the Curly Questions in Mental Health. Retrieved from
    http://www.maryohagan.com/
This publication and the website provide information about practical and personal ways to help
improve people's lives, including personal anecdotes of support and comfort.

Rosenberg, S. (ed.) (2016). Magical realism and the draft Fifth National Mental Health Plan.
    Croakey Health Media (website). Retrieved from https://croakey.org/magical-realism-and-
    the-draft-fifth-national-mental-health-plan/
This online essay, written in response to a draft release of Australia's National Mental Health
Plan, raises important questions about the role and function of primary care, hospital and tertiary
mental health care, and how they are designed, funded and evaluated.

Steen, M. & Thomas, M. (2016). *Mental Health Across the Lifespan: A handbook*. London:
    Routledge.
This summary of mental health and wellness concepts is suitable for health and human service
workers.

REFERENCES

Addis, J. & Gamble, C. (2004). Assertive outreach nurses' experience of engagement. *Journal of
    Psychiatric and Mental Health Nursing, 11*: 452–60.
American Psychiatric Association (APA). (2013). *Diagnostic and Statistical Manual of Mental Disorders
    (DSM)*. Retrieved from www.psychiatry.org/practice/dsm
Anthony, W. A. (1993). Recovery from mental illness: The guiding vision of the mental health service
    system in the 1990s. *Psychosocial Rehabilitation Journal, 16*: 11–24.
Australian Bureau of Statistics (ABS). (2007). *National Survey of Mental Health and Wellbeing:
    Summary of results*. Cat. no. 4326.0. Canberra: ABS.
——— (2018). *National Health Survey – First Results Australia 2017–18*. Cat. no. 4364. 0.55.001.
    Canberra: ABS.
Australian College of Mental Health Nurses (ACMHN). (2015). *What is Mental Health Nursing?*
    Retrieved from http://www.acmhn.org/about-us/about-mh-nursing
Australian Institute of Health and Welfare (AIHW). (2015). *The Health and Welfare of Australia's
    Aboriginal and Torres Strait Islander Peoples 2015*. Cat. no. IHW 147. Canberra: AIHW.
——— (2019). *Mental Health Services – In brief*. Cat. no. HSE 228. Canberra: AIHW.
——— (2021a). *Mental Health Services in Australia*. Retrieved from https://www.aihw.gov.au/reports/
    mental-health-services/mental-health-services-in-australia/report-contents/expenditure-on-
    mental-health-related-services/data-source#references
——— (2021b). *Australian Burden of Disease Study 2018: Key findings*. Australian Burden of Disease
    Study series 24. Cat. no. BOD 30. Canberra: AIHW.
Byrne, M. K. & Sullivan, N. L. (2006). Clinical optimism: Development and psychometric analysis of a
    scale for mental health clinicians. *Australian Journal of Rehabilitation Counselling, 12*: 11–20.
Carers Australia. (2012). *Carers Australia and Network of Carers Associations National Policy Position
    Statement: Mental health reform*. Retrieved from www.carersaustralia.com.au/publications/
    position-statements
Choudhry, F. R., Mani, V., Ming, L. C. & Khan, T. M. (2016). Beliefs and perception about mental health
    issues: A meta-synthesis. *Neuropsychiatric Disease and Treatment, 12*: 2807–18.
Cochrane. (2014). *Evidence-based Health Care and Systematic Reviews*. Retrieved from
    http://community-archive.cochrane.org/about-us/evidence-based-health-care
Commission on Social Determinants of Health. (2008). *Closing the Gap in a Generation: Health equity
    through action on the social determinants of health*. Geneva: World Health Organization.

Commonwealth of Australia. (2009). *National Mental Health Policy 2008*. Canberra: Commonwealth of Australia.

Correll, C. U., Detraux, J., De Lepeleire, J. & De Hert, M. (2015). Effects of antipsychotics, antidepressants and mood stabilizers on risk for physical diseases in people with schizophrenia, depression and bipolar disorder. *World Psychiatry*, *14*(2): 119–36.

Corrigan, P. (2004). How stigma interferes with mental health care. *American Psychologist*, *59*(7): 614–25.

Corrigan, P. W., Rafacz, J. & Rusch, N. (2011). Examining a progressive model of self-stigma and its impact on people with serious mental illness. *Psychiatry Research*, *189*(3): 339–43.

Council of Australian Governments (COAG). (2012). *The Roadmap for National Mental Health Reform 2012–2022*. Canberra: COAG.

Davidson, L. (2003). *Living Outside Mental Illness: Qualitative studies of recovery in schizophrenia*. New York: New York University Press.

Deegan, P. (1996). Recovery as a journey of the heart. *Psychiatric Rehabilitation Journal*, *19*: 91–8.

Department of Health. (2009). National Mental Health Policy 2008: Glossary. Retrieved from https://www1.health.gov.au/internet/publications/publishing.nsf/Content/mental-pubs-n-pol08-toc~mental-pubs-n-pol08-3

——— (2013). Capability 5A: *Supporting social inclusion and advocacy on social determinants*. Retrieved from https://www1.health.gov.au/internet/publications/publishing.nsf/Content/mental-pubs-n-recovgde-toc~mental-pubs-n-recovgde-app~mental-pubs-n-recovgde-app-5~mental-pubs-n-recovgde-app-5-a

Edward, K., Munro, I., Robins, A. & Welch, A. (2011). *Mental Health Nursing: Dimensions of praxis*. South Melbourne: Oxford University Press.

Elliott, D. E., Bjelajac P., Fallot, R. D., Markoff, L. S. & Reed B. D. (2005). Trauma-informed or trauma-denied: Principles and implementation of trauma-informed services for women. *Journal of Community Psychology*, *33*: 461–77.

Elliott, M., Maitoza, R. & Schwinger, E. (2011). Subjective accounts of the causes of mental illness in the USA. *International Journal of Social Psychiatry*, *58*: 562–7.

Felitti, V. J. (2002). The relation between adverse childhood experiences and adult health: Turning gold into lead. *The Permanente Journal*, *6*(1): 44–7.

Felitti, V. J., Anda, R. F., Nordenberg, D., Williamson, D. F., Spitz, A. M., Edwards, V., Koss, M. P. & Marks, J. S. (1998). Relationship of childhood abuse and household dysfunction to many of the leading causes of death in adults. *American Journal of Preventive Medicine*, *14*(4): 245–58.

Gardner, A., McCutcheon, H. & Fedoruk, M. (2010). Therapeutic friendliness and the development of therapeutic leverage by mental health nurses in community rehabilitation settings. *Contemporary Nurse*, *34*(2): 140–8.

Goffman, E. (1963). *Stigma: Notes on the management of spoiled identity*. New York: Simon Schuster.

Happell, B., Platania-Phung, C., Gray, R., Hardy, S., Lambert, T., McAllister, M. & Davies, C. (2011). A role for mental health nursing in the physical health care of consumers with severe mental illness. *Journal of Psychiatric and Mental Health Nursing*, *18*: 706–11.

Hellwig, K. (1993). Psychiatric home care nursing: Managing patients in the community setting. *Journal of Psychosocial Nursing and Mental Health Services*, *31*: 21–4.

Jeffs, S. (2009). *Flying with paper wings: Reflections on living with madness*. Carlton North, Vic.: The Vulgar Press.

Junghan, U. M., Leese, M., Priebe, S. & Slade, M. (2007). Staff and patient perspectives on unmet need and therapeutic alliance in community mental health services. *British Journal of Psychiatry*, *191*: 543–7.

Kaite, C. P., Karanikola, M., Merkouris, A. & Papathanassoglou, E. D. (2015). 'An ongoing struggle with the self and illness': Alpha meta-synthesis of the studies of the lived experience of severe mental illness. *Archives of Psychiatric Nursing*, *29*(6): 458–73.

Keleher, H. & Armstrong, R. (2005). *Evidence-based Mental Health Promotion Resource*. Melbourne: Public Health Group, Victorian Government Department of Human Services.

Killaspy, H., Johnson, S., Pierce, B., Bebbington, P., Pilling, S., Nolan, F. & King, M. (2009). Successful engagement: A mixed methods study of the approaches of assertive community treatment and community mental health teams in the REACT trial. *Social Psychiatry and Psychiatric Epidemiology*, *44*: 532–40.

Kirsh, B. & Tate, E. (2006). Developing a comprehensive understanding of the working alliance in community mental health. *Qualitative Health Research, 16*: 1054–74.

Lamont, E. & Dickens, G. L. (2019). Mental health services, care provision, and professional support for people diagnosed with borderline personality disorder: systematic review of service-user, family, and carer perspectives. *Journal of Mental Health*: 1–15.

Larkings, J. S. & Brown, P. M. (2018). Do biogenetic causal beliefs reduce mental illness stigma in people with mental illness and in mental health professionals? A systematic review. *International Journal of Mental Health Nursing, 27*(3): 928–41.

Link, B., Phelan, J., Bresnahan, M., Stueve, A. & Pescosolido, B. (1999). Public conceptions of mental illness: Labels, causes, dangerousness, and social distance. *American Journal of Public Health, 89*(9): 1328–33.

Longden, E., Read, J. & Dillon, J. (2018). Assessing the impact and effectiveness of hearing voices network self-help groups. *Community Mental Health Journal, 54*(2): 184–8.

Mendoza, J., Bresnan, A., Rosenberg, S., Elson, A., Gilbert, Y., Long, P., Wilson, K. & Hopkins, J. (2013). *Obsessive Hope Disorder: Reflections on 30 years of mental health reform in Australia and visions for the future. Summary report.* Caloundra, Qld: CoNetica.

Mental Health Council of Australia (MHCA). (2011). *Consumer and Carer Experiences of Stigma From Mental Health and Other Health Professionals.* Canberra: MHCA.

Michel, K. & Valach, L. (2011). The narrative interview with suicidal patient. In K. Michel & D. Jobes (eds), *Building a Therapeutic Alliance with the Suicidal Patient* (pp. 63–80). Washington, DC: American Psychological Association.

Ministry of Health. (2015). *Annual Updates of Key Results 2014/15: New Zealand Health Survey.* Wellington: Ministry of Health.

Mitchell, A. J., Vancampfort, D., Sweers, K., van Winkel, R., Yu, W. & De Hert, M. (2013). Prevalence of metabolic syndrome and metabolic abnormalities in schizophrenia and related disorders—a systematic review and meta-analysis. *Schizophrenia Bulletin, 39*(2): 306–18.

Morgan, V. A., Waterreaus, A., Jablensky, A., Mackinnon, A., McGrath, J. J., Carr, V. & Saw, S. (2011). *People Living With Psychotic Illness 2010: Report on the second Australian national survey.* Canberra: Commonwealth of Australia.

Muskett, C. (2014) Trauma-informed care in inpatient mental health settings: A review of the literature. *International Journal of Mental Health Nursing, 23*: 51–9.

National Association of State Mental Health Program Directors Centre for Trauma Informed Care (NCTIC). (2015) *NCTIC Reports: Resources.* Retrieved from http://www.nasmhpd.org/content/national-center-trauma-informed-care-nctic-0

Oakley Browne, M. A., Well, J. E. & Scott, K. M. (2006). *Te Rau Hinengaro: The New Zealand Mental Health Survey.* Wellington: Ministry of Health.

Our Consumer Place. (2010). *So you have a 'mental illness' … What now?* Melbourne: Our Community.

Parish, C. (2011). Mental illness reduces life expectancy: Research finds. *Mental Health Practice, 14*: 5.

Park, J., Joshanloo, M. & Scheifinger, H. (2019). Predictors of life satisfaction in Australia: A study drawing upon annual data from the Gallup World Poll. *Australian Psychologist:* 1–14.

Peris, T. S., Teachman, B. A. & Nosek, B. A. (2008). Implicit and explicit stigma of mental illness: Links to clinical care. *The Journal of Nervous and Mental Disease, 196*(10).

Pescosolido, B. (2013). The public stigma of mental illness: What do we think; what do we know; what can we prove? *Journal of Health and Social Behavior, 54*: 1–21.

Posselt, M., Galletly, C., de Crespigny, C. & Procter, N. G. (2014). Mental health and drug and alcohol comorbidity in young people of refugee background: A review of literature. *Mental Health and Substance Use, 7*(1): 19–30.

Priebe, S., Watts, J., Chase, M. & Matanov, A. (2005). Processes of disengagement and engagement in assertive outreach patients: Qualitative study. *British Journal of Psychiatry, 187*: 438–43.

Procter, N. (2008). Emergency mental health: Crisis and response. *Australasian Emergency Nursing Journal, 11*(2): 70–1.

Qu, L., de Vaus, D. A. & Australian Institute of Family Studies (AIFS). (2015). Life satisfaction across life course transitions. *Australian Family Trends, 8.* Melbourne: Australian Institute of Family Studies. Retrieved from https://aifs.gov.au/publications/life-satisfaction-across-life-course-transitions

Saha, S., Chant, D. & McGrath, J. (2007). A systematic review of mortality in schizophrenia: Is the differential mortality gap worsening over time? *Archives of General Psychiatry, 64*: 1123–31.

Schizophrenia Fellowship of NSW Inc. (2008). *Accommodation*. Retrieved from www.sfnsw.org.au/Mental-Illness/Quality-of-Life/Quality-of-Life-Accommodation#.Uh7KObxvSQk

Short, T., Thomas, S., Mullen, P. & Ogloff, J. R. P. (2013). Comparing violence in schizophrenia patients with and without comorbid substance-use disorders to community controls. *Acta Psychiatrica Scandinavia*, *128*(4): 306–13.

Stefanovics, E., He, H., Ofori-Atta, A., Cavalcanti, M. T., Rocha Neto, H., Makanjuola, V. … Rosenheck, R. (2016). Cross-national analysis of beliefs and attitude toward mental illness among medical professionals from five countries. *Psychiatric Quarterly*, *87*(1): 63–73.

Stewart-Harawira, M. (2005). *The New Imperial Order: Indigenous response to colonisation*. Wellington: Huia Publishers.

Stull, L. G., McConnell, H., McGrew, J. & Salyers, M. P. (2017). Explicit and implicit stigma of mental illness as predictors of the recovery attitudes of assertive community treatment practitioners. *The Israel Journal of Psychiatry and Related Sciences*, *54*(1): 31–7.

Vecchi, G. M., Van Hasselt, V. B. & Romano, S. J. (2005). Crisis (hostage) negotiation: Current strategies and issues in high-risk conflict resolution. *Aggression and Violent Behavior*, *10*: 533–51.

Von Lersner, U., Gerb, J., Hizli, S., Waldhuber, D., Wallerand, A. F., Bajbouj, M. … Hahn, E. (2019). Stigma of mental illness in Germans and Turkish immigrants in Germany: The effect of causal beliefs. *Front Psychiatry*, *10*: 46.

Wahl, O. & Aroesty-Cohen, E. (2010). Attitudes of mental health professionals about mental illness: A review of the recent literature. *Journal of Community Psychology*, *38*(1), 49–62.

Walker, E., McGee, R. E. & Druss, B. G. (2015). Mortality in mental disorders and global disease burden implications: A systematic review and meta-analysis. *JAMA Psychiatry*, *72*: 334–41.

Watts, J. & Priebe, S. (2002). A phenomenological account of users' experiences of assertive community treatment. *Bioethics*, *16*: 439–54.

Western Massachusetts Recovery Learning Community. (2020). Welcome to the Wildflower Alliance (Website). Retrieved from https://wildfloweralliance.org

Whiteford, H. A., Buckingham, W. J., Harris, M. G., Burges, P. M., Pirkis, J. E., Barendregt, J. J. et al. (2014). Estimating treatment rates for mental disorders in Australia. *Australian Health Review*, *38*(1): 80–5.

World Health Organization (WHO). (2012). *World Health Statistics. Part II: Highlighted topics*. Retrieved from www.who.int/gho/publications/world_health_statistics/EN_WHS2012_Part2.pdf

——— (2013a). *International Classification of Diseases (ICD)*. Retrieved from www.who.int/classifications/icd/en

——— (2013b). *Substance Abuse*. Retrieved from www.who.int/topics/substance_abuse/en

World Health Organization (WHO) & Calouste Gulbenkian Foundation. (2014). *Social determinants of mental health*. Geneva: WHO.

2 Trauma-informed care

Theory into practice

Helen P. Hamer, Debra Lampshire and Jane Barrington

LEARNING OBJECTIVES

At the completion of this chapter, you should be able to:

1 Understand how the Power Threat Meaning framework (PTMF) provides an alternative understanding of mental distress and extreme states.
2 Reflect on the interpersonal effects of trauma on people's mental health, and discuss the self-care required of practitioners when working with survivors of abuse.
3 Learn the skills required for trauma-informed care.

Introduction

This chapter discusses the knowledge, skills and confidence needed to provide a safe and compassionate environment through trauma-informed care (TIC). Many people have traumatic experiences outside of the safety of their family unit, such as bullying or sexual harassment. Therefore, we need to be cautious about blaming parents or caregivers without first establishing the situation and the context of the person's history of trauma.

Many people who present to mental health, addiction and disability services, however, report complex histories involving physical, psychological, emotional and sexual abuse (see Chapter 15). Evolving research recommends addressing complex trauma – as distinct from single-incident trauma (Kezelman & Stavropoulos, 2019) – which requires the practitioner to have a particular skill set in the provision of effective therapy. This chapter focuses on the fundamental skills needed to support people who disclose their trauma, particularly sexual abuse, and how practitioners can respond in ways that foster human connectedness.

The Power, Threat, Meaning Framework

This section of the chapter focuses specifically on issues related to power, the identification of patterns in emotional distress, unusual experiences and troubling behaviour, and presents an alternative to functional psychiatric diagnosis, described as the **P**ower, **T**hreat, **M**eaning Framework (PTMF) (Johnstone et al., 2018).

Moving away from the medicalisation of trauma and mental health, we need to understand how survivors of abuse and trauma make meaning of their experiences, within their social and relational environments as well as their life circumstances. The PTMF provides an evidence-based approach to collaboration with survivors, to identify and describe their patterns of distress and unusual experiences. Johnstone and colleagues (2018) assert that the PTMF provides a view of emotional distress and troubling behaviour as justifiable responses to a person's, experiences, circumstances and history. As Caruth (1995) proposes, it is the truth of the traumatic experience that forms the centre of psychological distress; therefore it is not a 'pathology of falsehoods or displacement of meaning, but of history itself' (p. 5).

Embracing the PTMF as an alternative view of trauma supports the practitioner to restore the link between the person's distress and the injustice of having their rights violated by the offender, and the continuing effects upon survivors' social and health outcomes (Tseris, 2020). The PTMF aims to increase people's access to power and resources, and promotes their social action as survivors. Further, the framework enables a dialogue that **validates** personal narratives to empower and inform people, groups and communities by repairing these links and meanings (Johnstone et al., 2018). As you read Debra's personal narrative, see if you can link the power, threat and meaning components in her life experiences.

validate – to affirm the truth in someone's statements or feelings; validation is important in every relationship, and it is thought that parental invalidation in the early stages of child development contributes to the emergence of borderline personality disorder

PERSONAL NARRATIVE

Debra's story – part one

When I was a new-born baby, circumstances meant my birthmother had to give me up for adoption. I spent the first year of my life with new parents. I did not meet the developmental milestones for my age and, as I had needed oxygen as a baby, the GP thought there was the remote possibility that I had sustained brain damage. The couple who fostered me decided not to proceed with adoption, and I was surrendered into state care. I was moved from home to home; a difficult child with behavioural issues. I was highly anxious and lived constantly in a state of fear of being removed from my 'family'.

Eventually I was placed into a stable environment and then became aware of a maternal voice that came to me at night, assuring me I was safe. I felt her presence and believed it was my birth mother trying to sustain a relationship with me. I felt secure in her existence – she was my secret and the only thing I had that was my own.

Going to school increased my feelings of insecurity and lack of belonging. I was bullied daily and retreated to the library, which was a sanctuary from the cruelty that overshadowed my life. Each day my anxiety grew more overwhelming and I felt more threatened, more vulnerable and more alone. I sank into sadness and anxiety. I had to prove that I was not 'brain damaged', that I was intelligent; that I was lovable and not something to be abandoned. I loved learning and reading about other places and ways of living. The bullying stole from me any pleasure, denied me the chance to grow socially and emotionally, and the ability to cultivate and sustain relationships. I had little self-esteem or sense of self. The only redeeming feature that helped me to endure was the maternal voice, which assured me that I was special and protected.

After a time, I began to hear negative voices that insulted and berated me. I frequently dashed out of classrooms as my fear multiplied exponentially, and I could no longer function. My decline, mentally and emotionally, reinforced my core belief that I was stupid and unlovable. It was a prerequisite to remain at school that I should see a psychiatrist but my behaviour there and at home became more worrying for my parents, and they were advised to admit me to the mental hospital and reluctantly they did so. I began my career as a mental health patient for many years.

The practitioners told my parents to cease all contact with me, and feelings of betrayal and abandonment consumed me. I delved deeper into so-called madness, which was a place of escape from the horrors that encapsulated me. It made my time there tolerable, not having to care for or about anyone. Over time, I formed friendships with other patients, and even love and laughter to fill the emptiness. But spending so much time in such a place comes at a huge cost and with little gains.

When the closure of the mental hospital began, I was discharged into my parents' care. We were strangers to each other due to our separation; it became untenable for me to stay with them, and I was moved to a community house with a group of fellow patients.

I spent all my days rocking in a chair, smoking cigarettes, with a monthly visit from a psychiatric nurse to make sure I was taking my medication. One day I had an unexpected encounter with a man who came to visit another person in the house. Finding me alone in the house, the man struck up a conversation with me. He said he was a panel beater and his hobby was restoring old cars. I was taken by his passion and wished that just once more I could feel those emotions of joy and excitement that had eluded me. From this brief but informative conversation I started to make connections to my own situation. I had never questioned why I was put on Earth but somewhere in the deep recesses of my being I knew it was not to rock back and forth in a chair all day and reside with disembodied voices.

REFLECTIVE QUESTION

Debra's narrative represents the many others' experiences, often relayed to practitioners, yet its importance is often overlooked. Consider how you would validate and affirm Debra to increase her sense of human connectedness.

Reading Debra's story through the lens of the PTMF reveals the traumatic aspects of her experiences, such as the injustices she faced within the psychiatric system, loss of power, threats to her well-being and her struggle to find meaning. The PTMF supports practitioners to develop a multifactorial and contextual approach to distress and extreme states by incorporating the social, psychological and biological factors. PTMF integrates many existing models and practices, rather than replaces them. It provides a conceptual resource for anyone to draw on. PTMF is not about narrow formulation but about broader narrative and meaning-making, and a framework for identifying broader patterns of distress and unusual experiences.

PERSONAL NARRATIVE

Debra's story – part two

My new friend asked questions I had never been asked before with great compassion and empathy, and he listened without judgement nor condemnation. Now, giving voice to my inner world I was able to make meaning and connections with past and present events, and the extreme anxiety that was so pervasive in my life. I wanted to take back my life, and together we developed a plan to reduce my constant state of fear and threat.

We worked on my anxiety, using the basic de-sensitisation techniques, and this alleviated my anxiety. It was a powerful and exhilarating process, and a time of great learning for me. I dedicated my time to focusing on my well-being and practising the new responses to stress and distress. This was the beginning of a new era. I had reclaimed my life and permission to be me.

I was aware that many of my peers had not fared as well and remained captive to the oppressive and controlling environment of mental health services. Through my experiences I decided to work alongside both service users and clinicians to challenge the old paradigm and enlighten people to a new understanding of mental distress – one embedded in compassion, empathy, curiosity and directed by service users. I involved myself in the service-user movement, taught clinicians and became involved in trauma research.

Reclaiming power, understanding the threat, and living the meaning

It is impossible to reconcile the person who sat for decades, rocking back and forth in a chair, with the person I am today. I maintain I was always that person but it took one person to question and not accept that that was all I was capable of, and to help me see my potential. I am forever grateful to that person; they chose not to be my rescuer but my 'friend'. They showed me what it is to be treated with dignity and to restore what I considered lost. They realigned me to my internal resilience and resourcefulness, and to understanding that I was courageous. They remained faithful to the adventure of self-discovery, they invigorated a broken heart and gave me the gift of knowing that the greatest limitations are those we place on ourselves.

REFLECTIVE QUESTIONS

- Debra described her resilience and resourcefulness. Consider the definition of each and their relevance to practice.
- Debra's turning point was learning to conquer her anxiety. What are some of the strategies you might use to help people overcome anxiety?

Debra's story – A textbook case?

In the following account, Helen provides a reflection on Debra's personal narrative to inform interprofessional practice.

Over the years of co-teaching with Debra in voice-hearing, trauma and now the PTMF workshops for practitioners, my understanding of her narrative has informed my practice in many ways. First, knowing that context is important. We need to be mindful of how easy it is to follow a single, pre-determined version of Debra's experiences. Without context and through our own need to make sense of her world we could inadvertently minimise the significance of her story. Looking back over Debra's description of her life, there are many examples of how she lost her personal sense of power during her school years and while in the mental hospital, and examples of the power and dominance of the biomedical model. By interpreting her experiences through this narrow lens, Debra was ascribed many psychiatric labels and symptoms, which precluded any exploration of the meaning of her experiences and their relationship to her distress.

Debra 'passed through so many hands' when she was a child, experiencing the different types of power wielded over her by adults, some teachers and the school bullies. These threats led to the disruption of the **attachment** (Bowlby, 1982) that young children need to enable their social and emotional development.

attachment theory – describes the emotional bond developed between an infant and the attachment caregiver in the first year of life, who provides comfort and protection when the child is distressed

I remember my early years as a student nurse in a large institution. I witnessed how the mental hospital was a place of power over the patients and staff. Debra became immersed in a place in which sharing power with practitioners was not evident; she had little opportunity to begin a collaborative journey of healing. Like during her school days, Debra went to the staff library for respite. This was an enduring pattern of resilience and resourcefulness that she developed to manage her trauma as she adapted to life as a psychiatric patient.

Not having a place or identity led Debra to construct her self-meaning on the basis of other people's beliefs and opinions. Again, without parents, and trying to survive as a teenager in the hospital, Debra needed to look to who held the power in the wards. She was now in the hands of psychiatrists and nurses whose questions were no longer about her, or her life experiences, but rather about gathering information to fit into the many diagnostic criteria.

To regain some personal power, Debra learned the signs and symptoms of the common psychiatric diagnoses of that era. Giving the language of psychiatric diagnoses back to the clinician was a way of connecting and an invitation to them to enter a dialogue and help her make meaning of her experiences. However, Debra saw that this was a trap, as once she fulfilled the list of diagnostic criteria the practitioner's interest and conversations ceased. No one was 'joining the dots' to create a sense of the whole meaning for Debra; they did not need to as they had now defined who she was – a 'textbook case'.

Stitching a life back together

The PTMF brings into focus to the power of Debra's narrative. Dorothy was the only nurse who would take Debra for walks and talks, even though this was a direct challenge to the powerful rules and norms of the wards. This small gesture by Dorothy is an example of the use of her professional power by subverting the institutional rules. It also helped Debra to begin stitching her life back together, inspired by this quote from writer Toni Morrison:

> ... she gather me, man. The pieces I am, she gather them and give them back to me in all the right order. (cited in Palladino, 2018, p. 142)

Perhaps Dorothy instinctively knew that the walks and talks would help Debra make meaning of the patterns in her life. Debra felt supported and cared for, which helped her on the journey of recovery from the trauma and abuse. Another turning point was her unexpected guest, the panel beater, who helped her to turn her life around. As practitioners we need to acknowledge and actively support people to engage with the safe attachments in their lives, such as family, friends and pets. As discussed earlier, being sensitive to the needs of these supporters is important, as the blame for the abuse is commonly lain at their feet.

When practitioners work in a trauma-informed way, it reduces the threat of further trauma, helps the person to make meaning and regain their personal power. We also continue to learn from the people we serve, and their stories of survival; we need to celebrate their lives that are now flourishing. Marsha Linehan, the author of dialectical behaviour therapy (DBT), based this therapeutic approach on her own experiences of surviving trauma and abuse and, like Debra, describes how she was 'desperate, hopeless, deeply homesick for a life she would never know' (Carey, 2011). As practitioners we can balance the many approaches to understanding distress by helping the person to find meaning through the cultural, the psychosocial and biological lenses. As we discuss later in this chapter, recovery from interpersonal abuse and trauma is considered as taking place in three sequential but overlapping stages (Herman, 2001). The third stage is helping people like Debra to reconnect with their social world.

REFLECTIVE QUESTION

Have we transcended the historical patterns of care in the institutions that Debra describes? If so, discuss some examples.

REFLECTIVE QUESTION

REFLECTIVE QUESTION

In pairs, discuss how you could facilitate conversations that help the person develop their own understanding of how power, threat and meaning play out in their lives.

The Power, Threat, Meaning Framework

People seek help from professionals because they are not sure 'what is wrong'. Therefore, a fundamental part of the practitioner's role is to help the person understand the challenges disrupting their life at that moment. The PTMF integrates many existing models and practices, rather than replaces them. Moving from the deconstructive approach of 'what's wrong with you?' to one that helps the person to reconstruct the meaning of their experiences can be elicited through the following questions (Johnstone et al., 2018):

- What has happened to you? (How is **power** operating in your life?)
- How did it affect you? (What kinds of **threats** does this pose?)
- What sense did you make of it? (What is the **meaning** of these experiences to you?)
- What did you have to do to survive? (What kinds of **threat responses** have you used/ experienced?)
- What are your strengths? (What access to **power resources** do you have?)
- What is your story? (How does all this fit together?)

REFLECTIVE QUESTIONS

- In pairs, choose two of the questions above and practise by asking these questions to each other. If this is a new approach for you, then reflect on your thoughts and feelings.
- In what way would this new information disclosed by service users inform how you write your clinical notes?

Interpersonal trauma and mental health

Self-care

As practitioners we bring our own experiences to our work, and few of us have not experienced the distress and trauma of bereavement, broken relationships or betrayal of trust. We also bring to our work our own human vulnerabilities, so before reading the following section on TIC, take a moment to think about self-care. Remember, it takes courage for people to tell us their stories – and courage for us to listen to them.

The following sections focus on how practitioners can create safe interpersonal spaces in which to engage with people and avoid their re-traumatisation. Developing a therapeutic relationship is a fundamental skill or technology in mental health practice. It creates a safe space within which the person can talk about their life, worries, current challenges and hopes and dreams for the future. The therapeutic relationship creates the place in which the unspeakable may be spoken, and in which the unspoken can be expressed in symbolic language or behaviour, and can be recognised and accepted. In listening to accounts of interpersonal abuse, the practitioner helps the person to find understanding, meaning, acceptance and compassion for themselves. It is the profound human connection between the person and the practitioner that enables a sharing and co-construction of a personal narrative that constitutes the work of recovery. For many people we work with, psychological distress often arises from terrible experiences of abuse caused by a known and often loved and trusted person. Our witnessing of these accounts is part of the work of the mental health practitioner.

Practitioners' care can be trauma-informed when they recognise the high prevalence of neurological, biological, psychological and social effects of abuse and trauma on a person's development. In this chapter we focus more on the psychological and sociopolitical aspects of trauma, and the importance that we hear the 'real-world' voice of the users of the services we provide.

Many people present to mental health, addiction and disability services with histories of physical, psychological, emotional and sexual abuse. Being with people whose reality is imploding or fragmenting, and who are overwhelmed with terror, is honourable but also very challenging work and can also trigger our own experiences of abuse. To sustain this work, we need to care for ourselves. Observe your own limits. Be aware of your own emotional and psychological well-being to minimise the potential for vicarious traumatisation (Puvimanasinghe et al., 2015) or compassion fatigue (Ledoux, 2015), which describes the erosion of our capacity to care and is associated with our exposure to accounts of another person's traumatic experiences. If you begin to feel vulnerable and out of balance, talk to a trusted colleague or a professional clinical supervisor about the support services that are available in your workplace or university. The following section focuses on the effects of sexual abuse.

The seminal work by Finkelhor and Browne (1985) conceptualised four core traumagenic dynamics in the sexual abuse of children. These are traumatic sexualisation, betrayal, stigmatisation and powerlessness. Practitioners encounter a range of expressions of these dynamics; for example, persistent anxiety, fearfulness, difficulties with trust and feeling safe in the world, passivity, loss of autonomy and loss of hope. The person may engage in unsafe behaviours such as unsafe sex, substance misuse or addiction, anti-social behaviour, and may experience difficulty with intimate relationships. The person may also re-experience their trauma in flashbacks, nightmares or psychotic episodes. The person may have a self-concept of being flawed or damaged, and may experience difficulty establishing an identity. The person may be filled with shame and self-stigma, and may isolate themselves from others or fail to reach their potential in many areas of life, including education and employment.

Traumatised people are more likely to have longer and more frequent admissions to acute mental health facilities, spend more time in seclusion, relapse more frequently, be given psychotropic medications and attempt suicide and engage in self-harm than the general population (Read et al., 2003; Wilson et al., 2017; Tasa-Vinyals et al., 2020).

The effects of abuse may be reduced by the presence of consistent, loving relationships; for example, with grandparents or pets, and by early disclosure of the abuse, where the child is believed, supported and protected. However, interpersonal abuse most often remains a secret as children can feel responsible for the abuse or fear the consequences of disclosure (Alaggia, Collin-Vézina & Lateef., 2019; Alaggia & Wang, 2020).

The longer-term, adverse effects of abuse are increased the younger the age of the person at the time at which it begins. These effects are closely associated with the severity and frequency of the abuse and the person's relationship to the abuser. If the abuser is a parent or carer, then this leads to a betrayal of trust. The seminal work by Berliner and Conte (1990, 1995) found that many abusers employ a technology of abuse involving deliberate strategies for grooming the child into the abuse, in order to decrease the child's resistance and increase compliance. The abuse may start out with pleasant events such as fun games, and gradually the games become sexualised. The abuser may use threats to ensure that the child keeps the secret, such as threatening to kill the child's pet. Herman (2001) suggested that because abuse often remains secret, traumatic events surface not as a verbal narrative, but as a cluster of symptoms that become transformed into diagnoses – for example, borderline personality disorder and schizophrenia.

Widespread understanding of the traumatic effects of interpersonal abuse has emerged only in recent decades, in response to social movements such as gay and lesbian rights and civil rights, and more recently by closer collaboration with service-users movements (Russo & Rose, 2013; Sweeney et al., 2018). This has created a space for the voices of survivors of abuse to be heard. The effects of intergenerational trauma on Indigenous populations are also of concern to practitioners. In Aotearoa New Zealand, McClintock and colleagues (2018) have developed a national approach to TIC for Māori that considers the effects of historical, cumulative, intergenerational and situational trauma, and an understanding of a pre-European Māori society in which *whānau* (family) violence was not acceptable nor common. Likewise, in Australia the Blue Knot Foundation (see Further reading) collaborates with Aboriginal and Torres Strait Islander service providers to provide culturally informed services.

Trauma-informed care

TIC is achieved when a human service program takes the step to become trauma-informed. Archer, Lau and Sethi (2016) reported that women with a serious mental illness were more vulnerable to abuse, exploitation, sexual harassment and assaults in acute care units. TIC aims to protect the traumatised person from further harm, such as labelling and shaming, powerlessness, invalidation, restraint, seclusion and other coercive practices. TIC aims to provide safe spaces in which people can begin to construct a narrative account of the events in their lives and make meaning of their distress or illness. As discussed in the PTMF, rather than focusing on the individual's flaws or deficits, TIC repositions the questions from the total focus on a deficit-based assumption of 'What is wrong with you?' to 'What happened to you?' (Bloom, 1997, 2014; Bloom & Farragher, 2013; Johnstone et al., 2018).

The following section describes the role of the practitioner working within a TIC paradigm, and the required knowledge, attitudes, skills and interventions that reduce further harm to the people we serve. Practitioners are likely to encounter people with histories of sexual abuse and trauma in acute settings (Hepworth & McGowan, 2013; Archer et al., 2016). However, in our clinical experience, many practitioners report feeling anxious about 'opening a can of worms' or 'stirring things up' for the person by talking about abuse and with no apparent benefit to the person in them doing so. Although some practitioners work as specialists in interpersonal trauma recovery, most are not specialised in trauma work and have had only brief periods of time working with a person; for example, during a period of hospitalisation when acutely ill. Following are some suggestions for implementing TIC and facilitating the person's recovery within any context in which that care occurs.

INTERPROFESSIONAL PERSPECTIVES

The disempowering forces of institutions (health, schools, prisons) often do not support people to tell their own stories, so life becomes fragmented. As Debra worked on reducing her anxiety, she took the opportunity to engage in therapy. Debra engaged with a psychologist and a psychiatrist; the latter collaboratively reduced her medication to therapeutic levels as Debra now had her first child. She also began her therapy with the psychologist. At an earlier time in therapy, the psychologist arrived late for their appointment; she rushed into the room and apologised to Debra saying, 'my new baby has kept me up all night and I feel a complete wreck'. Debra immediately validated her by praising her ability to even get to work! Debra relates this situation as the most memorable, powerful and normalising experience for her in therapy – concluding that 'she is just like me, so I am normal'. This spontaneous self-disclosure by the psychologist could be regarded as a blurring of therapeutic boundaries; alternatively, it is an example of how we, as practitioners, are human and can be the role models for survivors, because 'if you can't see it, you can't be it'. Debra is no longer angry at the institutional staff, acknowledging that they too were traumatised by the closed system. All the staff were doing the best that they could with the skills that they had at that time. However, the institutions were, and perhaps can continue to be, **spirit-breaking** environments for both staff and 'patients' (Deegan, 2000).

spirit breaking – a process of being dehumanised and de-personalised in a psychiatric institution

The fundamental role of the practitioner is to listen compassionately and to respond to the needs of the distressed person in that moment. Be aware that every experience of human connectedness is powerful and contributes to recovery. You do not need to 'fix' the person. The person will do the work of healing over time as they progress through recovery. Herman's (2001) seminal work asserts that recovery from interpersonal abuse and trauma is considered as taking place in three sequential but overlapping stages:

1 Safety and stabilisation
2 Trauma resolution: remembrance and mourning
3 Social reconnection.

The ways in which mental health practitioners can support the person's work at each of these stages are discussed in the following section.

Stage 1: Safety and stabilisation

Safety and stabilisation of the person's mental state and environment are the first therapeutic tasks. The provision of safe places and safe people to be with is paramount, as most highly distressed people are likely to be at this first stage of recovery. TIC requires the practice of universal precautions (Racine, Killam & Madigan, 2020; Raja et al., 2015). Just as we carry a high awareness of pathogens in physical health care in order not to spread them (think COVID-19), likewise practitioners are required to treat every person as though the person carries a history of interpersonal abuse and its effects. This assists us to avoid re-traumatising the person because we only know that there is no history of abuse once the person has a safe-enough relationship with us to tell us so.

The person must be asked about their experiences of abuse and trauma, but this should be done in the context of a wider assessment in which other information is being gathered, to position it as something that is important but not shameful (Read, Hammersley & Rudegeair, 2007). People often wait to be asked about their abuse history on the basis that when we are ready to ask the question, we are ready to hear the answer. To tell staff members who may disbelieve them, judge them or pathologise them is a huge risk for any person; therefore, it is important to note that even if a person says 'no' in the first instance, they may disclose later with someone trusted.

Once the person has been asked about their experiences (see Chapter 15 for the funnel technique), the details should be recorded in the person's notes, as it can be re-traumatising to be asked the same questions many times by people one has only just met. Use the skills of the therapeutic relationship, particularly respect, empathy and being non-judgemental. If someone decides to tell you about a painful experience it is appropriate to reply, 'I'm sorry that happened to you.'

Supporting the stabilisation and safety of the person is fundamental; it is only when a person feels safe enough in the present, has learned skills in managing stress and distress, and has been educated about trauma and the trauma-recovery process, that they are resourced and ready to venture back into the terrors of the past. If the person chooses to talk to you about painful experiences, let them take the lead on what and how much to disclose. This respects the person's autonomy, the pace of talking about their experiences and self-protection mechanisms.

It is this re-experiencing – known as exposure – that is central to healing from trauma for all people. Talking to you about their experiences is one of the ways the person may use the therapeutic relationship with you. A way to prevent the person from becoming overwhelmed is to proceed cautiously in these conversations. This pacing can be difficult to manage, so just do your best; sometimes the story and the feelings associated with the story simply tumble out. Going too far, too fast, is the greatest pitfall in TIC. The tortoise, not the hare, is the role model for trauma work!

Inform yourself about what is known about the person's trauma history from their clinical notes and by talking to your colleagues. Use this information sensitively to care for the person and to prepare yourself to talk to them about the abuse and its traumatic effects when – and if – the person opens the conversation. Let them tell their story, rather than you recounting it from their history. Your role is to listen compassionately. The person's role is to be the expert on themselves, and to do the work of recovery.

Let the person know that you are interested in helping them to achieve a sense of safety. You can ask general questions like 'Do you feel safe in your room, or in this unit?' or 'Is there anything we can do to help you feel safe and comfortable here?' Be aware of the person's safety strategies to manage their fear of being harmed again in an interpersonal situation; for example, needing to be near a door for a fast escape from a situation. By being aware of these needs you can assist the person to manage the environment within what is possible in that clinical setting and reduce their distress.

Use the least coercive practices possible. Draw on your practitioner skills in de-escalation, **sensory modulation** (Andersen et al., 2017; Hitch et al., 2020) and interventions that are set out in the person's advance directives or care preferences, to avoid restraint and seclusion. Being held down or locked up can be overwhelmingly re-traumatising for people who have experienced these events in their past. Anxiety and distress are very common among traumatised people and can manifest in many ways, including self-harm. It is important to understand the effectiveness of self-harm in its many forms – such as cutting, overdosing, and drug or alcohol abuse. Self-harm is helpful to people in different ways, including enabling their dissociation from painful memories and feelings or locating the pain in the physical body rather than in the heart or mind. Support the person to reduce their distress through self-soothing skills or medications they find helpful until the person's skill levels improve. Referral to structured therapies such as dialectical behaviour therapy (DBT) (Linehan, 2014) can provide effective skills for relief from symptoms of anxiety.

Be authentic and trustworthy; do what you say you are going to do. Trust feels like a dangerous risk if your life experience is one of betrayal by those who are supposed to nurture and love you. Take care not to judge the abusive people or their life experiences; it is for the person to do that if they choose. The work of making sense of loving someone while hating what they did to you takes time. Validate the person authentically. This means giving genuine feedback and care. Interpersonal abuse is a strong form of invalidation, so any form of validation is healing. Genuine, constructive feedback is usually very helpful to someone who is struggling with constructing an identity beyond 'shameful victim' or 'mad person', and in creating a narrative account of their life in which their strengths, character and talents can emerge and shine.

Use collaborative investigation and discovery, not of the details of the abuse but of abuse-related issues such as grief, anger or low self-esteem. The PTMF makes sense and meaning of the person's experience as part of the process of recovery, and them gaining understanding, processing anger and grieving for the many losses arising from their abuse.

Suspend your judgement about the truth of accounts of interpersonal abuse you may hear. Many health professionals find they are unable to believe that people can treat each other so cruelly, and question whether what they hear or read in clinical notes is indeed true. It is not our role to investigate the truth of these experiences; that would be the role of the legal system (Australian Government, 2017), based on the accounts of abuse of children in institutions.

Some people may want to report the abuse to legal authorities. This is often because the person wants to stop the offending and protect other children from the abuser. There are complex judgements to be made about how to proceed, so consult with your team and your supervisor if a person raises this with you. What most people want to resolve in their disclosure of traumatic experiences is acknowledgement that it happened, not denial and secrecy, and that it was the responsibility of the abuser, that it was harmful to them and that some repair is made such as acknowledgement and apologies from those who abused and those who failed to protect the person from abuse (NSW Health Education Centre Against Violence, 2013).

Safety is a paramount value in mental health practice. Be prepared to let the person know that if they tell you that they, or another person, is unsafe in some way, you will need to share

sensory modulation – 'the neurological ability to regulate and process sensory stimuli', which 'offers the individual an opportunity to respond behaviorally to the stimulus' (McClintock et al., 2018)

that information with others. Never try to deal with complex problems alone; consult with the team about how to proceed – this is where the wisdom of the team is needed – and check what current policies in your clinical area mandate on the reporting of abuse.

Consider ways in which you can increase your knowledge and skills in caring for abused and traumatised people. Reflect on accounts of interpersonal abuse in the news; understand the ways in which power plays out in interpersonal relationships and the attitudes and values that have led to them occurring. This provides a broader context for understanding the experiences of people and, indeed, ourselves.

Stage 2: Trauma resolution

Once a person has achieved safety and stability, they are able to move to the next stage: trauma resolution. In this stage, the person works with a trusted therapist to process their traumatic memories through graded exposure by telling and retelling their story within a safe, therapeutic space. The person is supported to make sense of their experiences; something they may have thought impossible because they consider themselves to be 'mad'. The person may have been told that they are mad by others as a way of keeping the abuse secret; constructing the teller of the story as 'crazy' and not to be believed. At this stage of recovery, the PTMF has supported the person to construct a narrative account that makes connections between past experiences, symptoms of mental illness and behavioural patterns.

The role of the practitioner in this stage is to support the work of therapy by following the plans of the DBT-trained psychotherapist, which guide the care and skill development of the person. You can make a great contribution to the person's recovery by being active and skilful in liaison and communication with their therapist or the crisis team, to help the health system to work smoothly and effectively.

Stage 3: Social reconnection

In this stage, the person reviews their social context and makes choices about whom to include in their life. They reconnect with education and employment and seek the ordinary joy and happiness of life. At this point many people experience freedom from their symptoms of psychological distress or mental illness because the source of these problems, past abuse and the trauma that ensued have been resolved. Many people make remarkable recoveries and contribute their knowledge of the experience of both abuse and recovery in the support of others on the recovery journey. This is known as the 'survivor mission'. As we heard from Debra, she has been on her mission to normalise distressing voices in the work she does with practitioners.

While TIC provides a pathway for recovery for many people, there are also people who do not wish to revisit their past or who do not attribute their current distress or problems to interpersonal life events. Each person has their own narrative account of experiences of mental ill health, which we must respect. Trauma-informed mental health practice is helpful for all people, regardless of how and where they experience their distress or illness. It respects their right to least-coercive care, is focused on the therapeutic relationship and empathic care, supports the development of skills for managing distress, and works for the creation of a narrative that makes meaning of the past in the present.

A practitioner's story

I recall the anxiety I felt as a new mental health nurse when I read a consumer's 'history' before working with them for the first time in the in-patient unit. Accounts of intense psychological distress and references to past abuse and chaotic life circumstances would often feel overwhelming to me. As a new nurse, what did I have to offer this person? Would I say the right things or make things worse? How would I meet my professional responsibilities as a mental health nurse? Over time I discovered for myself the wisdom of mental health nursing's focus on therapeutic relationships. The key to my anxiety as a new practitioner was learning how to create a safe therapeutic space. While 'history' can provide a helpful context for meeting the person, it is usually not written by that person. I needed to build a therapeutic relationship in which the person could speak of their hopes and needs.

The moment would come when I would need to introduce myself and explain my role. I would remind myself of the values of being authentic, respectful, non-judgemental, trustworthy and compassionate. I would take some deep breaths, greet the person, and listen to them with all my mind and heart. What had begun as a daunting professional challenge would become a conversation between two people grappling with the challenges of life, health and recovery. As time went by, I brought more knowledge and skills to my conversations with consumers; however, the foundation of the therapeutic relationship always remained essential and powerful. Experience helps us to build confidence but a little anxiety will always remain because we meet each consumer anew and afresh, and we are challenged to understand and engage with their uniqueness as a human being and with their unique recovery experience.

TRANSLATION TO PRACTICE

SUMMARY

This chapter has presented stories and information, supplemented with activities designed to deepen your understanding of:

- The *importance of supporting survivors of abuse* to make the links between their past and current experiences, and their distress. The PTMF contributes to the cultural and biological meanings of mental distress and extreme states experienced by the people we serve. Through the consumer narratives, we can begin to understand how we might facilitate a survivor's ability to stitch their lives back together again, as they continue on their journey of recovery from abuse and trauma.
- Our *own understandings and attitudes* towards trauma and how we can break the silence by asking and responding safely to those who have experienced trauma in some institutional care settings.
- How *working in a trauma-informed way* can decrease the risk of re-traumatisation in mental health settings and can increase practitioners' confidence and skills in delivering safe and effective care to survivors.

CRITICAL THINKING/LEARNING ACTIVITIES

1   In the TIC section we discussed the importance of recognising our own human vulnerabilities and the need to consider self-care as practitioners. Having reflected and discussed the above activities, pay attention to the helpful strategies that you are currently using, or could use in the future, that promote your own well-being.

2   Review the section on the PTMF and, when re-reading Debra's story, look for the experiences that demonstrate this theory within her narrative

3   Reflect on your current work or placement setting. How safe would it be for the people you serve to disclose their experiences of trauma and abuse?

4   Debra learned the medical textbook language to describe her experiences. Think about how you could collaboratively develop an alternative language that more effectively describes her experiences of trauma and abuse.

5   Practise the skill of validation with both service users and your colleagues.

LEARNING EXTENSION

The PTMF provides a lens through which practitioners might understand mental distress and extreme states, such as psychoses and dissociative experiences. Commonly, the 'hard science' of the biomedical model can dominate our understanding of these presentations, to the exclusion of the person's lived experience. The challenge for practitioners is to reconsider the focus and meaning of the latter – for example, is the person responding to the threat of negative voices, or is it part of a delusion? Is it part of how power and threat are operating in the person's life?

• Work systematically through the PTMF questions (Translation to practice – The Power, Threat, Meaning Framework) to guide you in exploring Debra's story again. Identify the meaning of the voices and/or her behaviours, and what recurring patterns there are in her life.

• Review some of the protocols in your unit to assess how trauma-informed they are, such as seclusion and restraint.

FURTHER READING

The Blue Knot Foundation: National Centre of Excellence for Complex Trauma (website). Retrieved from https://www.blueknot.org.au
This site provides a range of resources, guidelines and practitioner competencies for the clinical treatment of trauma and abuse, including guidelines for TIC and Aboriginal and Torres Strait Islander peoples.

British Psychological Society. (n.d.) *Power Threat Meaning Framework*. Retrieved from https://www.bps.org.uk/power-threat-meaning-framework
This site provides information on the PTMF, including an introduction, good practice examples, research and publications, and training materials and information on diversity, inclusion and anti-racism.

Family Action Network. (2015). *Balancing Acceptance and Change: DBT and the future of skills training*. Retrieved from https://www.youtube.com/watch?v=JMUk0TBWAScBorn

Watch this account of the development of DBT by Professor Marsha Linehan. DBT was developed for what practitioners described as the 'hard-to-treat' clients: people who presented with repeated self-harm and suicide attempts. DBT has revolutionised the approaches to people with such enduring problems.

Johnstone, L. (2019). Crossing cultures with the power threat meaning framework – New Zealand. *Mad in the UK* (Blog), 24 February. Retrieved from https://www.madintheuk .com/2019/02/crossing-cultures-with-the-power-threat-meaning-framework/

Lucy Johnstone, lead author of the PTMF, gives an account of the framework in the context of Aotearoa New Zealand.

McClintock, K., Haereroa, M., Brown, T. & Baker, M. (2018). *Kia Hora Te Marino– Trauma Informed Care for Māori*. Wellington: Te Rau Matatini. Retrieved from https://terauora.com/wp-content/uploads/2019/05/Kia-hora-te-marino-Trauma-Informed-Care-for-Ma%CC%84ori.pdf

This resource promotes the imperative that practices and implementation of a trauma-informed care approach for Māori be supportive for individuals, *whānau*, *hapū*, and communities, and that they consider intergenerational and historical trauma. Providing culturally safe trauma-informed care approaches that are cognisant of a Māori worldview and experiences, as Māori, that incorporate the values and beliefs expressed in the resource, is pivotal. Historical trauma is used in this context to encompass the profoundly negative and significantly harmful effects of colonisation on Māori health including physical, emotional, spiritual, social, cultural and economic well-being.

Te Rau Ora, Le Va, Werry Workforce Whāraurau & Te Pou. (2021). *Weaving Together Knowledge For Wellbeing – Trauma informed approaches*. Retrieved from https://www.tepou.co.nz/resources/trauma-informed-care-resources/877

These factsheets provide information on a range of trauma-informed resources, including resources to work with Māori.

REFERENCES

Alaggia, R., Collin-Vézina, D. & Lateef, R. (2019). Facilitators and barriers to child sexual abuse (CSA) disclosures: A research update (2000–2016). *Trauma, Violence, & Abuse, 20*(2): 260–83.

Alaggia, R. & Wang, S. (2020). 'I never told anyone until the #metoo movement'. What can we learn from sexual abuse and sexual assault disclosures made through social media? *Child Abuse & Neglect, 103*: 104312.

Andersen, C., Kolmos, A., Andersen, K., Sippel, V. & Stenager, E. (2017). Applying sensory modulation to mental health inpatient care to reduce seclusion and restraint: A case control study. *Nordic Journal of Psychiatry, 71*(7): 525–8.

Archer, M., Lau, Y. & Sethi, F. (2016). Women in acute psychiatric units, their characteristics and needs: A review. *Psychiatric Bulletin, 40*(5): 266–72.

Australian Government. (2017). *Royal Commission into Institutional Responses to Child Sexual Abuse*. Retrieved from https://www.childabuseroyalcommission.gov.au

Berliner, L. & Conte, J. (1990). The process of victimisation: The victim's perspective. *Child Abuse and Neglect, 14*(11): 29–40.

——— (1995). The effects of disclosure and intervention on sexually abused children. *Child Abuse & Neglect, 19*(3): 371–84.

Bloom, S. L. (1997). *Creating Sanctuary: Toward the evolution of sane societies*. New York: Routledge.

——— (2014). The sanctuary model of trauma-informed organizational change. *The Source, 16*(1). Retrieved from https://www.researchgate.net/publication/242222586_The_Sanctuary_Model_of_Trauma-Informed_Organizational_Change

Bloom, S. L. & Farragher, B. (2013). *Destroying Sanctuary: The crisis in human service delivery systems*. New York: Oxford University Press.

Bowlby, J. (1982). Attachment and loss: Retrospect and prospect. *American Journal of Orthopsychiatry*. https://doi.org/10.1111/j.1939-0025.1982.tb01456.x

Carey, B. (2011). Lives restored: Expert on mental illness reveals her own fight. *New York Times*, 23 June. Retrieved from http://archive.nytimes.com/www.nytimes.com/2011/06/23/health/23lives.html

Caruth, C. (ed.) (1995). *Trauma: Explorations in memory*. London: Johns Hopkins University Press.

Deegan, P. E. (2000). Spirit breaking: When the helping professions hurt. *The Humanistic Psychologist*, *28*(1–3): 194–209.

Finkelhor, D. & Browne, A. (1985). The traumatic impact of child sexual abuse: A conceptualization. *American Journal of Orthopsychiatry*, *55*(4): 530–41.

Hepworth, I. & McGowan, L. (2013). Do mental health professionals enquire about childhood sexual abuse during routine mental health assessment in acute mental health settings? A substantive literature review. *Journal of Psychiatric and Mental Health Nursing*, *20*(6), 473–83.

Herman, J. L. (2001). *Trauma and Recovery: The aftermath of violence – from domestic abuse to political terror*. New York: Basic Books.

Hitch, D., Wilson, C. & Hillman, A. (2020). Sensory modulation in mental health practice. *Mental Health Practice*, *23*(3), 10–16.

Johnstone, L., Boyle, M., Cromby, J., Dillon, J., Harper, D., Kinderman, P. … Read, J. (2018). *The Power Threat Meaning Framework: Towards the identification of patterns in emotional distress, unusual experiences and troubled or troubling behaviour, as an alternative to functional psychiatric diagnosis*. Leicester, UK: British Psychological Society. Retrieved from https://www.bps.org.uk/power-threat-meaning-framework

Kezelman, C. & Stavropoulos, P. (2019). *Complimentary Guidelines to Practice Guidelines for Clinical Treatment of Complex Trauma*. Sydney, Australia: Blue Knot Foundation. Retrieved from www.blueknot.org.au

Ledoux, K. (2015). Understanding compassion fatigue: Understanding compassion. *Journal of Advanced Nursing*, *71*(9): 2041–50.

Linehan, M. M. (2014). *DBT Skills Training Manual*, 2nd edn. New York: Guilford Press.

McClintock, K., Haereroa, M., Brown, T. & Baker, M. (2018). *Kia hora te marino – Trauma Informed Care for Māori*. Wellington, New Zealand: Te Rau Matatini. Retrieved from https://terauora.com/wp-content/uploads/2019/05/Kia-hora-te-marino-Trauma-Informed-Care-for-Ma%CC%84ori.pdf

NSW Health Education Centre Against Violence. (2013). *Recovering from Adult Sexual Assault: Navigating the journey*. Retrieved from http://www.ecav.health.nsw.gov.au/online-shop/booklets/recovering-from-adult-sexual-assault-navigating-the-journey/

Palladino, M. (2018). *Ethics and Aesthetics in Toni Morrison's fiction*. Leiden, The Netherlands: Brill Rodopi.

Puvimanasinghe, T., Denson, L. A., Augoustinos, M. & Somasundaram, D. (2015). Vicarious resilience and vicarious traumatisation: Experiences of working with refugees and asylum seekers in South Australia. *Transcultural Psychiatry*, *52*(6): 743–65.

Racine, N., Killam, T. & Madigan, S. (2020). Trauma-informed care as a universal precaution: Beyond the adverse Childhood Experiences Questionnaire. *JAMA Pediatrics*, *174*(1): 5–6.

Raja, S., Hasnain, M., Hoersch, M., Gove-Yin, S. & Rajagopalan, C. (2015). Trauma informed care in medicine. *Family & Community Health*, *38*(3): 216–26.

Read, J., Agar, K., Argyle, N. & Aderhold, V. (2003). Sexual and physical abuse during childhood and adulthood as predictors of hallucinations, delusions and thought disorder. *Psychology and Psychotherapy: Theory, Research and Practice*, *76*(1): 1–22.

Read, J., Hammersley, P. & Rudegeair, T. (2007). Why, when and how to ask about childhood abuse. *Advances in Psychiatric Treatment*, *13*(2): 101–10.

Russo, J. & Rose, D. (2013). 'But what if nobody's going to sit down and have a real conversation with you?' Service user/survivor perspectives on human rights. *Journal of Public Mental Health*, *12*(4): 184–92.

Sweeney, A., Filson, B., Kennedy, A., Collinson, L. & Gillard, S. (2018). A paradigm shift: Relationships in trauma-informed mental health services. *British Journal of Psychiatric Advances*, *24*(5): 319–33.

Tasa-Vinyals, E., Álvarez, M.-J., Puigoriol-Juvanteny, E., Roura-Poch, P., García-Eslava, J. S. & Escoté-Llobet, S. (2020). Intimate partner violence among patients diagnosed with severe mental disorder. *The Journal of Nervous and Mental Disease*, *208*(10): 749–54.

Tseris, E. (2020). *Trauma, Women's Mental Health, and Social Justice: Pitfalls and possibilities*. London and New York: Routledge.

Wilson, A., Hutchinson, M. & Hurley, J. (2017). Literature review of trauma-informed care: Implications for mental health nurses working in acute inpatient settings in Australia. *International Journal of Mental Health Nursing*, *26*(4): 326–43.

3

Māori mental health

Kerri Butler and Jacquie Kidd

LEARNING OBJECTIVES

At the completion of this chapter, you should be able to:

1 Understand the different ways of being Māori, and the importance of accurately identifying Māori mental health and cultural needs.
2 Consider how a practitioner's own ethnicity might influence their care of Māori *tangata whaiora*.
3 Explore how historical trauma and current health care practices have affected the mental health of Māori, and how health professionals can help to improve Māori health outcomes.
4 Develop skills in culturally safe assessment, including *whanaungatanga*.
5 Develop skills in facilitating the culturally safe care of *tangata whaiora* and *whānau*.

Whakatauki

Mā te rongo, ka mōhio; Mā te mōhio, ka mārama; Mā te mārama, ka mātau; Mā te mātau, ka ora.

Through perception comes awareness; through awareness comes understanding; through understanding comes knowledge; through knowledge comes life and well-being.

Mihi

This chapter was written by two women, each with different experiences of mental health, mental distress and being Māori. It also contains work and stories from Reina Harris, for which we are very grateful.

These are our ***pepeha***.

Ko Pukehaua ngā Pukehuia ngā maunga
Ko Toukahawai te awa
Ko Ngati Porou, ko Ngā Puhi, ko Ngati Pakeha ngā iwi
Ko Te Whānau a Hinerupe rāua ko Ngati Te hau ngā hapū
Ko Kerri Butler tōku ingoa

Ko Te Ahuahu tōku maunga
Ko Omapere tōku wai
Ko Ngāpuhi tōku iwi
Ko Te Uri Taniwha rāua ko Ngati Hineira ōku hapū
Ko Jacquie Kidd tōku ingoa

mihi – a speech, formally acknowledging, among other things, people you meet, the purpose of the meeting and the place where the meeting is being held, through protocols set by the *iwi* (tribe)

pepeha – a person's introduction, which includes the mountain, river, tribe and sub-tribe from which they have come

Introduction

There are many ways of being Māori. Ethnicity in Aotearoa New Zealand was historically assessed according to blood quantum (e.g. half-caste or quarter-blood) but has now moved to a more contemporary approach of self-identification, which assumes ethnicity is not static and predetermined. Instead, ethnicity and culture are viewed as intertwined aspects of a person's identity, influenced by our social environment, and therefore can change as we mature and our context shifts (Cormack, 2010; Kukutai & Didham, 2009). This means that any combination of physical features, cultural beliefs and ways of living can be found in people who self-identify as Māori.

PERSONAL NARRATIVE

Kerri's story – part one

I recall during one of my admissions being told by a Māori nurse that I had no right to talk about culture. She spoke to me in Māori and demanded that I translate it. I turned to her and said, 'You know I wasn't bought up in a Māori environment; I don't have to speak *te reo* to feel Māori'.

In short, it is not possible to assume that someone is Māori or non-Māori based on their appearance or lifestyle. Asking **tangata whaiora** (person seeking well-being) is the only way to be certain about someone's ethnicity and is a vital part of the first assessment.

For Māori, health and culture are intricately linked, so when a person identifies as Māori there are vital aspects of *te ao Māori* (the Māori worldview) that must be understood in relation to their mental health experiences in order to provide safe and effective care. In this chapter we discuss how practitioners from all cultural backgrounds can develop practices that engage with *tangata whaiora* and *whānau* in mental health and addiction settings. The chapter will be helpful for people practising in the Aotearoa New Zealand context, as well as those who encounter people of Māori descent in Australia or elsewhere. It will also assist practitioners to consider how institutional racism might influence their ability to care for Māori, and will encourage the exploration of personal cultural beliefs to transcend this. *Tūmata Kōkiritia* is a series of four interconnecting concepts that were developed by *tangata whaiora*; these will be presented as a framework for developing culturally safe practices.

> *Tūmata* means to ignite, to incinerate, to burn as getting rid of the old thinking. *Kōkiritia* means to champion, to promote, to lead and to advocate. *Tūmata Kōkiritia* therefore means igniting champions to lead, to advocate and provoke. (Butler & Te Kīwai Rangahau, 2017, p. 4)

Māori health

Māori in Aotearoa New Zealand have been subjected to a continuous process of colonisation since 1840, whereby land, language and traditions have been systematically removed and resulting in many Māori being displaced from the economic and social structures that had historically supported them. The consequences of colonisation can be seen in the continuing high levels of socio-economic deprivation and poor health status of many Māori (Ministry of Health, 2019).

Māori comprised 16.5 per cent of the population in Aotearoa New Zealand in 2018 (Stats New Zealand, 2020) and are a young and increasing population, with high proportions of young Māori people in every region of Aotearoa New Zealand.

Māori are disproportionately represented among those with the highest socio-economic need, which means that Māori have higher risks associated with poor mental health than non-Māori. Māori are also less likely to receive timely and effective health care than people from other cultures (Ministry of Health, 2019).

The only Aotearoa New Zealand national mental health survey was carried out in 2005. Of more than 12 000 households participating in the survey, more than 50 per cent of Māori experienced illnesses affecting their mental health at some time during their lives (Oakley Browne, Wells & Scott, 2006). The most common disorders identified by researchers were anxiety (31.3 per cent), substance-use disorders (26.5 per cent) and mood disorders (24.3 per cent), and many Māori had more than one diagnosable illness (Baxter et al., 2006). The most common diagnoses for Māori when hospitalised were schizophrenia and bipolar disorder. More than half of Māori who had a serious mental illness and about three-quarters who had a moderate illness also had no contact with health care providers for their mental health needs (Oakley Browne et al., 2006; Ministry of Health, 2008). Māori access to mental health care is often through the court and justice systems, with higher rates of overall hospitalisation and a higher likelihood of admission to forensic or secure units than non-Māori (Baxter, 2008). In 2012–14, young Māori men (aged 15–24 years) were more than twice as likely as young non-Māori men to die by suicide. Māori have higher incidence of mortality due to suicide than non-Māori; in 2012–14, Māori were over 1.5 times as likely as non-Māori to die by suicide (Ministry of Health, 2008, 2019).

While these statistics show a disturbing picture of Māori mental health, this is not the whole story. *Te ao Māori* provides an holistic approach to health and well-being that can be aligned with the philosophy of recovery. Effective mental health care requires practitioners to move beyond the deficit approach (a perspective that focuses on the negative aspects of health) towards a way of understanding *tangata whaiora* and *whānau* as people who have unique experiences, needs, strengths and stories of personal success. In the next section we discuss potential ways for clinicians to respond to Māori needs for health and wellness.

Kawa whakaruruhau (cultural safety)

The Nursing Council of New Zealand sets out competencies that require practitioners to practise in a manner that **tangata whenua** determine as being culturally safe, and to demonstrate the ability to apply the principles of the Treaty of Waitangi to nursing practice (Nursing Council of New Zealand, 2007).

The historical component of cultural safety is found in *te Tiriti o Waitangi*, which underpins the relationship between Māori and the settler government and legislation of Aotearoa New Zealand (Berghan et al., 2017). It is viewed as the foundational document for mental health service planning and delivery (Mental Health Commission, 2012). In summary:

- Article One requires the Crown to consult and collaborate with *iwi* (tribes) and **hapū** (subtribes) regarding the functions and operations of 'good government'. This includes the development and delivery of health services.
- Article Two 'guarantees Māori rights of ownership, including non-material assets such as *te reo*, **hauora** and **tikanga**' (Mental Health Commission, 2012).
- Article Three 'guarantees Māori the same rights of citizenship and privileges as British subjects, including the rights of equal access to mental health and addiction services, to equal health and well-being outcomes and to access mainstream mental health and addiction services that meet the needs of Māori' (Mental Health Commission, 2012).
- Article Four, which was a verbal addition to *te Tiriti* at the time of its first signing, guarantees religious freedom.

Early breaches of *te Tiriti* saw the theft of land through war, confiscation or subterfuge, which meant that *whānau, hapū* and *iwi* lost the means to support themselves economically, and lost places of great spiritual significance. These losses still affect the sense of *whānau* identity and individuals' ability to express themselves as belonging to a secure social structure. The transition from self-determination to powerlessness and poverty, in addition to the introduction of new strains of disease, reduced physical health further and affected the resilience of *whānau* (Jackson, 1992).

For mental health nurses, these Articles highlight the need to work together with Māori to improve health outcomes, support Māori participation in their own health care, recognise that health is a **taonga** (treasure) that is worthy of protection and facilitate equitable access to health care. The Articles of *te Tiriti o Waitangi*, along with education about Māori health, form the basis for *kawa* **whakaruruhau**, or cultural safety within the Māori context (Nursing Council of New Zealand, 2011).

---

tangata whenua – an inclusive term to indicate all the people who belong to a particular place; in the context of cultural safety it includes all people of Māori descent involved in care

hapū – a division of a Māori *iwi* (tribe), often translated as 'subtribe'; membership is determined by genealogical descent; a *hapū* is made up of a number of *whānau*

hauora – health, including social, emotional, spiritual and physical health

tikanga – the customs and traditions by which Māori live and practise within the environment; *Tikanga* also establishes the principle of **tino rangatiratanga**, ensuring autonomy and self-determination in Māori communities and organisations over their own property, assets and resources. In the mental health clinical context, *tino rangatiratanga* includes *tangata whaiora* and *whānau* autonomy.

tino rangatiratanga – self-determination, self-management, ownership, autonomy

taonga – a treasured object or idea; includes stories and tangible resources such as health and land

whakaruruhau – to protect, shield, shelter; *kawa whakaruruhau* is the term used in nursing for cultural safety

INTERPROFESSIONAL PERSPECTIVES

Cultural competence in the health professions

In Aotearoa New Zealand, all health professions make a commitment to cultural competence, as prescribed by the *Health Practitioners Competence Assurance Act 2003* and the Health and Disability Commissioner's Code of Rights. The aims of developing cultural competence include the provision of an accessible and welcoming service, and the ability to provide patients and their *whānau* with health information that they can relate to and understand.

The different disciplines have developed cultural competencies in their own distinct ways, but they are all interested in improving health equity for Māori.

There are two challenges in particular that can interfere with the delivery of culturally safe care. One is that, as practitioners and people, we are often not good at recognising how our culture influences our everyday attitudes and activities. Increased personal awareness is a way of opening our eyes to the cultural differences *tangata whaiora* and *whānau* might experience when they accept mental health care.

The second challenge is known as 'institutional racism', which means that Western-specific attitudes, processes and routines are embedded within the health system and create barriers that are detrimental to other cultures (Jones, 2000). Examples of institutional racism include staff attitudes and policies that do not recognise the value in *whānau* support of *tangata whaiora*, buildings and schedules that do not accommodate *pōwhiri* and **whanaungatanga** processes (greeting and connection processes, both of which are discussed later), professional codes of conduct that forbid the sharing of personal histories and the lack of provision of trained and acceptable translators.

whanaungatanga – from *whānau*, meaning family; Māori may share a common *whakapapa* with other people and therefore a strong sense of belonging, with common ancestral linkages. In another sense, *whanaungatanga* is about forming a connection with other people, which is not necessarily linked to *whakapapa*. The connection may be community, work, hobby or sports-related and acknowledges that there are other layers of *whānau*. This forms an important part of an holistic worldview within Māoridom.

PERSONAL NARRATIVE

Reina's story – part one

One of the key things that I can say with regard to working with Māori is to have an understanding of different worldviews. Essentially, the predominant worldview in the health sector is Eurocentric and with this worldview comes the tendency to place lesser emphasis on things that other cultures consider as extremely relevant. For Māori one of the key things that is relevant to well-being is spirituality.

REFLECTIVE QUESTION

What barriers to cultural safety can you identify in the education and health organisations of which you are a part?

Whānau ora

Whānau is the central structure in Māori society, so prioritising the health of *whānau* is a way of improving Māori health outcomes. The concept of *whānau ora* has been used widely within the public sector to describe an overarching goal in the development of Māori-specific programs, strategies and policies (Kara et al., 2011). *Whānau ora* happens when Māori families are supported to achieve their optimal health and well-being within both *te āo* Māori and the broader Aotearoa New Zealand society, and have control over their own destinies (Ministry of Health, 2002, 2008). The function of *whānau* is to provide strength, security, identity and nurturing. A *whānau* can have many shapes. A familiar one includes *tamariki* (children), *rangatahi* (youth), *pakeke* (adults) and **kaumātua/kuia** (grandparents/elders). *Whānau* can also include formal or informal adoptees, can arise through social structures such as school and church groups, and can emerge as organic networks based in shared experiences; for example, the *whānau* groups of *tangata whaiora*.

kaumātua – a male elder who is traditionally a guardian of genealogy, spirituality and Māori knowledge

kuia – a female elder who is traditionally a guardian of genealogy, spirituality and Māori knowledge

PERSONAL NARRATIVE

Kerri's story – part two

I remember my overnight stay at Sunnyside hospital after attending a conference. It sticks in my mind how amazing the staff were to involve my brother and sister-in-law. Instead of shunting them off with a 'Thanks, we'll take care of her now', the staff asked them to stay with me and to help them to encourage me to take the medication. I lay down and went to sleep with my family beside me. This was in vast contrast to less than a week later, in a different unit, when my husband was removed from the room and four or five staff lined up against a wall, ready to restrain and administer medication .

Whānau is the base structure from which *hapū* (wider *whānau* or subtribes) and *iwi* (tribes) are built, with the processes for connecting individual, *whānau*, *hapū* and *iwi* being as important as the structures themselves. Focusing on *whānau ora* has the potential to create ripples of health and well-being that improve health outcomes at every level of Māori society (Whānau Ora Taskforce, 2009).

REFLECTIVE QUESTIONS

- What shape is your *whānau*?
- Do you belong to more than one?

When working with Māori *tangata whaiora*, it is also important to recognise that *tangata whaiora* have individual voices. Some *tangata whaiora* have spoken of the distress they feel when their individual voice becomes 'lost' in the collective voice, especially if *whānau* adopt a caregiving role that focuses on symptom identification and management, and 'pathologises' reasonable responses to distress. Just as we identify the key roles a practitioner plays in recovery, we need to ensure that *whānau* are clear about the roles they can play in their loved one's life, and that *tangata whaiora* feel empowered to have a say in how that looks. Relationships can be severely damaged by health professionals who either expect *whānau* to monitor and manage their loved one or interfere with the healing role of *whānau* by excluding them.

PERSONAL NARRATIVE

Kerri's story – part three

I can remember an incident when I was walking around the open, low-stimulus area, asking if someone could please contact my mum. I can recall feeling like my head was fragmenting and the only thing I knew that would ground me was to speak to my mum. To be told 'We are not contacting her, she knows you are in here' was really distressing. I spoke to my mum about that, and she said, 'I never said that; I had no idea'.

I think about my own children and know that I would want to be there, no matter what time of night, if they needed me. First and foremost, *whānau* have to take care of themselves, but part of taking care of their own **wairua** is being there for their loved ones. There is a disjointedness that comes from being separated and left helpless when your loved ones are sick. This can damage relationships; while one is left to deal with the mental illness, the other is the *whānau*, who are left feeling like they have failed and let their loved one down.

wairua – spirit, soul, spirit of a person, which exists beyond death. It must also be acknowledged that not all *whānau* are healthy; some contribute to distress for the *tangata whaiora*. The principles of trauma-informed care can help to guide practitioners when this is identified.

oranga – well-being, in both material and non-material senses, including food, livelihood, welfare, health and living well; it may also refer to safety

Hauora (health) and *oranga* (wellness)

Hauora and **oranga** represent social, emotional, spiritual and physical health for Māori. With all these in a healthy balance, the *whānau* and individuals are able to participate in and enjoy their language, spirit and land. These are the cornerstones of a flourishing people (Blisset, 2011). These four concepts of social, emotional, spiritual and physical health have been drawn together in a model called *Te Whare Tapa Wha* (Durie, 1994), which views each concept as the side of a house. Each side is important to the structure and stability of the house; if one aspect of life is missing or unhealthy, the entire structure is at risk.

PERSONAL NARRATIVE

Reina's story – part two

In the Hokianga area, on the west coast of Northland, Māori cultural values are interlinked with the provision of health services. Why this works for *tangata whaiora* is that the service recognises the spiritual dimension of healing. *Mirimiri* is part of the 'package of care' wrapped around *tangata whaiora*. *Mirimiri* literally translates as 'massage', but it really means that a connection has to be made between the healer and the *tangata whaiora* on a spiritual level, for the treatment to have a greater effect ... a connection between energies ... I was not in a good place when I began *mirimiri*. I had my first session when my son was four days old, when things began to whirlwind out of control for me ... I remember walking blankly into the room and I just sat there with my baby in my arms and I just could not stop the tears. The healer just started to *mirimiri* me ... and when I left I felt lighter and centred within myself.

Wairua: Spirituality

Wairua (spirituality) is a fundamental part of *te ao Māori*. It is associated with more than religion. *Wairua* encompasses how a person is connected to their ancestors and to future generations, and also their connection to the environment: land, language, history, mythology and heritage. *Wairua* includes how a person communicates with their world, and what they have faith in.

PERSONAL NARRATIVE

Reina's story – part three

The way that I was taught is that the spirit world is closely connected to the living world. Māori will always acknowledge spirits as the essence of things. This worldview allows for little distinction between the world of the living and the spirit world. The reason I am talking about this is because, for me, when I am more 'sick' my connection with *te ao wairua* is more pronounced. I see things and hear things and am more aware of things.

Assessment of *wairua* in practice

It can be very difficult to find your way into an assessment of *wairua* in practice, particularly if it is viewed as an 'add on' to the assessment process. Often, it appears on an assessment form as a check box, or a space just big enough to write the name of a religion. Instead of waiting until you get to the space on the form, try starting your assessment by asking the person what is most important to them. You could share some of your own experiences, such as loving to walk on the beach, or how important your family is to you. Starting an assessment by identifying how a person enriches their *wairua* can give you a vitally important understanding of how they view the world.

TRANSLATION TO PRACTICE

Whanaungatanga: Engagement with *tangata whaiora*

The common biomedical understanding of an initial assessment includes the practitioner having a list of questions that the person in care needs to answer. The initial assessment of *tangata whaiora* and *whānau* requires a more human approach, with a focus on achieving connection, engagement and understanding first, before any probing questions are asked. It is important to note here that these processes are also quite likely to benefit *tangata whaiora* who do not identify as Māori. Culture is often presented as a boundary that divides people (Maddalena, 2009) but, in fact, people across the world have a similar need for connection and security. The processes we are describing here are taking a Māori worldview that is specific to meeting the needs of Māori, but need not be exclusive to Māori.

Whanaungatanga is a traditional Māori practice of connection and engagement, and has been identified as the single most powerful action health practitioners can bring into their practice with *tangata whaiora* and *whānau*, to uphold *kawa whakaruruhau* and improve Māori experiences of health care (Carlson et al., 2016; Slater et al., 2013). *Whanaungatanga* includes the whole care team and the whole *whānau*. It is usually begun with *karakia* to open and bless the space and the people involved. Following *karakia*, each person in turn shares information about the places that are important to them, their family connections and, for the clinicians, their professional qualifications and experience. Māori staff as well as *tangata whaiora* and *whānau* may share their *pepeha*, which are similar to the ones at the start of this chapter. *Whanaungatanga* is a transparent, caring, nurturing process that opens up a space for respectful communication to occur, and affirms the willingness of the health professionals to work in culturally safe ways.

Challenges for practitioners during *whanaungatanga* include having to work in buildings that were not designed for large groups of people to meet, the pressures of time for all health professionals and the need to produce large amounts of documentation within a very short period of the initial contact with mental health services. These issues can mean that *whanaungatanga* is limited to only a few people, is rushed, or is used for information gathering or assessment. A further challenge comes from the sector's worldview that health professionals should not share their own identities with patients, which acts as a barrier to establishing an authentic relationship with *tangata whaiora* and *whānau*.

After people are introduced to each other, the needs of *tangata whaiora* and *whānau* can be explored by inviting and respecting their stories. Nurses and other healthcare professionals tend to search for evidence of symptoms in people's stories, disregarding accounts that demonstrate values based on culture, personal achievements and their explanations about why they are distressed right now. When people are able to express their stories in a way that makes sense to them, it creates a feeling of empowerment. It communicates to them that their story matters, where they have come from matters and their sense of identity and 'self' matters. It is important to remember that storytelling is an important part of the process of *whanaungatanga*. Being too quick to offer explanations or to ask questions can stop the storytelling process, and the opportunity for connection may be lost. In our experience, giving *tangata whaiora* time to gather their thoughts and tell their stories in their own way usually results in people being more receptive to continuing contact with practitioners.

Engaging authentically involves putting aside our professional expertise in order to hear about the strengths, solutions and unmet needs of *tangata whaiora* and *whānau*. It allows *whānau* to be prioritised, rather than marginalised, through the expression of the *whānau* story, and gives us the tools to provide trauma-informed care.

Trauma-informed care (see Chapter 2) for Māori includes awareness of the dispossession and alienation associated with colonisation, as well as knowledge of the effects of socio-economic deprivation on rates of interpersonal violence, including sexual abuse (Marie & Fergusson, 2008). Historical trauma is associated with physical, mental, *whānau* and social problems that reoccur, and possibly worsen, from generation to generation (Pihama et al., 2014). Examples of historical trauma that continue to effect Indigenous peoples' lives include stress-related genetic conditions such as high cholesterol and high blood pressure, high cancer prevalence, deepening cycles of poverty and unresolved grief from the many losses they have experienced. Re-traumatisation can occur when an already traumatised person and/or *whānau* has their pain recreated through experiences in health settings (Herman, 1997). Having a respectful and caring process for listening to stories can help to create the profound human connection that enables the work of recovery from trauma to begin.

Opportunities to share stories

Listening to stories can seem like a very time-consuming activity, and when you are working in a highly pressured environment it can also be viewed as an addition to care rather than an essential part of care. However, some of the most effective ways to elicit and listen to stories involves making yourself available during ordinary activities. Going for a walk, sitting quietly together, tidying a bedroom, wiping down the kitchen bench and supervising a meal are all everyday activities in the mental health setting, and can all be storytelling and listening opportunities.

TRANSLATION TO PRACTICE

Listening carefully to the stories of *tangata whaiora* and *whānau* invites the purpose of the person's engagement with health services to be explored and therefore to recognise that their involvement with mental health and addiction services is purposeful, not a life sentence. Stories enable us to understand what needs to be done now to reduce distress, and what recovery looks like for this person and their *whānau* (Barker & Buchanan-Barker, 2004). It is the first step in planning for discharge, and it takes place in the very beginning of the relationship.

Once *whanaungatanga* has created a base of engagement, *tangata whaiora*, *whānau* and health care professionals can begin to work together. The collective commitment to connection and listening creates a united environment of support, expertise, shared insights and hope. This is the work of recovery.

The goal of recovery presents a challenge for practitioners to adapt to the adjustments and transformations experienced by *tangata whaiora* and *whānau* as distress resolves and new discoveries are made. Change for some people is a rapid process of revelations and new knowledge, while for others it is a slow progression that can span several years. During this time, it is easy for practitioners to become discouraged and either withdraw from care or become harsh (Caldwell et al., 2006), so being aware of our own mental health and job satisfaction is an important feature of being able to deliver culturally safe care.

PERSONAL NARRATIVE

Reina's story – part four

A well-known Māori *Tohunga* (expert) wrote about the connected nature of God, Man and Universe and, indeed, this is what I have been taught. Everything is connected and it is vital to make connections with regard to identifying yourself, your connections with the environment, mountains, rivers and land, and your connections to people, tribes and subtribes. It is these connections that can build or impinge on well-being. When I think back to the time when I became unwell (or depressed, as is the clinical term), I believe it is directly related to my loss of connection. I was brought up close to my tribal lands and I became unwell in the city, where I was estranged from my land. I am not saying that you can't move from your tribal area and be well, but I am saying that in my case I feel that being estranged from my tribal area contributed to my unwellness. Conversely, when I have difficulties, I have to go home; the water is very important to me so I go to this special place, a river where my ancestor healed his battle wounds.

Tūmata Kōkiritia: Shifting the paradigm

Research conducted in 2017 with *tangata whaiora* identified four key concepts to increase self-sufficiency for Māori health and well-being and to promote best practice approaches for *whaiora Māori* (Butler & Te Kīwai Rangahau, 2017). These concepts are *mātauranga Māori* (Māori knowledge), *mana* enhancing practices (respectful, uplifting practices), *tino rangatiratanga* (self-determination, autonomy) and *kotahitanga* (unity).

Mātauranga Māori is a source of healing, which includes practices such as *tohunga* (traditional healer), *kaumātua* and *kuia* (elders), *rongoā* (traditional medicine) and *romiromi* or *mirimiri* (traditional massage).

Mana-enhancing practices include cultural safety, being culturally responsive to the needs and aspirations of *tangata whaiora* and *whānau*, and valuing the knowledge and leadership of a Māori workforce who have lived experience. The process of *whanaungatanga* embracing the whole dynamics of a person, of forming relationships, are fundamental to health and well-being. The model of care with Māori must have less reliance on labels and diagnosis, and more on traditional interpretations such as the *Atua* (gods) and spiritual reconnections. Part of the healing is gaining self-identity.

Tino rangatiratanga means that the effectiveness of services should be evaluated by *tangata whaiora* and *whānau*; those with lived experience. The integration of mental health, physical health, spiritual health, cultural health, providing appropriate healing environments, offering choices and the creation of safe places are central to Māori autonomy. A healing environment that acknowledges culture encourages positive engagement and better health outcomes.

Kotahitanga creates spaces for Māori and *tangata whaiora* in decision-making, including policy. It emphasises the Māori worldview in all mental health care and ensures that funding for Māori solutions is equitable.

Tūmata Kōkiritia emphasises igniting, advocating and leading change. It shows how the mental health sector can be improved, not only for *tangata whaiora* and *whānau*, but for health professionals as well.

PERSONAL NARRATIVE

Mare's story – part one

I was the primary nurse for Mare, a young Māori woman who had developed puerperal psychosis following the birth of her first child, four weeks prior to her admission. Mare was brought to hospital by the police after a member of the public noticed the baby laying unattended on the front lawn. Mare believed that her child was sick and that she needed to be surrendered to *Papatuanuku* (Goddess of the Earth) for healing. From a Māori worldview, Mare's beliefs were consistent with a strongly traditional way of managing illness; however, the baby appeared to be healthy and meeting developmental milestones.

Mare's involvement with police, a mental health in-patient unit and social workers who were concerned for the welfare of the baby had increased her anxiety and separated her from her partner, mother and wider *whānau*. The processes of assessment and admission had removed from her the very people who could have explained her thought processes and relieved her anxiety.

I proposed that a *whānau hui* (meeting) be held and, in consultation with Mare's mother, organised a *hui* for Mare, her female relatives and a female psychiatrist. Mare's male relatives stepped back from this process because issues relating to childbirth are *tapu* (sacred) and are the domain of women. Mare's grandmother, a *kuia* (elder), opened the *hui* with a **karakia**, then provided support and spiritual protection for the *whānau* as they discussed what had happened.

An important process in this *hui* was for the psychiatrist and I to introduce ourselves with a high level of personal disclosure. I shared my *whakapapa* (genealogy), my nursing background and some information about my childbirth experiences, including that I had experienced severe postnatal depression following all my children's births. From this sharing of stories, the *whānau* came to see that I had a professional and personal history that enabled me to understand what Mare and the *whānau* might be experiencing.

by Jacquie

karakia – a prayer or incantation for a specific purpose, such as spiritual guidance or protection

REFLECTIVE QUESTIONS

- How does it make you feel to think about sharing personal information?
- How much is too much?

Mare's story – part two

The women of the *whānau* wanted to take responsibility for Mare and her baby, by taking them home and staying with them while Mare's symptoms resolved. The *whānau* revealed that Mare had been trying to get pregnant for almost two years before conceiving, and that even before the birth of her child she had been terrified that some harm would befall her baby. They felt that her anxiety had increased after the birth, and this had been exacerbated by a long labour and severely interrupted sleep over the previous month. Mare was getting up many times at night to check that the baby was breathing and warm. Mare's symptoms appeared to the *whānau* as a logical consequence of combined high levels of anxiety and fear with physical trauma from the birth and postpartum period, and a Māori worldview. They understood her desire to put her baby in close connection with the Earth Mother to assist with healing, although they were concerned about why and how she chose to do this, and the potential for harm to the baby.

The *whānau* discussed taking turns to stay with Mare and the baby, including Mare's mother taking leave from work to be available. In total, four of the women in the *whānau* committed to a roster, so that someone would be present in the house with Mare to support, monitor and help her with care of the baby. This included helping Mare and her baby to safely connect to *Papatuanuku* as a part of the healing process.

Daily visits from the Māori mental health service were organised, as well as weekly meetings with the psychiatrist to monitor Mare's progress. Social support services agreed to step back from the *whānau* on the condition that they received regular reports about Mare's care and the baby's progress. Mare's general medical practitioner was brought onto the care team to provide care for the *whānau* and to monitor the baby's health.

Mare and her baby were discharged from the mental health unit that day, and I had no further involvement in their care. Recovering from puerperal psychosis takes time and continuing treatment; for Mare and her *whānau* it took more than three months of care and support. Mare and her mother came to visit me six months after our meeting and brought along the baby for me to see her.

by Jacquie

Kerri's story – part four

I did not grow up with an attachment to my Māori roots, yet when I become unwell I discovered there is a connection. I sense my grandmother around me.

When I returned to the community after a particularly traumatising seclusion when I was six-and-a-half months pregnant, I knew all I wanted to do was to get back up north to where my grandmother was buried. I felt if I did, then everything would come right for me. The ward staff involved the Māori cultural team and I was given the most amazing support. They used to come and get me off the ward whenever I phoned and take me to the *whare*, which was a place of healing and sanctuary for me. More importantly, they helped me make connections and links to the people back 'home' in the north, so that when my baby girl was born we were able to take a trip back up north to bury her placenta at my grandmother's feet.

There was a huge sense of belonging. To this day, during times of turbulence and extreme distress I want to link back to my **turangawaewae** (land to which I belong). There's a feeling and sense of safety in 'coming home'.

During my most recent admission, after being secluded I wanted to have the seclusion rooms blessed, and to have a *taonga* (treasured object or idea). I was fortunate that the *Kaumātua* said 'Get your partner or *whānau* to bring something in for you'. I chose a football. My football was blessed and affectionately became known as 'Harry Hippo' to both me and fellow patients. I was allowed to dribble it around the unit sometimes, and I even slept with it. I became distressed and difficult to manage at those times when it was taken from me. It was a way I had of disconnecting from the trauma I was experiencing from being away from my *tamariki* (children) and my *whānau*. That ability to hold myself in the moment and create my own safe world was a powerful source of recovery or grounding for me.

turangawaewae – 'a place to stand'; places where we feel especially empowered and connected; our foundation, our place in the world, our home

REFLECTIVE QUESTIONS

In her story, Kerri has identified some important cultural needs, including feeling her grandmother around her when she's distressed, wanting to have the seclusion room blessed and keeping a *taonga* close to her. Changing the language of a story can completely change its meaning.

- Try rewriting Kerri's story from a medical perspective. How has it changed? What might those changes in language and meaning mean for your practice?
- Advocacy is an important part of our clinical role. Would you be brave enough to advocate for Kerri's football? What strategies could you use to gain acceptance from the rest of the clinical team?

SUMMARY

This chapter has presented stories and information, supplemented by activities designed to deepen your understanding of:

- The importance of not making assumptions about what looks, behaviours and beliefs are identifiable as Māori. People express their culture in many different ways, so the role of the mental health practitioner is to assess people's unique needs.
- How our own ethnicity and culture can shape how we experience the world, and therefore also can influence how we view Māori people in our care. Self-awareness is the principle underpinning our ability to provide culturally appropriate care.
- The strong connection between a history of economic and cultural loss and current mental health problems. This is compounded by the continuing institutional racism of many healthcare

organisations. Health professionals can influence the way care is planned, accessed and delivered, so are in a position to improve Māori mental health.

- The process of introducing ourselves and getting to know each other, which is fundamental to being able to conduct an effective assessment. We need to help people feel safe and understood before they share their stories with us, and then use our skills to elicit those stories that will help us to identify where their needs are and how we can best meet those needs.

- The aspects of care that help people feel safe and hopeful is the basis of culturally safe care. Our multidisciplinary approach to service delivery in the mental health setting provides the opportunity for the practitioners who know people best to advocate for their care to be individualised according to their cultural needs.

CRITICAL THINKING/LEARNING ACTIVITIES

1   In small groups, discuss the following:

   - When you think of your own ethnicity or culture, what are the most important aspects for you? These could include specific relationships, ceremonial occasions such as birthdays, weddings or Christmas, foods, or special places.
   - How often do these aspects of culture show up in your everyday life? Consider books, music, television, slang, and jokes.
   - Discuss how your own cultural outlook might manifest itself in your practice.

2   In small groups, list the benefits that come from having a regular, long-term source of income and place to live. Once you have completed your list, use *Te Whare Tapa Wha* to discuss the effects of losing these.

3   Role-play possible ways of working with *whanaungatanga* to establish engagement with clients. Consider how to arrange the environment, who should be present, who should speak and what should be shared.

4   In pairs, take turns to tell a story about a time in your life when you have felt distressed or traumatised. For the listener: how does it feel to listen to a story without interrupting, sharing your own story or providing solutions? For the storyteller: did you feel comfortable sharing this story? Why or why not?

5   In small groups, discuss your response to part two of Mare's story. What risk factors can you identify? Were all of these risk factors acknowledged in Mare's plan of care? What could have been done differently?

LEARNING EXTENSION

Aotearoa New Zealand has a diverse cultural population, including people who are Indigenous to other lands but who live here by choice or necessity. There are several Māori health models, some of which appear in the 'Further reading' section of this chapter. Choose one model that describes a Māori worldview and one from each of two other Indigenous cultures that are present in the region in which you live. Compare the similarities and differences in the approaches. Consider whether providing care that meets the competencies for *kawa whakaruruhau* might assist you in providing culturally safe care to people from other cultures.

FURTHER READING

Ministry of Health – Manatū Hauora. (2017). *Māori health models – Te Pae Mahutonga*. Retrieved from https://www.health.govt.nz/our-work/populations/maori-health/maori-health-models/maori-health-models-te-pae-mahutonga
A Māori health model that brings together elements of contemporary health promotion.

Ministry of Health – Manatū Hauora. (2017). *Māori Health Models – Te wheke*. Retrieved from https://www.health.govt.nz/our-work/populations/maori-health/maori-health-models/maori-health-models-te-wheke
A traditional Māori model of health that acknowledges the link between the mind, the spirit, the human connection with *whānau* and the physical world, in a way that is seamless and uncontrived.

NZ On Screen. (2017). *Waru* (trailer). Retrieved from https://www.nzonscreen.com/title/waru-2017
For this 2017 feature film, eight Māori women each directed a 10-minute segment of events, circling around the *tangi* of a boy named Waru. Each director had a day and a single shot to capture their take on the context behind a tragedy.

Te Pou. (n.d.). *Te Reo Hāpai – The Language of Enrichment*. Retrieved from http://www.tepou.co.nz/initiatives/te-reo-hapai-the-language-of-enrichment/169
The *Te Reo Hāpai* project aims to better accommodate the use of Maori language in the mental health and addictions sector.

Te Rau Matatini (n.d.). *He Manaaki Tangata: Tikanga Informed Guideline Adapted for Mental Health Services, and Acute Mental Health Units*. Retrieved from https://terauora.com/wp-content/uploads/2019/05/Manaaki-Tangata-Tikanga-Best-Practice-for-frontline-workforces.pdf
This practice guideline is a guide for health professionals who are supporting Māori *tangata whaiora* and their *whānau* in mental health services, and especially so in the acute mental health unit.

Ter Au Ora (Website). Retrieved from https://terauora.com/
This website provides the latest in Māori mental health research and projects.

REFERENCES

Barker, P. & Buchanan-Barker, P. (2004). Beyond empowerment: Revering the story teller. *Mental Health Practice, 7*(5): 18–20.

Baxter, J. (2008). *Māori Mental Health Needs Profile Summary: A review of the evidence*. Palmerston North, New Zealand: Te Rau Matatini.

Baxter, J., Kokaua, J., Wells, J. E., McGee, M. A. & Oakley Browne, M. A. (2006). Ethnic comparisons of the 12 month prevalence of mental disorders and treatment contact in Te Rau Hinengaro: The New Zealand Mental Health Survey. *Australian and New Zealand Journal of Psychiatry, 40*(10): 905–13.

Berghan, G., Came, H., Doole, C., Coupe, N., Fay, J., McCreanor, T. & Simpson, T. (2017). *Te Tiriti-based practice in health promotion*. Auckland: Stop Institutional Racism.

Blisset, W. (2011). *He Puawaitanga Mo Tatou Katoa. Flourishing for All in Aotearoa: A creative conversation to explore a Māori world view of flourishing*. Wellington: Mental Health Foundation.

Butler, K. & Te Kīwai Rangahau. (2017). *Tūmata Kōkiritia – Shifting the Paradigm*. Auckland: Te Rau Matatini.

Caldwell, B. A., Gill, K. J., Fitzgerald, E., Sclafani, M. & Grandison, P. (2006). The association of ward atmosphere with burnout and attitudes of treatment team members in a state psychiatric hospital. *American Journal of Psychiatric Rehabilitation, 9*: 111–29.

Carlson, T., Barnes, H. M., Reid, S. & McCreanor, T. (2016). Whanaungatanga: A space to be ourselves. *Journal of Indigenous Wellbeing: Te Mauri – Pimatisiwin, 1*(2): 44–59. https://journalindigenouswellbeing.com/media/2018/07/51.44.Whanaungatanga-A-space-to-be-ourselves.pdf

Cormack, D. (2010). *The Politics and Practice of Counting: Ethnicity in official statistics in Aotearoa/ New Zealand*. Wellington: Te Rōpū Rangahau Hauora a Eru Pōmare.

Durie, M. H. (1994). *Whaiora: Māori health development*. Auckland: Oxford University Press.

Herman, J. L. (1997). *Trauma and Recovery*. New York: Basic Books.

Jackson, M. (1992). The treaty and the word: The colonisation of Māori philosophy. In G. Oddie & R. Perrett (eds), *Justice, Ethics and New Zealand Society* (pp. 1–10). Auckland: Oxford University Press.

Jones, C. P. (2000). Levels of racism: A theoretic framework and a gardener's tale. *American Journal of Public Health, 90*(8): 1212–15.

Kara, E., Gibbons, V., Kidd, J., Blundell, R., Turner, K. & Johnstone, W. (2011). Developing a Kaupapa Māori Framework for Whānau Ora. *AlterNative: An International Journal of Indigenous Peoples, 7*(2): 100–10.

Kukutai, T. & Didham, R. (2009). In search of ethnic New Zealanders: National naming in the 2006 Census. *Social Policy Journal of New Zealand*, (36): 46–62.

Maddalena, V. P. (2009). Cultural competence and holistic practice: Implications for nursing education, practice, and research. *Holistic Nursing Practice, 23*(3): 153.

Marie, D. & Fergusson, D. M. (2008). Ethnic identity and intimate partner violence in a New Zealand birth cohort. *Social Policy Journal of New Zealand, 33*(March): 126–45.

Mental Health Commission. (2012). *Blueprint II: How things need to be*. Wellington: Mental Health Commission.

Ministry of Health. (2002). *He Korowai Oranga: Māori health strategy*. Wellington: Ministry of Health.

——— (2008). *Te Puawaiwhero: The second Māori mental health and addiction national strategic framework 2008–2015*. Wellington: Ministry of Health.

——— (2019). *Wai 2575 Māori Health Trends Report*. Retrieved from https://www.health .govt.nz/publication/wai-2575-maori-health-trends-report

Nursing Council of New Zealand. (2007). *Competencies for the Registered Nurse Scope of Practice*. Wellington: Nursing Council of New Zealand.

——— (2011). *Guidelines for Cultural Safety, the Treaty of Waitangi and Māori Health in Nursing Education and Practice*. Wellington: Nursing Council of New Zealand.

Oakley Browne, M. A., Wells, J. E. & Scott, K. M. (2006). *Te Rau Hinengaro: The New Zealand Mental Health Survey*. Wellington: Ministry of Health.

Pihama, L., Reynolds, P., Smith, C., Reid, J., Smith, L. T. & Te Nana, R. (2014). Positioning historical trauma theory within Aotearoa New Zealand. *AlterNative: An International Journal of Indigenous Peoples, 10*(3): 248–62.

Slater, T., Matheson, A., Davies, C., Tavite, H., Ruhe, T., Holdaway, M. & Ellison-Loschmann, L. (2013). 'It's whanaungatanga and all that kind of stuff': Maori cancer patients' experiences of health services. *Journal of Primary Health Care, 5*(4): 308–14.

Stats New Zealand. (2020). *2018 Census totals by topic – national highlights (updated)*. Retrieved from https://www.stats.govt.nz/information-releases/2018-census-totals-by-topic-national-highlights-updated

Whānau Ora Taskforce. (2009). *Whānau Ora: A whānau-centred approach to Māori wellbeing. A discussion paper*. Retrieved from www.msd.govt.nz/about-msd-and-our-work/publications-resources/planning-strategy/whanau-ora/index.html

The social and emotional well-being of First Nations Australians

4

Katrina D. Ward and Rhonda L. Wilson
With acknowledgement to Debra Hocking
for the previous editions

LEARNING OBJECTIVES

At the completion of this chapter, you should be able to:

1 Describe the concept of social and emotional well-being (SEWB).
2 Describe the determinants of SEWB in the context of colonisation.
3 Discuss priorities for closing the gap in the context of SEWB.
4 Discuss the application of cultural safety principles to SEWB and mental health practice.
5 Outline the cultural practice of *dadirri* as a strategy to promote and restore personal SEWB.

Introduction

This chapter is written by two Aboriginal women who are both experienced mental health nurses. We recognise that many First Nations Australians live with the challenges that stem from the legacy of the colonisation process (that is, past government policies), and the resultant and intertwined intergeneration trauma. Our perspective as First Nations women who work in the mental health context is that the Western, medicalised public-health delivery system does not always adequately accommodate the social and emotional well-being needs of First Nations people. This is a continuing challenge to effective and culturally safe mental health service delivery in Australia. We hope this chapter introduces you to some of the concepts that inform an understanding of social and emotional well-being in the mental health context.

social and emotional well-being (SEWB) – experienced individually and collectively, SEWB comprises experiences at the social, emotional and cognitive levels that resonate meaningfully as connectedness in the inner self with culture and spirit. SEWB is associated with a respect for the sacredness of land, sea, ancestry, spirituality, flora and fauna. It is experienced as an internalised sensation that is felt within the core of a person's or community's humanity and is outwardly expressed through relationships between culture and lore in a continuous cycle of life and death.

First Nations – a term denoting Indigenous peoples, used internationally. In the Australian context, First Nations and Indigenous peoples are also known as Aboriginal and/or Torres Strait Islander peoples. We recognise that Australia is a diverse multi-First Nations community, made up of over 500 Indigenous clans and nations.

We introduce the concepts of **social and emotional well-being (SEWB)** for **First Nations** people in Australia, from a First Nations standpoint, and in the context of mental health. In general, a mainstream understanding of health is applied when mental health (illness) presentations are considered, assessed and treated from a biomedical Western perspective and standpoint (Wilson & Waqanaviti 2021). A limitation of this approach is that services are designed and funded in a manner that frequently perpetuates the dominance and privilege of mainstream service users. It is apparent that not all individuals and groups who are eligible for public mental health services are able to access it equitably. Nurses and midwives throughout Australia have called for further action to promote culturally safe health care for First Nations people, as a mechanism to improve (mental) health service equity and to reduce the gap or disparity in health outcomes experienced by First Nations people in Australia (Geia et al., 2020).

This book presents a person-centred approach to mental health and is designed to support students to gain a practical understanding of the application of mental health caring strategies at the point of care. The SEWB and mental health needs of First Nations people can be considered from a person-centred approach. For many First Nations people, the term 'person' recognises that individuals are inseparable from their connections to family (past and present), Country and culture. These elements are intertwined into a singular, holistic expression of 'person'. Providing mental health care to First Nations people using a person-centred approach requires the adaption of Westernised, biomedically dominant approaches, to include a cultural knowledge that underpins the delivery of mental health care that is aligned with a cultural interpretation of personhood. For example, enabling the person and their families to be involved in the decisions about the planning, treatment and continuing care promotes an understanding of First Nations cultures as it endorses a consensus decision-making model, which is the accepted practice of First Nations peoples. This, in turn, can assist the individual in 'keeping well' as they feel valued and listened to on a wider scale.

The term 'First Nations people' is used throughout the world to refer to Indigenous peoples. In the Australian context, this includes people and communities who identify as Aboriginal or Torres Strait Islander First Nations peoples, who are recognised by the community in which they live, or who identify as Aboriginal and/or Torres Strait Islander. We have elected to use First Nations terminology in this chapter to encapsulate the Australian experience. This chapter aims to explore mental health through an alternative First Nations lens, that of SEWB. While there is a scarcity of national data that specifically measures the SEWB of

First Nations people, the data that is available paints a consistent picture: one of much higher rates of use of mental health services by First Nations people, compared to other Australians (Australian Institute of Health and Welfare (AIHW), 2009). To gain an understanding as to why First Nations people have higher incidence of mental distress, we must examine the historical and cultural factors that have affected, and continue to affect, the lives of First Nations Australians.

This chapter sets the context for further discussion regarding First Nations people and explores issues relating SEWB and mental health. Colonisation and its history are discussed, as well as the subsequent decimation and devastation that followed, and continue today. Government policies that were specifically designed to control the lives of First Nations people are discussed, and their effects revealed. The **resilience** and struggle that have taken place, along with cultural recognition and renewal, ultimately shape the present. While the present is explored in this chapter, the complexity and the effects of colonisation on First Nations peoples are so monumental that not all aspects are able to be covered within this chapter. For this reason, additional online resources are suggested for further reading and consultation.

resilience – an inner strength of spirit and capacity to bounce back from, and cope with, adversity

Social and emotional well-being

From a mainstream perspective, 'being socially and emotionally well means being able to realise your abilities, cope with the normal stresses of life, work productively and contribute to your community' (ACT Government, 2016, p. 46). However, from a First Nations' viewpoint, this is an overly narrow and impersonal definition because First Nations people extend the definition of SEWB to include the overall effects on the spiritual and cultural well-being of an individual (Wilson & Waqanaviti, 2021). The concept of mental health is derived from an illness, clinical or medical perspective and its focus is predominantly on the individual and their functioning in their environment. However, SEWB is a holistic concept that results from a network of relationships between self, family, kin and community (Wilson & Waqanaviti, 2021). SEWB, for First Nations people, also recognises the importance of connection to land, culture, spirituality, family and community, and how these affect the individual (Commonwealth of Australia, 2017a). A deficit in any of these domains can have a negative effect on the overall health and well-being of the individual. Deterioration in mental health and/or the development of mental illness is precipitated by a deterioration in SEWB.

The theme of connection

Many First Nations people identify rivers as a protective factor that enhances well-being. It is often said that 'a sick river leads to a sick community'. Traditionally, many rivers were identified as highways or boundaries of the many Aboriginal nations. Our ancestors would wander along the river systems and considered them a safe haven, providing a pathway to hunting and fishing. Rivers sides were also used as places for meeting and bartering, as well for ceremonies to be held.

> The river connected many tribes and many purposes for survival. During times of drought or flood, the ability of people to travel and connect along the rivers was reduced, hence affecting their own well-being as social connection was limited. When the rivers returned to their natural flow people returned to travel along the rivers, and their well-being improved as they became more active and engaged with activities the river provided. This is similar in many in rural areas, as a healthy river brings joy in provision of fresh food and recreational activities for young and old, which are simple ways of keeping well.

First Nations people also recognise that a person's SEWB has been, and continues to be, influenced by government policies and past events such as policies of assimilation, the legacies of the Stolen Generations and Aboriginal deaths in custody.

Determinants of social and emotional well-being

The First Nations population in Australia continues to experience significant inequity in accessing appropriate mental health services. This is expressed in the high incidence of poorer mental health, and other health conditions, experienced by First Nations people (Wilson & Waqanaviti, 2021). When antecedents are considered, we can observe that a range of ecological and political processes has underpinned mental ill-health in general.

colonisation – the forced act of establishing a colony or colonies, taking full political, social and economic control, and with disregard for existing peoples and cultures

British **colonisation** of Australia occurred very recently on the world calendar, only 233 years ago (1788). This led to a brutal era, with many massacres occurring throughout Australia, such as the Myall Creek massacre in 1838 (Friends of Myall Creek, n.d.), where First Nations people were killed in their tens of thousands. By way of further context, Australia's first prime minister was appointed to the role only 120 years ago (1901). Just 60 years ago, the Australian Parliament voted to accept the bill for the Assimilation Policy (Commonwealth of Australia, 1961, p. 1051), which aimed to force the assimilation of First Nations people into Australian society. In doing so, it relegated First Nations people to a status similar to children who required others to make responsible decisions for them. In 1962, Aboriginal people were permitted to register to vote in federal elections (National Museum of Australia, n.d.), but were not required (like other Australians) to vote until 1984. As recently as 1967, a referendum was held and Australians voted to recognise and count First Nations people in the national census; this event is within the living memory of many people today (Australian Institute of Aboriginal and Torres Strait Islander Studies (AIATSIS), n.d.). Before this time, the state had no higher regard for First Nations people than that of fauna, or perhaps a child or minor. In 1992, the High Court of Australia recognised for the first time that First Nations people had lived in Australia prior to colonisation, finding in favour of Eddie Mabo's challenge and resulting in the recognition that First Nations people are the Traditional Owners of Australian lands through provisions for Native Title land rights and claims (*Native Title Act 1993*; Commonwealth of Australia, 2017b). A far longer list could be generated than the small sample noted in these examples to highlight federal and state government policies and legislation throughout Australia that have resulted in discrimination against First Nations people since colonisation. Each of these have contributed to the collective deterioration of SEWB for First Nations people, with the intergenerational trauma consequences continuing to manifest today.

Tips for keeping well

The following are some tips that can help improve people's SEWB.

- Connect to self – tune in to who you truly are.
  - Become familiar with your senses to recognise 'how you feel':
    - listen to your body: aches, pains, churning, breath – fast/slow
    - feel the clothes against your skin: tight/loose, breath – hot/cold
    - identify smells around you: dull/sharp, sweet/odour
    - recognise tastes: dry, moist, salty, fresh.
- Connect to place and/or space.
  - Identify safe places to connect to land/Country:
    - feel the aura around you
    - sense your protective intuition.
- Find your rhythm.
  - Practise mindful breathing exercises:
    - feel the changes in body as you let out a deep breath – shoulders relaxing.
- Connect with family, loved ones or friends.
  - Spend time together:
    - share yarns, help each other, share quiet time
    - get active in sports or hobbies.
- Do things you enjoy – art, fishing, spend time with family or friends etc.
- Reduce substance misuse or abuse and increase healthy food choices.

There is a stark contrast between the proximity and trauma of colonisation in Australia, and the endurance and resilience of First Nations peoples with 60–65 000 years of their continuous cultural connection to land (Pascoe, 2014). On the one hand, colonisation has occurred in a relatively brief interval of time. On the other, First Nations people have cared for land, lore and each other for the longest interval of time of any peoples throughout the history of the world; one could say, since the Dreamtime. The cultural disruptions due to the impost of colonisation upon First Nations peoples have been severely limiting, with a deterioration in the determinants of SEWB apparent. The consequences are an enduring legacy of intergenerational trauma that has led to poor SEWB and significant mental ill-health for many people. It is unsurprising that this would be the case, based on our scientific understandings (both Western and Indigenous) of the determinants of SEWB and mental health, in general. In 2017, First Nations peoples gathered at Uluru, in a National Constitutional Convention. They noted that in 1967 First Nations people were counted in Australia; now the request was that they also be heard. The Uluru Statement from the Heart (see page 66) is an important outcome from the meeting and provides a narrative to propel change and nurture hope for a future free of systematic discriminations and disadvantage towards First Nations peoples throughout Australia. The Uluru Statement from the Heart urges 'truth telling' about Australian history, and calls for reconciliation in *makarrata*; that is, the coming together after a struggle.

Uluru Statement from the Heart

Our Aboriginal and Torres Strait Islander tribes were the first sovereign nations of the Australian continent and its adjacent islands, and possessed it under our own laws and customs. This our ancestors did, according to the reckoning of our culture, from the Creation, according to the common law from 'time immemorial', and according to science more than 60 000 years ago.

This sovereignty is a spiritual notion: the ancestral tie between the land, or 'mother nature', and the Aboriginal and Torres Strait Islander peoples who were born therefrom, remain attached thereto, and must one day return thither to be united with our ancestors. This link is the basis of the ownership of the soil, or better, of sovereignty. It has never been ceded or extinguished, and coexists with the sovereignty of the Crown.

How could it be otherwise? That peoples possessed a land for 60 millennia and this sacred link disappears from world history in merely the past 200 years?

With substantive constitutional change and structural reform, we believe this ancient sovereignty can shine through as a fuller expression of Australia's nationhood.

Proportionally, we are the most incarcerated people on the planet. We are not an innately criminal people. Our children are aliened from their families at unprecedented rates. This cannot be because we have no love for them. And our young people languish in detention in obscene numbers. They should be our hope for the future.

These dimensions of our crisis tell plainly the structural nature of our problem. *This is the torment of our powerlessness.*

We seek constitutional reforms to empower our people and take a *rightful place* in our own country. When we have power over our destiny our children will flourish. They will walk in two worlds and their culture will be a gift to their country.

We call for the establishment of a First Nations Voice enshrined in the Constitution.

Makarrata is the culmination of our agenda: *the coming together after a struggle.* It captures our aspirations for a fair and truthful relationship with the people of Australia and a better future for our children based on justice and self-determination.

We seek a Makarrata Commission to supervise a process of agreement-making between governments and First Nations, and truth-telling about our history.

In 1967 we were counted, in 2017 we seek to be heard. We leave base camp and start our trek across this vast country. We invite you to walk with us in a movement of the Australian people for a better future.

Source: The Uluru Statement (n.d.).

REFLECTIVE QUESTIONS

Read and reflect on the Uluru Statement from the Heart. Think about the phrase: 'This is the torment of our powerlessness'. What does this phrase mean to you? Can you think of an expression of such powerlessness that may have occurred for First Nations peoples? How might powerlessness intersect with the determinants for enjoying high levels of SEWB?

Suicide

We know that the incidence of suicide for First Nations people is high, at up to 2.3 times that of non-Indigenous people in Australia (AIHW, 2019a). In 2019, suicide accounted for 5.7 per cent of all deaths of Aboriginal and Torres Strait Islander peoples, compared to non-Indigenous Australians at 1.9 per cent (AIHW, 2019a). Suicide deaths per 100 000 people among First Nations Australians were 16.5 and 44.9 in those aged 0–24 and 25–44 years, respectively (AIHW, 2019a). From 2016 to 2019, almost a quarter (24 per cent) of deaths in First Nations Australians aged 0–24 was due to suicide, compared to 16.7 per cent in non-Indigenous Australians (AIHW, 2019a). These figures are staggering. The rates of suicide among First Nations people are disproportionately high within the Australian population. We know that improving cultural connectedness is a protective factor from suicide, and so there are some indications for ways forward to improve health outcomes. This will require a commitment from mainstream mental health services to recognise and apply culturally suitable, ecologically protective principles to underpin tailored mental health services, inclusive of SEWB services; mental health promotion campaigns; and suicide prevention interventions to ensure that outcomes improve (Gibson et al., 2021, Wilson, Wilson & Usher, 2015).

First Nation's Safety Plan

- Involve the suicidal person in making their safety plan.
- Identify protective factors, which may include:
  - connection to river /water
  - home / family
  - bushland
  - being on Country.
- Connect with a safe place, where the person feels emotionally safe.
- Identify people with whom the person feels comfortable and who are able to provide support during periods of unwellness.
- Agree to a suitable length of time the suicidal person will be able to cope before professional intervention is required. This will ensure the agreement can be achieved.
- Provide 24-hour contacts – family supports, suicide crisis line, counsellor or mental health worker.

TRANSLATION TO PRACTICE

REFLECTIVE QUESTION

What are five practical steps you can take at the point of care to help improve cultural connectedness for First Nations people as a protective factor for suicide? Discuss your suggestions with your peers.

First Nations storyteller – Rob Waters

Listen to spoken-word artist Rob Waters: '90.8' (https://soundcloud.com/rob-waters-11/908a)

Here, Rob asks, 'What will happen to First Nations people who are disconnected to their story … ? Their culture … ? The Stolen Generation … ? The children taken from their families and communities … ? Are they stuck in a limbo not sure who they are … "like a tree without roots" … ? disconnected to the 12 000 generations of storytellers that have gone before them … ?'

Rob aligns the trauma of the past and present with the inability to access hope for the future, and suggests that the 'tomorrow that waits for them [is] not too far from here' but without the necessary healing associated with SEWB, it is inaccessible. The trauma of their disconnection to culture and story prevents people from accessing hopefulness for the future. Thus, we see hopelessness calculated and recorded by the Australian Bureau of Statistics in the form of an Aboriginal and Torres Strait Islander suicide rate – that is *90.8 First Nations men per 100 000 population*. The retelling of statistics in this way reflects the sovereignty of First Nations people to be able to represent their stories from scientific data that is collected about them. That is, ensuring that the narratives derived from the data are the ones that arise from consultation or in partnership with First Nations people, not merely *about* them. In this sense, while the statistics from the Australian Bureau of Statistics quantifies the incidence of suicide, the retelling of story by a First Nations person in the oral tradition requires us to pay attention and to listen actively and mindfully, and this presents the powerful social narrative and authentic voice that completes the presentation of the data.

Closing the gap

The Australian government has set priority areas to address the disparity experienced by many First Nations people. The four priority reforms will:

- Strengthen and establish formal partnerships and shared decision-making
- Build the Aboriginal and Torres Strait Islander community-controlled sector
- Transform government organisations so they work better for Aboriginal and Torres Strait Islander people
- Improve and share access to data and information to enable Aboriginal and Torres Strait Islander communities make informed decisions. (Department of Prime Minister and Cabinet, n.d.)

While targets and monitoring are in place, the pace of change has been slow to date, and in many respects the gap is widening. A particular target relates to SEWB: 'Socioeconomic Outcome Area 14: Aboriginal and Torres Strait Islander people enjoy high levels of social and emotional wellbeing' (Productivity Commission, n.d.). While the aspiration is that the target for zero suicide should be achieved, it is also important to consider that SEWB is a holistic phenomenon, made up of many parts, and not limited to the absence of suicide. Enjoyment of high levels of SEWB will require a focus on a broader set of indicators. As defined earlier in this chapter, SEWB is a far wider attribute that cannot be limited to a singular association with the absence of suicide. It is critical that a broader approach than scientific measurement is utilised to engage meaningfully with First Nations people in developing solutions for extremely challenging problems, so that there is a shared understanding, a yarn or story, of an appropriate alignment of goals, interventions and outcomes. In doing so, it might be possible to achieve a holistic and strengths-based approach to SEWB success for First Nations people and contribute to closing the gap in the process. Closing the gap will require a concerted effort to eliminate systemic racism within our public institutions and to ensure that the workforces within these institutions (e.g. health, education, policing, social welfare and other government agencies) are adequately prepared and resourced to address disparity.

PERSONAL NARRATIVE

Kirra's story

Kirra is a 20-year-old First Nations woman who has recently moved to a flat (small apartment) of her own, having become eligible for social housing for herself and her young daughter. She has a history of depression and substance misuse (*yarndy*/cannabis) with her first use at 11 years of age. In the past Kirra has attempted suicide on several occasions but not since the birth of her daughter. She has worked hard to address her SEWB and mental health since the birth of her daughter and feels a sense of hope for the future, especially with settling into her new home and with stronger connections with her family. Culture is important to her, and she wants to raise her daughter with strong connections to family and culture. She is no longer in a relationship with her former partner, who is the father of her child. His poly substance misuse has been associated with anger and family violence. He is unhappy that Kirra has moved away from his community and his family. A member of his extended family has reported Kirra to police, alleging that Kirra has sent them an SMS outlining her suicidal ideation and plan.

Kirra is asleep, after a disrupted night caring for her 2-year-old daughter, Alina, who woke several times and needed to be settled. It is 6.00 a.m. on a Saturday morning. Three police cars arrive at Kirra's flat with lights and sirens blaring. She has no idea why they have arrived and is frightened as they enter her house uninvited and order her to lie on the floor with taser guns aimed at her. Kirra complies, even though she is wearing only a thin singlet and briefs. The commotion wakes her daughter, who is frightened and begins to cry unconsolably. The child is taken away by police and Kirra screams, asking not to be separated from her daughter. Kirra is placed in the back of a police 'paddy wagon' and transported to a mental health hospital for assessment under the State Mental Health Act. She is held for 24 hours under the Act and is not permitted visitors from her family, who are extremely worried for her welfare. During the mental state assessment interviews, Kirra denies she has any suicide ideation. She becomes distressed when no one can tell her where her daughter is and who she is with at this time. She punches walls, throws a water cup and yells profanities at staff. Security is called because there is a zero tolerance of violence in the hospital. Kirra is medicated and placed in a quiet, low-stimulation room for de-escalation purposes. The sedation causes her to sleep for several hours. When she awakes, Kirra is drowsy, her speech and cognition are slowed and she appears dishevelled. She has been offered hospital pyjamas to wear.

Later, it emerges that the allegations made by Alana's father's extended family were malicious and that no SMS indicating any suicide risk was ever sent by Kirra. She is released from hospital and reunited with her daughter.

REFLECTIVE QUESTIONS

Kirra's story is a confronting one; however, it is not unusual. What emotions does it stir within you as you read it? We know that cultural participation is a protective factor for SEWB and helps to mitigate risks of suicide, self-injury or mental ill health. Can you identify any protective factors in Kirra's story? Earlier in this chapter you were asked to think about the Uluru Statement from the Heart and to think about what might constitute the 'torment of powerlessness'. Can you draw any links from this statement in relation to Kirra's experiences?

Cultural safety

In mainstream discourse, culture is often referred to as 'religion', 'cuisine', 'dance', 'art' and 'dress code'. However, First Nations people experience culture as a much deeper inner spiritual experience, intrinsic to all aspects of life. It is a way of being in life that is scaffolded by respect, knowledge, and empathy for our fellow humans. In the delivery of competent health care and responsive mainstream services, it is important to be culturally respectful. The Australian Health Practitioner Regulation Agency (AHPRA) defines cultural safety as:

> Cultural safety is determined by Aboriginal and Torres Strait Islander individuals, families and communities. Culturally safe practice is the ongoing critical reflection of health practitioner knowledge, skills, attitudes, practising behaviours and power differentials in delivering safe, accessible and responsive healthcare free of racism. (AHPRA, 2021, para. 10)

AHPRA's Health Practitioner Codes of Conduct require that health care is delivered through culturally safe and respectful practice that:

- Acknowledge colonisation and systemic racism, social, cultural, behavioural and economic factors which impact individual and community health
- Acknowledge and address individual racism, their own biases, assumptions, stereotypes and prejudices and provide care that is holistic, free of bias and racism
- Recognise the importance of self-determined decision-making, partnership and collaboration in healthcare which is driven by the individual, family and community;
- Foster a safe working environment through leadership to support the rights and dignity of Aboriginal and Torres Strait Islander people and colleagues. (AHPRA, 2021, para. 11)

Culturally safe practice is now an imperative for all health practitioners. For example, nurses in Australia must confirm and endorse their agreement to abide by a Code of Conduct annually when they reregister. This includes several domains, values and principles that outline the practice requirements for the profession, with a significant number of these relating specifically to First Nations people. Nurses and students should familiarise themselves with the relevant code of conduct (Nursing and Midwifery Board of Australia (NMBA), 2021) and refine their practice to respond with adherence. In effect, this means that all nurses in Australia should be capable of delivering culturally safe practice to First Nations people. As such, it is an expectation that nurses in the mental health context are able to deliver culturally safe mental health nursing practice to First Nations people.

Challenges remain, even with such specific guidance. We know that racism is still experienced by First Nations people seeking (mental) health care, and this leads to the perpetuation of poorer health outcomes. For example, older First Nations people with mental health conditions experience amplified psychological distress when they also encounter racism in healthcare and other settings (Temple, Keleher & Paradies, 2020). While First Nations children who experience racism have poorer educational, social and health outcomes, this can be improved with affirmation of their ethnoracial identity (Macedo et al., 2019). Cultural safety and affirmation of culture are important mental health practitioner attributes that are helpful in promoting SEWB for First Nations people across the lifespan.

However, some SEWB and mental health commentators go further and suggest that culturally safe practice can only be achieved in the absence of systemic racism in health and educational institutions, and that this must be addressed with urgency (Geia et al., 2020). The context of intergenerational trauma for First Nations people is a further consideration, with calls for a requisite trauma-informed approach to cultural safety within mental health care to strengthen SEWB frameworks and address the disparity that exists for First Nations people (Tujague & Ryan, 2021).

Australian First Nations cultures are among the oldest surviving cultures in the world, and they are numerous and diverse, made up of hundreds of different kinship and language groups that have adapted to diverse living conditions throughout Australia over many thousands of years. First Nations cultures remain dynamic, are evolving and, for First Nations individuals and communities, form the context for the development of health and social policy (Pascoe, 2014). As traditional storytellers and oral communicators, with Elders as knowledge-keepers and teachers, many First Nations people are able to connect seamlessly, spiritually and culturally with respect towards each other and the natural environment, that is, with Country. A collective generosity exists whereby there is a reciprocity and an inherent responsibility to care for each other and Country. It is useful for mental health practitioners to pay particular attention and render respect towards the unique First Nations cultures that they encounter in the communities where they practice. While there are many cultural aspects that may overlap between cultural groups, great diversity also exists. One of the aspects that draws all First Nations people in Australia together is the unfinished business in relation to recognition within the Constitution, and until this is resolved, for many trauma and distress will remain a constant that undermines collective SEWB.

Story

Storytelling, through the traditions of yarning, song, art and dance, is an important communication pathway for many First Nations people. The passing on of knowledge, non-judgemental critique of information and problem-solving all respectfully occur using these mediums of narrative communication. The affirmation of cultural practices such as these can promote SEWB and facilitate the uptake of health promotion messages, and messages of strength, resilience and care. It also accommodates grieving, mourning (sorry business and sad news), truth-telling and reconciliation. Storytelling also enables the exploration of some traumatic topics (for example, dispossession of traditional lands) and provides an opportunity for First Nations people to express the depth of meaning this has for them, so it can be understood more fully by non-Indigenous people.

REFLECTIVE QUESTIONS

Read the poem and consider the cultural ramifications and the implications for poor SEWB experienced by First Nations people when non-Indigenous people fail to appreciate the depth of holistic, spiritual nuances that make up a cultural understanding of connection to land. In this context, how might this influence your development as a culturally safe mental health practitioner?

Stolen Land
There is no part of this place
that was not
is not
cared for
loved
by an Aboriginal or Torres Strait Islander nation
There are no trees
rivers
hills
stars
that were not
are not
someone's kin

Source: Kwaymullina (2021, p. 1).

In small groups (face to face or online), discuss your own culture:

* What aspects or influences of culture determine the way you live?
* Have you ever felt confronted or surprised by aspects of other cultures and, if so, what were they and why did you feel confronted?
* Compare your answers against the Lowitja Institute's *Cultural Determinants for Health* (Lowitja Institute, 2014).

The effects of child removals

It is difficult to overestimate the traumatic and harmful effects of the child removal policies of Australia between 1910 and the 1970s. Haebich (2000) described this era as perhaps the most brutal of government policies imposed upon First Nations peoples. The term 'Stolen Generations' originated in the *Bringing Them Home* report, which described the effects of trauma experiences as being widespread and enduring, and recurring across generations (Bessarab & Crawford, 2013).

Unfortunately, First Nations children continue to be over-represented in the Australian out-of-home care (OOHC) system (AIHW, 2019b). For First Nations children, the preferred placement is with other First Nations families, in accordance with the Aboriginal and Torres Strait Islander Child Placement Principle: a placement to ensure that children remain connected to their family, community, culture and Country. The principle has been adopted by all jurisdictions in legislation and policy (AIHW, 2019b; Secretariat of National Aboriginal and Islander Child Care (SNAICC), 2019). Yet, this remains difficult to achieve given the high rates of removal, highlighting the need for more to be done to urgently address the inequity and disadvantage experienced by many First Nations families, if high levels of SEWB are to be achieved in the future.

Formal apology to First Nations people

On 13 February 2008, Prime Minister Kevin Rudd delivered a speech to the nation with a formal apology to the Stolen Generations of Australia. The word 'sorry' was uttered many times, responsibility was finally take, and accountability was evident. The fact that it was not Mr Rudd's government that was responsible for the child removal policy and the actions that followed showed true leadership and sincerity on his part. The previous government, led by John Howard, had refused to apologise to First Nations people on the grounds that these events had not happened in his generation and therefore the government of that day was not responsible.

The speech delivered by Mr Rudd is reproduced here:

I move:

That today we honour the Indigenous peoples of this land, the oldest continuing cultures in human history.

We reflect on their past mistreatment.

We reflect in particular on the mistreatment of those who were Stolen Generations – this blemished chapter in our nation's history.

The time has now come for the nation to turn a new page in Australia's history by righting the wrongs of the past and so moving forward with confidence to the future.

We apologise for the laws and policies of successive Parliaments and governments that have inflicted profound grief, suffering and loss on these our fellow Australians.

We apologise especially for the removal of Aboriginal and Torres Strait Islander children from their families, their communities, and their country.

For the pain, suffering and hurt of these Stolen Generations, their descendants and for their families left behind, we say sorry.

To the mothers and the fathers, the brothers and the sisters, for the breaking up of families and communities, we say sorry.

And for the indignity and degradation thus inflicted on a proud people and a proud culture, we say sorry.

We, the Parliament of Australia, respectfully request that this apology be received in the spirit in which it is offered as part of the healing of the nation.

For the future we take heart; resolving that this new page in the history of our great continent can now be written.

We today take this first step by acknowledging the past and laying claim to a future that embraces all Australians.

A future where this Parliament resolves that the injustices of the past must never, never happen again.

A future where we harness the determination of all Australians, Indigenous and non-Indigenous, to close the gap that lies between us in life expectancy, educational achievement, and economic opportunity.

A future where we embrace the possibility of new solutions to enduring problems where old approaches have failed.

A future based on mutual respect, mutual resolve, and mutual responsibility.

A future where all Australians, whatever their origins, are truly equal partners, with equal opportunities and with an equal stake in shaping the next chapter in the history of this great country, Australia. (Rudd, 2008)

REFLECTIVE QUESTIONS

Using Figure 4.1 as a stimulus:

- Write a short statement that affirms high SEWB for First Nations people.
- Write a short statement that describes some characteristics of disparity for First Nations people when compared to non-Indigenous people.
- Write a short statement that proposes culturally safe SEWB and mental health care for First Nations people.

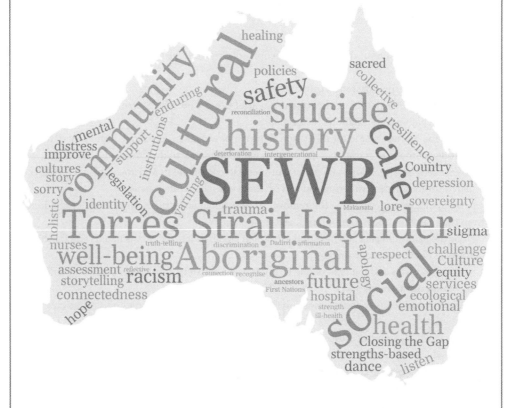

Figure 4.1 Word cloud relating to SEWB, derived from words in this chapter

The delivery of culturally safe health care requires health practitioners to challenge their own biases and assumptions, and to ensure that stigma and discrimination do not contribute to poor healthcare delivery. As discussed earlier in this chapter, the code of conduct (NMBA, 2021) for nurses, in particular, requires nurses to reflect on their practice so that they can support First Nations people to access timely health care and achieve healthy outcomes. The intersections between physical health conditions, mental health conditions and culturally safe practices can be complex, as Gail's story illustrates.

PERSONAL NARRATIVE

Gail's story

Gail is a 52-year-old Aboriginal woman who lives in remote New South Wales. She presents as a shy, softly spoken, underweight and undernourished Aboriginal woman who is pleasant but initially reluctant to engage with local services. As a child, Gail was removed from her maternal family and placed predominately 'off Country' at a young age. Her parents had a history of substance abuse and an inability to adequately care for her. Gail's teenage years and early childhood included physical and sexual abuse from several relationships, and she developed a dependence on substances as a form of self-medicating to mask the pain of her past traumas and continuing mental health problems. Gail also has poor literacy as well as high use of substances, so she is unable to secure employment, and this has led to her becoming financially dependent on others or Centrelink payments.

Gail has a daughter and teenage grandson who have also experienced physical and mental abuse, heighted during periods of substance abuse. Her daughter has found it difficult to secure meaningful employment and relies on Centrelink benefits to care for her young family. These issues further affect Gail, her daughter and grandson's mental health as they all exhibit symptoms of depression and anxiety. They express feelings of worthlessness and that they could never succeed at anything such as 'working or owning a car' – things most people take for granted. The transgenerational pattern of behaviour has been replicated from mother to daughter to grandson.

The area where Gail resides does not have an Aboriginal Medical Service close by and the only health care available is through mainstream services that do not provide culturally appropriate or safe environments, which often result in Aboriginal people not accessing medical treatment. Gail has developed a trusting rapport and a relationship with the SEWB Outreach Service where she is receiving ongoing support and counselling to reduce her alcohol and cannabis intake, to improve her overall outlook and her mental and physical well-being. Unfortunately, in her later life (which is still young) Gail displays symptoms of slurred speech, twitching and unsteady gait, which is often interpreted as her being 'drunk, charged up or under the influence'. When she attends mainstream medical service for assistance and assessment, she is usually turned away, being stigmatised as being 'another drunk black woman', and with no medical investigations occurring.

Through the support and advocacy from the SEWB worker, Gail is linked with an understanding doctor who diagnoses her with motor neuron disease. Although her symptoms mimic drunkenness, they have gone undetected for some time as a physical medical condition. Although the overall prognosis would not have changed, Gail's mental and social well-being could have been improved by having an earlier diagnosis and not being subjected to the additional stigma and racism many Aboriginal people endure.

REFLECTIVE QUESTIONS

- Create a mind map with some peers that explores the factors you consider have affected the historical, cultural, spiritual, social and psychological determinants of Gail's life.
- Brainstorm with your peers and suggest how recognition of Gail's cultural needs could be improved during her interaction with mainstream services.

INTERPROFESSIONAL PERSPECTIVES

Dadirri – Miriam-Rose Ungunmerr-Baumann

As we have indicated, SEWB intersects with a holistic perspective of mental health. It stands to reason that promoting SEWB will focus on establishing and maintain well-being. Doing so will incorporate a diverse range of practitioners and often include culturally suitable traditional healers and therapies. One example suitable to support SEWB is the traditional well-being practice of *dadirri*. Senior Australian of the Year in 2021, Dr Miriam-Rose Ungunmerr-Baumann AM, a Ngangiwumirr woman and esteemed educator, encourages the uptake of *dadirri* as a gift offered from First Nations communities for all people (First Nations and non-Indigenous). It is a SEWB self-care strategy designed to assist individuals to take a careful and focused time to listen quietly and deeply, using a technique to mindfully connect ourselves with our environment and those around us. The Miriam Rose Foundation (1988) has more details on the technique.

Dadirri

In essence, it is about taking a moment of quietness and stillness where you can focus on your breath, and to breathe slowly, or in harmony with another person if practised together. Within the resulting pause and quietness, the goal is to listen deeply within oneself and to connect to the 'sound of deep calling to deep ... the deep inner spring that is within us – we call on it, it calls on us' (Miriam Rose Foundation, 1988). While altering the pace of the world around us is often beyond our influence or control, it is still possible to steady oneself to the rhythm of pace that is the here and now. Being content to not race ahead of the present moment, nor linger behind in the past. In the present moment, we can commit to *seeing clearly, sitting strongly, and listening deeply*. In this way, we wait, taking time for growth to occur, and in doing so, Culture and healing of Country (and all it relates, to including us) will also grow. Dr Ungunmerr-Baumann says that *dadirri* is a gift to us all, using it will help us to grow in our experience of humanity and will act as an enhancement and maintenance of our SEWB.

TRANSLATION TO PRACTICE

SUMMARY

This chapter has presented some examples of the experiences of trauma and intergenerational trauma by First Nations people, from a First Nations standpoint. It has provided stories and information, supplemented by activities designed to deepen understanding of:

- The concept of SEWB.
- Some of the determinants of SEWB in the context of colonisation and associated intergenerational trauma.
- Continuing mental health and SEWB disparity and inequity in the context of priorities for Closing the Gap, with examples drawn from Australian Bureau of Statistics data, combined with the use of storytelling techniques to enhance relevance to First Nations.
- The application of cultural safety principles that underpin best practice SEWB and mental health practice. Case study examples have been used to translate the theoretical approach to the practical domain.
- The cultural practice of *dadirri* as an example of a traditional First Nations strategy to promote and restore personal SEWB.

It has only been possible to provide a brief introductory discussion about a complex topic area, and readers are encouraged to read more widely about the topic and to follow First Nations SEWB thought leaders in this rapidly evolving area of practice development and specialty. The authors hope that the chapter has been sufficient to inspire emerging mental health practitioners to consider carefully how they will draw alongside First Nations people in culturally safe practice to improve the SEWB and mental health outcomes of First Nations people in the future.

CRITICAL THINKING/LEARNING ACTIVITIES

1   Some First Nations people have become disillusioned by the inability of consecutive governments to address the gaps that exist between First Nations and non-Indigenous people in Australia. One way this may be expressed by some people is as an inherent right to collect some 'rent' due to them as traditional owners, because no treaty or agreement has ever been addressed in regard to ownership of land. Thus, a flipped alternative narrative may be that a social welfare payment represents one way in which some people might consider that the government is making a 'lease' payment to a traditional owner (i.e. a landlord) of the unceded lands. The flipped notion of social security conceptualised as a rental payment system challenges the mainstream discourse and the intention of government policies. Discuss.

    To help you in your discussion, consider: Have you ever leased a flat, apartment or house, as somewhere to live? Have you been obliged to agree to a lease agreement, with conditions or rules that you were uncomfortable with as a tenant, in order to achieve safe and secure housing for yourself or others? Did you agree with all the 'conditions' that the landlord or agent imposed upon you as a tenant? What power or influence did you have to challenge any of those conditions? How was your experience as that tenant? Can you align your own reflections on your own experiences as a tenant (or in discussions with others), with that of a First Nations person described above? If you were a landlord (traditional owner), how would you feel about tenants (colonisation) that damaged your property (e.g. sacred sites), failed to attend to the garden (e.g. care for the natural environment) by clearing the plants you valued and allowing exotic weeds to proliferate so that you could never return it to its former glory … or, even blowing up the back yard for mining purposes? What if your tenant decided to pay no rent, or minimal rent? What would you do? How would you feel?

2   First Nations adults make up approximately 2 per cent of the Australian population but disproportionally make up 27 per cent of the population of prisons in Australia, with two-thirds of this population receiving at least one mental health diagnosis. Additionally, since the 1993 Royal Commission into Deaths in Custody, on average, one First Nations person has died in custody every 22 days (Australian Law Reform Commission, 2017). Review The Uluru Statement from the Heart and consider what actions and conditions might be necessary to ensure that there is hope for the future for young First Nations people, as echoed by the authors of the Uluru Statement from the Heart.

3   Acknowledging the Elders past, present and emerging from the traditional Country where you live, work, study and travel is one way of strengthening your respect for First Nations people's cultures and Country. Affirmation of First Nations people is a valuable contribution within the health sector. Anyone (First Nations or non-Indigenous) can provide an Acknowledgement of Country at any time – for example, at a work or community function or meeting. When non-Indigenous people do this, and when it is offered from a place of their reflective deep respect of First Nations culture and place, it affirms First Nations people deeply. It is one way that non-Indigenous people can express a coming together to acknowledge the past and present, and demonstrate pride as an ally or accomplice of First Nations people. There is no singular right way to do this, and there is no singular phrase that is best to use. The main principles are that:
    a   It should always be the first activity of business.
    b   If esteemed Elder/s are present, it is important to First Nations people that you acknowledge them.

c Everyone should know something of, and appreciate something about, the Traditional Lands where they live and work. You can find out more about the Country you are on by using the AIATSIS Map of Indigenous Australia (AIATSIS, 1996), or by visiting your local Lands Council website, or https://www.indigenous.gov.au/.

d Your acknowledgement should express a sentiment that offers genuine respect 'from the heart' and invites others to join you in that sentiment.

Draft an Acknowledgement of Country and practise using it so you are able to contribute this to professional and community meetings and gatherings in the future.

LEARNING EXTENSION

Listen to another poem by storyteller Rob Waters, 'I Will Speak Now': https://soundcloud.com/rob-waters-11/i-will-speak-now

The powerful poem steps courageously to the forefront and demands that First Nations voice be heard:' I will speak now!' The time for truth-telling from a First Nations perspective has arrived. A retelling of truthful Australian history – a '600 Nations strong' history. It takes courage to tell the stories that have been concealed and for shame to be overcome. As First Nations people tell their truth, and non-Indigenous people join in the hearing, a reconciliation can emerge that empowers us to go forward together in trust and truth. As we go on this journey together in Australia, do you think it is possible that SEWB outcomes will improve? Justify your answer with evidence from the literature.

ACKNOWLEDGEMENT

The authors would like to thank Debra Hocking, who wrote the previous editions of this chapter, and Dr Janene Carey, for editorial assistance.

FURTHER READING

Print

Wilson, R. L. & Waqanaviti, K. (2021). Navigating First Nations social and emotional wellbeing in mainstream mental health services. In O. Best & B. Fredericks (eds), *Yatdjuligin: Aboriginal and Torres Strait Islander Nursing and Midwifery Care*, 3rd edn. Port Melbourne: Cambridge University Press.
Social and emotional well-being (SEWB) for First Nations people often occurs in the mainstream setting. Wilson and Waqanaviti offer a wider introduction to how SEWB is achieved in nursing and midwifery settings.

Online

Anthony, T. (2016). Deaths in custody: 25 years after the royal commission, we've gone backwards. *The Conversation*, 13 April. Retrieved from http://theconversation.com/deaths-in-custody-25-years-after-the-royal-commission-weve-gone-backwards-57109

This article discusses the 25th anniversary of the Royal Commission into Aboriginal Deaths in Custody, with a focus on whether the targets from the report have been met.

Australian Broadcasting Corporation. (n.d.) *Dust Echoes*. Retrieved from https://www.abc.net .au/education/collections/dust-echoes/

Dust Echoes is a series of 12 animated Dreamtime stories from Central Arnhem Land.

Australian Government. (2020). *Closing the Gap Report 2020*. Canberra: Commonwealth of Australia, Department of the Prime Minister and Cabinet. Retrieved from https://ctgreport.niaa.gov.au/sites/default/files/pdf/closing-the-gap-report-2020.pdf

Closing the Gap is a government strategy that aims to reduce disadvantage among Aboriginal and Torres Strait Islander peoples, focusing particularly on life expectancy, infant mortality rates, education and employment outcomes. This report monitors the efforts of the Council of Australian Governments.

Mental Health First Aid Australia. (n.d.). Aboriginal and Torres Strait Islander Mental Health First Aid Course. Retrieved from https://mhfa.com.au/courses/public/types/aboriginal

Mental health first aid (MHFA) training targets the public to support them to provide a first response to people they may encounter in the community with a mental health crisis, and to assist in supporting early navigation to appropriate mental health care when it is needed. A version of MHFA has been tailored for First Nations people in this resource.

Stolen Generations' Testimonies Foundation. (n.d.). Stolen Generations' Testimonies (Website). Retrieved from http://stolengenerationstestimonies.com/

This project shares the personal stories of survivors of Australia's Stolen Generations.

Film

Each of these films focuses on Indigenous narratives:

Bran Nue Dae (2010) – Directed by Rachel Perkins
The Emu Runner (2019) – Directed by Imogen Thomas
In My Blood it Runs (2019) – Directed by Maya Newell
Jindabyne (2006) – Directed by Ray Lawrence
The Last Wave (1977) – Directed by Peter Weir
Mabo (2012) – Directed by Rachel Perkins
Rabbit Proof Fence (2002) – Directed by Phillip Noyce
Samson and Delilah (2009) – Directed by Warwick Thornton
Ten Canoes (2006) – Directed by Rolf de Heer
The Tracker (2002) – Directed by Rolf de Heer

REFERENCES

ACT Government. (2016). *Guide to Promoting Health and Wellbeing in the Workplace*. Retrieved from https://www.healthierwork.act.gov.au/wp-content/uploads/2015/01/Guide-to-Promoting-Health-and-Wellbeing-in-the-Workplace-2016.pdf

Australian Health Practitioner Regulation Agency (AHPRA). (2021). *Aboriginal and Torres Strait Islander Health Strategy*. Retrieved from https://www.ahpra.gov.au/About-Ahpra/Aboriginal-and-Torres-Strait-Islander-Health-Strategy.aspx

Australian Institute of Aboriginal and Torres Strait Islander Studies (AIATSIS). (n.d.). *The 1967 Referendum*. Retrieved from https://aiatsis.gov.au/explore/1967-referendum

———— (1996). *The AIATSIS Map of Indigenous Australia*. Retrieved from https://aiatsis.gov.au/explore/map-indigenous-australia

Australian Institute of Health and Welfare (AIHW). (2009). *Measuring the Social and Emotional Wellbeing of Aboriginal and Torres Strait Islander Peoples*. Cat. no. IHW24. Canberra: AIHW.

———— (2019a). *Deaths by Suicide Amongst Indigenous Australians*. Retrieved from https://www.aihw.gov.au/suicide-self-harm-monitoring/data/populations-age-groups/suicide-indigenous-australians

———— (2019b). Child protection Australia 2017–18 (Child welfare series no. 70. Cat. No. CWS 65). Canberra: AIHW. Retrieved from www.aihw.gov.au/reports-data/health-welfare-services/child-protection/overview

Australian Law Reform Commission. (2017). *Pathways to Justice – An Inquiry into the Incarceration Rate of Aboriginal and Torres Strait Islander Peoples*, Final Report No 133. Canberra: Government of Australia. Retrieved from https://www.alrc.gov.au/sites/default/files/pdfs/publications/final_report_133_amended1.pdf

Bessarab, D. & Crawford, F. R. (2013). Trauma, grief and loss: The vulnerability of Aboriginal families in the child protection system. In B. Bennet, S. Green, S. Glibert & D. Bessarab (eds), *Our Voices: Aboriginal and Torres Strait Islander social work* (pp. 93–113). Melbourne: Palgrave Macmillan.

Commonwealth of Australia. (1961). Parliamentary Debates (Hansard), House of Representatives, 20 April 1961, *Native Welfare Conference*, p.1051. Retrieved from http://historichansard.net/hofreps/1961/19610420_reps_23_hor30/#debate-23

———— (2017a). National Strategic Framework for Aboriginal and Torres Strait Islander Peoples' Mental Health and Social and Emotional Wellbeing. Retrieved from: https://www.niaa.gov.au/sites/default/files/publications/mhsewb-framework_0.pdf.

———— (2017b). *National Native Title Tribunal*. Retrieved from http://www.nntt.gov.au/Pages/Home-Page.aspx

Department of Prime Minister and Cabinet. (n.d.). *National Agreement on Closing the Gap: At a glance*. Retrieved from https://www.closingthegap.gov.au/national-agreement

Friends of Myall Creek. (n.d.). *The Massacre Story*. Friends of Myall Creek. Retrieved from https://myallcreek.org/the-massacre-story/

Geia, L., Baird, K., Bail, K. … & Wynne, R. (2020). A unified call to action from Australian nursing and midwifery leaders: Ensuring that Black lives matter. *Contemporary Nurse*, *56*(4): 297–308.

Gibson, M., Stuart, J., Leske, S., Ward, R. & Tanton, R. (2021). Suicide rates for young Aboriginal and Torres Strait Islander people: The influence of community level cultural connectedness. *Medical Journal of Australia*, *214*(11): 514–18.

Haebich, A. (2000). *Broken Circles Fragmenting Indigenous Families, 1800–2000*. Fremantle: Fremantle Arts Centre Press.

Kwaymullina, A. (2021). *Living on Stolen Land*. Broome, Australia: Magabala Books.

Lowitja Institute. (2014). *Cultural Determinants of Aboriginal and Torres Strait Islander Health Roundtable: Report*. Retrieved from https://www.lowitja.org.au/content/Document/PDF/Cultural-Determinants-RT-Report-FINAL2b.pdf

Macedo, D. M., Smithers, L. G., Roberts, R. M., Haag, D. G., Paradies, Y. & Jamieson, L. M. (2019). Does ethnic-racial identity modify the effects of racism on the social and emotional well-being of Aboriginal Australian children?. *PLOS ONE*, *14*(8): e0220744.

Miriam Rose Foundation. (1988). *Dadirri: Inner deep listening and quiet still awareness*. Retrieved from https://www.miriamrosefoundation.org.au/wp-content/uploads/2021/03/Dadirri_Handout.pdf

National Museum of Australia. (n.d.). *Defining moments: Indigenous Australian's right to vote*. Retrieved from https://www.nma.gov.au/defining-moments/resources/indigenous-australians-right-to-vote

Native Title Act 1993 (Cth). Retrieved from https://www.legislation.gov.au/details/c2004a00354

Nursing and Midwifery Board of Australia (NMBA). (2021). *Professional standards*. Retrieved from https://www.nursingmidwiferyboard.gov.au/Codes-Guidelines-Statements/Professional-standards.aspx

Pascoe, B. (2014). *Dark Emu*. Broome, Australia: Magabala Books.

Productivity Commission. (n.d.). *Socioeconomic outcome area 14*. Retrieved from https://www .pc.gov.au/closing-the-gap-data/dashboard/socioeconomic/outcome-area14

Rudd, K. (2008). Apology to Australia's Indigenous Peoples, House of Representatives, Parliament House, Canberra, 13 February. Retrieved from http://australia.gov.au/about-australia/our-country/our-people/apology-to-australias-indigenous-peoples

Secretariat of National Aboriginal and Islander Child Care (SNAICC). (2019). The Aboriginal and Torres Strait Islander Child Placement Principle: A guide to support implementation. Retrieved from https://www.snaicc.org.au/wp-content/uploads/2019/06/928_SNAICC-ATSICPP-resource-June2019.pdf

Temple, J. B., Kelaher, M. & Paradies,Y. (2020). Experiences of racism among older Aboriginal and Torres Strait Islander People: Prevalence, sources, and association with mental health. *Canadian Journal on Aging / La Revue Canadienne Du Vieillissement, 39*(2): 178–89.

Tujague, N. A. & Ryan, K. L. (2021). Ticking the box of 'cultural safety' is not enough: why trauma-informed practice is critical to Indigenous healing. *Rural and Remote Health, 21*(3): 6411.

The Uluru Statement. (n.d.). *The Uluru Statemen from the Heart*. Retrieved from https://ulurustatement.org/the-statement

Wilson, R. L. & Waqanaviti, K. (2021). Navigating First Nations social and emotional wellbeing in mainstream mental health services. In O. Best & B. Fredericks *Yatdjuligin: Aboriginal and Torres Strait Islander Nursing and Midwifery Care*, 3rd edn. Port Melbourne: Cambridge University Press.

Wilson, R. L., Wilson, G. G. & Usher, K. (2015). Rural mental health ecology: A framework for engaging with mental health social capital in rural communities. *EcoHealth, 12*(3): 412–20.

Mental illness and narratives of experience

Nicholas Procter, Kirsty Baker, Monika Ferguson,
Lisa Hodge, Davi Macedo and Mark Loughhead

5

LEARNING OBJECTIVES

At the completion of this chapter, you should be able to:

1 Describe what mental illness is and have a general understanding of the
   mental health diagnostic process and diagnostic classification systems.
2 Become familiarised with the most common diagnoses for mental illness
   according to the Diagnostic and Statistical Manual for Mental Disorders
   (DSM) and understand the experience of people living with mental illnesses.
3 Discuss the limitations of diagnostic classification systems and present
   critical arguments on how diagnosis based solely on diagnostic criteria can
   be controversial.
4 Describe the likely effects of COVID-19 on the mental health and well-being
   of consumers, carers and practitioners, and the need for self-care.

Introduction

This chapter introduces the concept of mental illness and how it is diagnosed, and the main diagnostic classification systems used in health practice. The experiences and symptoms of people living with mental illness – according to criteria from the Diagnostic and Statistical Manual of Mental Disorders (DSM)-5 – are reviewed. It is emphasised that diagnostic criteria can be considered within an overall framework for conversation and engagement between practitioners, consumers and carers, with the overarching aim of exploring and understanding the best response to distress and treatment to promote recovery processes. Criticisms of diagnostic classification systems are also summarised. Finally, potential effects of the COVID-19 pandemic and its implication for people's mental health are presented.

Diagnosis of mental illnesses

mental illness – a set of clinically diagnosable conditions that manifest through distressing thoughts, emotions and behaviours and that may influence a person reaching their full potential and living a fruitful life

The constructs of mental health and **mental illness** can be understood on a continuum of adaptation and optimal functioning across life domains. Thus, mental illness can be understood as a set of clinically diagnosable conditions within the disciplinary context of psychiatry that may influence whether a person reaches their full potential and lives productively and fruitfully (World Health Organization (WHO), 2004). Mental illness is observed through patterns of often distressing thoughts, emotions and behaviours that frequently lead to substantial suffering and difficulties in everyday life. The diagnosis of mental illness is based on conventional classification systems, with the aim of creating a universal language. Uniform descriptions of mental ill health are designed to improve communication between health providers, consumers and researchers (Clark et al., 2017). A structured classification of symptoms is also thought necessary so that the mental health conditions people experience can be understood and monitored on different levels: within communities, cities, countries and globally (Clark et al., 2017; WHO, 2013).

The diagnosis of mental illness is characterised by a list of signs and symptoms documented at the time of interview and/or from collateral information obtained by the clinician from the person, their loved ones or others. The threshold for a diagnosis depends on the number and nature of the experiences reported. For example, for the diagnosis of major depressive disorder, five (or more) symptoms are required and at least one of them has to be loss of interest in activities or depressed mood. The consumer must report that these experiences are impairing their usual functioning and adaptation (American Psychiatric Association (APA), 2013). Some aspects of diagnosis are observations made by family members, the person themself and clinicians, particularly when symptoms are directly affecting the person's thinking, speech or behaviour (e.g. observation is used to assess experiences as delusions and hallucinations when a person is assessed as going through psychosis).

Contemporary diagnostic classification systems

The two main diagnostic manuals used to diagnose mental health illnesses are the International Classification of Diseases (ICD), developed by the World Health Organization (WHO), and the Diagnostic and Statistical Manual of Mental Disorders (DSM), created by the American Psychiatric Association (APA). The first edition of the DSM dates from 1952; mental illnesses were included for the first time in the 6th edition of the ICD, approved in 1948 (APA, 1952; Clark et al., 2017; WHO, 1949). The DSM is currently in its fifth edition, published in 2013 (APA, 2013), while the ICD-11 was released in 2018. The latter will only become current in 2022, to enable different countries to organise translations and prepare health professionals to use the new classification format.

Although diagnostic classification systems are subject to comprehensive critique (see subsequent sections), as a health worker it is helpful to have a good understanding of the **diagnostic criteria** for mental illnesses. This enables informed perspectives, which are sometimes necessary to assist in communicating with other professional groups within the health system, such as in organising specialist referrals and advocating within a health insurance benefits context. We recommend the symptoms described in the following sections are used as a guide to help identify potential experiences consumers might be going through.

diagnostic criteria – a list of signs and symptoms that, when present above a certain threshold and for a certain period, indicates the occurrence of a mental illness. To be diagnosed with a mental illness, a person must report experiences (symptoms) that resemble a given diagnostic category.

Common mental illnesses

Reflective of the mental health conditions most commonly experienced across the lifespan, an overview of mental illness based on the DSM-5 classification system are presented here. The DSM-5 is the diagnostic tool commonly referred to in healthcare practice (Khoury, Langer & Pagnini, 2014). The DSM-5 adopts the word 'disorder' as typically used in the discussion of mental illnesses and throughout the text (APA, 2013). However, many people with lived experience of mental health challenges may consider the term as stigmatising and marginalising of distress, and as creating shame. It is therefore recommended that you avoid terms that can reinforce stigma and exclusion (Hahm et al., 2020).

Where possible, and as much as possible, we use the term 'condition' rather than 'disorder' to emphasise the idea of mental illnesses as clusters of experiences along a continuum of functioning and adaptation, in a holistic understanding of health (WHO, 2004). Furthermore, working from a person-centred approach means recognising the importance of diagnostic classification systems but also validating the narratives of consumers beyond diagnosis. Information on prevalence rates is presented whenever available, according to the most recent sources of information. It is noteworthy that, together, mental illnesses and substance use are the second most-common cause of non-fatal burden of disease in Australia, especially in young people (15–30 years), and prevent the experience of a meaningful and productive life (Australian Institute of Health and Welfare (AIHW), 2015).

Anxiety conditions

Anxiety conditions generally involve chronic feelings of tension, distress or worry, expressed through psychological and physical symptoms. These can include diagnosis of generalised anxiety, social anxiety, panic disorder, agoraphobia, specific phobia and separation anxiety (APA, 2013). With generalised anxiety being the most commonly experienced anxiety condition, key diagnostic criteria include excessive and recurrent worrying about events or activities (e.g. work or school performance) for a minimum period of six months. The person has difficulty controlling the worry, which must occur in the presence of at least three of a range of symptoms including restlessness, fatigue, irritability, muscle tension, sleep disturbance and difficulty concentrating (APA, 2013).

anxiety conditions – characterised by recurrent experiences of tension, distress or worry that significantly impair functioning and hinder adaptation. A person might experience anxiety when thinking about different life domains and the future, such as when experiencing generalised anxiety.

Panic disorder is also a relatively common condition and often brings people to medical attention due to the associated anxiety about physiological symptoms. It is thus best demonstrated by recurrent, sudden and unexpected panic attacks – an unexpected surge of intense fear or discomfort that can be accompanied by palpitations, trembling, chest pain and fear of losing control and dying (APA, 2013). Additionally, the diagnosis includes the presence of recurrent worry about having other panic attacks and its consequences (e.g. having a heart attack). People with this condition are known to avoid activities that can provoke sensations such as panic, including exercising and climbing stairs (APA, 2013).

People with anxiety conditions often perceive situations in terms of risk and possible threats to safety, and can see others as being hypercritical or untrustworthy. Anxious thoughts may feel like a rollercoaster ride and often involve imagining worst-outcome scenarios. Examples of internal cues are physiological symptoms – such as when experiencing panic attacks – or cognitive stimuli, such as mental images that provoke distress, as in obsessive–compulsive disorder (OCD, described on page 87). These stimuli are thus linked with the emotional experience of fear, distress and anxiety.

Anxiety is the most common type of mental health condition in Australia and Aotearoa New Zealand, affecting 14–15 per cent of people aged 16–85 years, respectively (Australian Bureau of Statistics (ABS), 2008; Oakley Browne, Well & Scott, 2006). In both countries, women are more likely to have experienced anxiety than men (18 per cent compared to 11 per cent in Australia, and 19 per cent compared to 11 per cent in Aotearoa New Zealand) (ABS, 2008; Oakley Browne et al., 2006).

REFLECTIVE QUESTIONS

Anxiety and depression are two of the most common mental health conditions people experience in Australia and Aotearoa New Zealand. Have you or a person close to you ever experienced any of these symptoms? What are the signs that professional help is needed?

Affective conditions

affective conditions – include experiencing depressed or low mood, lack of motivation, changes in sleep and appetite, and loss of interest in previously enjoyed activities, for example. When these symptoms occur for at least two weeks, there might be indication of a major depression episode. When depression is accompanied by symptoms of mania, a bipolar affective condition might be present.

Affective or mood conditions involve a disturbance in mood or a change in affect, and diagnoses include major depressive condition, persistent depression (dysthymia) and bipolar affective illness (APA, 2013). Affective illnesses are experienced by 6.2 per cent of Australians aged 16–85 years, with a slightly higher prevalence in women (7.1 per cent) than men (5.3 per cent; ABS, 2008). Similarly, these conditions are more common among females (9.5 per cent) than males (6.3 per cent) in Aotearoa New Zealand and are most prevalent in the 16–24-year age bracket (12.7 per cent; Oakley Browne et al., 2006).

Major depression is characterised by the experience of five or more symptoms over a minimum period of two weeks, at least one of them being either depressed mood (e.g. feeling sad, empty, hopeless) or loss of interest or pleasure in previously enjoyed activities. These symptoms can include low self-esteem, fatigue, irritability, reduced energy and motivation, diminished ability to concentrate and feelings of worthlessness or inappropriate guilt (APA, 2013). Experiences congruent with depression symptoms can happen when a person has faced a significant loss (death-related loss, financial losses, serial medical illness). They can be understood as a natural human reaction to difficult circumstances. However, clinical judgement might consider whether the pattern of a person's responses and experiences has become an occurrence of major depression. The adequacy of such responses must be carefully weighed against the person's history and their sociocultural background (APA, 2013).

Postnatal depression is another affective condition experienced by some women in the postpartum period. It is also possible for men to experience depression in this period. Key diagnostic criteria are similar to those for major depression but may also include worries about leaving the home or about the baby's health and/or the mother's ability to cope with caring for the baby (APA, 2013). Women who experience postnatal depression may also feel high anxiety and experience intrusive thoughts about their confidence as a mother.

In general, people who experience depression exhibit a negative perception of themselves and feel hopeless about the future. Common thoughts a person experiencing depression might have include, 'I am worthless' and 'It is all my fault'. Consumers might feel they cannot escape their negative experiences and might be helpless about their abilities to cope ('What is the point of trying to get help?'). The intense negative-affect and rumination over past events are accompanied by a lack of energy, motivation and pleasure, further compromising quality of life. Practitioners must be understanding of the effects of depressive conditions on peoples' functioning, and that the negativity and helplessness are part of a cycle of dysregulation affecting the person at the biological, cognitive, emotional and behavioural levels.

Bipolar illness involves episodes of mania, either alone or with major depressive episodes (APA, 2013). Episodes of mania are characterised by a period of reduced need for sleep, increased activity or restlessness and disinhibited behaviour. A person going through mania may also experience increased self-esteem or grandiosity (that in many cases can resemble delusions), higher distractibility, intense loquacity or pressured speech, increase in goal-directed activities (e.g. long-term and unusual focus on social or work-related activities) and risky activities (e.g. unrestrained shopping, sexualised behaviour) (APA, 2013). When noticing that a person might be experiencing mania, an immediate response should be to seek support for the person and to prevent possible harm to self and others. Bipolar illness is divided into types 1 and 2, depending on the severity of the manic episode. When a person experiences at least one full manic episode (e.g. exceptional energy, feeling of euphoria), the condition is characterised as bipolar type 1. In this case, a depressive episode might be experienced or not. Bipolar type 2 consists of at least one hypomanic episode (a less severe experience of mania) and at least one two-week-long depression episode (APA, 2013). In the most recent Australian survey of mental health conditions, it was estimated that 1.8 per cent of Australians aged 16–85 years had symptoms of bipolar illness in the previous 12 months (ABS, 2008).

Obsessive–compulsive related conditions

Obsessive–compulsive related conditions involve the recurrent experience of intrusive and unwanted thoughts, urges, images or ideas that provoke an intense response of anxiety (**obsessions**). **Compulsions** are repetitive behaviours (including mental acts) performed with the intention of suppressing the thinking, or 'neutralising' it. Obsessive–compulsive conditions are thus characterised by the presence of obsessions or compulsions (most commonly both) that are recurrent and time-consuming, and can cause significant distress or impairment in personal, social or professional functioning. The person with OCD experiences obsessions that vary in content, such as ideas of contamination, harming or hurting someone, or breaking the law (e.g. excessive worries about proliferation of diseases, images about cheating

obsession – the recurrent experience of thoughts, images or urges that are uncontrollable and provoke anxiety or negative feelings (e.g. guilt, shame, fear)

compulsion – a repetitive behaviour performed to decrease anxiety provoked by obsessions

on a partner). These thoughts, urges or ideas are experienced with pronounced distress (e.g. horror or guilt when having thoughts about hurting someone) and the need to be suppressed or neutralised (Janardhan Reddy et al., 2017). People who experience obsessive–compulsive related conditions usually present rigid ideas and beliefs (e.g. 'a good person does not think about such things'), perfectionism ('things should be done this way or something bad will happen') and a high sense of responsibility ('if someone in my family gets sick, it is my fault'). These beliefs then lead to distress that the person feels must be alleviated through compulsive behaviours.

Trauma and stress-related conditions

Under the category of trauma and stress-related conditions, the two most relevant diagnoses are post-traumatic stress disorder (PTSD) and acute stress disorder. Both involve the previous experience of traumatic experiences such as threatened death, serious injury or sexual violence. The exposure to such events can occur in the form of personal experience, witnessing (in person) the event happening to others, learning that the traumatic event happened to someone close, or repeated and detailed exposure to details of the traumatic event, usually work-related (e.g. first responders after responding to a natural disaster; police officers exposed to details of violent crime) (APA, 2013).

For a PTSD diagnosis, the symptoms must be identified after a one-month period following the traumatic event and must include intrusive symptoms (e.g. memories, dreams and flashbacks; feelings that 'it is happening again'); avoidance of reminders of the trauma (e.g. efforts to avoid thoughts, places or activities that can bring the experience to attention); alterations in reactivity and arousal (e.g. hypervigilance, exaggerated startle response, anger outbursts) and negative alterations in cognitions and mood (e.g. increased experience of anger, guilt, or shame, exaggerated negative beliefs such as 'no one can be trusted' and feelings of detachment from others). Although some of the responses might begin immediately after the event, PTSD with delayed expression may be observed (criteria are met at least six months after the event). For the diagnosis of acute stress disorder, a constellation of the PTSD criteria is required (at least nine in total). The main differential is that such responses must happen in a period of three days to a month after the traumatic event (APA, 2013). In Australia, 12.2 per cent of adults aged 16–85 years reported experiencing PTSD in their lifetime (ABS, 2008).

When a person experiences a traumatic event, fundamental beliefs about oneself, others, the world and the future can be modified. The effects of trauma can lead to unhelpful beliefs about one's self-worth (e.g. 'I am "spoilt goods"'), and personal skills (e.g. 'I cannot trust my judgement'). Interpersonal relationships can also be hindered by beliefs such as 'if I try to trust others, they will end up hurting me'. The consequences of the trauma might be exaggerated and be always in focus (e.g. 'no one will ever want to be with me after this') (LoSavio, Dillon & Resick, 2017). People who have experienced trauma might be unsettled by uncertainty. Rumination over the past events and how negative outcomes could have been prevented is another marked feature associated with increased experience of PTSD, intrusion of memories and avoidance of reminders of the trauma (Seligowski, Rogers & Orcutt, 2016). Consumers may present with signs of confusion and may not be able to remember details of the events, due to potential feelings of de-realisation (the world is perceived as unreal, distant, dreamlike) and de-personalisation (feeling detached from one's mind or body, observing things as though from a third-person's perspective; APA, 2013).

Healthcare delivery within a trauma-informed framework

Practitioners working within a trauma-informed practice must be aware of such signs in order to avoid re-traumatisation. They must prioritise increasing the consumer's perception of safety and make the necessary referrals for the right support. Educating consumers about the effects of trauma can be helpful in decreasing their sense of confusion, normalise their experience and instill hope of working through symptoms. It can be beneficial to evaluate the need for medication, as well as discuss with consumers and carers the duration of treatment and potential side-effects. Involving carers in discussions can help them to understand the needs of their loved ones who have experienced trauma. It can assist them to appreciate that startled responses can be expected when the person is exposed to triggers and that communicating a sense of safety in these moments is important in helping their loved ones to cope and feel grounded in the present moment.

TRANSLATION TO PRACTICE

Schizophrenia spectrum and other conditions featuring psychosis

Schizophrenia is a condition that has profound effects on a person's social functioning and expression of self. Psychosis is a central feature in which the person's ability to think, feel and act in coherent ways is significantly affected. This condition is characterised by a range of cognitive, behavioural and emotional symptoms, with key diagnostic criteria including the presence of at least two of:

- delusions (that is, 'fixed beliefs that are not amenable to change in light of conflicting evidence' (Glasheen et al., 2016))
- hallucinations ('perception-like experiences that occur without external stimulus' (Glasheen et al., 2016))
- disorganised speech (frequent derailment or incoherence answers unrelated to questions being asked)
- grossly disorganised or catatonic behaviour (e.g. childlike responses, unpredictable agitation; maintaining a rigid inappropriate and bizarre posture)
- negative symptoms (diminished emotional expression).

Diagnosis also evaluates the affects of symptoms on functioning in major areas of life, such as work, interpersonal relations and self-care (APA, 2013). These symptoms must be present for at list six months. The DSM also lists variations of psychotic conditions, usually defined by reduced experience of symptoms (e.g. schizophreniform condition, brief psychotic condition; APA, 2013). Additionally, it is common to observe certain indicators of poor psychosocial functioning prior to the onset of the first psychotic experience. These include social withdrawal, limited interpersonal communication skills and difficulties in functioning outside the nuclear family (Lyngberg et al., 2015).

Although less common than anxiety and affective illnesses, schizophrenia is the most commonly psychotic related condition in Australia. It is estimated that 64 000 Australians between 18 and 64 years have had a psychotic illness and were accessing public mental health care services in the previous year (4.5 cases per 1000 population; Morgan et al., 2011). Males were more likely to present with a psychotic condition than females (5.4 males and 3.5 females per a 1000 population, respectively). Males aged 25–34 years presented with higher rates of a psychotic condition (7.4 per 1000 population or 11 975 persons). In both males and females, the first onset of symptoms occurred most commonly before the age of 25 years (Morgan et al., 2011). At present, no national data on the prevalence of psychotic-related conditions is available for Aotearoa New Zealand.

Schizophrenia and psychosis-related conditions are perhaps the most stigmatised mental health conditions. People with the condition of schizophrenia might experience the delusions or hallucinations as very frightening, going through further distress for not understanding their experience or not being able to share their distress with others. Consumers can benefit from medication but also from strategies that help them feel grounded and in contact with the present moment. The identification of events that frequently provoke distress and strategies to cope can be included in a safety plan to help decrease the effects of unexpected intrusive experiences. People living with schizophrenia can be supported to learn about aspects of experience as a part of a neurochemical and psychosocial condition, rather than being defined by stigmatised stereotypes, or solely by the illness.

Eating conditions

People with eating conditions experience persistent thoughts and disturbances related to eating, eating-related behaviour and body weight, and these are more commonly experienced by young women (APA, 2013). Although less prevalent than the other mental illnesses, eating conditions can bring people to the attention of medical professionals due to the associated physical symptoms and concerns. This is particularly true for anorexia nervosa, which is characterised by limited food intake, with key diagnostic criteria including restricted energy intake relative to physical requirements, resulting in significantly reduced body weight, intense fear of weight gain or persistent behaviour to prevent weight gain (APA, 2013).

Other eating conditions are bulimia nervosa, which involves recurrent episodes of binge-eating – or eating an amount that is larger than what would be normally consumed in a given interval. In bulimia nervosa, the person performs compensatory behaviours in an attempt to prevent weight gain (e.g. misuse of laxatives, inducing vomiting, intense exercising). These behaviours must be present at least once a week for three months. As in anorexia, the person's self-evaluation is highly influenced by body weight and shape (APA, 2013). These patterns of behaviour are thought to have developed within the person's response to manage distressing experiences. Dynamics of rejection, acceptance, approval and self-value can be mediated through perception of physical appearance. Eating conditions are often experienced with other comorbid mental health conditions, such as depression, anxiety and substance misuse (Keski-Rahkonen & Mustelin, 2016).

Substance misuse

Substance misuse conditions may be defined as dependence or harmful use of alcohol or other drugs. These conditions are slightly less prevalent than other types of mental illnesses, affecting 5.1 per cent of the adult population in Australia and 3.5 per cent in Aotearoa New Zealand (ABS, 2008; Oakley Browne et al., 2006). In Australia, substance misuse conditions are more common in men aged 16–24 years (13 per cent; ABS, 2008. Similarly, in Aotearoa New Zealand, these conditions account for 2 per cent of the female and 5 per cent of the male population, and are most common in the 16–24-year age bracket (9.6 per cent; Oakley Browne et al., 2006). Ten substance categories are listed in the DSM-5 substance use conditions (e.g. alcohol, caffeine, cannabis, opioid, tobacco). Examples of criteria are spending a large amount of time obtaining, consuming or recovering from the effects of the substance, and cravings or experiencing urges to use it. The person might also need increased amounts to experience the desired effects and may experience personal and interpersonal problems as a function of their substance use (APA, 2013).

Substance use conditions are likely the result of unhelpful coping strategies, often used to manage very difficult emotions and interpersonal difficulties people might have in different areas of life. In Australia, almost two-thirds (63 per cent) of people experiencing drug misuse indicated they also experienced mental illness in the previous 12 months (ABS, 2008). Empathetic understanding of a person's pattern of experiences and avoiding judgement of addictive behaviour are expected from health professionals, who must understand how a person's context and previous life experiences can shape their health-related behaviours.

Personality conditions

Personality conditions are defined as patterns of experiences and behaviours that are inflexible and are not in consonance with the expectation of a person's social and cultural backgrounds. In other words, the person differs markedly in the way they perceive themselves, others and social situations, and their experience of intense, inconstant emotions that might seem inappropriate responses to the context. The person's experiences and behaviours begin in adolescence and early adulthood, and can be observed across a range of settings; these can have a significant effect on the person's personal, social and professional functioning (APA, 2013).

One of the more well-known and frequently stigmatised conditions is borderline personality disorder (BPD). This is characterised by instability in a person's sense of self and relationships with others, intense emotional feelings, very high or low arousal and impulsive behaviour. The person experiencing borderline characteristics can make significant efforts to avoid rejection (real or imagined), present with impulsive behaviours and experience chronic feelings of emptiness. Intense anger can also be experienced, which is felt as difficult to control, and not appropriate to the situation as interpreted by others. People living with borderline experiences might also display self-harming behaviours thought to be associated with trying to relieve tension or be self-soothing, or to cope with intense emotions, as this can provide a sense of relief or control over difficult thoughts and feelings (Colle et al., 2020). People experiencing BPD may experience very high distress and suicidal crisis, with individuals and families seeking the support of emergency departments and other crisis services. Due to personality conditions being poorly understood by health practitioners, individuals and carers often receive stigmatised and minimising responses to distress (Acres, Loughhead & Procter, 2019).

personality conditions – patterns of emotional, cognitive and behavioural experiences that compromise a person's adaptation to their social context. The person can present responses that seem extreme and chaotic, and they often feel isolated from others.

Aaron's experience of receiving a mental health diagnosis

In high school, I was discovered as having mental health issues, through a school survey on mental health. I can't remember if I was having a particularly bad day; however, prior to this I had started self-harming with pins. I'd etch song lyrics into my arms and was quite amazed at how dead I felt inside; the scratching, which then turned into pencil sharpener blades and Stanley knives, didn't appear to hurt me greatly. I was 13 years old when I saw a psychiatrist, who prescribed an anti-depressant and said I had dysthymia. Things became really bad with self-harm; I eventually ended up in hospital and was admitted for a few days. The next diagnosis I received was borderline personality disorder (BPD). Many felt BPD was nonsense, a wastebasket diagnosis, and the next psychiatrist was determined to find out what was 'really wrong' with me.

I was misdiagnosed further with bipolar and schizophrenia, and placed on a myriad of medications: an anti-depressant, an anti-psychotic and a mood stabiliser. These medications enhanced a personal belief that I did have some form of a mood or psychotic disorder, and not BPD. I was 27 years old when I believed BPD may not be a 'wastebasket' diagnosis but this belief was enhanced in my 30s after I reviewed neuro-imaging literature that demonstrated BPD has a biological component in the brain. I was convinced BPD was no longer a wastebasket diagnosis as I had been told for many years. I had enormous trouble accepting a diagnosis, let alone being able to take one seriously.

REFLECTIVE QUESTIONS

Based on Aaron's lived experience, consider the following questions.

- What might be the effects of receiving multiple diagnoses over a period of mental health assessment or treatment? How can changes in diagnoses affect a person's understanding of their own experiences?
- How can receiving different diagnoses over time influence the choice of pharmacological treatment? Could medication side-effects make it harder for practitioners to distinguish what is an effect of the condition and what is medication-induced?

Why is the diagnosis of mental illness controversial? Critiques to classification systems

Although highly used in the healthcare context, the diagnostic classification system has faced significant criticism in specialist literature (Patel et al., 2018). The DSM-5 binary approach has also faced internal critics from members of the working groups established to update it (Khoury et al., 2014). This has led to the proposition of a dimensional approach to diagnosing by including the use of specifiers, subtypes and, more importantly, severity ratings, so as to provide a continuum view of consumers' experiences. Understanding the effects of experiences from the consumer's perspective might better assist practitioners to understand the gradients of a condition, which are not captured in a 'yes' or 'no' assessment (Boschloo et al., 2015; Regier, Kuhl & Kupfer, 2013). Despite this proposal, the alternative categorisation was not fully implemented. Furthermore, the threshold for several mental illnesses were reduced, potentially inflating the estimation of mental health conditions in the population (Frances, 2013; Khoury et al., 2014).

The criteria adopted to distinguish 'normal' from 'pathological' – such as number, frequency and duration of symptoms – are also suggested as being arbitrary. In the absence of biological or genetic markers to set such boundaries, the decision is highly influenced by cultural patterns of normality and the social acceptability of given behaviours. Therefore, mental health diagnosis might have the inherent characteristic of being based in values rather than facts. Expressions of discontentment or anger, for example, might be accepted or even instigated in certain cultural groups, while they are taken as a sign of poor adaptation in others. These norms also vary within a given society, as subgroups might develop their own sets of norms for expected behaviour and adaptation.

Another example is the inclusion of homosexuality as a pathological condition until 1972, which was changed following evidence from research and pressure from activists in the lesbian, gay, bisexual, transexual, intersex and queer (LGBTIQ) communities. In its current version, the DSM-5 lists transexual and intersex people as having a pathological condition, under the nomenclature of 'gender dysphoria'. Critics have argued that not every transexual and intersex person experiences distress and impaired functioning related to gender identity and that is necessary to de-pathologise their experiences as a way to reduce stigma and segregation (Davy & Toze, 2018).

Many consumers who have experienced the diagnostic process over time have also developed critical insights into the social construction of mental illnesses, and also the power dynamics involved in the diagnosis of illness as superior to other interpretations of distress and extraordinary experience, thereby rendering aspects of the self as pathological. Understandings of distress and diversity, offered by trauma-informed care, disability rights and neurodiversity, the lived experience and Mad studies movements, mean that consumers often understand their experience in much more diverse and broader narratives than as 'illness'.

PERSONAL NARRATIVE

Bonnee's story

I'm 34. Two years ago I became wobbly. I started to have anxiety that followed me everywhere. People who knew me didn't understand what I was experiencing and neither did I. My friends would say that I was in fear and needed to look at where the fear was coming from. It just got worse and worse. I'd be in safe spaces that were usually really comfortable but instead was feeling crippling anxiety. Also, I started sleeping less, I started to write a lot of poetry and my life story. I went to see a doctor as my GP was away on this day. The other GP prescribed me Zoloft for the anxiety.

After two days, this drug triggered me into a spiral of dissociation and distress. I was completely overwhelmed by severe anxiety. I would wake up in the morning and the thoughts in my head of dealing with life were so overwhelming that I would begin to cry in terror. It was like nothing I'd ever experienced before.

I went to see my original GP and as soon as I sat in her office I ended up having a mixed episode. Which was intense, hysterical laughter followed by intense crying. It was extremely scary and a very confusing time. I was kneeling on a chair in her office, and I asked her to sedate me as I knew I needed something to take the feelings away as my body and mind were not coping. I had a friend waiting outside the clinic. My GP invited my friend in and asked her to take me to the hospital to get evaluated by a psychiatrist. I was lucky I had a friend with me, otherwise – my GP told me later on – she would have needed to detain me. By the time I got to the hospital and was assessed, the olanzapine that my GP had given me was working and I was calm. I am a high-functioning and well-articulated woman, and when I spoke to the psychiatrist I would have presented well. The psychiatrist sent me home.

When I went to see my GP again she made a complaint and said that I needed respite. She was upset about the treatment I received. Anyway, what happened next was that I ended up in a manic episode for two weeks.

In the meanwhile, I was seeing a therapist who did a mental health assessment and diagnosed me with bipolar disorder in the same session. She then explained that I was too unstable to continue to have sessions with her and that I should come back into her care once I had stabilised. She had just diagnosed me with a mental illness. At the time, I felt rejected, abandoned, angry, very confused and – most of all – let down. It would have been helpful if instead this woman had sat down with me and explained why she diagnosed me with this condition. What would have been as important was if she had done it with kindness, care, gentleness and empathy.

My GP referred me to a community mental health organisation and had to call up and follow up on it, and I remember hearing her say to whoever she was talking to, 'Look, this girl is manic she needs help now,' so she was advocating on my behalf.

Only a few days later I had an appointment with a psychiatrist. I sat in a room with him and another woman who didn't do much talking but she was calm and smiled. Her presence alone was soothing. I was manic still, and this man just let me speak. I spoke for a good few hours. I was given the space to tell him the events that had taken place that had led me into that room that day. He nodded in all the right places, he paraphrased back to me, asked all the right questions, and I could tell that he was paying attention. If I could, I would find that psychiatrist and personally thank him. He gave me space to feel really heard and supported. He also took the time to help me understand that the things I was experiencing were symptoms of bipolar and that he wanted to start me on a mood stabiliser. When I left there I was still scared and this was all a lot to process. But I felt like I had some more understanding of what I was experiencing.

I kept seeing my GP regularly over this time and now every time I see her she gives me a hug as we've been through so much together. She was loving but firm. She told me she wanted me to stay on medication for at least a year. Actually, she was my first point of contact and has always been my biggest advocate. I feel very fortunate she has metaphorically held my hand throughout this journey with me.

Having people who took the time to reassure me, to guide me, to shine a torch and light the way with non-judgement, kindness and care has been what's helped me the most.

Also, I now have found it invaluable to connect with other people who identify with living with mental illness who have shared their own resilience and coping strategies with me, which fills me with hope and inspiration. I also work as a peer support person and use my story to connect with others when appropriate. I think the way people are spoken to and the language used is extremely important. And although it's taken me a while to process what I've been through, I now don't identify with labelling myself with bipolar. I believe that I had so many stressors at the time as well as past traumas that it was my brain's way of coping, as I didn't feel safe and or have the capacity to emotionally regulate all of life's circumstances.

REFLECTIVE QUESTIONS

Based on Bonnee's experience, consider the following questions.

- How might the person's own self-understanding and conceptualisation of distress be valued in the assessment process? Did this occur in Bonnee's initial experience at the hospital?
- What reflections do you have on the way the psychiatrist created space to hear Bonnee's experience in detail? What would it have felt like to be heard in that way?

Reflections on how to empathically respond to a person presenting with mental illness

It is common that busy routines and stressful work environments can switch practitioners' attention from the consumer's holistic needs to biomedically oriented tasks. Here are some examples of how to implement a person-centred approach and trauma-informed practice when delivering care for people who might be experiencing mental illnesses.

- When experiencing mental health challenges, people can feel overwhelmed, scared and disoriented. It is important to adopt a compassionate attitude, to hear the person's narrative and communicate that you are willing to help.
- Advocating for the person's well-being can produce long-lasting, positive effects in their life trajectory. Do your best to follow up on commitments. This can promote recovery and increase trust that health professionals are willing and prepared to help.
- Be aware of negative stereotypes and stigma associated with illness categories and symptoms. See the person, not just the illness. Enable space to hear diverse narratives from consumers.
- In your daily practice, reflect on how a person might be thinking and feeling; how they conceptualise their experience. Ask yourself 'What could be going through their head right now?' and 'How would I be feeling if I were going through a similar situation?'. Make this a habit to generate openness, empathy and respect.
- Trauma can affect people's lives in many ways and can have a long-lasting and deleterious effect. Be kind and compassionate, even when the person presents as difficult to engage with. Keep in mind that 'difficult' behaviour is a consequence of trauma.

TRANSLATION TO PRACTICE

COVID-19 and mental illness

The COVID-19 pandemic – the first outbreaks started in early 2020 – was challenging and unsettling for many people. Pandemics can create an overall sense of fear and uncertainty that both originates and reinforces the onset of distress. People with existing psychosocial and mental-health related conditions might be at increased risk of experiencing difficult thoughts, fear, distress and threat (Moreno et al., 2020). In the case of the COVID-19 pandemic, these can further exacerbated by the intensity of non-conclusive or conflicting information in the media (Brooks et al., 2020). The communication of pandemics can affect peoples' notion of what is predictable as it becomes challenging to identify patterns in the manifestation of disease (Moreno et al., 2020).

The overall climate created by a pandemic can make it especially challenging for those who find it difficult to cope with anxious thoughts (Yao, Chen & Xu, 2020). It is known that situations involving an unpredictable and prolonged sense of fear can lead some people to become hypervigilant (Steenblock et al., 2020). Hypervigilance and anxiety can contribute to the adoption of safety behaviours, from constant checking of information to binge-watching TV and the hoarding of essential goods (Moreno et al., 2020). People can also vacillate between believing everything is normal and behaving as though the pandemic does not exist, to the realisation that the situation is dangerous. Sleep disturbances, fatiguability and difficulties in self-regulation might also be noted as a sign of limited coping with the general feelings of uncertainty and unpredictability (Gao et al., 2020).

Health workers must be aware of the effects of pandemic in consumers and carers alike. It is important to be alert to sensitive information, such as feeling overwhelmed or being unable to tolerate distress. In people with a previous mental health diagnosis, identifying how the person's condition, use of medication, social and occupational impairment, drug use and suicidal ideation might have changed after the pandemic can offer insight into areas for intervention (Moreno et al., 2020).

REFLECTIVE QUESTIONS

Who are the people most likely affected by COVID-19 and its social and economic effects? Consider the potential burden to people's well-being, especially for those experiencing disadvantage. Do you think these effects could persist over time?

SUMMARY

This chapter has presented stories and information, supplemented by activities designed to deepen your understanding of:

- Mental illness or mental health conditions as clusters of experiences – thoughts, emotions and behaviours – that compromise a person' ability to live a meaningful life. Diagnosis is based on classification systems such as the DSM-5 and ICD-11.

- Some of the mental illness diagnoses most frequently observed in practice. It is important to build a trusting, caring relationship in the context of patterns of thinking, feelings and behaviours that people with a given mental illness might experience.
- Trauma, which can be associated with a range of mental health conditions, such as major depression and anxiety. Trauma changes the way people see themselves, others and the world around them. Trauma-informed care can help people to access the right support and avoid triggering of traumatic experiences.
- The need for health professionals to balance their knowledge of diagnostic criteria with approaches that are person-centred and trauma-informed, to focus on client's needs and reinforce resilience and potential for recovery.

CRITICAL THINKING/LEARNING ACTIVITIES

1 Think about the conceptions of narrative-approach, person-centred approach and trauma-informed practice, as discussed in Chapters 1 and 2. Sit with a colleague and discuss how reading through this chapter has helped you to understand the experiences of people with mental illness. What have you learned about people's experiences that came across as interesting or surprising?
2 Try to imagine yourself in a healthcare facility during your future professional practice. Can you foresee any difficulties in assisting a person with a given mental health condition? Which diagnoses might you consider challenging to discuss with people, their carers and other professionals, and why? How can you work towards reducing such discomfort?
3 Familiarise yourself with the mental health services located in your community. To which services would you refer someone in mental health-related distress? Make a list of emergency departments, mental health support helplines and community-based services in your area that would support people experiencing mental illness.

LEARNING EXTENSION

Audio and video recordings of lived experience can be easily found online. On the Black Dog Institute website, for example, you can find podcasts and written stories produced by people who live with depression, anxiety, PTSD, bipolar and eating conditions. Similar lived-experience accounts can be found on other websites, such as that of the Everymind organisation and the University of South Australia's Mental Health and Suicide Prevention Research and Education Group. To further expand your understanding, choose one podcast, video or written story and work on a distress conceptualisation report for the experience presented. Use the following questions as prompts.

- Describe the thoughts and emotions the person might have experienced during the course of their mental illness.
- How might these experiences affect everyday life?
- How did the person first respond to receiving a mental illness diagnosis? How might stigma have influenced what they shared with others in their family and community?
- What could have been some of the factors that contributed to the person's decision to reach out for help?

Suggested links:

- Black Dog Institute, Personal stories (Website). Retrieved from https://www.blackdoginstitute .org.au/resources-support/personal-stories/
- Everymind. Navigate your way to health and navigating their way to health (Website). Videos and podcasts retrieved from https://everymind.org.au/resources/navigating-your-way-to-health/videos-and-podcasts
- University of South Australia. Mental health (Podcasts). Retrieved from https://www.unisa .edu.au/research/mental-health-suicide-prevention/initiatives-resources/mental-health-podcasts/

FURTHER READING

Clayton, A. (2013). How person centred care helped guide me toward recovery from mental illness. *Health Affairs*, *32*(3): 622–6.

In this paper, the author describes her experience with depression and PTSD and the care received after attempting suicide. The author reflects on the care experiences she had in different hospital settings.

Jamieson, K. R. (1996). *An Unquiet Mind – A memoir of moods and madness*. New York: Vintage Books.

In this book, Dr Jamieson reflects on her experience of being diagnosed with bipolar affective condition, her first treatment experiences and how the condition affected her personal and professional life.

Murphy, M. A. (1998). Rejection, stigma, and hope. *Psychiatric Rehabilitation Journal*, *22*(2): 185–8.

This paper accounts for the lived experience of people with mental illnesses and their journey through psychosocial services.

Phoenix Australia. (2020). *Coronavirus (COVID-19) Practitioner self-care tips*. Retrieved from https://www.phoenixaustralia.org/wp-content/uploads/2020/04/Coronavirus-Practitioner-self-care-tip-sheet.pdf

This brochure provides useful tips for practitioners, to look after themselves in the context of the COVID-19 pandemic.

REFERENCES

Acres, K., Loughhead, M. & Procter, N. (2019). Carer perspectives of people diagnosed with borderline personality disorder: a scoping review of emergency care responses. *Australasian Emergency Care*, *22*(1): 34–41.

American Psychiatric Association (APA). (1952). *Diagnostic and Statistical Manual of Mental Disorders*. Washington, DC: APA.

——— (2013). *Diagnostic and Statistical Manual of Mental Disorders*, 5th edn. Washington, DC: APA.

Australian Bureau of Statistics. (2008). *National Survey of Mental Health and Wellbeing: Summary of Results*. Retrieved from https://www.abs.gov.au/ausstats/abs@.nsf/mf/4326.0

Australian Institute of Health and Welfare (AIHW). (2015). *Australian Burden of Disease Study – Impact and causes of illness and death in Australia 2015 – Summary*. Canberra: AIHW.

Boschloo, L., van Borkulo, C. D., Rhemtulla, M., Keyes, K. M., Borsboom, D. & Schoevers, R. A. (2015). The network structure of symptoms of the Diagnostic and Statistical Manual of Mental Disorders. *PLoS One*, *10*(9): e0137621.

Brooks, S. K., Webster, R. K., Smith, L. E., Woodland, L., Wessely, S., Greenberg, N. & Rubin, G. J. (2020). The psychological impact of quarantine and how to reduce it: rapid review of the evidence. *The Lancet*, *395*(10227): 912–20.

Clark, L. A., Cuthbert, B., Lewis-Fernandez, R., Narrow, W. E. & Reed, G. M. (2017). Three approaches to understanding and classifying mental disorder: ICD-11, DSM-5, and the National Institute of Mental Health's Research Domain Criteria (RDoC). *Psychological Science in Public Interest*, *18*(2): 72–145.

Colle, L., Hilviu, D., Rossi, R., Garbarini, F. & Fossataro, C. (2020). Self-harming and sense of agency in patients with borderline personality disorder. *Frontiers in Psychiatry*, 11: 449.

Davy, Z. & Toze, M. (2018). What is gender dysphoria? A critical systematic narrative review. *Transgender Health*, *3*(1): 159–69.

Frances, A. (2013). Saving normal: An insider's revolt against out-of-control psychiatric diagnosis, DSM-5, big pharma and the medicalization of ordinary life. *Psychotherapy in Australia*, *19*(3): 14.

Gao, J., Zheng, P., Jia, Y., Chen, H., Mao, Y., Chen, S. … Dai, J. (2020). Mental health problems and social media exposure during COVID-19 outbreak. *PLoS One*, *15*(4): e0231924.

Glasheen, C. Batts, K. Karg, R. Bose, J. Hedden, S. & Piscopo, K. (2016). *Impact of the DSM-IV to DSM-5 Changes on the National Survey on Drug Use and Health*, Rockville: Substance Abuse and Mental Health Services (SAMHSA).

Hahm, S., Muehlan, H., Stolzenburg, S., Tomczyk, S., Schmidt, S. & Schomerus, G. (2020). How stigma interferes with symptom awareness: Discrepancy between objective and subjective cognitive performance in currently untreated persons with mental health problems. *Stigma and Health*, *5*(2): 146–57.

Janardhan Reddy, Y. C., Sundar, A. S., Narayanaswamy, J. C. & Math, S. B. (2017). Clinical practice guidelines for obsessive-compulsive disorder. *Indian Journal of Psychiatry*, *59*(Suppl 1): S74–S90.

Keski-Rahkonen, A. & Mustelin, L. (2016). Epidemiology of eating disorders in Europe: prevalence, incidence, comorbidity, course, consequences, and risk factors. *Current Opinion in Psychiatry*, *29*(6): 340–5.

Khoury, B., Langer, E. J. & Pagnini, F. (2014). The DSM: Mindful science or mindless power? A critical review. *Frontiers in Psychololgy*, *5*: 602.

LoSavio, S. T., Dillon, K. H. & Resick, P. A. (2017). Cognitive factors in the development, maintenance, and treatment of post-traumatic stress disorder. *Current Opinion in Psychology*, 14: 18–22.

Lyngberg, K., Buchy, L., Liu, L., Perkins, D., Woods, S. & Addington, J. (2015). Patterns of premorbid functioning in individuals at clinical high risk of psychosis. *Schizophrenia Research*, *169*(1–3): 209–13.

Moreno, C., Wykes, T., Galderisi, S., Nordentoft, M., Crossley, N., Jones, N. … Arango, C. (2020). How mental health care should change as a consequence of the COVID-19 pandemic. *The Lancet Psychiatry*, *7*(9): 813–24.

Morgan, V. A., Waterreus, A., Jablensky, A., Mackinnon, A., McGrath, J. J., Carr, V. … Galletly, C. (2011). *People living with psychotic illness 2010 – Report on the second Australian national survey*. Canberra: Commonwealth of Australia.

Oakley Browne, M. A., Well, J. E. & Scott, K. M. (2006). *Te Rau Hinengaro: The New Zealand Mental Health Survey*. Wellington: Ministry of Health.

Patel, V., Saxena, S., Lund, C., Thornicroft, G., Baingana, F., Bolton, P. … UnÜtzer, J. (2018). The Lancet Commission on global mental health and sustainable development. *The Lancet*, *392*(10157): 1553–98.

Regier, D. A., Kuhl, E. A. & Kupfer, D. J. (2013). The DSM-5: Classification and criteria changes. *World Psychiatry*, *12*(2): 92–8.

Seligowski, A. V., Rogers, A. P. & Orcutt, H. K. (2016). Relations among emotion regulation and DSM-5 symptom clusters of PTSD. *Personality and Individual Differences*, *92*: 104–8.

Steenblock, C., Todorov, V., Kanczkowski, W., Eisenhofer, G., Schedl, A., Wong, M. L. ... Bornstein, S. R. (2020). Severe acute respiratory syndrome coronavirus 2 (SARS-CoV-2) and the neuroendocrine stress axis. *Molecular Psychiatry, 25*: 1611–17.

World Health Organization (WHO). (1949). *International statistical classification of diseases, injuries, and causes of death, 6th revision.* Geneva: WHO.

—— (2004). *Promoting Mental Health: Concepts, emerging evidence, practice: summary report.* Geneva: WHO.

—— (2013). *Mental Health Action Plan 2013–2020.* Geneva: WHO.

Yao, H., Chen, J.-H. & Xu, Y.-F. (2020). Patients with mental health disorders in the COVID-19 epidemic. *The Lancet Psychiatry, 7*(4): e21.

Assessment practices and processes in mental health

Mark Loughhead, Kate Rhodes,
Kirsty Baker and Davi Macedo

6

LEARNING OBJECTIVES

At the completion of this chapter, you should be able to:

1 Identify the key concepts and principles that inform high-quality assessment processes undertaken by mental health practitioners.
2 Identify and explore ethical issues relating to consumers' and carers' experiences of assessment practices.
3 Understand the importance of key therapeutic skills for ensuring the partnership of consumers and carers in the assessment process.
4 Identify and explore how assessment relates to recovery values, psychiatric diagnostic systems and contemporary mental health care.

Introduction

Assessment in the mental health field is a dynamic process of learning, using experience and applying multiple sources of knowledge and evidence. This chapter presents an overview of assessment practices and processes that are undertaken within formal mental health care, and discusses these within the context of consumer–health practitioner partnerships. We start by considering how assessment practices are a prominent feature of getting to know a person's situation and life context, and how these practices need to be based on the principles of person-centred care, trauma-informed care and cultural safety. We then outline the importance of engagement and therapeutic relationships skills for ensuring that consumers, carers and family members are meaningfully connected within a process for identifying the nature of the mental health problems the person is experiencing. Part of this awareness is reflecting on what it is like for a person to be assessed, and the power dynamics involved in naming experience, symptoms and diagnosis. The chapter then looks at the paradigm of comprehensive assessment, which is a broad biopsychosocial understanding of the features of a person's mental health and functioning within their life context. There are also specific discussions about strengths-based assessment, mental state examination (MSE) and the roles of different health professionals.

Approaching assessment: Understanding mental illness and mental health

This section begins by highlighting that assessment practices are usually the primary experience of consumers and carers when they first meet healthcare professionals. Assessment occurs on multiple levels and for several purposes. The most immediate is to understand the nature of distress being experienced by the person, and how the person is experiencing distress in terms of mood, thoughts, behaviours and relationships. There is a focus on discerning whether the person's distress is related to, or an expression of, a mental health condition. In clinical assessment, the emphasis is on self-reported and observable aspects of mood, cognition and behaviour, the period of time when the distress has developed and its effects on work, relationships and study. Within medical practice, there is also an assessment of the person's distress in the context of their physical health, and whether biological issues are affecting their mental state. Previous psychiatric history is also considered. Overall, the focus within the illness paradigm is on identifying whether the person's experiences are to be considered symptoms.

From a holistic mental health perspective, assessment practices seek information about a range of life areas, such as work, family history, personal values and meaningful activities. Further focus might include assessment of social relationships, access to housing and transport, prior and current experiences of trauma (Felitti et al., 1998, 2019; Muskett, 2014), or experiences of racism, homophobia or other discriminatory interactions. Health professionals often use the terms 'protective factors' and 'risk factors' when understanding the range of experiences that people may going through, and what supports or hinders mental health. The field of mental health promotion and prevention takes such a focus, highlighting that an individual's mental health reflects the interaction of biological, developmental, psychological, social, economic and cultural determinants (Allen et al., 2014).

The conceptualisation of mental health and illness is also informed by the growing presence of lived-experience writers and leaders in the **recovery** movement (Glover, 2012). Writers and leaders in the movement often provide different ways of viewing mental health-related distress. They may also critique the psychiatric language of disorder. An alternative paradigm of recovery has developed in Western countries, based on empowerment principles, inclusion and citizenship, peer support and the critique of psychiatry's influences on personal identity and social stigma. Many nations have a growing movement of peer workforce, organised within public mental health services, non-government services and consumer-run organisations. As we enter this chapter, we can see that assessment is shaped by the paradigms of mental illness and mental health, as well as lived experience. These foundations provide the conceptual foundations for understanding a person's distress and the aspects of life in which problems are situated.

recovery – can be understood as the establishment of a meaningful and fruitful life and a positive and autonomous identity of self. It is also about establishing or maintaining social connections and encouraging an inclusive society. The assessment process is a partnership between the health professional and the person seeking help, which identifies the person's strengths to build confidence and skills in managing distress, and to re-establish social roles and relationships.

Principles of care informing assessment: Strengths, cultural safety, trauma-informed and person-centred approaches

From the origins of person-centred care in the 1920s (Buber & Smith, 1958), and further developed by Carl Rogers in the 1950s (Rogers, 1961), today the concept is integral to the delivery of health care in Australia. Person-centred care transcends disciplines across medicine, psychology, nursing and throughout the human social sciences as one of the fundamental, 'consumer-centred' models of care recommended by the Australian Commission on Safety and Quality in Health Care (ACSQHC, 2010). As such, person-centred care has been adopted by the Australian Government Department for Health and Ageing (DHA, 2014) and is evident in local state health policy documents as a basis for best practice in health care. The central tenets comprise genuineness, non-judgemental caring and empathy (Raskin & Rogers, 2005), and underpin the way we interact with all people with whom we come into contact within our healthcare roles. Alongside this, and of equal importance, are cultural responsiveness and cultural safety. Cultural responsiveness refers to respectful care of people of diverse ethnicities and cultures, while cultural safety refers to respectful care of Māori and Aboriginal and Torres Strait Islander peoples (see Chapters 3 and 4) and acknowledges issues relating to colonisation specifically (Williams, 1999). Both cultural applications in health care include reflecting on one's own cultural beliefs and biases, and bear greater accountability in practice than simply cultural awareness. As a minimum, healthcare professionals respond to all people in their care using a person-centred and culturally responsive or safe manner.

Approaches to care are not one-size-fits-all models (see Figure 6.1). However, while we can adopt an overarching approach to care that is embedded in person-centred, culturally safe and responsive concepts at 'layer one', ultimately what follows at 'layer two' depends on the unique individual who presents before us. Figure 6.1 shows 'All people experiencing mental health problems' at the second layer, indicating an additional level of knowledge is needed to provide evidence-based mental health care to this group of people. Just as complex intergenerational trauma is experienced in some way by all Aboriginal and Torres-Strait Islander peoples, trauma at some level is, or has been, experienced by all people who have mental health problems (Felitti et al., 1998, 2019; Muskett, 2014) and therefore underpins a trauma-informed care approach towards all who come into contact with us as health professionals. Whether we are specialist mental health professionals or non-specialist health professionals, all people presenting to us with mental health issues need to be provided with interventions that understand trauma-informed care without them having to explain their historical past or current underlying traumatic circumstances.

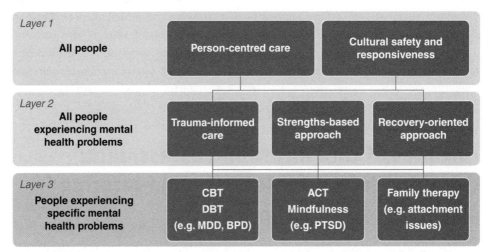

Figure 6.1   Multi-layered conceptual framework of models of mental health care informing assessment, therapeutic relationships and care planning

Providing mental health care to individuals is a multi-layered and unique undertaking (see Figure 6.1). While the first two layers in the diagram can be incorporated by health professionals in all disciplines, the third layer is utilised by mental health professionals with specific expertise in each specialty counselling area. What we focus on in this topic are the approaches that can be used by all health professionals because all health professionals encounter people experiencing mental health problems, either in managing general physical health issues or in mental health care specifically. Depending on the circumstances we are presented with, we adapt our approach to healthcare provision by drawing on the concepts and models of care that meet the person's particular needs. For example, an Aboriginal man experiencing a suicidal crisis who attends the emergency department needs all three of the layered approaches to care, including acknowledgement that social and emotional well-being (see Chapter 4) underpins his cultural understanding of mental health. Principles of person-centred, culturally safe, trauma-informed, recovery-oriented care combine in our approach for this individual at our first point of contact. In working with the person to assess the presenting mental health issues and to determine their unique needs in the present moment, a strengths-based approach is used to move forward with a plan of care. By asking what has helped in the past to overcome strong and similar emotional experiences, our stance is one of acknowledging the person is an 'expert-by-experience' (Happell et al., 2019) who has strengths that can also be called upon in the current crisis. Rather than 'doing for' the person, recovery-oriented principles espouse 'doing with', thereby utilising strengths to empower consumers in managing their symptoms or distress, with professional support alongside them.

In layer three, the figure shows some examples of more specific approaches to mental healthcare provision that further depend on the individual circumstances. Often, it is only once we have gotten to know a person better that we are able to advocate for more specialist services or therapy. There are three examples in the figure; however, there are an exponential number of needs that can be matched to appropriate services or expert care provision. The health professional's level of knowledge, skills, experience and attitudes will determine what happens at layer three. An individual experiencing mild psychosis and substance dependence may be referred for cognitive behavioural therapy (CBT) to manage auditory hallucinations, and drug and alcohol services for specific therapies such as motivational interviewing (Prochaska, Redding & Evers, 2015). Alternatively, an experienced mental health professional may have specialist skills to draw upon to aid in their assessment and may continue to work with the person. At layer three, a higher level of expertise is typically needed to adequately provide care for individuals presenting with specific mental healthcare needs.

Consumer experience of assessment and diagnosis

People seeking help for a mental health crisis can undergo very challenging situations in healthcare settings. Not only are they dealing with the crisis, but they also need to negotiate systems of care, including emergency department responses. In the following extract (BMJ, 2015), a consumer describes their assessment while experiencing psychosis:

> I am thinking fast; new fears flood in at the speed of perception. I'm noticing some things you – the interviewing doctors – do not. Yes hallucinations, some of them; fight or flight is also heightening my senses. Paranoid hypotheses are disproved and discarded; others take their place. Some will stay with me for months to come. But I don't know that there is any future. I am already passing through 'stages of grief' – much as someone would if awaiting execution. This figures – I believe I am facing execution. The thought, 'I'm experiencing psychosis' – terrifying when it comes – is unavailable; it's all too new for that. It follows that all talk of 'doctors', 'treatment', or 'admission' feels like so much persecution and deceit.
>
> In my case I was looked at by two emergency departments within 36 hours. In between the two I was put to bed at a relative's home and soon enough put my fist through a second floor window. But after treating the hand injury, the doctors in the second emergency department were still vacillating between home treatment and hospital admission ... All in all, I was inter-viewed by more than a dozen doctors ...

The insights of this writer reveal the inner experiences of coping with psychosis as well as help-seeking. Imagine the difficulty in being participating in discussions about your mental health when you are trying to manage internal responses such as these, are sleep deprived and interviewed multiple times by sometimes detached and tired health professionals. This is what it can be like seeking help when in a mental health crisis.

It is good practice for everyone involved in mental health services to reflect on consumer experience. It can help to illustrate the patterns of distress that people are going through as well as the meanings they give to distress and other areas of life. Narrative accounts of consumer experience and personal recovery also reveal the effects of service environments and preferable communication with professionals (Llewellyn-Beardsley et al., 2019).

It is important to consider a range of perspectives that consumers may have about engaging in assessment processes, depending on previous experience and contact with mental health professionals. Consumers are 'assessing' as well. People who have had positive experiences of services and treatment may feel more trusting towards the clinical language and processes of assessment and diagnosis, while those who have had negative experiences of care may be critical of these aspects of psychiatry (Daya, Hamilton & Roper, 2020).

Many consumers with experience of public mental health services are aware of the provisions of mental health legislation and how this shapes the power relationships in assessment and diagnosis. To engage with services is to engage with the latent powers of treatment orders. This awareness often shapes a person's sense of safety and trust in sharing their experience and feelings. Some consumers have experienced trauma within services, including trauma resulting from practices of restraint and seclusion. Fears about the coercive power of public services also affect their feelings of trust and safety.

Apart from legislative powers, there is another dynamic in the assessment process that is unequal. This relates to the presumed expertise of professionals about lived experience. The traditions of the biomedical model establish the health practitioner as the knower of objective knowledge about illness and treatment, while the patient is the known, and assessment is the process by which the clinician gains subjective and objective observations of the person's health. A person undergoing assessment can therefore feel that their sense of self and personhood are objectified through clinical discourses and knowledge, and are translated from grounded experience into diagnostic language they do not understand or have a background in. Consumers may feel that the assessment is one-sided, whereas their many years of lived experience are not asked about or taken into account. Or they might feel shame, as diagnosis can feel inseparable from stigma and negative imagery; the 'spoilt identity' of having parts of the self that are seen as disordered. These features of power and diagnosis can affect trust and how a person with lived experience may disclose. Carers may experience similar yet also distinct dynamics in the assessment process.

As mental health conditions are enduring and life-changing for the person, lived experience and sociological critiques have highlighted that the biomedical model and its processes are intrinsically reductionist, disempowering, and that they encourage a passive definition of self and capability (Glover, 2012; Karter & Kamens, 2019).

Recovery narratives are often critical of psychiatry. They depict positive changes occurring outside formal mental health care (Llewellyn-Beardsley et al., 2019). A pro-recovery approach to assessment should be a process of recognising lived experience and a practice of knowledge sharing. Assessment should support a person's sense of agency, and awareness of their skills and strengths (Shepherd, Boardman, Rinaldi, & Roberts, 2014). This is not the same as suggesting that people do not need support and connection because they already know everything that is happening. When a person is in crisis, it can be difficult for them to remember their experience and to feel grounded and in control. A recovery focus seeks personal knowledge and preferences that have been hard-won through lived experience and recognises that a person's autonomy as well as support are critical. For instance, a person may only want to express their situation or seek a crisis response and may not want to be 'fixed'. Their personal beliefs may be different but not delusional. A high mood may be something that's important and enjoyable, not a symptom. Expression of harm-based thoughts may be about sharing pain, rather than someone whose risks need to be managed. A lived-experience perspective would ask whether 'assessment' can recognise a diversity of viewpoints and alternative possibilities for the helper's response. Being mindful that in mental health each individual's experience – even of the same diagnosis – will be different. These points illustrate that it is important for nurses and other health professionals to recognise that there are diverse perspectives in health care. Consumers have a distinct set of interests in accessing care, and their voice and perspective will be different to a health practitioner perspective.

REFLECTIVE QUESTIONS

- How can the person's agency be fostered during assessment?
- What questions are important to include to make sure you are not adopting a 'need-to-fix' lens?
- How can health workers reduce the power differential between professionals and people receiving care?

Mental health diagnosis

For some people, receiving a diagnosis can offer an explanation for their experience of symptoms and this might come as a relief when first diagnosed (Rose & Thornicroft, 2010). Symptoms can be understood and normalised so the person feels less confused by what is happening to them. Common treatment options and therapies used to treat the diagnosed mental health condition can be explored using evidence-based research to guide decision-making. Yet, with the growing understanding of the lived experience of people with mental health conditions, we begin to recognise the flaws within a biomedical approach that can be characterised by poor health outcomes despite the use of psychotropic medication (Deacon, 2013). For many, a mental illness diagnosis does not adequately reflect the lived experience of their mental health condition, and it can diminish their social identity. Older consumers may have experienced significant stigma, as well as a prognosis that has reduced their sense of self and hope for the future. Negative messages about illness and self-capacity are often internalised (Ben-Zeev, Young & Corrigan, 2010). Using a person-centred approach, we are able to see past the diagnosis and support the individual in using their strengths, abilities and supports to promote recovery, regardless of symptoms.

PERSONAL NARRATIVE

Aaron's experience

The biggest thing that stuck out for me was being told for years that I didn't have a mental illness. I often watched psychiatrists engage in rhetorical banter about whether borderline personality disorder (BPD) is a mental illness. Psychiatrists were completely oblivious to the suffering I was experiencing, the self-harm, the impulsive moods and inability to function. At stages, these problems were passed off as 'attention-seeking' or 'manipulative', as if to infer that I gained some form of pleasure in making others' lives miserable. I was often told I could 'switch on and off' my symptoms. I was a teenager against so-called mental health professionals. This drove a lot of bitterness I held towards the mental health profession for many years. I let this go after realising any bitterness I held did not affect anyone else except myself. Sometimes, mental health responses from telehealth services would be like a sledgehammer. For example, I would often endure police and ambulance services turning up at the family home at 2.00 a.m., waking my parents up and carting me off to hospital. My mental health issues started to feel like a competition with the attitudes of clinicians, who asserted there was nothing wrong. Denial was commonplace with BPD in the early 1990s. Often, this denial was the cause of escalated tension and trauma. I felt bad prior to presenting, only for trauma to be amplified with the disproportionate responses of police, ambulance and some mental health staff who treated me as a nuisance. I wanted help, not judgement.

REFLECTIVE QUESTIONS

- How might experiences of diagnosis vary depending on assumptions about the condition and what a person is experiencing?
- What are the important aspects of working with a person's own understanding of distress and ensuring assessment is a meaningful process for them?
- What questions would you ask a person and their family or carer to check in about their experience of assessment and diagnosis?

Help-seeking and engagement

A person may be seeking help for a variety of reasons, and it is important to ascertain from them exactly what the reason is. This helps the mental health professional to prepare their approach to the assessment, with the aim of facilitating the process of meeting the person's needs. The person may have been experiencing a problem that has occurred over a long period and which they are no longer able to cope with, or the problem may be new to them. In any case, it is essential that the mental health professional carries out a full assessment to gain a sound understanding of the person's experiences and what has been the trigger or stressor prompting their help-seeking.

Triggers or stressful life events can often cause a person's mental health to deteriorate and may prompt them to seek help. Common reasons people experience an acute stress reaction are related to stressful events that can be experienced by anyone, such as relationship difficulties, financial stress, loss of employment, withdrawal from substances, exacerbation of pre-existing symptoms, uncertainty about the future and loss of a loved one or pet. When people have a secure support network of family and friends and strong resilience, being able to cope with these major stressors is achievable. However, when all supports have been exhausted and a sense of hope has been lost, the person's coping might become limited. It is essential during a first encounter that the mental health professional does not minimise or dismiss the person's distress and reason for seeking help. An open, non-judgemental attitude communicates genuine care and attention.

How the mental health professional opens the discussion sets the scene for the person and can influence their sense of safety and trust. First, the mental health professional introduces themself by their name and professional background. Then they describe purpose of the assessment clearly so the person is informed of the process and is able to offer consent to engage. Too often, people are confused and kept in the dark about why they are expected to speak to so many different people about the same problem. To ensure transparency the consumer must be informed every step of the way. This promotes awareness and understanding, which help the person to feel safe in the knowledge of what is happening now and what is planned to occur.

Lived expertise in assessment

Consumers often have considerable knowledge of:

- issues relating to helping-seeking: e.g. emotional responses, preferences, barriers
- living with the effects of psychotropic medicines
- recent stressful and supportive events
- accessibility and suitability of mental health services
- preferred language in describing their experience – e.g. effects of labels
- recovery and therapeutic practices that are effective for them.

TRANSLATION TO PRACTICE

To facilitate an open conversation, the mental health professional needs to consider how to elicit personal information in a safe and supportive way. It is recommended that they use open and broad, non-judgemental questions that seek to understand why the person has sought help. Examples include the following.

What has happened to bring you here today?
Can you tell me what happened before coming in today?
Can you tell me why you have come to find help today?
How can I best help you today?

These responses offer an opportunity for the person to begin to explain their reason for seeking help. These questions imply something has happened to the person, rather than something is wrong with the person. They do not dismiss the person or blame them for their distress but rather seek to understand the reason for the distress. Often, people feel shame and embarrassment about seeking help (Clement et al., 2015) and having to explain to a stranger what has happened to them. Some people have been exposed to discrimination by health professionals who have been dismissive of their distress, and this is experienced as invalidating and creates mistrust of the health system (Clement et al., 2015). The mental health professional must be aware of these fears and possible past traumatic experiences so they can promote a safe space for the person to disclose their story in a supportive and therapeutic way. Often, people are referred to mental health services by a concerned family member, friend or allied health professional, and the person may disagree with their reason for referral. In this situation it is important to gather collateral information from the referrer about their concerns and explore these with the person, by openly using a therapeutic approach that is sensitive to the person's emotional state.

Meeting needs and assistance

Once the person has decided to seek help, the mental health professional should explore the person's hierarchy of needs, using a comprehensive mental health assessment.

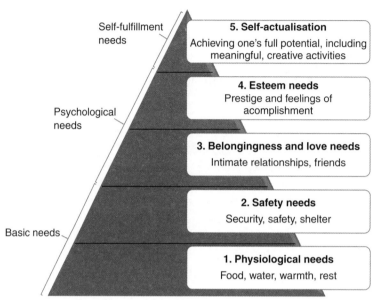

Figure 6.2   Maslow's hierarchy of needs

Source: Adapted from Maslow (1943).

Maslow's hierarchy of needs is presented in Figure 6.2. It proposes that people are motivated to fulfil their basic needs before moving onto more advanced needs and desires (Martin, Carlson & Buskist, 2013). A person may present in great distress and express serious thoughts of hopelessness, which is often a reaction to a stressful incident that has occurred. The person's psychological needs of safety and security are not met in this situation, and they are highly distressed. Before any other needs are met, the person requires assistance to express their emotions in a safe environment before the emotional distress can be stabilised. The mental health professional allows the person time and space to express their thoughts and feelings before intervening with a therapeutic intervention to stabilise emotional dysregulation. This process requires the mental health professional to walk alongside the person, to listen and understand their distress and validate their experience. In this situation, listening is the therapeutic tool provided to the person in distress. Throughout this process the mental health professional considers questions such as the following.

What are the needs of the person?
Do they need me to listen?
Do they need me to help them calm down now?
Do they need validation of their distress?
Do they need some practical assistance to respond to the trigger to their distress?

Once the person has reached a less distressed emotional state the interaction can then focus on the assessment of the person's needs to begin the process of care planning.

Comprehensive mental health assessment

A **comprehensive mental health assessment (CMHA)** is an essential process used to gather information from a person, in order to evaluate their mental health state. The aim is to understand the person's lived experience and develop a plan of care that best supports their needs. The therapeutic relationship is developed throughout this process by using active listening skills and a non-judgemental approach when asking sensitive questions. This might be communicated through the use of body language, facial expressions and the tone of voice when speaking. How you respond to the person's story must convey empathy and understanding, and must let them know that you believe what they are experiencing. The act of listening without judgement and offering validation to the person is therapeutic in and of itself. You are not expected to provide solutions or answers in this context but simply to ensure you are focused on what the person is saying.

comprehensive mental health assessment (CMHA) – a broad, biopsychosocial understanding of the features of a person's mental health and functioning within their life context. It involves collecting information on social determinants of mental health, mental illness history, triggers, coping strategies, neuro-vegetative symptoms and elements of current mental state (e.g. thought processes, perception, insight, mood).

Timing of the CMHA

Consider the timing of the CMHA. The person may not be prepared to openly disclose their story or experiences straight away. Allowing the person time and a private space to share their story is essential in providing a safe environment the person feels comfortable in. This may not always be possible if the assessment is conducted during a crisis or in a busy hospital setting but acknowledging you care about the person's comfort and safety communicates that you are aware of the challenges and that you are sensitive to the person's needs.

Consider whether it is absolutely necessary to carry out a full CMHA when the person may be scheduled to see another clinician who will be asking the same questions. Repeating one's story to health professionals is often reported by consumers as repetitive and traumatising (Blanch et al., 2012). Minimising the number of times one is expected to disclose personal information should be considered by health professionals prior to conducting a CMHA.

Core components of the CMHA

The core components of the comprehensive mental health assessment include (Queensland Health, 2019):

- Personal details – name, age, gender, address, employment status, family structure
- Presenting problem – reason for seeking help, reason for referral from health professional or family
- Stressors or triggers – these often stem from difficulties with relationships, employment, finances, accommodation, forensic issues, visa requirements, exacerbation of existing mental illness
- Substance use – type of substance used, current amounts used, method of use and historical use
- Medical conditions – physical health status, new or existing medical conditions, BMI, exercise, diet
- Current medications – prescribed and over the counter, side-effects, allergies, historical medications prescribed and their effectiveness
- Supports – health professionals, general practitioner, community supports.

History

A person's developmental history is usually available in their medical file, and it is recommended this information be accessed prior to the CMHA, to avoid asking repetitive questions. This will minimise the risk of re-traumatisation and the person having to repeat their history. For a first presentation, the following historical information may be required:

- history of mental illness – current diagnosis and any previous diagnosis, course of illness, current status
- developmental history – family structure growing up (genogram), experience of abuse or neglect, educational achievement, employment
- family history – including mental illness, drug/alcohol use or suicide.

TRANSLATION TO PRACTICE

Involving carers in assessment

A carer is a family member or friend who is identified by the consumer as a person providing support to them. Mental health services most often operate on an individual therapeutic or treatment model, in which the primary relationship is between the consumer and health practitioner, and their team. Many carers have felt excluded from assessment and treatment discussions on this basis, often describing how practitioners tend towards a default of excluding them due to privacy and confidentiality regulations. Recent policy supports the appropriate inclusion of carers as key partners in healthcare decision-making, and encourages practitioners to support carers in their own experience (*Carer's Recognition Act 2005* (SA) s 5). Appropriately including carers is an important area of practice and skill for health practitioners. Here are some key points to consider in your learning.

- Include support people or carers as identified by the consumer. If a carer has played a role in help-seeking, ask the consumer for permission to include them, or to share non-confidential information with them.
- Be mindful of conflict, hurt and guilt in situations where a carer has acted against the consumer's wishes in arranging help. Consumers may be estranged from family members and definitely *do not* want them involved.
- Identify or learn about cultural patterns of family decision-making. For many Māori and Aboriginal and Torres Strait Islander families, the carer role needs to be seen in the context of kinship networks and may involve non-direct relatives who are considered family.
- Most mental health legislation provides guidance for the inclusion of carers and confidentiality.
- Carers often have valuable insights into the consumer's recent situation and life stresses. They are likely to provide support in the future.
- Carers often have many questions about mental health and illness, and benefit from education and information on treatment options and services.
- Carers can be stressed, anxious and or exhausted, and may appreciate attention and support for their well-being. Remember to refer them to local carer support networks.
- Carer peer workers can provide helpful support and information and help to engage carers in assessment or planning discussions.
- Remember potential legal implications; provide carers or family members with legal information and status changes regarding involuntary treatment.

Mental status examination

When completing a mental health examination, practitioners should consider (Norris, Clark & Shipley, 2016; Soltan & Girguis, 2017):

- Appearance – assess the person's physical characteristics and dress, including age, gender, hair style, weight, clothing, hygiene and grooming, scars or tattoos
- Behaviour – how is the person behaving? Assess their posture and body language, their level of engagement, motor activity
  - Example: psychomotor agitation or retardation
- Conversation – describe the person's speech including quantity, volume, rate and flow
  - Examples: softly spoken, loud and pressured, stuttered with paucity of speech
- Thought processes – observe the person for any evidence of thought disorder
  - Examples: flight of ideas, derailment, ideas of reference, tangential thoughts
- Thought content – assess what the person is saying to you and the themes of the conversation
  - Examples: delusions, suicidal ideation, depressive and nihilistic themes, grandiose ideas
- Affect – observe the person's emotional expression. Is this congruent with the situation and their conversation?
  - Examples: reactive, flat, blunted, restricted, euphoric, elevated, euthymic
- Mood – assess the emotional state described by the person and whether this has an effect on their perception of their environment
  - Examples: calm, serene, depressed, anxious, angry, ecstatic
- Perception – look for evidence of sensory alterations experienced by the person or observed by others. These relate to the senses:
  - Visual (example: seeing a person or object that does not exist)
  - Auditory (example: hearing voices or sounds, which may express the person's thoughts or feelings but which are interpreted by the person as outside of themselves and not heard by others)
  - Olfactory (example: smelling odours that are not present, including smoke)
  - Tactile (example: strange physical sensations to the skin such as bugs crawling)
  - Gustatory (example: a taste that is not present, such as poison)
  - Illusions (example: mistaking real stimuli for something else, such as mistaking a pen for a syringe, a shadow for a person)
- Cognition – assess whether the person is orientated to person, place and time, and whether there is evidence of cognitive impairment requiring mini-mental state examination, intellectual disability assessment or specialist dementia assessment for memory impairment (long-term and short-term)
  - Examples: being unable to describe the correct year, the building they are in, or what their real name is, unable to recall recent long-term or short-term events
- Insight – assess the person's understanding of the nature of their difficulties, the causes and solutions required to improve their mental health
  - Example: what is their awareness of the effects of risk-taking behaviours on their safety?
- Judgement – assess the person's capacity to make sound and responsible decisions to improve their mental health

– Example: is the person willing to minimise their engagement in risk-taking behaviours to improve their safety?

• Rapport – assess the person's engagement with the mental health professional conducting the assessment

– Examples: tenuous, established easily, not established (Soltan & Girguis, 2017).

Neuro-vegetative symptoms

Neuro-vegetative symptoms are changes that occur in function necessary to maintain life and often occur in people experiencing mood disorder. These changes can increase or decrease in severity.

• Appetite – obvious change in appetite evidenced by weight gain or loss
• Sleep – interrupted or disturbed sleep, total hours of sleep per night and day, initial, middle or late insomnia, rumination affecting sleep
• Energy – may present as psychomotor retardation with excessive sleep or rest, or psychomotor agitation with increased energy and less need for sleep
• Concentration – impaired, difficult to concentrate on simple activities, becomes distracted and unable to complete tasks, affect on occupational functioning
• Interest – lacks interest in once pleasurable activities, anhedonia associated with low mood (Queensland Health, 2019).

INTERPROFESSIONAL PERSPECTIVES

Different professions are likely to be involved in the assessment of people experiencing mental health conditions. The scope of practice of each occupation can influence its focus and goal during assessment. As discussed, mental health nurses engage in a comprehensive mental health assessment, collecting information on the person's developmental history, previous experience of mental illness, current symptoms, stressors, neuro-vegetative symptoms and mental state (e.g. affect, mood and perception, as per the mental status examination).

Psychologists, in turn, are focused on identifying patterns of experience that can be understood as a cluster of symptoms. The assessment process is thus focused on checking people's experience against diagnostic criteria (e.g. DSM or CID; see Chapter 5) that would characterise a mental illness. In the process, information is usually collected through validated scales (e.g. Depression and Anxiety Stress Scale; PTSD Checklist for DSM-5). The assessment results will guide the choice of intervention. The psychologist might then refer the person for further evaluation, start psychological intervention (e.g. CBT; dialectical–behavioural therapy) and suggest engagement with other services and professionals (e.g. social welfare services; group-based therapy).

When couples or families are seeking assistance, the professionals involved (e.g. counsellors, psychologists, social workers) evaluate the dynamics within the couple or family system and investigate patterns that contribute to the problem. This process involves collecting information to refine the main directions for change and talk with the person or family about other interventions (e.g. improve parenting skills; anger management).

Psychiatrists engage in a similar assessment process, aiming to identify the presence of a given cluster of symptoms. The assessment informs the decision to prescribe medication, which medication is more likely to be beneficial and the need for collaboration with other professionals (e.g. referral for individual, couple, family therapy, or community mental health-care coordination). Psychiatrists and psychologists may collaborate when assisting people in recovery, as medication might be necessary to achieving goals in psychological therapy and to promote life changes.

Mental health nurses monitor the effects and potential side-effects of prescribed medication, and administer medications safely. Some medications are delivered by long-acting injectables that are given in hospital, at clinics or by home visits. Some medications require regular blood tests that mental health nurses also attend to. Psychologists and mental health nurses may consult with the consumer about whether a medication dose needs to be adjusted or reduced, depending on their recovery goals and current well-being.

Peer support workers are a key part of mental health teams and offer opportunities for consumers to meet with a person who has lived experience of recovery and specialist support skills. Peer support workers work from a values base of hope, mutuality, respect, empathy, openness, equal power-sharing and honesty. Their role is to offer support and to purposefully use their lived expertise in ways that are helpful for the person. They work with the expressed interest and perspective of the consumer in voluntary situations. They do not evaluate or assess the person from a clinical standpoint; rather, they operate from a transparent, mutual support model that is complementary to clinical services. A further role of peer support workers is to help the consumer identify their strengths and challenge injustices they experience (National Association of Peer Supporters, 2013).

All professions involved in healthcare provision are responsible for assessing risk and referring for appropriate intervention (e.g. safety planning when suicide risk is identified). Community mental health teams are tertiary services that comprise psychiatrists, psychologists, mental health nurses, social workers, peer support workers and occupational therapists. Interdisciplinary approaches to care are common in tertiary, community and in-patient settings, whereby all professions contribute to care planning and recovery according to the unique needs of the individual.

Assessment of risk

Recognising and managing risk in people accessing mental health care is an essential component of the mental health assessment and is upheld by standards of practice and national mental health policy, including the National Safety and Quality Health Service Standards (ACSQHC, 2017), The National Practice Standards for the Mental Health Workforce (National Mental Health Strategy, 2013) and The Fifth National Mental Health and Suicide Prevention Plan (National Mental Health Strategy, 2017). The approach used in conducting a risk assessment is varied across practices but maintains an overall common approach that aims to be able to understand the person's risk as 'the likelihood of an event happening with potentially harmful or beneficial outcomes for self or others' (Morgan, 2004). This assessment informs decisions for the actions required of the healthcare team, which address the risks identified (ACSQHC, 2018a, 2018b). Clinicians follow a validated formatted risk assessment tool, used to guide questioning focused on assessing the person's acuity level and risk to themself and/or others.

Key assessments of risk factors within tools include:

- risk to self
- risk to others
- risks from others, exploitation or vulnerability
- self-neglect
- social circumstances and personal factors
- substance misuse, including alcohol and other drugs
- safeguarding child and adult (National Confidential Inquiry into Suicide Safety in Mental Health (NCISH), 2018).

According to the NCISH (2018), types of risk factors considered in risk assessment tools include:

- Dynamic Factors, which are present at a point in time but may fluctuate in duration and intensity, such as feelings of despair, hopelessness, or substance use.
- Stable Factors, which do not change, such as supports, and current diagnosis.
- Static Long-term factors, which are likely to endure for many years, or that do not change, such as age and gender, history of self-harm.
- Future Factors, which can be anticipated and may occur from changing circumstances, such as future distress, or access to means (NCISH, 2018).

The risk assessment tool is used as a guide and in conjunction with a deep conversation with the person about their state of mind, psychosocial factors, protective factors (SANE, 2016) and own decisions regarding the management of their safety. This assessment enables an interpretation of the person's symptoms and behaviours, informing the risk or safety management plan. The safety management plan identifies specific interventions that aim to minimise the person's risk and improve their health outcomes (Higgins et al., 2016). This plan is designed in a collaborative way, whereby health professionals work in partnership with the person, their families and carers to develop an effective plan of care that is responsive to the person's changing condition (ACSQHC, 2017).

The concept of dignity of risk requires the mental health professional to ensure the person's dignity is afforded in support of their personal growth and quality of life (Ibrahim & Davis, 2013). This promotes respect and trust, and the belief in the right to self-determination and autonomy (Marsh & Kelly, 2018) when risk factors are present. Balancing a duty of care with the notion of enabling autonomy can be extremely difficult (Marsh & Kelly, 2018) in a structured healthcare system but should be incorporated into a safety management plan that aims to promote human rights and ethical practice in supporting people in their recovery. Practitioners should be mindful also that a constant focus on risk can become a dominating feature of interactions and planning, as experienced by many consumers seeking help for suicidal crisis. Dignity of risk acknowledges that a balance between opportunity and risk is needed, and that support is offered for people to move through the crisis.

Use of therapeutic skills and connection in assessment

Engagement skills

Layered models of care (refer to Figure 6.1) can be incorporated by any health professional, ranging from novice to expert. However, engagement with a person goes beyond the health professional's knowledge and skills. True engagement occurs with the development of a therapeutic relationship with a person. This is based on the trust developed between two people that creates a safe space for a person to share their innermost thoughts and feelings. True engagement is genuine and meaningful. It can develop in the early phase of the assessment process, at the first contact with a person, by showing empathy (discussed later) and authenticity. The discussion is gently guided but in an organic process that is unique to every individual person, rather than a structured question-and-answer format. In eliciting a person's story, the mental health professional draws out the salient points to craft an assessment of the person's mental health problems. During the narrative, much of the mental status examination, for example, can be noted for recording afterwards. Thus, the experience for the person seeking help is one of a non-confrontational, safe and reassuring conversation with a health professional who is able to offer effective support and facilitate care planning with the person.

Connecting: Empathy

Empathy occurs when someone is immersed in the experience of another. As a health practitioner, depending on our own cultural identity, social and developmental experiences and even our socio-economic status, all of these factors can affect the extent to which empathy is felt towards others. Therefore, it is paramount to reflect on our capacity for empathy by exploring the influencing factors that have shaped our own lives and, where necessary, to improve our knowledge, skills and attitudes.

It is important to consider that in multicultural societies such as Australia and Aotearoa New Zealand, First Nations and diverse ethnicities co-exist in the one population (ABS, 2017). Therefore, the health practitioner needs to consider others' perspectives and understandings of mental illness, which may vary greatly from our own. Health practitioners in Australia typically come from a variety of cultural and disciplinary backgrounds to share in an interdisciplinary team approach to mental health care. This brings to the healthcare setting a wide heterogeneity in people's social construction of mental health issues. Stereotypical social constructs of mental health can be challenged by facilitating reflection and developing an awareness of the collective human aspect of mental distress.

empathy – the competence of engaging with another person to understand their experiences and feelings from their perspective. Empathy occurs when someone faithfully recognises and validates the feelings and interpretations of another.

Responding to distressed consumers or family members in assessment

When supporting people seeking access to mental health care, there are many opportunities for stressful events to occur that can cause consumers or family members to become distressed, upset and angry. Mostly this occurs when a person's freedom is restricted and they are required to remain in hospital against their will. Or when a person's needs are perceived to be ignored by others. Situations in which people can lose control of their emotions and behaviour can result in serious injury to others. How do health practitioners respond in ways that recognise the person's feelings and reduce the risk of the situation becoming unsafe?

- Recognise that the person may have a background of personal trauma and therefore may be experiencing very powerful emotions.
- Maintain personal space.
- Talk openly about the situation.
- Keep calm and demonstrate respect to the person using your communication skills.
- Ask the person how they are feeling about the situation.
- Listen carefully to the person and their perspective.
- Offer an alternative approach that can meet the interests of the person, and talk with them about this.
- Set clear boundaries and offer choices and options to the person.
- Note changes to the person's emotional state and expression as you talk. If indicators of risk are evident after the interaction, plan your approach as a team.
- If you feel unsafe, leave the situation immediately and seek other staff to support the person.

When working at layer two, this concept can be highlighted further using a trauma-informed framework in mental health care. For example, childhood trauma increases the likelihood of developing a mental health condition in adult life (Felitti et al., 1998, 2019). However, the disconnect between the origin of childhood trauma and the time taken to present with mental illness as an adult often means the history of trauma is not at the forefront of primary mental health care. Childhood coping strategies can be considered maladaptive when these same behaviours persist into adulthood. Subsequently, health professionals' misinterpretation of coping behaviours as being intentionally 'difficult' can occur when people present in crisis for help – with negative outcomes for those who are help-seeking. However, a trauma-informed approach to care means understanding that the person in crisis knows no other way of coping and needs to learn how to cope in more adaptive ways (which can occur in layer three care, using CBT at a later time, for example). When we enquire into the experiences of people, coupled with our enhanced knowledge in the area, only then can empathy truly develop. With knowledge comes understanding, and with true understanding comes empathy. The experience of empathy by the help-seeking person means that it is more likely that they will seek help in the future should a crisis occur.

REFLECTIVE QUESTIONS

- Based on what you have learned about trauma-informed practice, how can previous experience of trauma influence how people disclose information?
- What are some examples of person-centred and trauma-informed practices that can increase the person's sense of safety and comfort to disclose personal information during assessment?

Normalising mental illness experience

When overwhelmed by negative emotions, such as high anxiety or strong feelings of failure, people may think that their experience is unique to them and they project it as: 'I am going mad', 'I am completely hopeless', 'I have lost everything'. Thoughts can be distorted or catastrophic; a sense of doom floods their outlook. Normalisation of a person's response to a stressful event or experience can help to reduce the person's sense of anxiety and provide reassurance that how they are feeling is to be expected given the situation. Rationalising the experience of distress helps the person feel less out of control and aware that how they are feeling is normal under the circumstances. This reassurance can stabilise the person's perspective and facilitate a practical discussion to focus on a plan for recovery. For example, Ashley is a man who is ashamed by his appearance and poor self-care that has developed after an exacerbation of his major depressive condition. He is embarrassed, he has no motivation to shower and fears he will never be able to return to work. Normalising Ashley's experience means offering a rational explanation for his distress. For example, you might respond with 'Ashley, I understand what you are saying, and lacking motivation to care for yourself is a common symptom of depression that many people experience when feeling as low as you do. You have felt this way before, and you've been able to find ways over time to improve your self-care. What has helped you in the past?'

Validation

For people who are sharing their story, the simple act of being offered **validation** of their experience can be powerful and can communicate that you believe what they are saying. Validation is chiefly within the domain of psychology. It describes the condition of feeling valued or worthwhile, and that one's feelings and opinions have validity, truth or worth. Providing validation promotes strength and self-worth (Oxford English Dictionary, 2020). The mental health professional listens and communicates to the person that they understand what has happened and that their response makes sense within the situation. This can be considered when similar events or experiences occur in the lives of others and the response is like that of another. The person's responses are taken seriously by the mental health professional and are accepted, and this is reflected to the person using language that is affirming. Validation means seeing the person as meaningful, giving them attention and acceptance (Linehan, 1997). This genuine care and interest in the person strengthens the therapeutic relationship as trust is developed.

validation – the understanding and acceptance of one's perception and emotional experience. It is the communication that a person's response to a situation is appropriate and acceptable. The person's experience is not contested – on the contrary, it is re-affirmed through acceptance and empathy.

Reflections on how to respond to people experiencing alternate beliefs

A person experiencing delusions or hallucinations is likely to also experience a wide range of corresponding emotions. What are some of the strategies that can be useful when interacting with someone experiencing symptoms of psychosis?

- Remember that each experience is unique to the individual and very real to them. Show genuine concern when listening to their story by listening with empathy and understanding. Identify and validate the person's feeling state. For example, if a person tells you that an alien is living in their roof,and they are scared, you could say 'That must be very frightening for you.'
- Be patient and be mindful that people experiencing acute psychosis might be attending to internal stimuli that we are not outwardly aware of. This can make it difficult for the person to concentrate on what you are saying. Give time for the person to provide answers to each of your questions. In conversation, gently re-orient the person to the here and now without engaging in argument or having a contrary stance about their present beliefs and experience.
- Sometimes, just remaining calm and present is all that is needed. Assuring the other person that you are simply there with them can alleviate anxiety while simultaneously being mindful of their need for sufficient personal space.
- When entering into conversation with the person, assure them you are there to help in their current distressed state. Ask what their most pressing concerns are and offer solutions that might alleviate some of their distress (e.g. if they have arrived at a hospital, letting a trusted loved one know they are safe, asking a carer to check that their house is locked or making sure their pet is cared for). This can help to develop a rapport with the person so that you can assist further.
- Think broadly in terms of another person's reality. Cultural variations arising from diverse spiritual beliefs that might differ from our own can contributing to their present state of mind. If relevant, find out whether a family member is available to help you understand the person's typical cultural beliefs and any symptoms that go beyond cultural social norms.
- Consider the factors that may have contributed to a presentation with these symptoms, such as stress, recent losses, grief, substance use such as illicit drugs or alcohol, or relapse of a psychotic disorder due to running out of regular prescribed medications. This information may be needed for documentation in your assessment.
- Plan the next steps to ensure the person's safety and consider what interventions might be necessary to assist the person in the immediate next phase of their recovery process. Does the person require urgent review by their community psychiatrist or a mental health in-patient admission? Do notifications to mental health teams or private psychiatry need to be made for more information about the person's baseline presentation and usual level of functioning? Does the person have a mental healthcare plan you can refer to for more information? Is there a family member or carer available to help or support the person safely at home? What other supports might be needed in the community setting?

Language when describing peoples' experience

When communicating in the clinical setting and between health professionals, it is best to focus on the objective symptoms reported and associated experiences of the person. A summary of the person's reason for presentation and mental health symptoms can be used when providing a clinical handover. For example, 'Ashley is a 45 yr old man with bipolar disorder and suicidal thoughts' lacks detail essential to understanding what is happening to Ashley and the unique experience he is presenting with. Alternatively, a health professional might add that 'Ashley's symptoms are extreme low mood with a lack of sleep for 3 nights due to stress, related to his loss of employment along with escalating anxiety and feelings of hopelessness for the future. He has suicidal thoughts and fears that he might take an overdose if he can't get help'. Here, the focus is not on Ashley's diagnosis but instead on his symptoms and the context of his problems. This provides the mental health professional with specific background information relating to Ashley's distress.

REFLECTIVE QUESTIONS

- How can previous experiences in health settings affect how people respond to health professionals during assessment?
- Can you think of any examples of professional conduct that can compromise trust in the assessment process?

Strengths-based assessment

As discussed, assessment must encompass cultural safety principles and trauma-informed, person-centred and **strengths-based approaches**. A strengths-based approach to mental health assessment seeks to understand the person's life experience to explore the strengths, abilities and talents inherent within them (Rapp & Goscha, 2012). It is common within a mental health assessment that professionals immediately identify the deficits or problems they are seeking to change. An example of a strengths-based approach: a person experiences anxiety and can no longer leave their home without a support person by their side. The person and the mental health professional take the time to understand the issues faced by the person. The history of the situation is explored: 'When did this start? What was happening to you when this began?' The mental health professional has a deep understanding of how the problem began and how well the person coped prior to the problem developing. Inherent, individual strengths and capabilities are explored and the narrative changes to one that is positive and upholds values conducive to a strengths-based approach. How much work and effort are possible for the person right now? Is their mental health and motivation in early stages of recovery? Is it about developing strength in the person, step by step, to build the person up enough so they might tackle bigger goals? A stepped approach is guided by the person, to build on personal strengths as achievements are made. Communicating hope for the future and having an optimistic outlook is a fundamental quality that mental health professionals can provide the person in care. This sentiment must be central to the care plan, with the overall aim being to support personal recovery and control over one's future.

strengths-based approach – in assessment, a strengths-based approach refers to working in collaboration with the person to identify personal interests, talents, assets and resources that can help to generate effective coping strategies and recovery for the person. Practitioners should assist people to find strategies and supports that are meaningful for the person's life context and preferences.

Shared decision-making

Finally, a recovery-centred and strengths-based approach is only achieved by the active participation and collaboration of the person receiving care and the mental health professional delivering the care. This shared decision-making process is further discussed in Chapter 9. In summary, the two have a common goal of making a mutually agreed-upon decision that will benefit the person to meet their mental healthcare needs. There are three key components that contribute to the definition of shared decision-making: information sharing between the person accessing mental health care and the mental health professional, a discussion about treatment options and a care plan that is mutually agreed upon by both parties (Eliacin et al., 2015).

Care planning

As discussed, a diagnosis of mental illness should not be seen as the essential defining feature of a person (Rose & Thornicroft, 2010) but rather as a working label for which treatment is offered, and this is guided by a psychiatrist or general practitioner. The mental health professional's role in supporting the person living with illness is to walk alongside them, to understand their experiences and reflect genuine care while promoting choices for evidence-based treatment as well as other actions meaningful for recovery. A care plan is developed in partnership with the person and their family or carers identifying the most important needs first, as described by the person in their own words. These needs are often different from that of the mental health professional, whose perspective is often guided by a biomedical approach. It is essential that this approach informs only part of the care plan, which is led by the person-centred, recovery approach promoted in health care today.

TRANSLATION TO PRACTICE

Therapeutic skills in trauma-informed care

Engaging with people experiencing different conditions contributes to practising the therapeutic skills of genuine engagement and empathetic listening. The more experiences you encounter, the more natural it becomes to normalise and validate people's experiences. Adopting a person-centred approach means practising the attitude of seeing the person and their experience: not just seeing symptoms of illness or a cluster of diagnostic criteria. This open attitude will help to reduce the influence of bias and stigma on assessment outcomes. As you focus on assisting people to see their conditions as part of the human experience, you can help them to identify personal strengths and promote autonomy and support. People will guide you on what type of response they need, whether it might be validation, crisis response or referral to services in the health and community sectors.

Pandemics and mental health assessment

Pandemics such as COVID-19 can alter standard health services' procedures. Services, for example, might adopt safety measures to prevent transmission of disease and may use telehealth for assessment and review purposes. It is important to inform consumers throughout the process about why measures are in place and what to expect next. It is common for people to experience anxiety, to have difficulty in regulating their emotions and to be hypervigilant to threat. Practitioners must communicate an empathetic response and validate people's experiences. Actively listening to the person's conceptualisation of their distress and enquiring how the person is coping with social isolation and other safety measures can help to identify areas for support. Sharing information can be useful in reducing stress. People benefit from information about what services are available through technologies such as smartphone apps and websites, and on the importance of maintaining social relationships. These might also include lived-experience telephone supports and online conversations. A safety management plan could be created or reviewed if risk is identified. Care must be delivered based on the person's preferences, promoting autonomy and respect. Involving carers and keeping in contact through are options for supporting the person's safety and well-being.

SUMMARY

This chapter has presented stories and information, supplemented by activities designed to deepen your understanding of:

- Strengths-based, recovery-oriented and trauma-informed approaches in the mental health assessment process. The person receiving care is considered 'an expert by experience', which recognises their personal journey and knowledge.
- A comprehensive mental-health assessment involving these principles to generate information on the person's understanding of the presenting problems, characteristics of mental health and functioning within their life context and risk levels.
- Assessment as an unequal interaction for consumers, whereby the health practitioner asks questions and the consumer is expected to disclose. Practitioners should seek to reduce power differentials in communication, respect the vulnerability of the person and encourage their agency in the process.
- The need for practitioners to connect with people in a genuine manner, practising therapeutic skills such as empathy, validation and normalising people's experiences and language regarding symptoms and diagnostic criteria.
- The importance of practitioners assisting people in identifying their strengths, to manage distress while using professional experience to facilitate person-centred care planning and crisis responses.

CRITICAL THINKING/LEARNING ACTIVITIES

1   What do you think can be some of the barriers practitioners might face in connecting with people in a non-judgemental and empathetic way? How could you overcome these barriers in practice?
2   Consider Aaron's case. How did the health professional's attitudes influence his view of the healthcare system?
3   If Aaron had presented to you and reported his lack of trust of the mental health system, how would you engage with him? How would you display empathy and validate his experience?

4   What might be some of the reasons people find it difficult to discuss their reasons for seeking help? How can you provide a trusting, transparent process for a person's disclosure?

5   How might you identify and consider a person's strengths within the assessment process? What methods would you use for accomplishing this?

LEARNING EXTENSION

Choose one of the consumer personal narratives presented throughout the book. With a colleague, talk through the possible assessment scenarios in the narrative. Identify the person's presenting problem and explore what questions you would be interested in asking the person. These might be about potential stressors, mental health history, experience of trauma, family, substance use and medical history. Role-play using your therapeutic skills to ask questions or offer effective responses based on empathy, normalising, validation and recognising strengths. Draw on skills for being transparent and encouraging the person's inclusion in the process. Consider how your skills might enable a positive, respectful and affirming experience for the person.

FURTHER READING

Isobel, S., Wilson, A., Gill, K. & Howe, D. (2020). 'What would a trauma-informed mental health service look like?' Perspectives of people who access services. *International Journal of Mental Health Nursing.* https://doi.org/10.1111/inm.12813.
This qualitative study explores the perspectives of mental health services users in Australia in relation to the question 'What would a trauma informed mental health service look like?'

Jacob, K. S. (2015). Recovery model of mental illness: a complementary approach to psychiatric care. *Indian Journal of Psychological Medicine, 37*(2): 117–19.
The paper explores the concept of recovery-oriented approach and contrasts it with the biomedical psychiatric approach of mental health.

Mental Health Coordinating Council. (2018). *Recovery Oriented Language Guide,* 2nd edn. Retrieved from https://mhcc.org.au/wp-content/uploads/2019/08/Recovery-Oriented-Language-Guide_2019ed_v1_20190809-Web.pdf
This publication presents useful guidelines for adopting person-centred and trauma-informed use of language when discussing mental health

Mind Australia, Helping Minds, Private Mental Health Consumer Carer Network (Australia), Arafmi Mental Health, Carers Australia and Mental Health Australia. (2016). *A Practical Guide for Working with Carers of People with a Mental Illness.* Retrieved from https://www.chiefpsychiatrist.wa.gov.au/wp-content/uploads/2017/04/A-Practical-Guide-for-working-with-people-with-a-mental-illness-February-2016-1.pdf
A publication on involving carers and family in fostering recovery across the lifespan.

REFERENCES

Allen, J., Balfour, R., Bell, R. & Marmot, M. (2014). Social determinants of mental health. *Internatiional Review of Psychiatry, 26*(4), 392–407.

American Psychological Association (APA). (2013). *Diagnostic and Statistical Manual of Mental Disorders,* 5th edn. Washington, DC: APA.

Australian Bureau of Statistics (ABS). (2017). 2016 Census QuickStats. Retrieved from https://quickstats.censusdata.abs.gov.au/census_services/getproduct/census/2016/quickstat/036.

Australian Commission on Safety and Quality in Healthcare (ACSQH). (2010). *Australian Safety and Quality Framework for Health Care*. Retrieved from https://www.safetyandquality.gov.au/sites/default/files/migrated/Australian-SandQ-Framework1.pdf

——— (2017). *National Safety and Quality Health Service Standards,* 2nd edn. Retrieved from https://www.safetyandquality.gov.au/sites/default/files/migrated/National-Safety-and-Quality-Health-Service-Standards-second-edition.pdf

——— (2018a). *Implementing the Comprehensive Care sSandard – Approaches to person-centred screening, August 2018*. Retrieved from https://www.safetyandquality.gov.au/sites/default/files/migrated/Implementing-Comprehensive-Care-Approaches-to-person-centred-risk-screening-Accessibility-PDF.pdf

——— (2018b). *User guide for health services providing care for people with mental health issues*. Retrieved from https://www.safetyandquality.gov.au/sites/default/files/2019-05/nsqhs-standards-user-guide-for-health-services-providing-care-for-people-with-mental-health-issues_0.pdf

Ben-Zeev, D., Young, M. & Corrigan, P. (2010). DSM-V and the stigma of mental illness. *Journal of Mental Health, 19*: 318–27.

Blanch, A., Filson, B., Penney, D. & Cave, C. (2012). *Engaging Women in Trauma-informed Peer Support: A guidebook.* Washington, DC: National Centre for Trauma Informed Care.

British Medical Journal (BMJ). (2015). Psychiatric assessments: How much is too much? *BMJ, 351*: h3503.

Buber, M. & Smith, R. G. (1958). *I and Thou: With a postscript by the Author*, 2nd edn. Edinburgh, UK: T&T Clark.

Carer's Recognition Act 2005 (SA). Retrieved from https://www.legislation.sa.gov.au/LZ/C/A/CARERS%20RECOGNITION%20ACT%202005/CURRENT/2005.55.AUTH.PDF

Clement, S., Williams, P., Farrelly, S., Hatch, S. L., Schauman, O., Jeffery, D. ... Thornicroft, G. (2015). Mental health–related discrimination as a predictor of low engagement with mental health services. *Psychiatric Services, 66*(2): 171–6.

Daya, I., Hamilton, B. & Roper, C. (2020). Authentic engagement: A conceptual model for welcoming diverse and challenging consumer and survivor views in mental health research, policy, and practice. *International Journal of Mental Health Nursing, 29*(2): 299–311.

Deacon, B. J. (2013). The biomedical model of mental disorder: A critical analysis of its validity, utility, and effects on psychotherapy research. *Clinical Psychology Review: 33*(7), 846–61.

Department of Health and Ageing (DHA), South Australian Safety and Quality in Health Care Consumer and Community Advisory Committee. (2014). *Staff Information on Respecting Patients' Privacy and Dignity with Patient Centred Care Principles*. Adelaide: SA Health Safety and Quality Unit.

Eliacin, J., Salyers, M. P., Kukla, M. & Matthias, M. S. (2015). Patients' understanding of shared decision making in a mental health setting, *Qualitative Health Research, 2*(5): 668–78.

Felitti, V. J., Anda, R. F., Nordenberg, D., Williamson, D. F., Spitz, A. M., Edwards, V. ... Marks, J. S. (1998). Relationship of childhood abuse and household dysfunction to many of the leading causes of death in adults – the Adverse Childhood Experiences (ACE) Study. *American Journal of Preventive Medicine, 14*(4): 245–58.

——— (2019). Reprint of: Relationship of childhood abuse and household dysfunction to many of the leading causes of death in adults: the Adverse Childhood Experiences (ACE) Study. *American Journal of Preventive Medicine, 56*(6): 774–86.

Glover, H. (2012). Recovery, lifelong learning,empowerment & social inclusion: is a new paradigm emerging? In P. Ryan, S. Ramon, & S. Greacen (eds), *Empowerment, Lifelong Learning and Recovery in Mental Health: Towards a new paradigm*. London: Palgrave.

Happell, B., Waks, S., Bocking, J., Horgan, A., Manning, F., Greaney, S., ... Biering, P. (2019). 'I felt some prejudice in the back of my head': Nursing students' perspectives on learning about mental health from 'Experts by Experience'. *Journal of Psychiatric and Mental Health Nursing, 26*(7–8): 233–43.

Higgins, A, Doyle, L., Morrissey, J., Downes, C., Gill, A. & Bailey, S. (2016). Documentary analysis of risk-assessment and safety-planning policies and tools in a mental health context. *International Journal of Mental Health Nursing, 25*(4): 385–95.

Ibrahim, J. E. & Davis, M. C. (2013). Impediments to applying the 'dignity of risk' principle in residential aged care services. *Australasian Journal on Ageing, 32*(3): 188–93.

Karter, J. M. & Kamens, S. R. (2019). Toward Conceptual Competence in Psychiatric Diagnosis: An Ecological Model for Critiques of the DSM. In S. Steingard (ed.), *Critical Psychiatry: Controversies and Clinical Implications* (pp. 17–69). Cham: Springer International Publishing.

Linehan, M. M. (1997). Validation and psychotherapy. In A. C. Bohart & L. S. Greenberg (eds), *Empathy Reconsidered: New directions in psychotherapy* (pp. 353–92). Washington, DC: American Psychological Association.

Llewellyn-Beardsley, J., Rennick-Egglestone, S., Callard, F., Crawford, P., Farkas, M., Hui, A. … Slade, M. (2019). Characteristics of mental health recovery narratives: Systematic review and narrative synthesis. *PLoS One, 14*(3): e0214678.

Marsh, P. & Kelly, L. (2018). Dignity of risk in the community: a review of and reflections on the literature. *Health, Risk & Society, 20*(5–6): 297–311.

Martin, G. N., Carlson, N. R, & Buskist, W. (2013). *Psychology*, 5th edn. Pearson Education.

Maslow, A. H. (1943). A theory of human motivation. *Psychological Review, 50*(4): 370–96.

Morgan, S. (2004). Positive risk-taking: an idea whose time has come. *Health Care Risk Report*: 18–99.

Muskett, C. (2014). Trauma-informed care in inpatient mental health settings: A review of the literature. *International Journal of Mental Health Nursing, 23*(1): 51–9.

National Association of Peer Supporters. (2013). National Practice Guidelines for Peer Specialists and Supervisors. Retrieved from https://www.peersupportworks.org/resources/national-practice-guidelines/

National Confidential Inquiry into Suicide and Safety in Mental Health (NCISH). (2018). *The Assessment of Clinical Risk in Mental Health Services*. Manchester, UK: NCISH.

National Mental Health Strategy. (2013). *National Practice Standards for the Mental Health Workforce*. Victorian Government Department of Health. Retrieved from https://www1.health.gov.au/internet/main/publishing.nsf/content/5D7909E82304E6D2CA257C430004E877/$File/wkstd13.pdf

——— (2017). *The Fifth National Mental Health and Suicide Prevention Plan*. COAG Health Council. Retrieved from http://www.coaghealthcouncil.gov.au/Portals/0/Fifth%20National%20Mental%20Health%20and%20Suicide%20Prevention%20Plan.pdf

Norris, D. R., Clark, M. S. & Shipley, S. (2016). The mental status examination. *American Family Physician, 94*(8): 635–41.

Oxford English Dictionary. (2020). Retrieved from https://www.oed.com/view/Entry/221193?redirectedFrom=validation#eid

Prochaska, J. O., Redding, C. A. & Evers, K. E. (2015). The transtheoretical model and stages of change. In B. R. K. Glanz & K. Viswanath (eds), *Health Behavior: Theory, research, and practice*. San Francisco, CA: Jossey-Bass.

Queensland Health. (2019). *Mental Illness Nursing Documents for Nurses and Midwives*. Retrieved from https://www.health.qld.gov.au/clinical-practice/guidelines-procedures/clinical-staff/mental-health/guidelines

Rapp, C. & Goscha, R. J. (2012). *The Strengths Model: A recovery-oriented approach to mental health services*, 3rd edn. New York: Oxford University Press.

Raskin, N. J. & Rogers, C. R. (2005). Person-centered therapy. In R. J. Corsini & D. Wedding (eds), *Current Psychotherapies*, pp. 130–65. Thomson Brooks/Cole Publishing.

Rogers, C. R. (1961). *On Becoming a Person: A therapist's view of psychotherapy. Boston*, MA: Houghton Mifflin.

Rose, D. & Thornicroft, G. (2010). Service user perspectives on the impact of a mental illness diagnosis. *Epidemiologia e Psichiatria Sociale, 19*(2): 140–7.

SANE Australia. (2016). *Suicide Prevention and Recovery Guide – A resource for mental health professionals*. Retrieved from https://www.sane.org/images/PDFs/2779_SANE_SPRG_2016_06.pdf

Shepherd, G., Boardman, J., Rinaldi, M. & Roberts, G. (2014). *Supporting recovery in mental health services: Quality and Outcomes*. London: Implementing Recovery Through Organisational Change.

Soltan, M. & Girguis, J. (2017). How to approach the mental state examination. *British Medical Journal, 357*: j1821

Williams, R. (1999). Cultural safety – what does it mean for our work practice? *Australian and New Zealand Journal of Public Health, 23*(2): 213–14.

Person-centred care in suicide and self-harm distress

Nicholas Procter, Davi Macedo and Monika Ferguson

7

LEARNING OBJECTIVES

At the completion of this chapter, you should be able to:

1 Understand definitions of suicide and self-harm, and discuss aspects to consider in the language used to communicate about suicide.
2 Understand how pervasive the problems of suicide and self-harm are, some of the factors that can predispose people to self-harm and suicidal behaviour, and identify which groups are most vulnerable.
3 Discuss the interpersonal theory of suicide.
4 Reflect on how to respond to suicide and self-harm behaviours in a compassionate and person-centred way, how to include carers when responding to suicide distress, and explore initiatives such as the Connecting with People approach and the use of safety planning as key in suicide prevention.
5 Reflect on how the COVID-19 pandemic has influenced self-harm and suicidal behaviours, and how to adapt a care response in the context of a pandemic.

Introduction

Suicide is a significant national and international public health concern. Each year an estimated 3300 Australians and 650 New Zealanders die by suicide. Suicide is a behaviour, not an illness, and it can occur in the absence of mental illness. The determinants and precipitants of mental illness and suicide are interrelated and frequently associated with one another. The aim of this chapter is to discuss and describe the demographic characteristics of suicide, key definitions and drivers of suicide, suicide risk factors, and the lived experience of suicide and suicide-related harms through first-person accounts. As with other forms of mental distress, people in suicide and self-harm crisis can be helped through compassionate and person-centred approaches.

Defining suicide and self-harm

The nomenclatures of suicide and related behaviours are the subject of continuing debate, and definitions are being advanced by the international field of suicidology (Silverman & De Leo, 2016). The key terms for discussion are suicide, suicide attempt, suicide ideation and self-harm.

self-harm – behaviours that involve causing pain or injury to oneself, usually not accompanied by suicide ideation (willingness to die); they can vary in form and purpose

suicide – self-initiated and potentially injurious behaviours directed towards causing one's own death. When the behaviour (e.g., overdose, hanging, self-cutting) results in death the term 'death by suicide' is most appropriate. A suicide attempt occurs when the behaviour does not result in death.

Self-harm corresponds to any behaviour that involves deliberately causing pain or injury to oneself (e.g. cutting, burning or hitting oneself, head-banging, scratching, starving, binge-eating or putting oneself in dangerous situations) (Lifeline, 2020). Self-harm may be associated with some degree of intent to die – something greater than zero. It may also be associated with ambivalence towards death, and the acting out of inner turmoil, self-soothing and/or tension relief.

Suicidal behaviours are those accompanied by suicidal ideation: the thought of ending one's life. Suicide ideation can be passive (expression of a wish that 'it would all end') or active (effective planning of circumstances and means) (Silverman et al., 2007). Suicidal behaviours are thus self-initiated and potentially injurious behaviours adopted with the intention to die (World Health Organization (WHO), 2014). When a suicidal behaviour does not result in death, it is considered a suicide attempt. Death by suicide, or simply 'suicide', is the term used when suicidal behaviour results in death (Silverman et al., 2007). Regardless of the intention associated with self-harm or suicidal behaviour, it is critical that each person, regardless of the motivational elements associated with self-harm or attempted suicide, must be comforted, validated and supported with compassion. In some instances, motivational elements associated with suicide and self-harm can change (e.g. tension relief upon onset or worsening intense emotions; to 'feel something' when feeling 'empty') (Stone et al., 2020).

Language and communication are critical aspects of suicide prevention, and when discussing suicide it is important to avoid words that promote stigmatisation, trigger distress or discourage help-seeking (Padmanathan et al., 2019). A recent study involving people with experience of suicide (either their own experience, or that of someone they know), found that terms such as 'suicide attempt', 'took their own life' and 'death by suicide' had high acceptability, and were perceived as accurate, clear and neutral (Padmanathan et al., 2019). In contrast, it is widely accepted in the suicide prevention community that the term 'committed suicide' should be avoided, given the associated criminal undertones. At all times, it is important to ensure that language is non-judgemental, to avoid stigmatisation, validate emotions and be respectful of the person's experiences (Padmanathan et al., 2019).

How widespread is suicide?

Suicide is a significant global public health concern. It is estimated that approximately 800 000 people die by suicide globally every year (WHO, 2019a). The global average rate was 10.5 per 100 000 people in 2016 (WHO, 2019b). It is noticeable that 52 per cent of global suicides occurred before the age of 45 years (WHO, 2019b). The effects of suicide are pervasive and substantial. It is estimated that for everyone who dies from suicide, up to 135 people are exposed (knew the person) (Cerel et al., 2019).

In 2019, 3318 Australians died by suicide, representing an average of nine people per day. The age-standardised mean suicide rate in 2019 was 12.9 deaths per 100 000 population (ABS, 2020). Overall, suicide was the leading cause of death among Australians aged 15–49 years in 2019 (ABS, 2020). Similarly in Aotearoa New Zealand, the mean suicide rate in 2019–20 was 13.1 per 100 000 (654 deaths; Coronial Services of New Zealand – CSNZ, 2020).

Like global trends, suicide deaths in Australia are largely accounted for by relatively young people and by males. In 2019, the mean age at death for suicide was 43.9 years and more than half of the rates of suicide deaths (55 per cent) occurred in people aged 30–59 years. In comparison, 24 per cent of deaths by suicide occurred among those aged 15–29 years (ABS, 2020). This suggests that, although suicide rates among young people are concerning, the highest rates are observed among people in their forties. Overall, more than three-quarters (75.4 per cent) of the deaths registered by suicide occurred in males. The highest rates observed were in men aged 45–49 years, and 85 years and over. Among females, the highest age-specific suicide rate was observed among those aged 40–44 years (9.7 per 100 000) (ABS, 2020). While males are more likely to die by suicide, rates of hospital admission due to self-harm are higher among females (64 per cent of intentional self-harm hospitalisations in 2016–17) (AIHW, 2020). A similar pattern is observed in Aotearoa New Zealand. Young males (25–34 years) presented the highest rates (33 per 100 000). Among females, most deaths happened among those aged 15–19 years (15 per 100 000) and 80–84 years (13 per 100 000) (CSNZ, 2020).

Recent data also reveal high prevalence rates of suicide in regional and rural Australia. The age-standardised suicide rate in the Northern Territory in 2019 was the highest observed in the country, at 21.0 per 100 000 population, followed by Tasmania (19.5 per 100 000, the highest in the past 10 years) (ABS, 2020). Especially vulnerable to suicide risk are farmers under 35 years, both living and working at a farm, experiencing financial hardship and living in outer remote or very remote regions (Austin et al., 2018).

Self-harm and suicidal behaviour is also common among people who belong to minority groups. Due to stigmatisation and discrimination, people who identify with certain minoritised groups are susceptible to increased experiences of mental illness and suicidal behaviour. In Aboriginal and Torres Strait Islander communities, for example, the age-standardised suicide rate was two-fold that of non-Indigenous Australians (27.1 compared to 12.7 per 100 000 in 2019; ABS, 2020). In Aotearoa New Zealand, rates among Māori were at 20.2, compared to 13 per 100 000 among non- Māori (CSNZ, 2020). This is considered as reflecting the historical processes of segregation and stigmatisation initiated and perpetuated through colonisation (Paradies, 2018) in both countries. See Chapters 3 and 4 for a comprehensive discussion.

Members of the lesbian, gay, bisexual, transgender, queer and intersex (LGBTQI) communities are also at increased risk of self-harm and suicide. It is estimated that 33 per cent of people identifying as LGBTQI and aged 16 to 27 years reported having ever self-harmed; 41 per cent had thoughts of harming themselves; and 16 per cent reported having attempted suicide (Robinson et al., 2014). Previous suicide attempts were also reported by 48.1 per cent of transgender and gender diverse people aged 14 to 25 years (Strauss et al., 2017).

Risk factors for suicide behaviour

Several risk factors have been identified for the onset of suicidal behaviour. Nonetheless, it is important to highlight that a person might still be at risk of experiencing suicide even when they are not assessed as being in a so called 'high-risk' group. In other words, while demographic factors might help us to understand trends in rates of suicide at the population level, there is a national and international move away from the discredited risk-assessment approach, to newer risk formulations. There is no reliable indicator of (singular or clustered) risk factors for the onset of suicidal behaviour (Stone et al., 2020). A person might fall within a group considered more likely to be at risk of suicide even when not presenting any of the known risk factors; similarly, it cannot be assumed that all members of a 'more likely' group are equally vulnerable. Instead, risk factors may be useful for identifying people who may benefit from an intervention, and the type of intervention that may be most useful, rather than being useful for predicting which individuals will die by suicide (Stone et al., 2020). Among the most-commonly identified risk factors for suicide are:

a Demographic and social factors: being a young adult (particularly between 15 and 29 years) or elderly (above 80 years); male; experiencing a lack of social support, social isolation or stressful events (e.g. unemployment, financial worries, family conflict); and being part of an ethnic minority (e.g. Māori; Aboriginal and Torres Strait Islander) or LGBTQI group (Stone et al., 2020; Van Orden et al., 2010).

b Psychosocial and clinical history: having a previous history of mental illness, especially when accompanied by recent relapse or discharge from mental health care service; past suicide attempts or self-harm; impulsivity or diagnosis of personality disorder; long-term medical conditions, aggravated by recent discharge or experience of pain; substance misuse; having lost someone close through suicide (family history); and access to lethal means (e.g. pesticides, firearms) (Stone et al., 2020; Turecki & Brent, 2016; Van Orden et al., 2010).

c Current mental state and suicidal thoughts: having experience of emotional pain, especially when related to hopelessness, guilt and shame; sense of being trapped, boxed in or unable to change current circumstances; increase in suicidal ideas; suicidal ideas with a well-designed plan or preparation; and symptoms of psychosis (e.g. persecutory hallucinations, hearing command hallucinations) (Hor & Taylor, 2010; Stone et al., 2020; Turecki & Brent, 2016; Van Orden et al., 2010).

Although suicide is a behaviour, not a mental illness, mental health conditions are among the most important precipitants of suicide behaviours. It is estimated that people with a mental illness are at approximately an eight-fold increased risk of suicide compared to individuals without a mental health condition (Too et al., 2019). Among the common mental health conditions linked to suicide attempts are major depression, bipolar affective condition, borderline personality, eating conditions, schizophrenia and substance use (Turecki & Brent, 2016; Tyrer, Reed & Crawford, 2015; Van Orden et al., 2010). Having a diagnosis of depression was shown to be associated with two-fold the odds of having suicide ideation and attempting suicide (Ribeiro et al., 2018). Similarly, among people experiencing a bipolar condition, recent mood episodes were identified as a risk factor for death by suicide (Hansson et al., 2018).

General risk factors are identified across conditions, such as physical illness, depressive states, hopelessness, social isolation, unemployment, criminal conviction, drug use and previous history of suicide attempts (Hansson et al., 2018; Hor & Taylor, 2010; Popovic et al., 2014). This highlights the importance of drivers and context for the onset and worsening of suicidal behaviours. Interactions between individual and contextual-level risk factors can contribute to the onset of suicidal thoughts, planning, and execution of suicidal behaviours. It is important to have a working understanding of risk factors for suicidal behaviour, to be able to know potential points at which to intervene and support people, rather than to predict the likelihood of suicide. Health professionals' practice must be guided by the premise that people experiencing thoughts of suicide need to be always validated and supported in keeping themselves safe.

REFLECTIVE QUESTIONS

- What are some of the risk factors leading to self-harm and suicidal behaviours, and how can this affect people's experiences and emotions at the time of professional intervention?
- What are some of the misconceptions about mental health conditions, suicide and self-harm behaviours we might encounter in the work environment?

Another drawback of relying solely on risk-factor identification is that suicide ideation has been shown to fluctuate. These findings are based on the ecological momentary assessment method, which involves participants recording data on suicidal ideation multiple times per day (Bentley et al., 2019). Suicide ideation, for example, was shown to vary dramatically within a short period of time – such as 4–8 hours – and over the course of days (Kleiman et al., 2017). Individuals' perceptions of loneliness, burdensomeness and hopelessness – known risk factors for suicide – also varied considerably over just a few hours (Kleiman et al., 2017). In this manner, more important than assessing the presence of risk factors or how serious suicide ideation might be, it is necessary to support fluctuations of suicide risk over time (Brodsky, Spruch-Feiner & Stanley, 2018), assisting people to navigate through suicidal urges while in safety.

The interpersonal theory of suicide behaviour

Several theories exist to explain suicidal behaviour. A widely accepted theory is one developed by Joiner and collaborators: the Interpersonal Theory of Suicide (Van Orden et al., 2010). This theory is based on the premise that two interpersonal processes influence thoughts and

thwarted belonginess
– perception of the complete absence of a meaningful and reciprocally caring relationship, impairing the satisfaction of a need for connection and belonging

perceived burdensomeness
– perception of being a burden to one's family and friends. The person experiencing suicide ideation believes their loved ones would be better off in their absence.

actions towards suicide risk: **thwarted belongingness** and **perceived burdensomeness** (Van Orden et al., 2010).

Thwarted belongingness reflects a person's perception of loneliness and the absence of a reciprocally caring relationship ('I care for others and others care or need me'). This is a dynamic process, which might depend on the person's social network, confidence and capability to engage with others. The theory highlights the role of severe thwarted belongingness; that is, the perception that these connections are completely absent. Perceived burdensomeness, in turn, relates to the self-perception of being a burden to oneself, family and significant others, which can be further exacerbated by psychosocial stressors such as homelessness, unemployment and incarceration. Perceived burdensomeness worsens when the person has feelings of self-hatred, self-blame, shame and poor self-esteem (e.g. 'I hate myself', 'I am useless') (Van Orden et al., 2010). People experiencing heightened burdensomeness might see the solution to their troubles as requiring self-sacrifice for the sake of their loved ones (e.g. 'They will be better off without me') (Joiner et al., 2015).

The combined elements of feeling a state of not belonging, not being part of a meaningful and caring (reciprocal) relationship and as a burden to others can be triggering of suicide ideation (e.g. 'I wish I was dead'). The theory further posits that, when combined with hopelessness about one's prospects of change, passive suicide ideation progresses to active ideation; an active phase of planning and concrete action. Hopelessness about these states thus marks the transition from passive to active desire for suicide (Chu et al., 2017).

A third component of Joiner's interpersonal theory of suicide is acquired capability. There is, in this context, a fearlessness towards suicide and death, and simultaneous tolerance to provocative acts. The factors associated with having the capability to die are therefore lowered fear of suicide or death and increased tolerance to physical pain (Chu et al., 2017; Van Orden et al., 2010). People presenting these characteristics might be more prone to attempting suicide by lethal or near-lethal means. Factors such as previous suicide attempts, impulsivity, childhood maltreatment and combat exposure can contribute to increasing a person's tolerance to threat, to their survival, and can influence their choice for lethal or near-lethal means when attempting suicide (Van Orden et al., 2010).

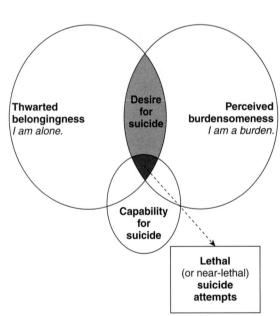

Figure 7.1 Assumptions of the interpersonal theory of suicide

Source: Van Orden et al. (2010).

PERSONAL NARRATIVE

Sarah's experience

My name is Sarah. I am an 18-year-old woman with a history of depression and anxiety. I first started to feel 'not quite right' around the age of 17. Prior to this I was doing well in school and spending free time hanging out with friends. I was popular at school and had a good friendship group with about four close friends that I spent most of my time with. Around the time of my 17th birthday, I started to feel a bit different. The first thing I noticed was that I started to become nervous about going to parties. I found myself not able to socialise like I used to.

And for the first time I felt nervous talking to people.

Not long after this experience, I was out shopping with my close friends and suddenly felt overwhelmed by the busy shopping centre. I told my friends that we needed to leave and that I didn't feel safe. My friends said I was being 'crazy' and should just chill. This didn't help so I decided to leave by myself. When I got home, I felt completely overwhelmed and scared by what had just happened, and kept asking myself 'What the hell was that? Why did I feel that way? Am I losing it?'

From this point forward I didn't want to hang out with friends anymore as I was scared it would happen again. I found myself spending more and more time at home, and even at school I just wanted to be alone. Things got worse and I started needing to take sick days regularly and had problems studying. My parents took me to see a doctor as they too were concerned about my changes in mood. After I told the doctor how I was feeling, he told me that I was suffering from depression and anxiety. This scared me at first, but I was also happy to know what was going on and agreed to see a psychologist and try an antidepressant.

After about six weeks and a few sessions with the psychologist I started to feel a bit better and to feel like my normal self again. A few months later I found out someone I knew at school had died by suicide after being depressed for some time. This hit me hard, and I started to get anxious and really depressed again. As it got closer to my 18th things got a lot worse and I became isolated. My family encouraged me to go out and see my friends, but I told them that I didn't want to see anyone, and that they did not understand how it felt. My parents said things like 'you will get through this – you're just having a bad time, plus it has passed before'. This didn't help and I started to think no one understood me. A week went by and I started feeling so alone and depressed thinking: 'This will never get better and not even my parents understand how I feel'.

One bad night I just wanted it to end so I took an overdose thinking 'I and everyone else would be better off if I died'. Luckily my parents found me passed out on the floor and called an ambulance. I woke up in the emergency department. I asked the doctor what had happened, and she told me that I had attempted suicide. I looked at my parents and the look on their face was of being so worried and scared. They said to me, 'Why did you do that?' and 'Why didn't you talk to us?' I replied, 'I just want this pain to end'. The doctor asked to speak to me alone. At first, I was worried that she would judge me and not understand. I was surprised when I told her how I was feeling that the doctor was very understanding and acknowledged that it must have been tough for me. She asked some questions in a compassionate way including:

- How has your life changed?
- What are some of the things you are finding hard to do in life?
- How long have you been feeling this way?
- Is there anything that helps you to feel better?

The doctor also told me that depression can be hard, but it can be treated and suggested a change to my medication. After about an hour of talking to the doctor I felt for the first time that someone understood me and didn't tell me I was 'just being crazy'. I asked if I had to stay in the hospital and the doctor said she thought I was feeling better and was happy for me to go home. She asked to see me the next Monday for a follow up. I agreed. I was happy to see the doctor again as I felt she really understood me.

REFLECTIVE QUESTIONS

Sarah had a relapse of depression and anxiety symptoms after knowing someone at school had recently died by suicide. What are some of the thoughts that might have occurred to her? How could this awareness have triggered her suicide attempt? What could have been done to prevent it?

Responding to suicide with a person-centred approach

The Connecting with People program

Sarah's story aligns with increasing recognition that all suicidal and self-harming behaviour should be taken seriously, and that all people experiencing these feelings should be offered a compassionate, person-centred response. Connecting with People is a suicide and self-harm mitigation and prevention program that has been recognised internationally. The program has been adopted by different countries worldwide, including Australia (Tasmanian Government Department of Health, 2020).

The approach outlined by Connecting with People is a paradigm shift in the way suicide is considered, as it assumes that suicide is preventable and can be avoided when practitioners have access to necessary tools and are able to confidently intervene using appropriate skills. It focuses on clinicians undertaking comprehensive, person-centred assessment, safety planning and suicide mitigation by using evidence-informed and peer-reviewed clinical tools to identify and respond to suicide risk. It requires practitioners to engage with the person in a compassionate, person-centred manner to identify potential risks, distress triggers, needs and strengths, thereby encouraging them to seek and accept support and feel hopeful. The Connecting with People approach is strongly based on the practice of safety planning, as it is considered best practice for suicide risk mitigation, internationally. A safety plan document is co-created by a consumer and clinician, aiming to mobilise a collaboration between consumers, carers, families and other support systems to increase safety when suicide distress arises (Life in Mind, 2018).

TRANSLATION TO PRACTICE

Reflections on how to respond to a suicide crisis

Having a caring conversation with a person in suicide-related distress can be lifesaving in a critical moment. What are some of the strategies that can be useful when interacting with someone in a suicidal crisis?

- Enter into the person's conceptualisation of their distress. Try to understand the experience from the person's perspective and what ideas and interpretations the person is carrying.
- Enquire in a gentle and empathetic way. Demonstrate genuine interest and concern. Work towards helping the person feel understood and validated.
- Remember that people at the time of their suicide attempt might be facing numerous compounding stressors.
- Consider interventions that might be necessary to assist the person in the recovery process. Are they receiving adequate mental health support? Are referrals needed? Does the person have a safety plan?

Safety planning

One internationally recognised intervention is the **Safety Planning** Intervention (SPI) (Mann, Michel & Auerbach, 2021). Developed by Stanley and Brown (2012), it involves the co-creation of a personalised list of coping and support strategies that people can use to support themselves during the onset or worsening of suicide-related distress (Stanley & Brown, 2012). A safety plan typically includes six core components: 1) recognising individual warning signs for an impending suicidal crisis; 2) identifying and employing internal coping strategies; 3) using social supports to distract from suicidal thoughts; 4) contacting trusted family or friends to help address the crisis; 5) contacting specific mental health services; 6) reducing access to and use of lethal means (Stanley & Brown, 2012).

A major benefit of the SPI is that it is a flexible intervention – it can be incorporated with other treatment approaches, such as follow-up phone-calls and home visits. It can also be delivered by a range of health professionals and is suitable in various care settings, including emergency departments and community care, as well as individual and group treatment. Further, a safety plan is a living document. It should be one that is used and revised as needed. The person should also be encouraged to keep the safety plan in a readily accessible location, such as their wallet or car, provided that they feel comfortable to do so.

There is growing evidence to support the SPI as a suicide prevention strategy. Studies primarily conducted with veterans in the United States have found that it is associated with reduced suicidal behaviour and hospitalisations, improved treatment attendance (Stanley et al., 2015; Zonana, Simberlund & Christos, 2018), and is acceptable and feasible to both consumers (Kayman et al., 2015; Stanley et al., 2016) and clinicians (Chesin et al., 2017). There is also emerging evidence linking the quality of safety plans to reduced hospitalisations (Gamarra et al., 2015) and suicidal behaviour (Green et al., 2018). While promising, more research is required to understand the effect of safety planning on other populations.

In addition to being used in a therapeutic context, the SPI has been the basis for several freely available safety planning resources, such as the Beyond Now safety planning application (Beyond Blue, 2020). While this resource can be accessed and worked through by individuals

safety planning – an intervention for suicide prevention that consists of elaborating a personal document to list one's triggers and internal and external coping strategies to help resolve the suicide crisis. A safety plan must be readily available (e.g. kept in one's wallet) to assist in navigating suicidal urges.

on their own, it is recommended that it is done in collaboration with a trusted person, such as a family member, elder or health professional.

Integrating the person's family and support persons

Family members and support persons accompanying loved ones who have engaged in self-harm or suicidal behaviours often report difficulties when accessing emergency care. Carers of people with personality conditions – such as borderline personality – often present to emergency departments in the absence of appropriate specialised services to help them manage their loved one's suicide-related behaviours (National Health and Medical Research Council (NHMRC), 2012). Qualitative studies suggest that instead of the appropriate care and understanding they would expect, carers of people experiencing suicide ideation report being excluded from the intervention process (Acres, Loughhead & Procter, 2019b; McLaughlin et al., 2016).

Carers report that health professionals with patronising and stigmatising attitudes towards mental health conditions – for example, who assume that presentation is a behavioural issue – is not uncommon, and that stigma acts as a barrier to the offer of appropriate care and compassion (Acres et al., 2019a). Lack of respect for the individual's privacy is also observed, with carers reporting their loved ones are often asked about their self-harm and suicide attempts in the presence of others, with triage sometimes taking place in crowded waiting rooms (Acres et al., 2019b). Unsupportive professional attitudes add to the stressors that carers often face, such as feelings of responsibility, worries about their loved ones, secrecy, shame, helplessness and guilt (McLaughlin et al., 2014).

Carers expect nurses to provide support and minimise distress. Simple actions, such as referring them to the companions' waiting room, offering a cup of tea and updating them on the status of their loved ones can be perceived as enough to help carers to feel understood and cared for (Acres et al., 2019b). Acting in accordance with a person-centred approach often requires simple attitudes, based on empathising with carers and consumers' distress. Communication and respect for confidentiality are fundamental. However, in many circumstances, ethical issues regarding confidentiality must be weighed against the benefits of involving carers in the assessment process, as often they can contribute with valuable insights into history of mental health and suicide, what works best to soothe their loved ones and keep them safe (Acres et al., 2019b; NHMRC, 2012).

TRANSLATION TO PRACTICE

How to include loved ones when responding to a suicide crisis

Explore your preconceptions about self-harm and suicide and how they can affect your engagement with consumers and carers. Do you feel anxious or overwhelmed about approaching the support person of someone who engages in suicidal behaviour? Remember that carers need compassionate support. Provide information about the status of their loved ones whenever possible (e.g. 'We are doing all we can to keep them safe and comfortable'). Maintain clear communication and inform them of any updates (e.g. notice of discharge).

Carers want to feel their loved one's presentation is approached in the same neutral and professional way reserved for physical health issues, and that their distress is considered (Acres et al., 2019b). It is necessary to keep in mind that when taking care of a cherished person, carers are also in crisis and need validation and information, and to be supported and valued in a respectful and collaborative way. Carers often want to communicate with staff but feel stigmatised (McLaughlin et al., 2014). Contact with health professionals who enquire about how carers are coping and who offer emotional support for their current distress can be highly beneficial. Providing information on available resources and support for the family, and information on how to provide care in the home setting are others ways in which health professionals can involve carers in the recovery process (Acres et al., 2019b; McLaughlin et al., 2016; NHMRC, 2012).

INTERPROFESSIONAL PERSPECTIVES

Laura – A mental health nurse's perspective

I have been working as mental health nurse in a hospital emergency department (ED) for approximately 12 years now. As a member of the psychiatric consultation team, I work with psychiatrists and other mental health nurses in responding directly to individuals with acute mental health presentations. In addition, our team provides guidance to other team members (e.g. general practitioners and registered nurses) on how to respond to people experiencing mental illnesses. In my day-to-day practice, I always have to manage different stressors and to balance out the needs of consumers and colleagues with varied professional backgrounds and experiences.

At the ED, we often see people with mental health concerns waiting for a long period for admission into one of our intensive care units. These overflow moments are usually stressful for consumers and practitioners alike. Part of my job is to attend to consumers' basic needs in these moments. I try to prevent escalation of symptoms by providing information about waiting times, making sure they are eating, being looked after and in contact with support systems. Validating their perceptions of stress and assuring them we are doing everything within our reach to provide admission is also helpful. During these waiting times, we also need to validate the perceptions of colleagues from the ED teams. Psychoeducation is often required to help them understand that presentations are symptomatic and not simply inappropriate behaviour. Communicating how a consumer might be feeling (e.g. scared or threatened when experiencing psychotic symptoms) might assist them in understanding consumers' needs and that there are effective ways of managing the often-challenging situations we see. A calm and professional attitude can help to communicate a sense of shared responsibility. We are experiencing distress because we all want the best outcomes for the people we are working with.

Acknowledging consumers' feelings is a helpful strategy across scenarios. When a person is feeling agitated or distressed, seeing through the underlying risk factors assists me to act in a person-centred and trauma-informed approach. Often, challenging presentations reflect previous traumatic experiences and signal the presence of triggers for that person. Through an open-listening attitude we can remove triggers when possible, or at least communicate willingness to do so. Communication of empathy is essential. People respond well to acknowledgement of how they might be feeling and of our intention to help. This validating and empathetic approach can prevent re-victimising responses, often seen when the situation escalates (e.g. forceful restraining and injection of medication).

Another example is when a person is admitted after a suicide attempt. In my experience, cases of overdosing precipitated by a current stressor (e.g. relationship conflict, financial problems) are not uncommon. When deciding whether to admit or discharge a consumer we mostly focus on what precipitated the current episode and how the person is feeling at present. We investigate their levels of ideation, what supports are available and strategies that prevented suicide behaviours in the past, consistent with safety planning principles. We focus on what might be different this time and what can mostly contribute to keeping the person safe at present. We can review previous safety plans and make additional suggestions that might help. People are often honest when they are still having suicidal thoughts and we often communicate with community mental health team members in care for that person and other support systems when making a decision.

Throughout my practice, I have learned that it is important to cultivate a compassionate understanding of consumers' presentations. I understand that individuals are often highly emotional and in a very stressful situation, but I know this is just one moment in their lives; that is when they hit 'rock bottom'. But it helps me to remind myself that they are human and are usually coping better than this when they are not so unwell. They are just vulnerable at the moment and that is when they need help the most. When this attitude encompasses your practice, it translates into the mutual communication between you, the consumer and the team you are working with. That is when you feel supported by your team members too, when you know everyone is working towards professionals and consumers' safety and well-being.

REFLECTIVE QUESTIONS

Laura is an experienced professional working in a multidisciplinary team in a hospital ED.

- What are some examples on how to maintain a compassionate attitude towards people experiencing mental health symptoms and suicide ideation? What is most important to communicate to consumers and support persons?
- How might Laura ensure she maintains her own well-being when working with often challenging scenarios?

COVID-19 effects on self-harm and suicidal behaviours

The COVID-19 pandemic's unprecedented conditions have led to worsening of symptoms among people experiencing mental illness and has contributed to development of new symptomatology such as anxiety, depression and PTSD (Gunnell et al., 2020; Rogers et al., 2020). Frontline care workers have also been affected by the distress imposed through increased workloads, fear of contamination and sensitive decision-making processes involved in responding to cases (Holmes et al., 2020). It was concerning that the most critical COVID-19 prevention strategy was social distancing, as social isolation and loneliness are known risk factors for suicide (Chu et al., 2017; Reger, Stanley & Joiner, 2020). Among the general population, pandemics also have the potential to exacerbate other risk factors, such as financial distress, domestic violence, drug misuse and sense of entrapment (Gunnell et al., 2020).

Among people who are vulnerable are those who are in confined spaces, such as prison populations and immigrants being held in refugee centres (Center for Migration Studies (CMS), 2020). Furthermore, people from refugee backgrounds might be easily triggered when required to isolate (e.g. enhancing the sense of confinement) or when facing the socio-economic consequences of a pandemic (limited resources, lack of medical care, difficulties in providing support to one's family) (Kooy, 2020). Increased risk of suicide might be also observed among other vulnerable groups, such as females, ethnic minorities, single young adults, people with previous mental illness and people experiencing food insecurity (Fitzpatrick, Harris & Drawve, 2020).

Therefore, mental healthcare responses during a pandemic period should include reducing the effects of social isolation on people's mental health, with special attention paid to vulnerable groups. Whether suicide rates increased during the COVID-19 pandemic is still being investigated. Nonetheless, suicide has the potential to become a pressing concern as pandemics evolve and affect general populations and economies (Gunnell et al., 2020). Care must be delivered in different ways to reach those who need help the most. Digital modalities for suicide prevention and interventions must be tested and implemented (Gunnell et al., 2020). Safety plans can be modified to accommodate coping strategies within pandemic conditions while preserving its original function (e.g. substituting going to the gym to using an online exercise program) (Pruitt, McIntosh & Reger, 2020).

SUMMARY

This chapter has presented stories, information and activities designed to deepen your understanding of:

- Nomenclature for suicide and the need to avoid using derogatory terms that can undermine person-centred approaches in responding to suicidal behaviour
- Suicide as one of the leading causes of death among young people, with most of deaths by suicide occurring before the age of 45 years. Several characteristics can predispose people to the risk of suicide, including history of mental illness, substance misuse, experiencing psychosocial stressors and minority group status.
- The interpersonal theory of suicide, which explains the role of thwarted belongingness and perceived burdensomeness in the onset of suicidal behaviours. When people perceive these states to be unchanging, suicide ideation might switch from passive to active.
- Safety planning, which involves identifying distress triggers, ways of responding safely to the onset or worsening of suicidal urges, and internal and external coping strategies that can help to mitigate and prevent suicide.
- The need for all people presenting with suicidal thoughts or behaviours to be validated and treated in a compassionate way. Carers and loved ones are also under considerable distress and, where possible, should be included in health practitioners' compassionate responses.

CRITICAL THINKING/LEARNING ACTIVITIES

1   Think about the most common terms people can use to refer to suicide. What are some of the terms to be avoided? How might using these terms affect people who have experienced suicide ideation in the past, or have family or friends who have lost a loved one due to suicide?

2   Take a moment to think about a situation in your life that might have been moderately traumatic or especially difficult. Was there a moment where you felt you were losing hope? Was it easy to talk openly about the situation and reach out for help? How do you imagine a person experiencing suicide ideation might be thinking and feeling?

3   How can a person-centred approach to mental health care assist people experiencing suicide ideation? What are some of the barriers to adopting a person-centred approach in daily practice?

4   Join with a colleague and take a moment to think about ways to assist a loved one experiencing suicide ideation or in suicide or self-harm crisis. Discuss your thoughts and experiences. What could be the experience of friends and family members when a loved one presents to the emergency department after attempted suicide?

5   What are some potential ways in which health practitioners can involve carers when assisting people experiencing suicidal behaviours? What are some examples of practices that should be avoided?

LEARNING EXTENSION

Safety planning has been shown to be an effective intervention in preventing suicidal behaviour. One potentially useful resource is the Beyond Now Safety Planning software application, which is available for free (beyondblue.org.au). Take a moment to download the application and browse through the distinct phases of creating a personalised safety plan.

Reflect on some other examples that can be included in each section of a safety plan. What might be helpful to assist people in navigating suicide ideation while in safety?

FURTHER READING

Lees, D., Procter, N. & Fassett, D. (2014). Therapeutic engagement between consumers in suicidal crisis and mental health nurses. *International Journal of Mental Health Nursing*, *23*(4): 306–15.

This paper focuses on the views and experiences of both mental health nurses and people recovering from a suicidal crisis. It summarises some of the challenges faced in care provision in public mental health settings from a multimethod study conducted in Australia. The findings were based on interviews with mental health nurses who recently provided care for people who attempted suicide and consumers who recently experienced suicidal urges. The results highlight the importance of therapeutic interpersonal engagement and provide recommendations for professional practice.

McLaughlin, C., McGowan, I., Kernohan, G. & O'Neill, S. (2016). The unmet support needs of a family member caring for a suicidal person. *Journal of Mental Health, 25*(3): 212–16.

This paper summarises common experiences of family members caring for a person with experience of suicidal behaviour and their role in suicide prevention. Qualitative findings for the support needs of carers include feeling acknowledged and included, and consistency of support is discussed.

Stanley, B. & Brown, G. K. (2012). Safety planning intervention: A brief intervention to mitigate suicide risk.*Cognitive and Behavioural practice, 19*(2): 256–64.

The paper presents the background of safety planning research as an intervention strategy for suicide prevention and discusses in detail the components included in safety planning. An example of a safety plan is presented to illustrate how the strategy can be implemented.

REFERENCES

Acres, K., Loughhead, M. & Procter, N. (2019a). Carer perspectives of people diagnosed with borderline personality disorder: A scoping review of emergency care responses. *Australian Emergency Care, 22*(1): 34–41.

——— (2019b). *Please talk to me. Please include me. I want nurses to understand – A report on carer perspective on emergency department nursing practices for a person with borderline personality disorder.* Retrieved from https://www.unisa.edu.au/contentassets/ 65b73cb620f64e6ba564256a70f72c99/bpd-carers-views-report.pdf

Austin, E. K., Handley, T., Kiem, A. S., Rich, J. L., Lewin, T. J., Askland, H. H. … Kelly, B. J. (2018). Drought-related stress among farmers: Findings from the Australian Rural Mental Health Study. *Medical Journal of Australia, 209*(4): 159–65.

Australian Bureau of Statistics (ABS). (2020). Causes of death, Australia. Retrieved from https://www .abs.gov.au/statistics/health/causes-death/causes-death-australia/2019#intentional-self-harm- suicides-key-characteristics

Australian Institute of Health and Welfare (AIHW). (2020). Suicide and intentional self-harm. Retrieved from https://www.aihw.gov.au/reports/australias-health/suicide-and-intentional-self-harm

Bentley, K. H., Kleiman, E. M., Elliott, G., Huffman, J. C. & Nock, M. K. (2019). Real-time monitoring technology in single-case experimental design research: Opportunities and challenges. *Behaviour Research and Therapy, 117*: 87–96.

Beyond Blue. (2020). *Beyond Now – Suicide Safety Planning.* Retrieved from https://www.beyondblue .org.au/get-support/beyondnow-suicide-safety-planning

Brodsky, B. S., Spruch-Feiner, A. & Stanley, B. (2018). The zero suicide model: Applying evidence- based suicide prevention practices to clinical care. *Frontiers in Psychiatry, 9*: 33.

Chesin, M. S., Stanley, B., Haigh, E. A., Chaudhury, S. R., Pontoski, K., Knox, K. L. & Brown, G. K. (2017). Staff views of an emergency department intervention using safety planning and structured follow-up with suicidal veterans. *Archives of Suicide Research, 21*(1): 127–37.

Chu, C., Buchman-Schmitt, J. M., Stanley, I. H., Hom, M. A., Tucker, R. P., Hagan, C. R. … Joiner, T. E. (2017). The interpersonal theory of suicide: A systematic review and meta-analysis of a decade of cross-national research. *Psychological Bulletin, 143*(12): 1313–45.

Center for Migration Studies. (2020). *Immigrant detention and COVID 19: How a pandemic exploited and spread through the US Immigrant Detention System.* Retrieved from https://cmsny.org/ wp-content/uploads/2020/08/CMS-Detention-COVID-Report-08-12-2020.pdf

Cerel, J., Brown, M., Maple, M., Singleton, M., Van de Venne, J., Moore, M. & Flaherty, C. (2019). How many people are exposed to suicide? Not six. *The American Association of Suicidology, 49*(2): 529–34.

Coronial Services of New Zealand (CSNZ). (2020). *Suicide.* Retrieved from https://coronialservices .justice.govt.nz/suicide/annual-suicide-statistics-since-2011/

Fitzpatrick, K. M., Harris, C. & Drawve, G. (2020). How bad is it? Suicidality in the middle of the COVID-19 pandemic. *Suicide and Life-Threatening Behaviour, 50*(6): 1241–9.

Gamarra, J. M., Luciano, M. T., Gradus, J. L. & Stirman, S. W. (2015). Assessing variability and implementation fidelity of suicide prevention safety planning in a regional VA healthcare system. *Crisis, 36*(6): 433–9.

Green, J. D., Kearns, J. C., Rosen, R. C., Keane, T. M. & Marx, B. P. (2018). Evaluating the effectiveness of safety plans for military veterans: Do safety plans tailored to veteran characteristics decrease suicide risk? *Behavior Therapy, 49*(6): 931–8.

Gunnell, D., Appleby, L., Arensman, E., Hawton, K., John, A., Kapur, N. … Yip, P. S. F. (2020). Suicide risk and prevention during the COVID-19 pandemic. *The Lancet Psychiatry, 7*(6): 468–71.

Hansson, C., Joas, E., Palsson, E., Hawton, K., Runeson, B. & Landen, M. (2018). Risk factors for suicide in bipolar disorder: A cohort study of 12 850 patients. *Acta Psychiatrica Scandinavica*, *138*(5): 456–63.

Holmes, E. A., O'Connor, R. C., Perry, V. H., Tracey, I., Wessely, S., Arseneault, L. … Bullmore, E. (2020). Multidisciplinary research priorities for the COVID-19 pandemic: a call for action for mental health science. *The Lancet Psychiatry*, *7*(6): 547–60.

Hor, K. & Taylor, M. (2010). Suicide and schizophrenia: A systematic review of rates and risk factors. *Journal of Psychopharmacology*, *24*(4 Suppl): 81–90.

Joiner, T., Hom, M., Hagan, C. & Silva, C. (2015). Suicide as a derangement of the self-sacrificial aspect of eusociality. *Psychological Review*, *123*(3): 235–54.

Kayman, D. J., Goldstein, M. F., Dixon, L. & Goodman, M. (2015). Perspectives of suicidal veterans on safety planning. *Crisis*, *36*(5): 371–83.

Kleiman, E. M., Turner, B. J., Fedor, S., Beale, E. E., Huffman, J. C. & Nock, M. K. (2017). Examination of real-time fluctuations in suicidal ideation and its risk factors: Results from two ecological momentary assessment studies. *Journal of Abnormal Psychology*, *126*(6): 726–38.

Kooy, J. V. (2020). *COVID-19 and Humanitarian Migrants on Temporary Visas: Assessing the public costs*. Retrieved from https://www.refugeecouncil.org.au/wp-content/uploads/2020/07/COVID-19-van-Kooy-.pdf

Life in Mind. (2018). *Suicide Prevention Insights – Connecting with people in South Australia*. Retrieved from https://lifeinmind.org.au/news/suicide-prevention-insights-connecting-with-people-in-south-australia

Lifeline. (2020). What is self harm? Retrieved from https://www.lifeline.org.au/get-help/information-and-support/self-harm/

Mann, J. J., Michel, C. A. & Auerbach, R. P. (2021). Improving suicide prevention through evidence-based strategies: A systematic review. *American Journal of Psychiatry, 178*(7): 611–24.

McLaughlin, C., McGowan, I., Kernohan, G. & O'Neill, S. (2016). The unmet support needs of family members caring for a suicidal person. *Journal of Mental Health*, *25*(3): 212–16.

McLaughlin, C., McGowan, I., O'Neill, S. & Kernohan, G. (2014). The burden of living with and caring for a suicidal family member. *Journal of Mental Health*, *23*(5): 236–40.

National Health and Medical Research Council (NHMRC). (2012). *Clinical Practice Guidelines for the Management of Borderline Personality Disorder*. Retrieved from https://bpdfoundation.org.au/images/mh25_borderline_personality_guideline.pdf

Padmanathan, P., Biddle, L., Hall, K., Scowcroft, E., Nielsen, E. & Knipe, D. (2019). Language use and suicide: An online cross-sectional survey. *PLoS One*, *14*(6): e0217473.

Paradies, Y. (2018). Racism and Indigenous Health. *Oxford Research Encyclopedias Global Public Health*. Retrieved from doi:10.1093/acrefore/9780190632366.013.86

Popovic, D., Benabarre, A., Crespo, J. M., Goikolea, J. M., Gonzalez-Pinto, A., Gutierrez-Rojas, L. … Vieta, E. (2014). Risk factors for suicide in schizophrenia: Systematic review and clinical recommendations. *Acta Psychiatrica Scandinavica*, *130*(6): 418–26.

Pruitt, L. D., McIntosh, L. S. & Reger, G. (2020). Suicide safety planning during a pandemic: The implications of COVID-19 on coping with a crisis. *Suicide and Life-Threatening Behavior*, *50*(3): 741–9.

Reger, M. A., Stanley, I. H. & Joiner, T. E. (2020). Suicide mortality and coronavirus disease 2019: A perfect storm? *JAMA Psychiatry*, *77*(11): 1093–4 .

Ribeiro, J. D., Huang, X., Fox, K. R. & Franklin, J. C. (2018). Depression and hopelessness as risk factors for suicide ideation, attempts and death: meta-analysis of longitudinal studies. *British Journal of Psychiatry, 212*(5): 279–86.

Robinson, K. H., Bansel, P., Denson, N., Ovenden, G. & Davies, C. (2014). *Growing Up Queer: Issues facing young Australians who are gender variant and sexuality diverse*. Retrieved from https://www.twenty10.org.au/wp-content/uploads/2016/04/Robinson-et-al.-2014-Growing-up-Queer.pdf

Rogers, J. P., Chesney, E., Oliver, D., Pollak, T. A., McGuire, P., Fusar-Poli, P. … David, A. S. (2020). Psychiatric and neuropsychiatric presentations associated with severe coronavirus infections: a systematic review and meta-analysis with comparison to the COVID-19 pandemic. *The Lancet Psychiatry*, *7*(7): 611–27.

Silverman, M. M., Berman, A. L., Sanddal, N. D., O'Carroll, P. W. & Joiner Jr, T. E. (2007). Rebuilding the tower of Babel: a revised nomenclature for the study of suicide and suicidal behaviors.

Part 2: Suicide-related ideations, communications, and behaviors. *Suicide and Life-Threatening Behavior, 37*(3): 264–77.

Silverman, M. M. & De Leo, D. (2016). Why there is a need for an international nomenclature and classification system for suicide. *Crisis, 37*(2): 83–7.

Stanley, B. & Brown, G. K. (2012). Safety planning intervention: A brief intervention to mitigate suicide risk. *Cognitive and Behavioral Practice, 19*(2): 256–64.

Stanley, B., Brown, G. K., Currier, G. W., Lyons, C., Chesin, M. & Knox, K. L. (2015). Brief intervention and follow-up for suicidal patients with repeat emergency department visits enhances treatment engagement. *American Journal of Public Health, 105*(8): 1570–2.

Stanley, B., Chaudhury, S. R., Chesin, M., Pontoski, K., Bush, A. M., Knox, K. L. & Brown, G. K. (2016). An emergency department intervention and follow-up to reduce suicide risk in the VA: Acceptability and effectiveness. *Psychiatric Services, 67*(6): 680–3.

Stone, H., Barret, K., Beales, D., Das, S., Deshpande, M., Gibbons, R. … Witharana, D. (2020). *Self-harm and Suicide in Adults – Final report of the patient safety group*. Retrieved from https://www.rcpsych.ac.uk/docs/default-source/improving-care/better-mh-policy/college-reports/cr229_self-harm-and-suicide.pdf

Strauss, P., Cook, A., Winter, S., Watson, V., Wright Toussaint, D. & Lin, A. (2017). *Trans-Pathways – The mental health experiences and care pathways of trans young people. Summary of results*. Retrieved from https://www.telethonkids.org.au/globalassets/media/documents/brain–behaviour/trans-pathways-report.pdf

Tasmanian Government Department of Health. (2020). *The Connection with People (CwP) Approach*. Retrieved from https://www.dhhs.tas.gov.au/mentalhealth/suicide_risk_and_prevention/connecting_with_people

Too, L. S., Spittal, M. J., Bugeja, L., Reifels, L., Butterworth, P. & Pirkis, J. (2019). The association between mental disorders and suicide: A systematic review and meta-analysis of record linkage studies. *Journal of Affective Disorders, 259*: 302–13.

Turecki, G. & Brent, D. A. (2016). Suicide and suicidal behaviour. *The Lancet, 387*(10024): 1227–39.

Tyrer, P., Reed, G. M. & Crawford, M. J. (2015). Classification, assessment, prevalence, and effect of personality disorder. *The Lancet, 385*(9969): 717–26.

Van Orden, K. A., Witte, T. K., Cukrowicz, K. C., Braithwaite, S. R., Selby, E. A. & Joiner, T. E., Jr. (2010). The interpersonal theory of suicide. *Psychological Review, 117*(2): 575–600.

World Health Organization. (2014). *Preventing Suicide – A global imperative*. Retrieved from https://apps.who.int/iris/bitstream/handle/10665/131056/9789241564779_eng.pdf;jsessionid=B77D496E4CA51F924CC0DA666FF5E19D?sequence=1

——— (2019a). *Suicide – Key facts*. Retrieved from https://www.who.int/news-room/fact-sheets/detail/suicide

——— (2019b). *Suicide in the World – Global Health Estimates*. Retrieved from https://apps.who.int/iris/bitstream/handle/10665/326948/WHO-MSD-MER-19.3-eng.pdf?sequence=1&isAllowed=y

Zonana, J., Simberlund, J. & Christos, P. (2018). The impact of safety plans in an outpatient clinic. *Crisis, 39*(4): 304.

8

Mental health in the interprofessional context

Anne Storey and Denise McGarry

LEARNING OBJECTIVES

At the completion of this chapter, you should be able to:

1 Describe the roles of members of the interprofessional mental healthcare team.
2 Identify different roles of the practitioner within the interprofessional mental healthcare team.
3 Discuss the changing nature of professionals who contribute to mental health care.
4 Recognise the preparation and expertise brought to mental health care by different professions.
5 Understand regulation and standards governing the mental health workforce.
6 Recognise what contributes to an effective interprofessional team and appreciate the contribution of self-care to the professional outcomes.

Introduction

Regardless of the setting of mental health care, an **interprofessional** or **multidisciplinary** approach is a sound response to the multifaceted problems faced by people with mental health problems. Staff may contribute different expertise. Through collaboration with consumers, the needs of the person experiencing mental health problems can be comprehensively met.

The examples and discussion in this chapter draw extensively from the context of mental health services in New South Wales, Australia. Service details vary between services in different locations, but the examples provided offer a range of approaches that clearly illustrate common underlying possibilities across many jurisdictions.

Extensive engagement of an interprofessional model of care does have drawbacks. At times, the extent of overlap may result in the blurring of roles. Responsibilities may be uncertain or unclear. Consumers and their carers may find it difficult to identify whom to approach, especially if care is delivered across service organisations. Mental health services have responded with the development of several roles based on the function performed rather than the preparation for practice undertaken. Team leaders and case managers are examples of such roles.

An interprofessional workforce involves a range of professions and other staff with different educational backgrounds. These are broadening, increasingly, from the traditional professions employed in provision of mental health services – medical, nursing, social work, psychology and occupational therapy – to embrace other workers with skills to contribute. They may be drawn from increasingly diverse educational backgrounds. Some of these workers are subject to regulation through their professional bodies and national regulatory authorities. Others working with the mental health workforce are not subject to such authority or regulation. This has supported the development of standards for the mental health workforce in Australia and Aotearoa New Zealand, in order to provide uniform and consistent guidelines to govern everyone working with people experiencing mental health problems.

> **interprofessional** – of, relating to or involving two or more academic disciplines that are usually considered distinct, to undertake a task together
>
> **multidisciplinary** – 'combining or involving several academic disciplines or professional specialisations in an approach to a topic or problem' (Baltic Organisations' Network for Funding Science, 2014)

Historical professional precedents

Until the late 19th century, care for people experiencing mental health problems was usually delivered outside of the medical paradigm. Families, religious and criminal justice systems played significant roles at different times. Today, their roles continue under various guises and to differing extents, and their influence continues to be felt. It is not infrequent that these outdated models are perpetuated in the popular media, particularly in film.

Late in the 19th century, care for people with mental health problems was assumed by the medical profession. The medical profession was experiencing marked growth in expertise across a range of clinical areas, in part due to its adoption of the scientific model. It was hoped that advances in medical science would also apply to the problems of mental health. Luminaries in the field, including Sigmund Freud, did much to promote the notion of mental health problems being amenable to medical intervention.

The two great wars of the 20th century can be argued to have been instrumental in the alignment of mental health care with a medical paradigm. Large numbers of young people from the nations of the world experienced mental health problems following their exposure to the trauma of war.

The nursing workforce in traditional mental health services has evolved from the role of 'asylum attendants'. During the early 20th century, localised training programs became formalised and, by the mid-20th century, had developed into a separate and equivalent nursing certificate, subject to regulation and professional nursing standards.

Social workers, occupational therapists and psychologists were later additions to the mental health workforce, becoming established during the middle of the 20th century. It would be negligent not to acknowledge the continuing role of religious institutions, whether formalised or not. Some mental health services, such as those delivered by St John of God Health Care, continue to be delivered by religious orders that have a long history of supporting those with mental health problems.

The interprofessional mental health workforce

Under the auspices of the World Health Organization, a committee was convened to consider issues of interprofessional education and workforce collaboration (Health Professions Networks, Nursing & Midwifery & Human Resources for Health, 2010). This committee is testament to the recognition given to the notion of interprofessional work, and its report was titled, in part, 'A framework for action'. The message of this report was to promote an interprofessional workforce as a key response to an impeding global crisis in the health workforce. Further, the committee asserted that a health workforce characterised by interprofessional education and collaboration could deliver improved health outcomes for consumers but concluded that this would represent a challenging cultural change for health services.

The composition of the mental health workforce

This section reviews the principle professional disciplines that work within mental health services.

Nursing

Nursing has a dominant position in mental health services in terms of numbers. In Australia, there were 85.8 full-time equivalent (FTE) nurses per 100 000 population working in mental health services in 2017 (see Figure 8.1) – an estimated 22 159 nurses, registered and enrolled (Australian Institute of Health & Welfare (AIHW), 2019).

In Aotearoa New Zealand, the adult mental health and addiction workforce in 2014 was about 7 per cent of the total health workforce, at around 9071 FTE positions. This workforce is distributed between public (District Health Board) mental health services, with around 52 per cent of the workforce, 32 per cent in non-government organisation (NGO) mental health services, 7 per cent in public addiction services and 9 per cent in NGO addiction services (Ministry of Health, 2018, p. 11). In Aotearoa New Zealand, nurses form a smaller proportion of the mental health workforce than in Australia. Around 28 per cent of the workforce comprises nurses, and there is a much greater representation of support workers.

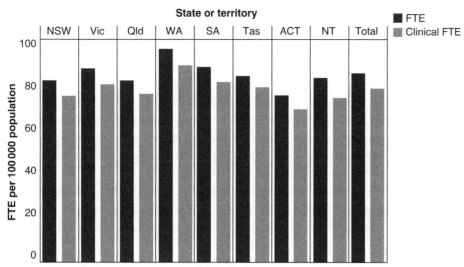

Figure 8.1   Employed mental health nurses, FTE and clinical FTE per 100 000 population, Australian states and territories, 2018

Note: State and territory mental health nurse workforce estimates should be treated with caution due to low response rates in some jurisdictions.

Source: AIHW (2019).

The non-regulated workforce consists of both a community support worker role (CSW) and the lived experience workforce, commonly known as 'consumer advisors' or 'peer support specialists'. The latter workforce is more likely to be contracted into public health services by NGOs (see Figure 8.2).

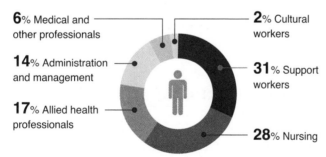

Figure 8.2   Percentage of each professional group working in Vote Health-funded adult mental health and addiction services, Aotearoa New Zealand

Source: Ministry of Health (2018, p. 12).

The preparation and composition of nurses have changed over the past 30 years in Australia, and continue to change. The registered nurse (RN) became the initial nursing preparation for employment in the health workforce from 2010. This may be a comprehensive undergraduate nursing degree delivered through Australian and Aotearoa New Zealand universities, or a graduate degree following completion of a prior undergraduate degree; it qualifies graduates for practice as beginning health practitioners across all clinical environments. All courses include mandated theoretical subjects in mental health nursing.

Clinical placement experiences are not compulsory in the Australian context; while some universities do ensure placements in mental health services, others do not. The extent of this component is quite varied between different universities, in part due to the difficulty in securing sufficient numbers of high-quality clinical placements and mental health nursing academics to support them (Australian College of Mental Health Nursing (ACMHN), 2018; Mental Health Nurse Education Taskforce (MHNET), 2008).

Aotearoa New Zealand prepares comprehensive registered nurses by a Bachelor program overseen by the Nursing Council of New Zealand. In these programs, clinical placement in mental health services is required to qualify for registration, including both acute and rehabilitation, or continuing care settings.

Mental health nursing remains a contested specialty in nursing. The professional bodies, the Australian College of Mental Health Nurses (ACMHN) and the New Zealand College of Mental Health Nurses (NZCMHN), provide a credentialled award that recognises nurses with advanced qualifications in mental health nursing.

Postgraduate courses are run by several tertiary education providers in mental health nursing. These courses do not bestow a different professional or clinical award as is done in medicine. Instead, the qualifications can support promotion to positions such as Clinical Nurse Specialist or Clinical Nurse Consultant.

scope of practice – in the health context, this refers to the range of work practices and activities undertaken by health professionals, according to the competence of the practitioners, education and training of the practitioners and regulatory authorities, and health-related legislation overseeing the practitioners; a 'scope of practice' is neither a job description nor a list of tasks or set of procedures (ACMHN, 2013)

Nurse practitioners (NPs) have a **scope of practice** regulated by the Australian Nursing and Midwifery Accreditation Council (ANMAC) and the Australian Health Practitioner Regulation Agency (Ahpra) following completion of a specific postgraduate program of study, endorsed by Ahpra and successful application for a designated nurse practitioner position within a mental health service. NPs are expert nurses who practice both collaboratively with other health professions and in independent practice. The NP role is a unique blend of clinical leadership, scholarship, research, planning and advocacy. In Australia and Aotearoa New Zealand, the NP's scope of practice includes authorisation to prescribe medications. In Australia, NPs make up only a small part of the nursing workforce.

INTERPROFESSIONAL PERSPECTIVES

Geraldine – nurse practitioner

I became an NP in 2007, after 9 years of practice in CNS, CNC and NUM roles. The role of NP has enabled the care and treatment of clients to be given by one clinician in an equal partnership with the client, while utilising other professions as needed. Clients talk of the benefit and reliability of this model, and while nurses have greatly increased work responsibilities, this has resulted in increased satisfaction. Anecdotally, there has been talk of the increased compassion NPs feel towards their clients.

It is rewarding to see the work of nursing elevated and the professional practice of expanded nursing given appropriate professional recognition. It is also rewarding to see the implementation of this care and the consequent positive effects on client outcomes. It is to the betterment of the profession that autonomy and independent practice become integral to the nursing profession.

The challenge to other professions to regard nurses and NPs as independent and autonomous practitioners who collaborate with other health professionals is to give the science of nursing its proper place.

For me, the pinnacle of becoming a mental health NP is that the human-to-human relationship becomes the focal point of care and treatment, and lies at the foundation of the philosophy of nursing.

REFLECTIVE QUESTION
What are the benefits for the consumer of a NP?

Enrolled nurses (ENs) have been employed in small numbers across mental health services for many years. Their scope of practice must be supervised by an RN and includes administration of medication. Educational preparation for this role is ordinarily at an undergraduate diploma level, obtained through the Tertiary and Further Education (TAFE) or the vocational education sector. These courses do not include mandated mental health nursing curricula or clinical placement, although many individual institutions do include this preparation.

Although not strictly part of the nursing workforce, Assistants-in-Nursing (AINs) is another group in the mental health workforce. Some people employed in this role may be engaged in current studies towards a Bachelor of Nursing (BN). Alternatively, a formal qualification as an AIN can be obtained in the TAFE sector or from the vocational education sector. There is not yet a dedicated preparation for work in mental health services, but this does not preclude employment in these services with this qualification.

Specialist RNs working in the interprofessional context

Mental health services are comprised of a variety of teams, and especially so in the community. These include services for:

- perinatal mental health
- eating disorders
- child and adolescent mental health (CAMHS)
- early intervention in psychosis services (EIPS)
- acute care services (Crisis Teams / Community Mental Health Emergency Teams (CoMHET), Police Ambulance Clinical Early Response (PACER) – see NSW Health, 2019)
- case management / care coordination
- assertive outreach teams (AOT)
- in-patient services
- aged care psychiatry, including the older person mental health services (OPMHS)
- forensic mental health, including court liaison services
- consultation liaison
- dual diagnosis – mental health, drug and alcohol, and mental health and intellectual disability (see specific chapters in this text).

Services for people using illicit substances and misusing alcohol or prescription drugs are often provided as separate interprofessional services. RNs working within these teams

Emily's experience as a clinical nurse consultant in drug health services

There are many benefits for patients admitted to mental health services, including access to specialist drug and alcohol services while in hospital. At times people may use tobacco, alcohol, cannabis or other illicit substances to cope with their feelings, stress and worries. Some patients with mood disorders also use tobacco and other substances to cope or self-manage manic or depressive symptoms. In the short term this may act to self-medicate or provide some relief; however, in the medium to longer term it can worsen outcomes for the patient.

For the nurse, being able to take an alcohol and substance use history when a patient is admitted to hospital is a key part of identifying risk factors and providing patient-centred care. Being aware of the services available to support our patients and how to make a referral is important in optimising care.

Many local health services have access to drug and alcohol consultation and liaison services. These services have two main aims:

1   To provide advice on the clinical management of patients who are known or considered to have alcohol and substance use disorders, with the goal of optimising care.
2   To increase the knowledge, skills and confidence of staff and to complement the professional practice of healthcare professionals working in hospital settings who deliver care to people living with substance-use disorders.

Hospital consultation liaison drug and alcohol services may include nursing, medical and allied health services and face-to-face or phone support. The clinicians have expertise and skills in engagement, comprehensive assessment, management of withdrawal and intoxication, review of diagnostic results and case formulation. They may also provide support in health education, harm-minimisation, referral and discharge planning.

A range of intensive treatment options is available to optimise patient outcomes:

1   Counselling services – these primarily focus on harm-reduction and relapse-prevention skills that are tailored to the patient's goals.
2   In-patient and ambulatory withdrawal – provide medically supported and supervised treatment of patients' physical withdrawal symptoms.
3   Mutual support groups – recovery focused groups that provide social, emotional and practical support, including:

    a   12-step groups such Alcoholics' Anonymous (AA), Narcotics' Anonymous (NA) and Marijuana Anonymous (MA; GROW n.d.).

    b   Self-Management and Recovery Training (SMART) recovery groups are based on cognitive behavioural therapy (SMART Recovery Australia, 2021)

4   Residential rehabilitation programs – an intensive and supportive living environment in which people who are working towards recovery from substance use live together.
5   Involuntary drug and alcohol treatment (IDAT) under the NSW *Health Drug and Alcohol Treatment Act 2007* provides treatment and medical care for the withdrawal and treatment of people with serious substance use problems who have not responded to less restrictive care and would be likely to benefit from short-term involuntary treatment.

provide a variety of interprofessional care, including counselling, assessment and clinics (e.g. methadone dispensing). People referred to as having a 'dual diagnosis' – experiencing problems due to both mental health illness and another condition or illicit drug use – are often cared for by these services.

People with an intellectual disability and a mental health problem are provided with specialist services, but often fail to receive care they require, perhaps because of diagnostic overshadowing, which is the tendency for comorbid conditions to be ascribed to the individual's initial presenting problem.

Medicine and psychiatry

Medical professionals working within mental health services include doctors, psychiatrists and registrars. Registrars are enrolled in postgraduate medical studies in psychiatry. They rotate through compulsory placements including child and adolescent mental health (six months), consultation liaison (six months) and rural placement (three months), and complete 12 months' delivery of psychotherapy to an individual under the supervision of a specialist psychotherapist. The usual course for a registrar is three years for a basic psychiatric registrar and at least two years as an advanced trainee (AT), in which the registrar can specialise in areas such as perinatal or older persons' mental health. Psychiatrists have completed their postgraduate studies and are registered as a separate division of medicine by the regulatory authority (Ahpra). Their professional body, the Royal Australian and New Zealand College of Psychiatrists (RANZCP), plays a central role in their regulation, standards and delivery of training.

Assistants in Medicine is a recent addition. These positions are for final-year medical students to support simple procedural tasks such as cannulation and help with administrative tasks such as report writing. It serves to introduce these students to the interprofessional workplace and offers them a paid means to expand their learning prior to registration as a medical practitioner.

Social work

In mental health care, social work is a specialised field of practice that focuses on the social contexts and consequences of mental ill-health. Social work practice in mental health aim to promote recovery, to restore individual, family and community well-being, to assist individuals to develop power and control over their lives and to advance principles of social justice. Social workers are employed in treatment and rehabilitation services across the public, private and NGO mental health service sectors, as well as in primary health care (Australian Association of Social Workers (AASW), 2020). Social workers are not currently regulated under Ahpra, but there is a campaign by the professional association to investigate possible forms of regulation for the profession. Aotearoa New Zealand is moving toward registration for social workers by 2021.

Occupational therapy

Occupational therapists (OTs) work to improve the functional performance of a person in order to achieve maximum independence. Their work is with people of all ages, aiming to overcome barriers to participation in occupations and activities. Occupational therapists work in a wide range of mental health services, including in-patient and community settings. They also focus on how a person's lifestyle can support mental health and improve quality of life (Occupational Therapy Australia, 2020).

OTs typically complete a four-year undergraduate program accredited by the Australian Association of Occupational Therapists (OT Australia) and it is a regulated profession. The degree program requires clinical placement as a component of educational preparation but this may not be in mental health services. The Occupational Board of New Zealand (OTBNZ) is the regulatory board for this profession in Aotearoa New Zealand.

Psychology

Psychologists undertake a four-year undergraduate degree. They are required to undertake clinical hours with supervision to become a registered psychologist. Clinical psychologists are frequently employed in mental health services. They have specialist training in the treatment of mental ill-health. Clinical psychologists undertake a masters or doctoral program in clinical psychology in order to be eligible for membership of the Australian Psychological Society's (APS) College of Clinical Psychologists. Psychologists are regulated health practitioners under Ahpra.

PERSONAL NARRATIVE

Phil – peer worker

I began my long involvement with the local health district in November 1999. We were then called Consumer Consultants and all of us were part-time casuals with our office and workplace in Rozelle Hospital. We were a small team of about six to eight consultants, a coordinator and a manager. Our role was to ensure consumer rights were upheld and to run some groups (e.g. creative writing, men's groups and joint groups with OTs). At Rozelle we worked in the three acute wards, one observation ward, an intensive psychiatric care unit and the long-term rehabilitation ward. We visited the wards daily and gave hope to the consumers, listened to their stories and empowered them in their recovery. Our motto was to walk in their shoes and provide an opportunity to be heard, to provide non-clinical care and walk beside the consumer without judgement.

Rozelle Hospital was the first facility to employ consumers in 1993. A group of consumers met before then and devised a training program and a set of expectations for the new workforce. It included training on the Mental Health Act, patient rights, active listening and the history of patient activism, among other things. At first it was limited to in-patient care, whereas now it is predominately in the community setting.

Then, the records of interactions were only informal and much of our work was in Ward 28 West – a long-stay unit. I think there was a clear line between consumer and clinician, and a power differential. Unlike today, we were not attached to teams in the community and our training was organised by ourselves, not by the service. Now, we are expected to do the same training as clinicians and we also do electronic medical records on our occasions of service. The advantage is that we are more accountable and can better lobby for more positions, based on our statistics. The disadvantage is losing our independence as a team and the edge of challenging the status quo.

Personally, I began my work after a job interview on site and 5 years' experience of sitting on consumer committees set up in 1995.

We attended a two-week training program run by consumers at Royal North Shore Hospital. As a diagnosed voice hearer, I had experienced long periods of unemployment, a couple of decades of being on a pension and receiving care coordination. My worst period was in the 1970s, when I relapsed twice, had periods of hospitalisation and at times was bereft of hope. My recovery took off in the 1980s when I achieved stable accommodation, volunteer work and support through local community centres.

At Rozelle I was able to achieve paid work and use my lived experience to support and care for other consumers. I built up a friendship with my coordinator and was able to debrief with her nearly every day. Now, I have a clinical supervisor and also have peer-group supervision.

Currently, the theme of recovery, strength-based care, trauma-informed care and a more optimistic view of the consumer's journey is prevalent. When the consumer consultants were employed in 1993 it was very much rights-based and about empowerment and challenging the medical model. This was underpinned by a consumer movement that had great advocates who pointed out the discrimination and unfairness, and there were some who developed an 'us versus them' approach, which could become confrontational. The consumer consultants worked together and talked together and told their stories. Now, the net has widened, and the experience of mental distress could be an entry point to a peer-worker job.

I often wonder about what makes peer work, with its rich history in Sydney, so powerful. It is, I think, because it gives people hope in crisis, it is democratic and inclusive. Peers and consumers tell each other their stories and both benefit from this. We are experts of lived experience and can use our times of distress to help others on their journey.

Peer work, to me, is meaningful and I learn something new every week about myself and about others. The role offers additional opportunities along the way.

Some of my achievements include attending conferences, public speaking, facility planning, research and writing peer-reviewed articles, systems advocacy, memberships of boards, committee memberships etc. But the greatest thrill is to watch a person improve and know that in some small way you have made a difference to that person. That was the hope in 1993 and, although I have detailed some of the history and changes, I think this common thread remains to this day.

As a consumer, my involvement in peer work has benefitted my recovery by hearing the stories of others; lifting my self-esteem; providing meaning in my life; developing problem-solving skills; encouraging self-care – physical and emotional; making a difference; having choices in my life; feeling part of a wider community; helping deal with adversity with resilience; becoming more confident; having employment and more income; and having a better life.

I would like to acknowledge the many hundreds of consumers I have worked with and talked to. And the clinicians who have gone the extra yards to support me.

The consumer movement has grown in many ways. We are more confident and switched on. We are social-media savvy. We are an important part of clinical teams. Our voices matter. Mental health is a growing industry and many more peer workers will be employed in the public mental health sector. Our perspectives matter and we are not shy to express them. I feel I have found myself and my voice. I feel I have come out the other end after much adversity. And the one thing I never thought would happen when I was 20 years old: I have a good job and I no longer hear voices.

Throughout New South Wales, each health district has developed its own team of peer workers and we have a statewide steering committee with a consumer manager in the Ministry of Health and a public workforce of over 150.

REFLECTIVE QUESTION

How can tokenism be avoided in a peer workforce?

The evidence base for the value of peer workers has grown. The position of consumer consultant has been phased out in favour of a new model of peer workers that is embedded within multidisciplinary teams in community mental health services, and some in in-patient units. These workers use their lived experience to support consumers who access these services. The support of the peer workers includes assisting clinical staff in maintaining a recovery focus during clinical discussions, and peer workers have championed the adoption of strengths-based care review practices.

Peer workers report to community mental health team managers on an operational level, and seek learning, development and peer supervision through their professional lead, the district senior peer worker.

The qualification to work as a peer worker in mental health is a lived experience of mental health issues and a Certificate IV Mental Health Peer Work. This qualification has been available since 2013. Peer workers are part of an unregulated sector of the mental health workforce.

PERSONAL NARRATIVE

Jemima – senior peer worker (an oxymoron)

The day I was diagnosed with bipolar disorder, I felt like my spirit was crushed under the weight of the nothingness – like nothing I had dreamt of could ever become real, or maybe nothing I thought was real. I ended up talking to someone who reminded me that I was a person called Jemima – a caring, loving person, an artist and a thinker, a sister, a friend, a persistent activist for change in the mental health services space. They reminded me of myself and saved my life by helping me restore my identity. This is the role of peer workers in mental health.

I work across five community health centres and two hospitals as a senior peer worker. This is a role that echoes the hierarchy in other professional groups; for example, a senior social worker or senior occupational therapist.

I provide supervision, training and strategic direction to the peer workforce group, systemic advocacy within the mental health service and group and individual peer work with consumers using our service.

What is a peer worker? A person with lived experience who works to use their experience for the benefit of others. A person who is aware of power dynamics and makes a conscious effort to subvert them, giving the consumer more power and leadership in the mental health journey.

Being a senior peer worker could be described as an oxymoron. A peer worker is someone who is of equal status to the person they are working with. This is problematic in a similar way to being a peer worker. Are we a person's peer if we have the key to the hospital door? We can walk away, and they are left behind, locked inside. We must vocalise this power dynamic at all levels. We cannot pretend that the imbalance is not there. We must help people to get free of the cycle of dependence on mental health services.

Essentially, peer work is about being part of a learning community and a listening tribe. We use our life experiences to learn from each other. Peer work is about listening and providing space for different experiences that are commonly labelled as mental illness. A space where we can find like-minded folks to have open discussions. We tell our stories to shine a light in the darkness of discrimination and stigma against people like us. To help us regain our proper place in community as healers, teachers and radical change-makers.

REFLECTIVE QUESTION

Jemima identifies power imbalance as an issue and indicates a responsibility to address this. Given the legal context of involuntary treatment, how could this be effectively done?

INTERPROFESSIONAL PERSPECTIVES

Michael – security services

Security services work in well with nurses, doctors and mental health practitioners.

We see our security service as the friendly but assertive person who helps in times of crisis; we manage people, not circumstances. As security, we understand that people may be distressed or angry about issues pertaining to their stay in hospital, and our approach to these situations is to strike a calm and empathetic tone.

Hospital security is more than the standard 'bouncer' position. The hospital security staff work side by side with the clinical team to ensure patient and staff safety, which is the foundation of our service delivery. We have evolved our approach to security in the healthcare environment, using tools such as de-escalation, a key component in the management of aggression.

You would also note this in our appearance, which is tailored to be more approachable and customer-service orientated, and this assists us with patients who are elevated. Instead of a hostile approach we utilise our experiences and speak with people to try and find a common ground so that staff, security and the patient stay safe.

Security falls under a clinical structure, and we form part of the clinical management of patients. We are included in the team discussions about the safety of staff, patients and others.

Security has the mindset of talking with someone to gain compliance, instead of going directly to a restraint that has the potential to injure both the patient and other staff.

REFLECTIVE QUESTION

The use of security can differ between general hospital settings and mental health services. Describe the differences.

Dietitians

A small but growing part of the mental health workforce, dietitians are making contributions to helping with preventative and treatment approaches to the lives of people who experience mental health problems. This is particularly important in eating disorders, and addressing the metabolic syndrome that is increasingly experienced. Dietitians are part of an unregulated workforce, prepared by a university program. Mental health is not a compulsory component of this bachelor's degree, although some students may undertake a mental-health specific clinical placement.

Speech pathologists

Expertise in swallowing and speech provides skills that are useful in particular for people experiencing mental health problems. Dysphagia is a common experience of consumers being treated with anti-psychotic medications. Speech disorders are also prevalent. Speech pathologists undertake preparation at university through an undergraduate program. Not all students undertake mental health placements, but mental health theory is covered in most of these courses. Speech pathology is not a regulated profession in the health workforce.

Clergy

As historical providers of mental health services, the religious, or clergy, continue as part of the workforce in mental health. There is some resurgence in engagement by clergy, now utilising a multi-denominational model that reflects the spiritual allegiances of consumers of mental health services.

Police

The police force performs a critical role in mental health services as the first point of contact of many people experiencing distress. Under the mental health legislation of many jurisdictions, police officers are given power to transport people involuntarily to designated places for assessment of their mental health. Police officers are educated through a mix of training provided within the police force, in the community and at university level. Education about mental health problems is variable.

Mental health nurses work with police in various jurisdictions to provide assessment and support for people in distress. Recent pilot studies in New South Wales (NSW), for example, are being expanded due to successful evaluation to 10 police-area commands and districts. NSW police reports around 55 000 mental health referrals annually (Smith, 2020). The Police, Ambulance and Clinician Emergency Response (PACER) program offers expert mental health nurse support to police and ambulance officers who are called to mental health emergencies in NSW, Australian Capital Territory (ACT) and Victoria.

Paramedics

The education of the paramedic workforce has undergone transition from training within the ambulance service to education within a university structure. As first responders in the health workforce, paramedics also perform this role in mental health services. In Australia, special powers are conferred upon paramedics under mental health legislation to transport people involuntarily to mental health services for assessment (see, e.g. section 20 of the *Mental Health Act 2007* (NSW)). In 2018, paramedics became a regulated workforce in Australia following a period of transition.

INTERPROFESSIONAL PERSPECTIVES

Tara – paramedic

The responsibilities of paramedics when treating people with acute mental ill-health have changed dramatically over the past 20 years. Over this time, ambulance legislation has moved away from the paternalistic 'protection' of individuals experiencing acute mental ill-health to focus on the recognition of people's civil rights (Parsons, O'Brien & O'Meara, 2011; Townsend & Luck, 2009). Community-based services such as local assessment and support services are vastly inadequate, which leaves people within the community with no other option other than to call an ambulance when they are unwell (Bradbury et al., 2017; Roberts & Henderson, 2009; Roggenkamp et al., 2018). Approximately 10 per cent of all ambulance calls are for mental health-related presentations (Roggenkamp et al., 2018).

The *Mental Health Act 2007* (NSW) accommodated increased responsibility and intervention of paramedics when treating acute mental ill-health. Paramedics became the preferred responders to people with acute mental distress (Townsend & Luck, 2009).

Paramedics in NSW are now able to perform de-escalation of high-risk situations, restrain people when all other options are exhausted and sedate for acute behavioural disturbance with midazolam and droperidol (Nambiar et al., 2020; Townsend & Luck, 2009). Droperidol has been shown to have fewer side-effects and a shorter time to sedation (Page et al., 2018). Implementation of these growing responsibilities have highlighted the need to build skills and support through advanced education (Emond, O'Meara & Bish, 2019). The paramedic role has now been expanded to include community assistance, with specialist nurses and paramedics working together (Faddy et al., 2017).

Hospital and community pharmacists

Specialist mental health pharmacy professionals are not commonly employed in the mental health sector, except in large population centres. This regulated health workforce makes critical contributions to interventions in mental health care. Within the hospital environment, it could probably be argued that the contribution of pharmacists is more specialised, due to the extensive role of psychopharmacology in supporting consumers' recovery. The medication reconciliation function that pharmacists add to care is essential. Community pharmacists have an important collaborative role to help maintain a consumer's well-being. They are a mainstay for people's continuing support, and work collaboratively with the consumer and multidisciplinary teams (MDTs). Clozapine-dispensing rights illustrate this clearly. Pharmacists are prepared with an undergraduate bachelor's degree.

INTERPROFESSIONAL PERSPECTIVE

Sarah – pharmacist

Mental health pharmacists provide great benefits in the pharmacological management of consumers by ensuring quality use of medicines. This includes 'choosing suitable medicines if a medicine is considered necessary and using medicines safely and effectively' (Australian Diabetes Educators Association, 2004). For example, they work as clozapine coordinators involved in registration of patients, blood-test monitoring, dispensing clozapine and guiding the appropriate dose for initiation, or re-initiation if there was interruption to therapy. They follow up with patients' round to provide support in case they are experiencing problems with medication. These interventions can range from assessing the appropriate dose of psychotropic medicines, changing medicines following adverse drug effects or serious drug-to-drug interaction or drug-to-disease interaction and providing drug information, to organising discharge medications with dose-administration aids.

REFLECTIVE QUESTION
What skills and knowledge would specialist mental health pharmacists bring to the MDT?

Exercise physiologists

Exercise physiologists (EPs) hold a four-year university degree and are allied health professionals who specialise in the delivery of exercise for the prevention and management of chronic diseases and injuries. Currently, EPs are not a regulated health workforce in Australia or Aotearoa New Zealand.

Accredited persons

Under the provisions of the *Mental Health Act 2007* (NSW) and amendments, and legislation in other jurisdictions, there is the capacity for experienced mental health workers from relevant clinical settings to gain recognised qualifications that enable them to utilise the compulsory assessment provisions of the relevant Acts. These individuals must be nominated by their employer to confirm this is part of the role and must undergo a specific course that qualifies them for a specific period (three years in New South Wales). Their performance is audited, and re-qualification is required to maintain these powers.

The roles of accredited persons provide a degree of flexibility in the implementation of the Acts, allowing its compulsory assessment provisions to be brought to bear in circumstances in which medical staff are absent or unavailable. This is particularly evident in rural and remote settings but is also witnessed in metropolitan community settings. The role of the accredited person can assist in avoiding the use of police or paramedic groups, who also have independent powers under the Acts, and may provide greater continuity in care and perhaps lessen stigmatising outcomes.

Ro's story – accredited person

I work as a clinical nurse specialist and accredited person on a busy community mental health acute care service (ACS), in metropolitan Sydney. Before moving to community mental health about 8 years ago, I worked as an in-patient registered nurse in mental health. I've been an accredited person for most of my time in the community.

An accredited person under the *Mental Health Act 2007* (NSW) is a non-medical health clinician with at least 5 years' experience as a mental health practitioner. We are nominated by our employer to undertake accreditation. My initial training was through a course run by the Royal Institute of Psychiatry at Cumberland Hospital. The course is now offered by the Health Education and Training Institute (NSW) at several locations annually throughout NSW. Unlike a medical officer, an accredited person is required to pass a triannual online examination to maintain their accredited status.

At work, most of our referrals for mental health assessments are from police or family members but they also come from community mental health teams, education providers, other health clinicians and the public. We assess clients at home, in police stations, in public places such as parks and transport hubs, and at the health centre. We do this, 7 days per week, with two shifts per day.

Treating a client in the community is always our preferred option. The assessment is comprehensive and includes a review of their mental health history, family history and physical well-being.

When a client cannot be treated at home, the least restrictive option, due to factors such as risk (to self and others), distress, disorganisation, insight, judgement and likelihood of further deterioration, is further assessment in hospital. The client may agree that they need hospitalisation, and further assessment and an admission can be arranged.

When further assessment is necessary but the client refuses or lacks the capacity to agree due to their mental state, an accredited person can write both Mentally Ill (S19) and Mentally Disordered (S19.31) Schedules (as distinct from police and ambulance, who write only Mentally Disordered Schedules). Almost all schedules written by accredited persons are upheld. The schedule itself is a document requiring involuntary, further assessment at a gazetted facility. It is an onerous responsibility to compel someone against their will, and frightening or disempowering for the person scheduled.

Sometimes a client will be scheduled on the initial assessment, other times after a failed community engagement, with an escalation of risks and deterioration in mental state. When clients are scheduled to hospital, they may need to be medically cleared by the emergency department, where both their mental and physical health are assessed.

Where possible, the schedule is an inclusive act, with the welfare of the person scheduled considered paramount. Their dignity and privacy must be safeguarded. Their questions must be answered and the process explained.

There is a Memorandum of Understanding with emergency services, and where possible we transport clients in our car. The next option is a police officer with us in the car or by ambulance. Clients are seldom transported in a police vehicle. Carers and family are consulted where possible, and collateral information obtained. A comprehensive mental health assessment is completed for all admissions from the community and accompanies the client who has been scheduled.

This is vital for the client, their family and carers, but it is also essential for continuing care. Working as an accredited person in the community means that when clients are discharged from hospital they are referred to community mental health for post-discharge follow up.

REFLECTIVE QUESTION

What principles would guide you to employ the involuntary provisions of mental health legislation?

Counsellor

Counsellors are part of the mental health workforce that is unregulated and their educational training can be extremely varied. Some undertake formal, assessed programs but essentially this is not a requirement to self-described as a counsellor. Approaches and interventions can widely vary. Employment is primarily within non-government organisations (NGOs).

Welfare worker

This non-regulated health practitioner has a similar role to counsellors, with varied educational preparation. The NGO sector is the primary employer of these workers in mental health services.

Mental health services

Private sector

Private mental health services offer care for a broad range of issues, but only for people with a voluntary status under the *Mental Health Act 2007* (NSW) or equivalent. The availability of services is often greater than in public services, and admission can be arranged by mutual convenience. Staff assessment of risk may prevent admission to these services in some circumstances as private mental health services may not be equipped to support consumers considered at high risk of harm to self or others. In such circumstances, consumers may be admitted to public services.

INTERPROFESSIONAL PERSPECTIVE

Kathryn – NGO delivery of mental health services

NGOs play an important role in the person-centred recovery of individuals living with mental health issues. NGOs provide non-clinical, government-funded and community-based psychosocial services for individuals. The level of support is dependent on the individual's need, and the fundamental aim is to provide a coordinated-care approach to ensure that individuals receive the right level of care at the right time (Australian Government Department of Health, 2019).

NGOs operate within the National Stepped Care approach to mental health (Australian Government Department of Health, 2019), which allows individuals to move within the different levels of mental health care as required. NGOs offer a range of services, from early intervention to acute services. The ability to move between services enables consumers to take responsibility and control of their recovery, recognise signs and symptoms of deteriorating mental health and respond to the episodic nature of their mental illness by accessing the most appropriate support at the right time (Australian Government Department of Health, 2019). NGOs are linked with clinical services, forming a multi-agency care plan approach to working together in assisting consumers to assess their recovery progress and identify any deterioration with their mental health. This enables individuals to proactively transition to higher-intensity or lower-intensity services as required to meet their needs (PHN Western NSW, 2017).

A key element within person-centred recovery is the active involvement of people with lived experience in the co-design of services. Co-design enables consumers to utilise their expert knowledge of their lived experience to shape the types of support they would like to participate in and that will assist in increasing their personal capacity, increase their confidence and self-reliance on their strengths, and enhance their ability to self-determine and self-manage their recovery (Commonwealth of Australia, 2013a).

NGOs provide support to individuals with significant and permanent disability to test or retest their eligibility for National Disability Insurance Scheme (NDIS) funding, should they wish to (HNECC PHN, 2019). The multi-agency care approach creates pathways to access, supporting documentary evidence required for applications. A planned and coordinated approach to collating supporting evidence has been a key challenge in recent years, resulting in a lower-than-anticipated rate of successful NDIS applications among people living with psychosocial disability (Hancock et al., 2019). Coordinated care between NGOs, clinical services and individuals living with mental health issues removes barriers to accessing the required documentation and applying for NDIS funding. Funding through the NDIS allows individuals access to NDIS-funded psychosocial support.

Psychosocial services assist individuals to build capacity within their social support networks with family and community; assists in their recovery and supports their well-being; increases capacity in daily living skills; enables access to support to maintain employment and housing; assists in maintaining physical health and well-being; and provides psychoeducation and support for family, carers and individuals living with mental health issues (HNECC PHN, 2019).

For further discussion of the NDIS see Chapter 16.

Public sector

As in other health services, public mental health services provide for a wide variety of mental health needs across different settings. Provision of service is available for all problems; however, admission may not be readily available for less pressing problems. Mental health services in the public sector have the entire responsibility under mental health legislation. General public sector hospital services provide complex care when consumer needs involve more than mental health.

PERSONAL NARRATIVE

Rachael's story – mental health in general medical wards

Working in a general medical ward with mental health consumers has given me numerous challenges. Most consumers I work with often present after experiencing a crisis and require continuing medical treatment for the effects of overdoses or injuries from self-harm episodes. However, I also work with consumers who are experiencing a psychotic episode and require medical care. My first few months working in this field were spent trying to figure out if I was providing appropriate supportive care to the consumer or if there were aspects that were missing. With medical treatments, we know which steps treatment should follow, we know the treatment end points. In managing mental health consumers, the treatment course is not as certain, and this can create a lot of concern for the ward nurses. One of the biggest challenges I have faced is trying to ensure that there is consistency in the care provided to consumers.

Stigma continues to be attached to mental health crises, and trying to develop therapeutic relationships with consumers when other people can easily overhear conversations in a public ward can be difficult.

I have worked with colleagues in mental health to try and better understand the needs of the consumers and to make sure that we have as supportive an environment as we possibly can. We want to be able to help people, and there can be many different triggers for consumers on a general ward when compared to specialist units. There are very limited areas for consumers to seek respite from the noises of the wards so they can try to self-regulate. It becomes very important for me to be able to work with the consumer to identify their triggers and the interventions we can put in place to help them. We now have a mindfulness activity box on the ward for consumers, to try and help them with any anxiety and stress that they are feeling, and this has helped. Despite all the challenges, it is still incredibly rewarding.

REFLECTIVE QUESTION

What are the challenges you could face while supporting a patient with mental ill-health during a physical health admission?

Forensic mental health services

Forensic mental health services is an example of a specialist mental health service provided only by public health systems.

INTERPROFESSIONAL PERSPECTIVES

Carlie – forensic services

Forensic mental health services support the assessment and treatment of people who are in contact with the criminal justice system or who are at risk of offending behaviour. In Australia, depending on state or territory legislation, mental health care may be delivered in a secure hospital or within the prison environment. The environment can add complexity to practice, particularly within the prison environment, where correction officers are responsible for maintaining safety and control. Clinicians working in this environment have the added focus of supporting mental health within the security constraints. Secure hospitals do not typically have corrections officers but may have security staff to support the environment. Clinicians also support maintenance of the safe environment and rely heavily on relational security to do so. Relational security describes the knowledge and understanding a clinician has of the person they are working with and uses this information to form appropriate responses and care within the environment (Department of Health (UK), 2010). This relies heavily on the development of rapport and the therapeutic relationship, which is central to care delivery to support recovery.

Delivery of collaborative care involves close liaison with several professionals, including (but not limited to) other health professionals such as psychologists, occupational therapists, social workers and consumer consultants, to provide members of the Mental Health Tribunal (*Mental Health Act 2014* (Vic.)) or the consumer to obtain and navigate legal representation. Partnerships also exist with other mental health services and services within the community, to ensure the needs of the person are being met.

Interprofessional practice is not without its challenges. There are at times 'grey areas' in relation to disclosure of information to and between different members of the interprofessional team; challenges associated with balancing risk, safety and recovery; as well as varying levels of knowledge, skills and experiences between team members, which may influence their practice.

Regulation of the mental health workforce

The *Health Practitioners Competence Act 2003* legislates the health regulatory authorities in Aotearoa New Zealand. These authorities are 'responsible for the registration and oversight of practitioners in specified health professions' (Ministry of Health, 2014), which includes outlining the profession's scope of practice, prescribing qualifications necessary for practitioners to register, registering practitioners, issuing annual practising certificates and setting standards of competence. Each regulatory authority can investigate the competence and conduct of individual practitioners through professional conduct committees.

Australia commenced a national registration scheme for the pre-existing 14 registered health professions in 2010, and announced the intention to extend registration to include others progressively over time. The body created to coordinate this scheme is the Australian Health Practitioners Registration Authority (Ahpra). Each profession has a national board that is supported by Ahpra and is charged with the primary role of protection of the public. Ahpra manages the registration of health professionals and students around Australia. It is the body to which any member of the public may make a **notification** about a health professional or student. On behalf of the national boards, except in New South Wales, where the Health Professional Councils and Authority and the NSW Health Care Complaints Commission perform the role, Ahpra manages investigations into professional conduct, performance and the health of registered health professionals. It also publishes national registers of health professionals in a manner accessible to the public. Ahpra works with the individual boards in development of registration standards, codes and guidelines.

notification – conveying facts with the intention to apprise a person of a proceeding in which their interests are involved, or informing them of some fact the informer has a legal duty to communicate

Registered health professionals are those legally able to practice, within the scope of their registration. The current regulated health professions are 'Aboriginal and Torres Strait Islander health practitioners, Chinese medicine practitioners, chiropractors, dental practitioners, medical practitioners, medical radiation practitioners, nurses, midwives, occupational therapists, optometrists, osteopaths, paramedics, pharmacists, physiotherapists, podiatrists and psychologists' (Gillam et al., 2020).

Some of these professions, including dental practitioners, medical practitioners and nurses, have divisions into which are grouped specialties or health practitioners with different scopes of practice or preparation.

Professional associations

These groupings are organised by the professionals themselves to further the interests of that profession and the individuals engaged in the profession, and to protect the public. The roles of these associations are multifaceted but share as a central tenet the self-regulation of the professions' scope of practice. This control of the profession is powerful and is closely linked with the professional bodies' roles in protection of the public. In some ways these aspects of professional associations are in conflict. Protection of the public is addressed by standards of practice, ethics and education. However, professional associations also have characteristics of trade unions in their roles to promote the interests of their members and profession. In this way, professional associations can be charged with promoting self-interest and control of the profession.

In mental health nursing, the professional associations in Australia and Aotearoa New Zealand (ACMHN and NZCMHN) can be seen as embodying this contradiction. They are involved in protection of the public by developing standards for practice in this specialist field. They are also involved in policy development to establish the educational preparation standards recognised for practice in this field. Although intertwined with protection of the public, such an argument can also be interpreted as an effort to control this part of the health workforce.

REFLECTIVE QUESTION

What contribution to professional practice might membership of a professional association provide?

Professional standards for practice

Mental health nursing in Australia has a set of practice standards (2010) and a scope of practice (2013) devised by its professional body (ACMHN, 2010). However, these standards are voluntarily adopted by nurses practising in mental health and have no formal regulatory authority. Nursing practice in the field is also guided by competency standards administered by the Nursing and Midwifery Board of Australia, which are recognised by Ahpra (Nursing and Midwifery Board of Australia (NMBA), 2016). Overarching standards for the mental health workforce have been developed by the Australian government to guide all health practitioners, irrespective of their profession (Commonwealth of Australia, 2013b). As with the mental health nursing practice standards, the national practice standards for the mental health workforce (2013) do not have formal regulatory status but carry much informal weight in circumstances in which professional practice is called to account. The substance of the national standards for the mental health workforce is to provide guidelines for the development and implementation of appropriate practices.

The Ministry of Health in Aotearoa New Zealand is the government agency concerned with health policy, regulation and monitoring, among other functions. *Te Pou o te Whakaaro Nui* is the National Centre for Mental Health Research, Information and Workforce Development. The development of the first national mental health strategy in Aotearoa New Zealand was fundamental to the growth and quality improvement until 2005. *Te Tahuhu: Improving Mental Health 2005–2015: The Second New Zealand Mental Health and Addiction Plan* (Ministry of Health, 2005) augments the plan, which is titled *Looking Forward and Moving Forward Together with TeKokiri: The Mental Health and Addiction Action Plan 2006–2015* (Ministry of Health, 2006).

'Let's get real' is the mandated government framework since 2005 (Ministry of Health, 2005) and most recently renewed in 2018. It sets out the standards expected of people working within mental health and addiction services, irrespective of the type of organisation, profession or consumer group. 'Let's get real' comprises seven 'real skills' that are interrelated (Ministry of Health, 2011). The development of 'Let's get real' and the 'real skills' emerged from competency frameworks for mental health and addiction treatment services within Aotearoa New Zealand (Ministry of Health, 2011). The workforce in mental health services has a program of reform in line with these plans (Ministry of Health, 2018). The plan emphasises the social determinants of health by equipping the workforce with requisite skills across sectors including justice, housing, social sectors and health.

Effectiveness of interprofessional workforces

Historically, consumers of mental health services have been passive recipients of care, with minimal input into care. Recovery-based care emerged from a growing consumer movement in the 1970s–80s, designed to increase consumer involvement in care planning and treatment (Deegan, 1988). In the literature, recovery is depicted as a movement, paradigm, model and philosophy. Recovery is difficult to define, and every individual's journey is self-defined and unique, with the consumer considered an expert on their own needs and experience. All journeys of recovery are highly individual but the recovery model of mental health has as its underpinning a philosophy of empowerment, hope and therapeutic optimism.

Within the National Practice Standards for a Mental Health Workforce, a recovery-based approach to service delivery is emphasised (Commonwealth of Australia, 2013b), with recovery stated as a sense of hope, meaning and purpose in life, and an understanding of one's abilities and disabilities alongside a personal and social identity. The term 'consumer' refers to a person who has engaged with mental health services. Implicit in the notion of recovery is the position that the consumer is active in their treatment plan, and that the treatment is a partnership between the consumer and the interprofessional team (IPT).

The concept of recovery has changed the ways in which mental health services are now structured. Consumer and carer participation have been important aspects of government policy for more than 30 years, requiring consumer input into mental health service planning and delivery. An underpinning principle of the National Practice Standards for a Mental Health Workforce is that consumers should educate mental health professionals while also having an active role in planning, implementation and evaluation of mental health services (Commonwealth of Australia, 2013b). This can be seen as a positive move for inclusive, recovery-based mental health services.

Team work

Teams matter in mental health, given the increasingly complex, knowledge-rich environment in which mental health professionals work. The IPT comprises a range of professionals from different agencies or organisations, working together to deliver comprehensive, consumer-centred care. This care is delivered under the umbrella of the IPT and can convey benefits to the consumer with specialised expert advice while also providing efficient use of resources. As the consumer's circumstances change, the IPT needs to adjust recovery plans with the consumer. The IPT composition should also reflect the consumer's changing needs.

New, evidence-based therapies are constantly emerging; pharmaceuticals are changing while changes in policies can have a direct effect on a consumer's finances or ability to work. No single professional group can be versed in all areas of a consumer's recovery. For a team to work effectively, there needs to be collaboration along with respect and shared leadership centred on the consumer. This can be on the basis of knowledge and experience, not necessarily of roles. For an IPT to function effectively, the team needs to work together and independently, relying on each other's knowledge and expertise to carry out tasks required to achieve the desired goal.

co-dependence – a psychological condition or a relationship in which a person is controlled or manipulated by another who is affected with a pathological condition (such as an addiction to alcohol or other substances); broadly, dependence on the needs of or control by another

This way of working can be daunting for many members of the IPT, as it challenges the traditional, biomedical model of mental health care in which the medical doctor has been the team leader. The recovery model requires a shift in IPT values and attitudes, but mostly it requires a fundamental shift in the power base. Recovery shifts power to the consumer, thereby challenging all IPT members' roles. Recovery challenges the IPT to develop practices that are less formal, enables the consumer to take risks and encourages independence, not **co-dependence**. This requires the function and values of the IPT to change with more discussion than direction, strengths-based, not psychopathology, and autonomous rather than paternalistic values. Empowerment of the consumer represents the civil right to autonomy and addresses power inequalities.

Barriers to implementation of IPT

Barriers to implementation of a recovery based IPT stem from the biomedical approach to mental health. Traditionally, many mental health professionals have worked within the custodial form of mental health, with the biomedical approach being the dominant model of care. This has led inadvertently to dependence on the biomedical approach to care, with many consumers only receiving care within the hospital setting. Unfortunately, this directly affects the effectiveness of the recovery and needs to be addressed if the recovery approach is to be authentically engaged.

With a blurring of roles within the IPT, mental health practitioners are at times unclear about the role they are to perform. It can be challenging for members of the IPT to have a thorough understanding of each team member's role. The consumer can find it even more difficult to know who is responsible for their housing concerns, or medication issues, for example. Lack of role clarity extends to many mental health practitioners who are unsure of their roles and have difficulty describing mental health practice.

Practitioners' stigmatising attitudes towards mental illness can directly affect the functioning of the IPT when they are unable to acknowledge the person behind the distress (a Bháird et al., 2016; Storm, Hausken & Mikkelson, 2010). Some mental health practitioners nominate caring, counselling and alleviation of distress as their main roles within the IPT, whereas others talk of maintaining control and administering medications (Smart et al., 2018).

Reciprocal interdependence is defined as individuals working together while actively coordinating care, in collaboration with the consumer (Bharwani, Harris & Southwick, 2012). This can only occur if the team members have appropriate expertise and are able to speak safely, freely, openly and meaningfully with each other. Recovery for any consumer requires a well-functioning IPT, yet skills required for the team to work together are rarely addressed. These challenges need to be communicated, acknowledged, discussed and explored if the IPT is to work in the true sense of the recovery model (Smart et al., 2018).

Each IPT has a different approach, although every team should be based on sharing roles, power and knowledge. Leadership has emerged as a dominant theme in studies of IPTs (Aufegger et al., 2019; Lingard et al., 2012). Due to the structures of many medical models within the Australian and Aotearoa New Zealand healthcare systems, consumers may only be referred to another professional by a medical doctor, and many diagnostic tests may only be ordered by medical doctors. Therefore, regardless of the model that defines an IPT, it will still operate within a larger system in which a medical doctor's authority is required for certain procedures, such as involuntary admission, seclusion, discharge, ordering tests and referring consumers. This confers a special position upon medical doctors, with rights and responsibilities in the health system in part due to insurance arrangements. Although this may not be problematic, it does create a tension and a power imbalance within the IPT team. Due to their medico-legal responsibilities, medical doctors may be obliged to take control or be responsible for the team. With each healthcare worker expected to be part of the team, ultimately medical doctors may bear the responsibility and accountability in greater measure.

Looking after yourself

Healthcare work can be one of the most stressful occupations. Support systems such as mentoring, clinical supervision and preceptorship are essential for all healthcare workers. Mental health care is reliant on therapeutic communication skills, humanistic philosophy and knowledge of psychological therapies; therefore, traditional models of mentoring and preceptorship may not be adequate to address these needs. The development of clinical supervision is ideally suited to staff in mental health services. Clinical supervision incorporates a skills-based approach (reflection), which is often lacking in other forms of mentoring. It is a formal mentoring arrangement that enables practitioners to discuss their work.

PERSONAL NARRATIVE

James – rural and regional mental health

Engaging in rural and remote areas can pose many difficulties, but can also offer a great deal of job satisfaction. Working in a centralised telehealth service, we primarily were staffed by registered nurses and psychiatrists. The team worked as a virtual consultation liaison team for many small, low-resourced sites, day and night. These towns, however small, are often rich in character.

Working so far away from population centres, it is important to have a sense of where the person is presenting, to understand the identity of the place. This helps you practically by enabling the assessment of resources, access and capacity to work with the person accessing services. To have true outcomes though, you need to immerse yourself in that place, in the local team and engage in an interprofessional way.

Working in a place like Brewarrina, we would work with the local hospital staff, engaging in a plan that met the needs of the crisis. We would engage the local community mental health team, a social worker who understood the local needs and knew how to access services. We would work with the local Aboriginal Medical Service and talk to the Aboriginal Health Worker, who understood what general health options were available, knew the family of the consumer as well as who and how to engage in a culturally appropriate way. We would engage the local GP and community health nurses to ensure the medication offered was prescribed and given, and that the general health needs of the consumer were being met.

People with mental health needs are people with multifaceted requirements, necessitating complex responses from multiple sources. As you can see, in my work, working with others is not an option: it is the only way.

REFLECTIVE QUESTION
What are the challenges of rural settings for consumers and health professionals?

SUMMARY

This chapter has presented stories and information, supplemented with activities designed to deepen your understanding of:

• The most common disciplines and professions contributing to the mental health workforce. Students can examine the preparation, regulation and skills of the different members to attain an understanding of their roles.

- The importance for the consumer of a cohesive interprofessional mental health team. The strengths and the blurring of roles and subsequent uncertainties were explored in a critique of this model of health provision. This exploration of preparation, regulation and skills supports the students' recognition of the preparation and expertise brought to mental health care by different professions
- The emerging trends in the mental health workforce. The traditional mental health care professions were described, thus facilitating an appreciation of the magnitude of recent changes in the nature of professionals contributing to mental health care.
- The role of regulation for the mental health professions. The standards applying to the mental health workforce were explored. This content supports the understanding of the role that both regulation and standards play in the mental health workforce.

CRITICAL THINKING/LEARNING ACTIVITIES

1   Is goodwill sufficient preparation to work in the mental health workforce?
2   What minimal levels of educational preparation should be required for the (specialist) mental health workforce?
3   Explore the provisions and regulations addressing the support and mandatory notification for the mental health workforce if they experience mental health difficulties; for example, the health assessment for health practitioners or students if they experience an impairment that does or may adversely affect their capacity to practice.

LEARNING EXTENSION

When does a peer worker's allegiance to consumer advocacy change to organisational loyalty? Does payment, the nature of the employment body, or participation in policy development influence this?

Prepare a class debate to explore these issues, addressing the proposition: The concept of peer workers is doomed to failure as peer workers cannot pay allegiance to both an employer and their peers.

FURTHER READING

Australian College of Mental Health Nurses Inc (ACMHN). (2010). *Standards of Practice for Australian Mental Health Nurses 2010*. Canberra: ACMHN. Available from https://www .cambridge.org/highereducation/isbn/9781108984621/resources
The standards are concerned with the performance of mental health nurses across a range of clinical environments and include professional knowledge, skills and attitudes (attributes).

Australian College of Mental Health Nurses Inc (ACMHN). (2013). *Scope of Practice of Mental Health Nurses in Australia 2013*. Canberra: ACMHN. Available from https: www .cambridge.org/highereducation/isbn/9781108984621/resources
The standards clarify the scope of practice of mental health nurses, mental health policy and procedural frameworks, health systems and structures.

Australian Clinical Supervision Association (Website). Retrieved from http://clinicalsupervision.org.au/
This website is an Australia-wide resource from an association that supports clinical supervision for health practitioners.

Commonwealth of Australia. (2013). *National Practice Standards for The Mental Health Workforce*. Retrieved from https://www.health.gov.au/resources/publications/national-practice-standards-for-the-mental-health-workforce-2013

The standards outline capabilities that all mental health professionals should achieve in their work and complement discipline-specific practice standards and competencies in nursing, occupational therapy, psychiatry, psychology and social work.

Te Ao Māramatanga New Zealand College of Mental Health Nurses. (2012). *Standards of Practice for Mental Health Nursing in Aotearoa New Zealand*, 3rd edn. Retrieved from https://nzcmhn.org.nz/about-us/our-standards-of-practice-for-mental-health-nursing/

These standards underpin quality mental health nursing practice for all mental health nurses in Aotearoa New Zealand.

Te Pou. (2009). *National Guidelines for the Professional Supervision of Mental Health and Addiction Nurses*. Auckland: Te Pou, The National Centre of Mental Health Research, Information and Workforce Development.

These guidelines are intended to set a national direction for professional supervision.

REFERENCES

a Bháird, C. N., Xanthopoulou, P., Black, G., Michie, S., Pashayan, N. & Raine, R. (2016). Multidisciplinary team meetings in community mental health: A systematic review of their functions. *Mental Health Review Journal, 21*(2): 119–40.

Aufegger, L., Shariq, O., Bicknell, C., Ashrafian, H. & Darzi, A. (2019). Can shared leadership enhance clinical team management? A systematic review. *Leadership in Health Services, 32*(2): 309–35.

Australian Association of Social Workers (AASW). (2020). Accredited Mental Health Social Workers. Retrieved from https://www.aasw.asn.au/information-for-the-community/accredited-mental-health-social-workers

Australian College of Mental Health Nurses (ACMHN). (2010). *Standards of Practice for Australian Mental Health Nurses 2010*. Canberra: ACMHN.

——— (2013). *Scope of Practice 2013 and Standards of Practice 2010*. Canberra: ACMHN.

——— (2018). *National Framework for Mental Health Content in Pre-registration Nursing Programs 2018: Survey summary data and results*. Canberra: ACMHN.

Australian Diabetes Educators Association. (2004). *Managing Insulin Therapy in Ambulatory Care Settings: Guiding Principles*. Chifley: Australian Diabetes Educators Association.

Australian Government Department of Health Primary Health Network. (2019). PHN primary mental health care flexible funding pool programme guidance: Psychosocial support services for people with severe and episodic mental illness. Retrieved from https://www.health.gov.au/sites/default/files/documents/2021/04/primary-health-networks-phn-primary-mental-health-care-guidance-services-for-people-with-severe-mental-illness-primary-health-networks-phn-primary-mental-health-care-guidance-primary-mental-health-care-services-for-people-.pdf

Australian Institute of Health & Welfare (AIHW). (2019). *Mental Health Services in Australia*. Retrieved from https://www.aihw.gov.au/reports/mental-health-services/mental-health-services-in-australia/report-contents/mental-health-workforce/mental-health-nursing-workforce

Baltic Organisations' Network for Funding Science (BONUS). (2014). Strategic research agenda 2011–2017, update 2014. *The Joint Baltic Sea Research and Development programme*. Finland: BONUS.

Bharwani, A. M., Harris, G. C. & Southwick, F. S. (2012). Perspective: A business school view of medical interprofessional rounds: transforming rounding groups into rounding teams. *Academic Medicine, 87*(12): 1768–771.

Bradbury, J., Hutchinson, M., Hurley, J. & Stasa, H. (2017). Lived experience of involuntary transport under mental health legislation. *International Journal of Mental Health Nursing, 26*(6): 580–92.

Commonwealth of Australia. (2013a). A National Framework for Recovery-oriented Mental Health Services: Policy and theory. Retrieved from www.health.gov.au/internet/main/publishing.nsf/content/B2CA4C28D59C74EBCA257C1D0004A79D/$File/recovpol.pdf

——— (2013b). *National Practice Standards for a Mental Health Workforce 2013*. Canberra: Commonwealth of Australia.

Deegan, P. (1988). Recovery: The lived experience of rehabilitation. *Psychosocial Rehabilitation Journal*, *11*(4): 11–18.

Department of Health (UK). (2010). Your guide to relational security: See, Think, Act. Retrieved from https://assets.publishing.service.gov.uk/government/uploads/system/uploads/attachment_data/file/320249/See_Think_Act_2010.pdf

Emond, K., O'Meara, P. & Bish, M. (2019). Paramedic management of mental health related presentations: a scoping review. *Journal of Mental Health*, *28*(1): 89–96.

Faddy, S. C., McLaughlin, K. J., Cox, P. T. & Muthuswamy, S. S. (2017). The mental health acute assessment team: a collaborative approach to treating mental health patients in the community. *Australasian Psychiatry*, *25*(3): 262–5.

Gillam, M., Leach, M., Muller, J., Gonzalez-Chica, D., Jones, M., Muyambi, K., Walsh, S. & May, E. (2020). Availability and quality of publicly available health workforce data sources in Australia: A scoping review protocol. *BMJ Open*, *10*(1) Retrieved from https://bmjopen.bmj.com/content/bmjopen/10/1/e034400.full.pdf

GROW. (n.d.). *Grow: Mental wellbeing programs*. Retrieved from https://www.grow.org.au/

Hancock, N., Gye, B., Digolis, C., Smith-Merry, J., Borilovic, J. & De Vries, J. (2019). Commonwealth Mental Health Programs Monitoring Project: Tracking transitions of people from PIR, PHaMs and D2DL into the NDIS. Final Report. Sydney: University of Sydney & Community Mental Health Australia.

Health Professions Networks, Nursing & Midwifery & Human Resources for Health. (2010). *Framework for Action on Interprofessional Education & Collaborative Practice.* Geneva: World Health Organization.

Hunter New England and Central Coast Primary Health Network (HNECC PHN). (2019). Psychosocial support program (PSP) FAQs. Retrieved from https://hneccphn.imgix.net/assets/src/uploads/resources/Psychosocial-Support-Program-PSP-FAQs.pdf

Lingard, M., Durrant, M., Fleming-Caroll, B., Lowe, M., Rahotte, J., Sinclair, L. & Tallett, S. (2012). Conflicting messages: Examining the dynamics of leadership on interprofessional teams. *Academic Medicine*, *87*(12): 1762–7.

Mental Health Nurse Education Taskforce. (2008). *Final Report. Mental Health in Pre-Registration Nursing Courses*. Melbourne: Mental Health Workforce Advisory Committee. Retrieved from www.nhwt.gov.au

Ministry of Health. (2005). *Te Tahuhu: Improving Mental Health 2005–2015: The Second New Zealand Mental Health and Addiction Plan*. Wellington: Ministry of Health.

——— (2006). *Looking Forward and Moving Forward Together with TeKokiri: The Mental Health and Addiction Action Plan 2006–2015*. Wellington: Ministry of Health.

——— (2011). *Mental Health and Addiction Services for Older People and Dementia Services: Guideline for district health boards on an integrated approach to mental health and addiction services for older people and dementia services for people of any age*. Wellington: Ministry of Health.

——— (2014). *Professional and Regulatory Bodies*. Retrieved from https://www.health.govt.nz/new-zealand-health-system/key-health-sector-organisations-and-people/professional-and-regulatory-bodies

——— (2018). *Mental Health and Addiction Workforce Action Plan 2017–2021*, 2nd edn. Wellington: Ministry of Health.

Nambiar, D., Pearce, J. W., Bray, J., Stephenson, M., Nehme, Z., Masters, S. … Fatovich, D. (2020). Variations in the care of agitated patients in Australia and New Zealand ambulance services. *Emergency Medicine Australasia*, *32*(3): 438–45.

NSW Health. (2019). *PACER – Police, Ambulance, Clinical, Early, Response*. NSW Health. Retrieved from https://www.health.nsw.gov.au/innovation/2019awards/Pages/pacer.aspx

Nursing and Midwifery Board of Australia (NMBA). (2016). *Registered Nurses' Standards for Practice*. Canberra: NMBA.

Occupational Therapy Australia. (2020). About Occupational Therapy (Website). Retrieved from https://otaus.com.au/about/about-ot

Page, C. B., Parker, L. E., Rashford, S. J., Bosley, E., Isoardi, K. Z., Williamson, F. E. & Isbister, G. K. (2018). A prospective before and after study of droperidol for prehospital acute behavioral disturbance. *Prehospital Emergency Care, 22*(6): 713–21.

Parsons, V., O'Brien, L. & O'Meara, P. (2011). Mental health legislation: An era of change in paramedic clinical practice and responsibility. *International Paramedic Practice, 1*(1): 9–16.

PHN Western NSW, (2017). Western NSW PHN stepped care approach for mental health. Version 1, April.

Roberts, L. & Henderson, J. (2009). Paramedic perceptions of their role, education, training and working relationships when attending cases of mental illness. *Australasian Journal of Paramedicine, 7*(3).

Roggenkamp, R., Andrew, E., Nehme, Z., Cox, S. & Smith, K. (2018). Descriptive analysis of mental health-related presentations to emergency medical services. *Prehospital Emergency Care, 22*(4): 399–405.

Smart, C., Pollock, C., Aikman, L. & Willoughby, E. (2018). Power struggles in MDT meetings: Using different orders of interaction to understand the interplay of hierarchy, knowledge and accountability. In C. Smart & T. Auburn (eds), *Interprofessional Care and Mental Health: The language of mental health* (pp. 97–121). Palgrave Macmillan.

SMART Recovery Australia. (2021). *Smart Recovery: Life beyond addiction*. Retrieved from https://smartrecoveryaustralia.com.au/

Smith, A. (2020). Mental health nurses to be based at police stations. *Sydney Morning Herald*, 10 June. Retrieved from https://www.smh.com.au/politics/nsw/mental-health-nurses-to-be-based-at-police-stations-20200609-p550yf.html

Storm, M., Hausken, K. & Mikkelson, A. (2010). User involvement in in-patient mental health services: Operationalisation, empirical testing and validation. *Journal of Clinical Nursing, 19*: 1897–907.

Townsend, R. & Luck, M. (2009). Protective jurisdiction, patient autonomy and paramedics: The challenges of applying the NSW Mental Health Act. *Australasian Journal of Paramedicine, 7*(4).

Use of psychotropic medicines in mental health care

Mark Loughhead, Simon Bell,
Davi Macedo and Nicholas Procter

9

LEARNING OBJECTIVES

At the completion of this chapter, you should be able to:

1   Discuss consumer and community perceptions of the use of medicines in mental health care and the effects of these perceptions on patterns of help-seeking, consumer experience, medicine concordance and health outcomes.
2   Identify the major types of psychotropic medicines used in mental health care and the indications for which they are prescribed.
3   Understand the concept of shared decision-making as a means for assisting consumers, carers and families to be informed and involved in treatment decision-making.
4   Explore the limitations of the available evidence for the efficacy of psychotropics.
5   Identify common side-effects and adverse events associated with the use of psychotropic medicines, and link these with the appropriate selection of medicines, effective monitoring, consumer experiences and safety considerations.
6   Discuss the role of the mental health worker in the context of medicine use, including through partnerships with consumers, carers, pharmacists, medical specialists, general practitioners and support service providers.
7   Identify changes to the protocols for psychotropic administration and monitoring during the COVID-19 pandemic.

Introduction

This chapter provides an overview of the common medicines prescribed within mental health care and explores the ways in which personal narratives and social expectations can influence the experience of taking medicines. The chapter also looks at concepts and practices that influence the management of medicines and encourage safe and high-quality use of medicines. These concepts include consumer experience, concordance and shared decision-making. Facilitating a positive experience of medicinal use requires quality communication and team work, whereby nurses, psychologists, occupational therapists, dietitians, medical practitioners and pharmacists work in partnership with the consumer and their carers.

Why do I need to know about the use of medicines?

psychotropic medicine – a medicine that affects mental functioning, perception, emotions and behaviour

Psychotropic medicines are commonly used in medical treatment of many mental health conditions. Most health practitioners come into contact, on a daily basis, with people taking psychotropic medicines. Providing safe and high-quality health care requires you to understand the concepts and themes expressed within the learning objectives. This learning will help you to understand why the prescription of psychotropic medicines is linked to community attitudes and stigma towards mental illnesses, and why many consumers may be hesitant to take these medicines or may wish to discuss their experience of them. From a safety perspective, in this chapter you will learn about the side-effects of psychotropic medicines and how you can assist in identifying adverse events and monitor the health risks for consumers. The chapter also introduces the concept of shared decision-making, which is a framework that includes consumers and carers in treatment planning and helps them to understand and express their wishes and preferences regarding treatment. This, along with the focus on quality use of medicines, will encourage you to ensure that your healthcare practice is inclusive of consumers' needs and has a deep appreciation of person-centred care.

PERSONAL NARRATIVE

Sarah and Angela's story

Sarah: When I was 18 years old, I experienced a very difficult period after starting university. I was unsure about whether I really wanted to be at uni, and felt isolated and lost. After finding some new friends, I had fun smoking cannabis with them and then found myself smoking at parties at the weekends and also on campus. One day, while waiting for a class to start, I had a terrible reaction where I had disturbed thinking and paranoia. I kept thinking I knew people around me and had these feelings of 'rushes' racing down internally, from my head to my body. I panicked but felt I couldn't move and was stuck in this experience for some time. Eventually, I got up and spent hours walking through the city, wanting these feelings and thoughts to disappear – which they did.

Some weeks later, these experiences returned. I had intrusive, negative thoughts with suicidal and threating themes, and a running mental commentary on my behaviour and what I was thinking, which didn't seem to be 'me'. I was stuck in a highly anxious state. I was horrified of being mentally ill and found that my own thoughts and fears about my future would trigger panic attacks. After three days of pacing about the house, I agreed to go to the local doctor with my mother. We talked about the panic attacks and anxiety, and their relationship with my distressing experience after smoking marijuana. The doctor asked lots of questions about whether I was still smoking, or going to university, whether I was sleeping. He outlined the different types of medicine used to treat anxiety, and that we may need to consider if things didn't improve for me in the following few weeks. I was glad he also talked about other strategies, including relaxation, exercise and learning how to manage panic attacks. He asked us to come back for another appointment, as it was still too early to consider medicines.

Angela (Sarah's mother): I had strong reservations about medicines. Years earlier, my husband had been prescribed various antidepressants and benzodiazepines (Valium™ and Mogadon™) and these, along with my husband's alcohol use, had contributed to a number of upsets and crises. Also, I wondered whether something spiritual was happening to Sarah: our family are Spiritualists, so I took her to one of our leaders, who did a healing on her. That seemed to help Sarah, and the leader advised her about dealing with anxious thoughts and gave her some visualisation exercises.

Sarah: For me, it was like I had already made a decision about medicines without knowing much about their positive effects. To be medicated, I would have to be really sick, and I didn't want to be sick. In subsequent visits with the doctor, I talked about not wanting to use medicines, and we talked about other things I would do to cope. I wouldn't really tell him about the disturbing stuff in my head and I focused instead on the anxiety. After a while, I had longer gaps between seeing the doctor and pursued meditation and self-help resources.

REFLECTIVE QUESTIONS

- What are the roles of prior experience and health beliefs in shaping how a family responds to the use of medicines to treat mental illness?
- If you had met Sarah and Angela, as a health practitioner how would you engage them in discussion about the role of medicines, psychological therapies and lifestyle practices in the treatment of distress?

Community beliefs and understandings of psychiatric medicines

When consumers and their families are offered psychotropic medicines to treat a mental illness, they are drawn into a social context of beliefs and stereotypes about medicines and mental illness. As mental health and mental illness have traditionally been stigmatised topics, treatment with medicine can also elicit meanings or behaviours that reflect stigma. While many people benefit from medicines and have positive and open views about treatment, there is also uncertainty and doubt within the wider community and some consumer circles.

These views may stem from the controversial history of some specific groups of medicines regarding safety, side-effects, misuse or efficacy. Health professionals may also hold stereotypes about certain medicines, which can inadvertently reinforce stigma and negative community views.

For instance, anti-psychotic medicines may be seen to be stigmatised medicines due to the history of undesirable side-effects. This would include concerns associated with first-generation anti-psychotics such as **extra-pyramidal symptoms**, and also side-effects common to the second-generation anti-psychotics, such as weight gain and obesity (Sajatovic & Jenkins, 2007). Antidepressant medicines may also reflect perceptions about depression itself, in terms of beliefs about personal inadequacy and blame. There has been controversy regarding the selective serotonin re-uptake inhibitors (SSRIs, e.g. fluoxetine) and whether the medicine is associated with increased suicidal thoughts and behaviours in a small percentage of consumers (Marshall, Georgievskava & Georgievsky, 2009). A third group of psychotropic medicines, benzodiazepines, also has generated mixed views in the community. These include views that benzodiazepines can be over-prescribed, and that they are misused by people for recreational purposes. There are also concerns about physical dependence and withdrawal reactions (Marshall et al., 2009; Rosenbaum, 2005). Debates within the discipline of psychiatry continue regarding the appropriate use of benzodiazepines in treating different conditions (Starcevic, 2014).

While there remains uncertainty in the community, Australian surveys conducted by Jorm and colleagues (2007) indicate that in general the community is becoming more familiar with the role of medicines in treating mental health conditions. In Jorm and Wright's (2007) survey of the beliefs of young people and parents about effective interventions, medicines such as anti-psychotics and antidepressants received the most negative ratings for effectiveness when compared with other forms of help (e.g. counselling, informal supports, relaxation and physical activity). Less than 50 per cent of respondents rated the medicines as likely to be helpful, with 32–44 per cent rating antidepressants as helpful for depression and 21–28 per cent believing that anti-psychotics would assist a person experiencing psychosis (Jorm & Wright, 2007). A similar survey conducted four years later suggested that public belief in the effectiveness of these medicines was improving. While respondents continued to give higher ratings to counselling, informal care and lifestyle practices, a greater proportion believed that medicines for depression would be effective (59 per cent for depression, 63 per cent for depression with suicidal thoughts). Similarly for schizophrenia, more respondents believed that anti-psychotics would be an effective intervention (48 per cent for early schizophrenia, 52 per cent for chronic schizophrenia). More recently, a systematic review of surveys conducted globally showed that the use of psychotropics was recommended by 80 per cent of respondents for the treatment of psychotic-related conditions and by 70 per cent for depression. Although the review suggests there was an increased belief in the efficacy of psychotropics for these specific mental health conditions, psychologists and psychotherapists are preferred for the treatment of depression, particularly in Europe and the United States (Angermyer et al., 2017). Overall, these studies suggest that gaps between community understandings and recommended professional treatment can lead to delayed help-seeking, can influence treatment choice or cause issues with low 'adherence' (Reavley & Jorm, 2011).

Literature from the social sciences describe how consumers draw on their belief systems and other meanings when prescribed medicines. These meanings may be shaped by personal experience and community narratives. Smardon (2008) explores how both positive and negative narratives, including those from friends and the media, influence the

extra-pyramidal symptoms – reactions caused by the effects of early generation anti-psychotic medicines in the extra-pyramidal system of the brain; the medicine can lower the transmission of dopamine, causing symptoms such as tremors, restlessness, muscle spasms, rigidity and slowness

adherence – a term reflecting clinical perspectives on the extent to which a consumer follows the treatment recommendations (e.g. taking medicines or following dietary advice) of a healthcare professional

decisions and practices of consumers regarding antidepressants, or telling others about their use. Britten, Riley and Morgan (2010) synthesised the results of 12 qualitative studies, which indicated that the use of medicines emphasised the seriousness of the person's illness and 'serves as a daily reminder of their socially devalued status' (Britten et al., 2010, p. 216). Accordingly, many consumers work to minimise their use of medicines. The study also suggested that consumers worried about psychological dependence, side-effects and harms from long-term use.

INTERPROFESSIONAL PERSPECTIVES

What is the view of your profession?

Different professions in health care, such as nutrition and dietetics, medicine, nursing, occupational therapy, pharmacy, psychology and social work, may have different perspectives about the role of medicines in improving mental health status. The individual professions have diverse paradigms within which human functioning and the basis of therapeutic interventions are perceived.

Social workers are likely to emphasise the role of the social environment in contributing to mental distress, as well as being a site for intervention. Some professionals may be critical of the biomedical model, suggesting that it places too great an emphasis on disease, over the social determinants of health (Moses & Kirk, 2006).

Psychologists and psychotherapists tend to be focused on learning new skills and the connection between cognition, emotions and behaviours. Mindfulness and cognitive behavioural therapy (CBT) have an established evidence base as effective interventions for depression and anxiety. Evidence is emerging for these therapies in assisting people experiencing symptoms of psychosis (Morrison et al., 2012). Some psychologists (e.g. Breggin, 2016) are critical about psychotropic medicines and the influence of pharmaceutical companies on research and practice.

REFLECTIVE QUESTIONS

What is your profession's relationship with psychotropic medicines? Are there relevant clinical perspectives or areas of research?

Studies of consumer beliefs and perceptions by social scientists and clinicians suggest that consumers need to have clear information about the intention, mechanism, effects and risks associated with particular medicines. Research by Desplenter, Simoens and Laekeman (2006) indicated that educational interventions that aim to inform and educate consumers about the evidence for particular medicines can result in higher rates of commitment and understanding about medicines. The authors' systematic review noted that education based on the combination of oral and accessible written information had the greatest effect on consumer understanding (Desplenter et al., 2006).

Medicines used in mental health care

This section provides summaries of key groups of medicines used in mental health care. Anti-dementia medicines are included due to their relevance to mental health care of older people.

Where to find information

There is a large volume of information available about medicines used in mental health care. This information is of variable quality and should be critically appraised prior to use in practice or care. Highly reputable sources of information about medicines include the *Australian Medicines Handbook* (2020), *eTG Complete* by Therapeutic Guidelines (2020) and the *NPS MedicineWise* website (2020b). NPS MedicineWise also publishes the *Australian Prescriber*, a peer-reviewed journal for health professionals providing critical commentary on drugs (NPS MedicineWise, 2020a). Evidence about the benefits and risks of medicines changes as new research becomes available. It is important to check the publication dates of books, websites and clinical practice guidelines. Outdated information about medicines should be used cautiously (Day & Snowden, 2016). Pharmacists in Australia often supply consumer medicines information (CMI) leaflets when dispensing medicines. CMI are produced by the pharmaceutical companies that market these products according to requirements of the Therapeutic Goods Administration.

Antidepressants

Antidepressants are among the most widely prescribed medicines in Australia. Common types of antidepressants include SSRIs, tricyclic antidepressants (TCAs) and other antidepressants (e.g. mirtazapine, venlafaxine and reboxetine). Antidepressants are prescribed for a range of indications in addition to major depressive disorders, including anxiety disorders, eating disorders and neuropathic pain.

Antidepressants have similar effectiveness across these conditions, although consumers may respond differently to different agents. Selection of the antidepressant type is guided by the person's previous response to a particular antidepressant (past response predicts future response), comorbid illness, adverse event profile, likelihood of drug-to-drug interactions and safety in overdose (Australian Medicines Handbook, 2020).

SSRI antidepressants are generally considered first-line therapy for the treatment of major depression in adults. The recommended dose is dependent on the prescribing indication. Higher doses of antidepressants are not necessarily more effective than standard doses for treating depression. When prescribing higher doses of SSRIs for depression, small benefits in effectiveness may be partly offset by a higher incidence of adverse effects (Jakubovski et al., 2016). Higher doses of SSRIs are typically prescribed for eating disorders such as bulimia nervosa (Australian Medicines Handbook, 2020).

Antidepressants do not provide immediate relief of depressive symptoms. This may be one reason rates of antidepressant discontinuation and non-adherence are high immediately after commencing treatment. People prescribed antidepressants for the first time should be counselled that the full therapeutic effect may take six to eight weeks to be achieved, although improvement is often observed within the first three weeks. Approximately 50 per cent of adults with moderate-to-severe major depression respond to antidepressant treatment, and antidepressants are generally continued for four to 12 months following an episode of major depression (Australian Medicines Handbook, 2020).

Many people do not achieve the desired therapeutic response or may experience intolerable side-effects to the first antidepressant that they are prescribed. For this reason, antidepressant discontinuation or switching is common. Antidepressants are best discontinued gradually, to avoid **discontinuation syndromes** (Haddad, 2001). Switching strategies are dependent on the specific antidepressants prescribed. Switching may involve gradual **dose tapering** and a 'washout' period prior to starting the new antidepressant (Keks, Hope & Keough, 2016). In some cases, rapid antidepressant switching may involve cross-tapering, which is when the new medicine is started before the previous medicine is discontinued. Significant care is needed when adopting this approach, in order to avoid toxicity. Antidepressant monotherapy is generally preferred to antidepressant **combination therapy**. Combining antidepressants can increase the risk of adverse events there is no clear evidence for greater effectiveness of this strategy (Galling et al., 2015).

Depressive symptoms are highly prevalent in older people, including those with dementia. A Cochrane systematic review concluded that there is no strong evidence that antidepressants improve depression symptom scores in people with dementia, especially when used for periods longer than 12 weeks (Dudas et al., 2018). Although antidepressants remain widely prescribed in this patient population, antidepressants may be associated with a higher incidence of adverse events.

The role of antidepressants in treating major depression in children and adolescents is widely debated. Non-pharmacological approaches are considered first-line, and antidepressant prescription for children and adolescents is usually performed by psychiatrists (Australian Medicines Handbook, 2020). A network meta-analysis suggested that, despite a lack of high-quality evidence, fluoxetine with or without CBT may be the most appropriate in treatment of moderate-to-severe depression (Zhou et al., 2020). The decision to prescribe should be made on an individual-consumer basis and should be balanced against the risk of adverse events, including suicidality.

Evidence for the effectiveness of antidepressants for treating major depression in people with conditions such as cancer and epilepsy is limited (Maguire et al., 2015; Ostuzzi et al., 2018). In the absence of specific evidence, prescription is generally based on an individualised assessment of likely benefits and risks, based on evidence for effectiveness in the general population.

discontinuation syndrome – the onset of a group of symptoms that occur shortly after stopping a drug (antidepressant); these are resolved when the drug is restarted. Symptoms may occur across somatic (e.g. headache, lethargy), equilibrium (dizziness), sleep disturbance, gastrointestinal and affective (mood) groups.

dose tapering – the gradual reduction in the dosage of a drug over a planned period

combination therapy – the use of two or more drugs to treat a particular illness

Anti-dementia medicines

Anti-dementia medicines include the cholinesterase inhibitors (donepezil, rivastigmine and galantamine) and memantine. It is important for practitioners and carers to be aware that none of the currently available anti-dementia medicines has been shown to prevent Alzheimer's disease (AD) nor to modify AD pathology, and each have similar efficacy and safety (Tan et al., 2018). Anti-dementia medicines have been associated with only modest improvements in cognitive function; they may not improve neuropsychiatric symptoms (Blanco-Silvente et al., 2017). Treatment tapering and discontinuation should be considered as part of a shared decision-making approach in individuals who do not benefit, who are no longer experiencing benefit, and who are in severe or end-stage dementia (Reeve et al., 2019). Structured approaches to recognising and managing pain have shown promise in reducing the behavioural symptoms in people with dementia in aged-care facilities (Husebo et al.,

2011). However, recent European guidelines recommend against the routine prescribing of analgesics for behavioural symptoms, given that analgesics may also be associated with adverse effects (Frederiksen et al., 2020).

Side-effects of cholinesterase inhibitors and memantine include gastrointestinal symptoms (e.g. nausea, vomiting and diarrhoea), dizziness, drowsiness, bradycardia and syncope (Tan et al., 2018). There is little evidence that prescribing anti-dementia medicines for people with mild cognitive impairment affects progression to dementia (Russ & Morling, 2012). Complementary and alternative medicines (CAMs) are often taken to maintain or improve memory in people with dementia. In considering the evidence regarding effectiveness, *Ginkgo biloba* extract appears to be well tolerated, while evidence is mixed regarding its effectiveness in stabilising cognitive decline in people with established dementia (Birks et al., 2009; Tan et al., 2018).

Anti-psychotics

Antipsychotics are indicated for the management of psychotic disorders, including schizophrenia and bipolar disorder. Anti-psychotics can be classified into first-generation (e.g. haloperidol, chlorpromazine) and second-generation agents (olanzapine, risperidone, aripiprazole).

Non-adherence to anti-psychotic medicines is a leading cause of treatment relapse in people with psychotic disorders (Alvarez-Jimenez et al., 2012). Practitioners play an important role in encouraging continuing use of medicines. Long-acting, injectable formulations of anti-psychotics are associated with a 20–30 per cent risk of re-hospitalisation when compared to the use of oral formulations only (Tiihonen, Tanskanen and Taipale, 2018). Consumers taking anti-psychotic medications often report having unmet needs for information about the medication. Practitioners should be encouraged to provide verbal and written information to consumers and their carers.

Network meta-analyses of randomised controlled trials suggest that different anti-psychotics have similar efficacy in terms of reducing overall symptom scores in people with multi-episode schizophrenia (Huhn et al., 2019). However, clozapine has been demonstrated to have superior efficacy over other non-clozapine, second-generation anti-psychotics in cohort studies (Masuda et al., 2019). Newer anti-psychotics may be more effective in managing the negative symptoms (reduction in capacity and usual functioning such as blunted expression, decreased speech and slow movement) (Australian Medicines Handbook, 2020). The selection of medication is usually guided by the individual consumer's experience of effectiveness and adverse events. It is common for consumers who are prescribed anti-psychotics to treat psychotic disorder to switch between anti-psychotics in order to maximise treatment effectiveness and minimise adverse events. Clozapine is often prescribed for treatment-resistant schizophrenia (Siskind et al., 2016). Anti-psychotic monotherapy is preferred to anti-psychotic poly pharmacy, except when switching between anti-psychotics.

Despite having similar efficacy, the adverse-event profile of anti-psychotics varies from agent to agent. First-generation anti-psychotics are generally associated with a higher incidence of extra-pyramidal side-effects, when compared with the second-generation antipsychotics. However, second-generation anti-psychotics have been associated with clinically relevant weight gain and diabetes (Hirsch et al., 2017; Alonso-Pedrero, Bes-Rastrollo and Marti, 2019). Other adverse events may include sedation, anti-cholinergic side-effects, QT interval prolongation, orthostatic hypotension and an increase in prolactin (Australian

Medicines Handbook, 2020). Consumers prescribed clozapine in Australia are required to undergo regular blood tests and other monitoring because clozapine has been associated with infrequent, but potentially serious, adverse events including agranulocytosis and myocarditis. Neuroleptic malignant syndrome is a rare but potentially fatal adverse reaction associated with anti-psychotic use (Kaplan & Fisher, 2005).

Anti-psychotics are also prescribed to treat a variety of other mental and neurological conditions. This includes the behavioural and psychological symptoms (BPSD) of dementia. Widespread prescribing of anti-psychotics for the purposes of 'chemical restraint' has been highlighted by the *Interim Report of the Royal Commission into Aged Care Quality and Safety* (Royal Commission into Aged Care Quality and Safety, 2019), and the conclusions are that the risks outweigh the benefits in most circumstances. Anti-psychotic medication use in people with dementia has been associated with only modest improvements in behaviour, but an increased risk of adverse events, including stroke and all-cause mortality (Ma et al., 2014). Australia's *Clinical Practice Guidelines and Principles of Care for People with Dementia* (National Health and Medical Research Council Partnership Centre for Dealing with Cognitive and Related Functional Decline in Older People, 2016) highlight the importance of engaging in a full discussion with the person with dementia and their carers about possible treatment benefits and risks before initiating anti-psychotics. Many people prescribed anti-psychotics to manage BPSD can discontinue taking them without detrimental effects on behaviour (Declercq et al., 2013). Evidence does support the use of anti-psychotics to manage insomnia (Thompson et al., 2016). Similarly, there is currently insufficient evidence to support the prescription of anti-psychotics for the in-hospital treatment or prevention of delirium (Neufeld et al., 2016).

Benzodiazepines

Benzodiazepines are often prescribed to manage insomnia and anxiety. However, non-pharmacological approaches are preferred to pharmacological approaches for these conditions. The need to take a benzodiazepine should be carefully considered on an individual basis.

Benzodiazepine use is associated with moderate improvements in sleep duration but minimal improvement in sleep latency (Holbrook et al., 2000). However, benzodiazepines have been associated with a range of adverse events, including falls, fractures, oversedation and confusion (Australian Medicines Handbook, 2020). Benzodiazepines have also been associated with an increase in all-cause mortality (Parsaik et al., 2016), although this finding has not been consistent across all studies and settings (Gisev et al., 2011). For many consumers, the benefits associated with taking a benzodiazepine may not outweigh the risks.

If benzodiazepines are used to manage insomnia, then they are best used intermittently, for a short duration (2–4 weeks) and as part of a broader treatment plan (Australian Medicines Handbook, 2020). While guidelines recommend intermittent and short-term use, people often use benzodiazepines on a regular and long-term basis. Benzodiazepine withdrawal is often possible (Reeve et al. 2017) although abrupt cessation of benzodiazepines can produce withdrawal symptoms (e.g. rebound insomnia, irritability and anxiety) (Brett & Murnion, 2015). Withdrawal symptoms may occur among consumers who have used benzodiazepines on a regular and long-term basis. Withdrawal should be based on an individualised withdrawal plan, with the rate of dose-tapering based on the dose, duration, risk of relapse and how well tapering is tolerated (Brett & Murnion, 2015). Short-acting benzodiazepines can be less likely to cause residual sedation, particularly among people with renal impairment. However, both long and short-acting benzodiazepines have been associated with falls (Xing et al., 2014), and short-acting benzodiazepines may be more likely to cause acute withdrawal symptoms (Australian Medicines Handbook, 2020). Benzodiazepines are also prescribed for other indications, including seizures, alcohol withdrawal and acute agitation. The use of benzodiazepines for each of these indications is associated with a special range of considerations that are beyond the scope of this chapter (for more information, refer to the Australian Medicines Handbook, 2020).

REFLECTIVE QUESTION

A consumer asks you whether a certain medicine is safe to take and is known to be effective. Where would you go to find further information to support their decision-making?

Mood stabilisers

Medication treatment for bipolar disorder includes the treatment of acute mania and depressive episodes, and the prevention of mania and depressive symptom relapse (Khoo, 2012).

While evidence for medicine choice in bipolar disorder is limited, lithium is often considered the first-line mood stabiliser and the prophylaxis and treatment for acute mania, and is also considered moderately effective in the depressive phase of illness (McKnight et al., 2019; Australian Medicines Handbook, 2020). Lithium is often combined with an anti-psychotic medication for treating acute mania, with the combination associated with better change on mania rating scales than either lithium or anti-psychotics alone (Glue & Herbison, 2015). Valproate is also considered an alternative to lithium for treating mania, especially among consumers for whom lithium is unsuitable or not effective (Australian Medicines Handbook, 2020).

Approximately one-third of consumers with bipolar I disorder remain clinically well over the long-term on lithium monotherapy (Malhi & Outhred, 2016). However, there are no biological measures to predict which consumers will remain well. Continuous monitoring and dose adjustment are required. Consumers prescribed lithium are required to undergo regular blood tests. The dose required to reach the target therapeutic range varies considerably between individuals, with lower doses generally required in older people and those with renal impairment (Khoo, 2012). Consumers should be counselled on the signs of lithium toxicity (e.g. extreme thirst and frequent urination, nausea and vomiting) (Australian Medicines Handbook, 2020). The risk of lithium toxicity may be increased during periods of illness, excessive sweating or low fluid intake. Lithium is also associated with a range of other adverse events including tremor, hypothyroidism, weight gain and sedation (Khoo, 2012).

Other mood stabilisers and anti-psychotics have demonstrated efficacy for acute and maintenance treatment, although a range of additional factors need to be considered with the use of these medications. Despite being widely prescribed in bipolar disorder, evidence does not suggest that antidepressants act as mood stabilisers (Khoo, 2012). There is also a risk that antidepressants may induce mania or rapid cycling (Australian Medicines Handbook, 2020).

Opioids

Prescription of opioid analgesics used to be primarily restricted to the treatment of cancer pain. However, there has been a rapid increase in prescription of opioids for non-cancer pain, with more than 3 million Australians using and 1.9 million initiating opioid analgesics each year (Lalic et al., 2019). The reasons for this are likely to be multifactorial. Possible reasons include the tendency to initiate treatment at the level of analgesia corresponding to a person's level of current pain, to more aggressively treat acute pain and in an attempt to prevent chronic pain. This is due to the awareness that pain has been historically under-recognised and undertreated in specific settings, such as residential aged care (Tan et al., 2015).

Examples of opioids include oxycodone, morphine, fentanyl, buprenorphine, tramadol and codeine. A range of formations of opioids is available, including tablets, capsules, liquids and lozenges for oral administration, and patches. Patches are not suitable to treat acute pain because safe dose titration is not possible (Australian Medicines Handbook, 2020). Fentanyl patches should not be used in consumers who are opioid naive.

When using opioids, the provision of adequate analgesia needs to be balanced against the risk of adverse events. Common adverse events include nausea, drowsiness and constipation. Regular laxative use is indicated if a person is using opioids on a continuing basis. A serious adverse event is respiratory depression, and opioids should be used with caution in people with respiratory disease (Australian Medicines Handbook, 2020). Some opioids and their active metabolites can accumulate in people with renal impairment, and so dose reduction or prescription of an alternative opioid or non-opioid analgesic may be necessary (Bell et al., 2013).

Misuse of prescription opioids has emerged as a major public health concern in countries including Australia and the United States, and has been associated with fatal and non-fatal overdose, increased health-service utilisation, injection-related injuries or diseases, and criminal activity (Lalic et al., 2019). People seeking opioids with the intention to misuse do not necessarily display stereotypical drug-seeking behaviours (James, 2016). Opioid misuse is not restricted to prescription-only opioids such as oxycodone, fentanyl or buprenorphine. The misuse of codeine has also been associated with considerable harm.

PERSONAL NARRATIVE

Nino's story

In my late teens my world changed. Prior to this time, I was going well in school, getting good grades and had an active social life, which included great friendships and training in martial arts. At this time, around the end of high school, like many young people I started to experiment with drugs, mainly marijuana and later other substances. Many unusual experiences soon followed, which would change my life significantly. It started with me having difficulty sleeping and was soon followed by paranoid thoughts – thinking my family and friends were out to get me. This was then followed by racing thoughts, confusion, problems concentrating and what seems to be a complete change in who I thought I was. I started not trusting important people in my life, getting into verbal and at times physical fights with my friends and family because of paranoia.

I experienced increased anxiety and loss of interest in all areas of my life. This meant that I started to push away the people who had been so important in my life, and relationships broke down. I also found I couldn't relax and my mind felt like it was running at a million miles an hour. This led to increased drug use, which at first I thought would help my mind slow down, but soon became a major part of my life, with daily use as a form of self-medication that was only making things worse. I began to think I couldn't take this anymore and I started to have suicidal thoughts.

My family was really worried about me, and after much convincing I agreed to see my local GP for help. After a review by my GP and then a psychiatrist I was diagnosed with bipolar affective disorder, and it was recommended I start medication. This included an anti-psychotic to treat the mania and psychosis I was experiencing, a mood stabiliser and an antidepressant to control the depression and suicidal thoughts. I was so shocked that, firstly, I had been diagnosed with a major mental illness and, secondly, that it might mean I need to take medication for the rest of my life, or at least a long period. I knew very little about mental health at that time and so did my family. I saw this diagnosis as 'my life was over' and that I was crazy, which made me think I didn't have a future to look forward to and to question my life.

I now had to take medication for something I didn't understand, with one medication being an anti-psychotic. All I could think of was that 'psychotic' is what you see in the movies, being dangerous and out of control. This worried me because if I were thinking this I could only imagine what friends, partners and family would think. When I filled the script I was given an information sheet on the medications and all of them had possible, massive, side-effects, which I naturally thought I would experience many if not all of. This led me to not take the medication or to take it only when things got really bad.

For several years my life spiralled downwards, including hospital admissions and suicide attempts. In my most recent admission, I had a doctor and treating team who really helped me. For the first time, I agreed to take the medication and to learn how to manage my illness and address my drug use, which had become a major problem. I asked lots of questions about my treatment and found out that I may experience some side-effects but that these could be managed through regular monitoring and appointments with my doctor. I soon found that the medication really helped to control my manic and depressive episodes, and helped me to maintain a more normal life, including sleeping better and reduced anxiety, depression and psychosis. My family also received education about my condition, and this really helped them to help me and find the support they also needed.

Eventually, after years of torment, pain and also suffering, I started to turn my life around. A lot of this was due to education and learning about my illness and treatment. Today, I work full-time in a job I love, go to university part-time, have great relationships with my friends, family and wife, and enjoy a life that I didn't think was possible with a mental illness.

REFLECTIVE QUESTIONS

What would have made a difference in Nino's life when he was first diagnosed? What information would have been helpful to encourage him to accept treatment?

Shared decision-making in mental health treatment

Shared decision-making is a specific approach or model of practitioner–consumer decision-making that is gaining prominence across all of health care. It involves informed and facilitated decision-making when practitioners and consumers, including carers, are considering which treatment options to pursue, including surgery or specific medicines.

The emphasis in shared decision-making is on considering the best available evidence on the efficacy or benefits and costs of a particular treatment, when compared to other treatments or no treatment at all. Another emphasis is on involving consumers, in terms of their views, needs, preferences and experiences in the difference steps of decision-making and action. An example of these steps is provided in Table 9.1.

Table 9.1 Essential steps in shared decision-making

Essential steps	Key processes
Step 1: Seek the consumer's participation. Communicate that they have a choice and invite the consumer to be involved in decisions.	• Summarise the health problem, provide options, encourage participation, involve family and carers.
Step 2: Help the consumer explore and compare treatment options, including no treatment. Discuss the benefits and harms of each option, using evidence.	• Identify the consumer's knowledge, list options in plain language and communicate risks, benefits and unknown factors. • Use visual aids and information to illustrate evidence. • Use teach-back technique. For example, ask the consumer to explain the available options in their own words.
Step 3: Identify the consumer's values and preferences. For example, what matters most to them?	• Ask open-ended questions and listen with empathy.
Step 4: Reach a decision with the consumer. Decide together on the best option and arrange for a follow-up appointment.	• Assist in decision-making – is the consumer ready? • Confirm the decision and organise treatment.
Step 5: Evaluate shared decisions. Support your consumer so the treatment decision has a positive effect on their health outcomes.	• Monitor the consumer's treatment experience and assist them to manage barriers. • Revisit the decision with the consumer.

Source: Adapted from Agency for Health Care Research and Quality (2014).

One aspect of shared decision-making includes the use of **decision aids**. These are pamphlets, booklets, pictograms and other ways to present information and evidence about the treatment being discussed. Decision aids often help consumers to understand the context of their decision and the likely benefits, risks and costs (including side-effects) of using

decision aids – information tools that enable and encourage consumers to make informed decisions about their treatment options; information is provided about different options and likely benefits and costs, and can be used to support shared decision-making

a treatment. They can help consumers and families to identify how their own needs and preferences will matter in the decision. Part of the challenge of this approach is producing up-to-date decision aids that build in the most recent evidence from clinical trials, related research and consumer experience. Examples of decision aids in mental health care include the pamphlets 'Depression: Should I take antidepressants while I am pregnant?' (Healthwise, 2015) and 'Considering the role of antipsychotic medicines in my recovery plan' (US Department of Health & Human Services, 2015). Dr Patricia Deegan (a well-known consumer advocate based in the United States) has developed decision-making resources to assist consumers to identify and document their experiences and feelings prior to their medical consultations. These help consumers to be more prepared, knowledgeable and involved in care planning (MacDonald-Wilson et al., 2013).

Shared decision-making as a practice is promoted within Australia's National Safety and Quality Framework (Australian Commission on Safety and Quality in Health Care, 2010). This means that there is an expectation that our public and private health services will integrate the approach as standard practice across all areas of care. In the mental health context, there is a particular range of issues that make shared decision-making more complex but also more compelling. The central concern involves treatment decisions when consumers are acutely unwell and may not have the cognitive capacity to make informed decisions. This is a consideration in the legal context of care and possible treatment orders. There is also the history of consumers not readily being invited to participate in decision-making about their treatment, even when they may have stabilised and regained legal capacity (after experiencing psychosis).

Consumer experience and decisions about medicines

Dr Patricia Deegan is a lived-experience academic who has worked extensively to promote consumer rights and involvement in decision-making. Her study of consumer recovery stories illustrate that consumers often experience the negative effects of medicine, which confound their own life interests, such as pursuing education and hobbies, or affect their sexual relationships (Deegan, 2007). Consumers reported many side-effects, including sedation, 'foggy' thinking, weight gain and shaking, which limited these activities. Consumers often saw medicines as useful but also needed medicines that acted to support activities that provide meaning and purpose. Deegan coined the term 'personal medicine' to refer to the activities and practices that consumers felt contributed to their recovery. She argues that 'pill medicine', as prescribed by medical practitioners, needs to support the life interests of consumers rather than restricting or creating barriers to enjoying life (Deegan, 2007).

compliance – the extent to which a consumer's treatment behaviour complies with medical directions or orders

concordance – the idea that a consumer and their treating physician should make treatment-related decisions together and reach agreement regarding a treatment plan

Deegan also criticises the use of the term **compliance** in medicine use, as it refers to client's medicine-taking behaviour and does not value consumers' agency and autonomy. The term **concordance** has been proposed in the literature, as it refers to the nature of interaction between health professional and consumer. A concordant interaction may, in some cases, involve the health professional respecting a consumer's decision not to take a prescribed medicine. This reflects shared decision-making, which is based on both consumer experience and clinical knowledge (Bell et al., 2007). In most contexts, consumers will decide whether to continue with medicines, based on their experience of whether the medicine works for them, and concordance involves respecting this decision. This is evident in the statistic that approximately 50 per cent of consumers decide to continue anti-psychotic medicines, while 50 per cent do not (Aldridge, 2012).

Australian consumer experiences with medicines have been documented by several studies (Happell, Manias & Roper, 2004; Mental Health Commission of New South Wales, 2015: Salomon, Hamilton & Elsom 2014). Qualitative evidence on the experience of consumers taking anti-psychotic medicine suggests people often have significant information needs that need to be addressed, including information about side-effects, reasons for prescription and the time period or duration of treatment (Happell et al., 2004). When these needs are neglected a person's commitment to treatment is compromised. In Salomon and colleagues' (2014) investigation of consumers' discontinuation of anti-psychotic medicines, commonly cited reasons included consumers' dislike of the adverse effects of medicines and of the idea of being on medical treatment over the long term. Other reasons included 'feeling better in my life and didn't need them' and that 'they were not useful' (p. 920).

The literature suggests that unsafe withdrawal heightens the risk of relapse and rehospitalisation, whereby consumers who withdraw have a 50-per-cent relapse rate (Morken, Widen & Grawe, 2008). Consumers in the study by Salomon and colleagues (2014) reported common withdrawal symptoms as including problems sleeping, mood changes, increases in anxiety and agitation, increases in hallucinations and delusions, paranoia, headaches, memory loss, nightmares and nausea (p. 920). Psychiatrists, friends, family and counsellors/psychologists were cited as sources of support when deciding to stop taking medicine (Salomon et al., 2014).

Trust between consumers and mental health practitioners is supported by the qualities of effective and clear communication, listening, choice and empathy (Maidment, Brown & Calnan, 2011). Consumers report experiences in which their sense of trust is either strengthened by these qualities or undermined when communication is limited (e.g. a practitioner's lack of disclosure about medicines) or that choices are limited (compulsory treatment). A further issue is people's perceptions of uncertainty as the receivers of treatment, and practitioners not listening to concerns (Maidment et al., 2011).

A recent report on the mental health system in the state of Victoria points out that consumers often perceive mental healthcare practice as focused on risk management and crisis response. Thus, medicines are frequently used as the service's perferred treatment while other psychosocial resources and support services are often neglected. People seeking treatment and their families report that the support received in these services was overly focused on medicines without consideration of the person's further needs, and did not contribute to ameliorating people's well-being in the medium and long terms. (Armytage, Cockram, Fels & McSherry, 2019).

To seek insights into consumer's concerns and needs, a study by the Mental Health Commission of New South Wales (2015) undertook consultations and sought submissions from consumers, families, organisations and practitioners. It summarised several key issues regarding consumer experiences:

- Medicine as a complementary treatment option: people want prescription to occur in 'conjunction with non-pharmacological therapies' (p. 6).
- Living with the side-effects of medicine: consumers told of the various negative effects of medicines. Some consumers felt the benefits of medicines outweighed the negative side-effects, and this enabled them to continue. Others reported the effects to be debilitating.
- Positive experiences: medicines have helped many consumers to return to work and study, and to be more active with family and the community. 'They said medication could help them become well and stay well when it was part of broader treatment – and when they were involved in meaningful discussions about personal recovery goals' (p. 7).

Decision-making amid complex evidence for psychotropic medication use

Anti-psychotic use

Anti-psychotic medicines are seen as playing a major role in reducing distressing symptoms associated with psychosis. In the past 25 years, second-generation drugs have also increased the range of effective treatments available and have avoided the side-effects and negative outcomes associated with earlier treatments. However, second-generation drugs have also been associated with increased risks of metabolic-related illnesses, posing further challenges for consumers and mental health care (Nguyen, Brakoulias & Boyce, 2009).

For anti-psychotic medicines, a complex context of appraisal is emerging, given the diversity of studies reporting on longer-term health outcomes for people living with psychosis-related illness, and the role that both medicines and service design play in these outcomes. Editorials in psychiatric journals by Morrison and colleagues (2012) and Gordon and Green (2013) have summarised a range of study outcomes that offer challenges to the professions' consensus views that anti-psychotic drugs are central to effective treatment of schizophrenia and early psychosis. These studies relate to positive mental health outcomes from innovative service models across the European context, which place emphasis on psychosocial and community supports and reduced long-term use of medicines (see Bola & Mosher (2003) on the Italian Soteria project and also Gordon and Green (2013) on the Finnish Open Dialogue service model). Harrow, Jobe and Faull (2012) indicated that consumers living with schizophrenia who were not on medicines for long periods had increased periods of recovery, reduced rates of relapse and better internal resources for coping.

Health outcomes of anti-psychotics

A further area of evidence relates to negative health outcomes associated with some types of anti-psychotics. With the use of second-generation anti-psychotics there are increased health risks due to factors associated with metabolic syndrome: weight gain and hyperglycaemia, hypertension and hyperlipidaemia. More recently, a meta-analysis has suggested that anti-psychotic use raises mortality rates across all patient groups. The authors analysed data on 359 235 people using anti-psychotics. Among the most important findings was that the risk of mortality for consumers with dementia using anti-psychotic drugs is two-fold that of non-users. A similar high risk was also observed among consumers without dementia. The findings highlight that risk of all-cause mortality increases with greater doses. The authors recommend that anti-psychotics use should be closely monitored by nurses and other authorities (Ralph & Espinet, 2018).

The association between anti-psychotic exposure and increased mortality was not evident in a larger Finnish retrospective study (Fin11) published by Tiihonen and colleagues (2009). This work examined mortality (all-cause, including cardiovascular disease and suicide) within a very large cohort of consumers (66 881) in comparison to the country's overall population of 5.2 million. This study found that long-term, cumulative treatment (7–11 years) with any anti-psychotic treatment is associated with lower mortality when compared with no anti-psychotic treatments (Tiihonen et al., 2009).

Complex evidence on the efficacy of antidepressants

The mixed evidence on the effects of antidepressants is another example of the complexity involved in using psychotropic medicines for the treatment of mental health conditions. A meta-analysis of studies that highlight the superiority of antidepressants over placebo have been criticised and the clinical relevance of findings questioned (Jakobsen, Gluud & Kirsch, 2020). Criticism that we only know how antidepressants affect mental health in the short-term as evidence for antidepressant effectiveness is mostly based on 6-to-8-week clinical trials (Cipriani et al., 2018; McCormack & Korownyk, 2018). Furthermore, interpretations of a recent meta-analysis suggest that only 10–12 per cent of people in the treatment groups would benefit from antidepressants, compared to placebo treatment. This could mean, according to the authors, that 80 per cent of participants who get better are not improving because of the drug (McCormack & Korownyk, 2018).

Other authors hypothesise that depressive symptoms might improve naturally over time – as they might be the result of life experiences and contextual factors (Cipriani et al., 2018; McCormack & Korownyk, 2018). These critiques suggest that other options need to be considered with consumers when informing them about treatment options, including psychotherapy, sleeping habits, diet and exercise, and addressing psychosocial determinants of mental health (Jakobsen et al., 2020). When medication is the chosen therapy, it might be important to start with low doses and systematically re-evaluate the need for continuing treatment after a response is achieved (McCormack & Korownyk, 2018).

Clinical practice and experience of medicines

This context of evidence presents a challenge for consumers and practitioners when making decisions over which medicine-based treatment to choose. Given the heterogeneity of possible outcomes of medicines, the principle of individualised care and choice is heightened. The ability of both professional and consumer to build their literacy in understanding evidence is central. Consumers and families can make gradual, informed choices, in collaboration with practitioners. Also, given that choice may mean choosing not to take medicines, services need to be designed so that consumers continue to be offered psychosocial supports and therapies.

In their discussion of consumer experience and continuing use of medicines, Aldridge (2012) suggests that services adopt a position of 'non-adherence harm-reduction'. This includes service provision that widens the range of psychosocial supports available to consumers.

Aldridge (2012) also discusses the role of mental health nurses. Nurses can play a central role in supporting the autonomy of consumers, in recognising their capacity for choice. Listening to what consumers know about their medicine use and working to support their informed decision-making are key considerations. The advocacy role becomes important in assisting the consumer to have a voice, helping to document and express challenges that consumers may experience in their use of medicines, and encouraging effective problem-solving. Taking a non-judgemental stance is another practice highlighted by the authors. These roles can enhance engagement and encourage consumers to continue shared conversations about medicines rather than withdrawing from care.

PERSONAL NARRATIVE

John's story

In my early 20s I was diagnosed with schizoaffective disorder along with anxiety. To treat this the doctor recommended a range of medications, including regular antidepressants, mood stabilisers and anti-psychotics. He also recommended Valium for occasional use, to treat anxiety. My father had a mental illness so I was prepared to try medication because my dad was always better when he was receiving treatment. When he prescribed the medication, the doctor told me about possible side-effects and that I would need to have regular blood tests to monitor them. He also gave me some information on each medication and said to contact him if I had any questions or concerns. I started the medication but found I quickly developed some side-effects. The first was always being tired. I was used to having a fair bit of energy, and all of a sudden I felt like a zombie and found I was often late to work due to sleeping in. I also found that it was really hard to concentrate, especially in the mornings, which affected my university studies. I spoke to the doctor and he told me this was common and would improve a bit but would not go away completely. I was, however, really worried about getting very sick, so I kept going and just tried to have earlier nights and take my medication earlier in the day.

After being on medication for a little while I noticed that I felt really thirsty all the time and one very hot day I got really dehydrated, which led to a short hospital admission to get my fluids up. What I didn't know was that this was because of the lithium, which was my mood stabiliser, and I had to keep my fluids up and be careful on very hot days. The hospital staff also told me I should have blood tests to check my lithium levels every three months, as toxic levels can lead to kidney damage. I was okay with this but I was starting to feel a bit overwhelmed with it all and especially the kidney damage, as my grandfather had had kidney disease.

Not long after this I went through a period during which my anxiety got really bad so I ended up taking Valium pretty regularly and that seemed to help. However, I started to notice after a little while it wasn't working as well. I needed higher doses and I also started to feel that I couldn't cope without it. I chatted to my doctor and he said that I had been using too much and had built up a dependence. The doctor suggested I needed to stop using Valium and try some other medication but advised me that I may experience some withdrawals and to take it slowly. The doctor had told me, when it was first prescribed, that it could be addictive and to try not to use too much, but I didn't think this would happen so easily.

In addition to these side-effects, I started to put on weight and noticed that I was always hungry and particularly craving junk food. Soon I was 10 kilograms heavier. Once again I spoke to the doctor as he had said this could happen, and he suggested exercising more and trying to improve my diet, which was hard work. I managed to not put on much more weight but really struggled to get back to my previous weight.

I worked with my doctor on all these things and got them under control; when starting treatment, I didn't think there would be so many things I needed to address. The final, unexpected surprise was the cost of medications. After I started working full-time, I wasn't able to receive a healthcare concession card, and the costs increased significantly. Each script was over $30 and I was getting four scripts per month. Unfortunately, there wasn't anything I could do about this, and I was feeling much better on medication so I didn't want to stop.

REFLECTIVE QUESTIONS

• What are some of the problems John did not expect along with taking medications?
• How would you assist John in better managing his treatment?
• Considering John's experience, what could have happened if the doctor did not talk to him in detail about his treatment?

How can health practitioners assist consumers and carers to be more involved in treatment decision-making?

• Take an active interest in the person's experience of medicine use and what they see as the benefits and costs of using a particular medicine.
• Encourage the consumer to learn about the medicine they are taking. This includes finding written information from consumer sources such as NPS MedicineWise or by talking to a pharmacist.
• Listen to any complaints or negative comments about medicines and build trust. A consumer's experience is most often a valid one. If the consumer does not agree that they have an illness or need treatment, or if they are being treated involuntarily, then this is a different level of conversation. Here, you might note that others have identified that the person requires treatment but that you also appreciate that the consumer is dissatisfied with this. You can also focus on ways of helping the medicine use to be easier for the person. Consumers may be able to consider a longer-term plan for coming off medicines, in consultation with their medical practitioner.
• Encourage the consumer to prepare for medical consultations ahead of time. This can involve the consumer preparing a written summary of points and questions in advance. These can be about the drug's side-effects in the context of the consumer's lifestyle or to ask about practical strategies on how these can be reduced (see e.g. Therapeutic Guidelines, 2020).
• Encourage the consumer and their family to consider medicines in the context of a framework of benefits and costs. Benefits are likely to include reducing the effects of symptoms and enabling a focus on recovery activities.

TRANSLATION TO PRACTICE

Quality use of medicines and medicine reviews

In recent decades, Australia has developed an organised movement towards the quality use of medicines. *The National Strategy for Quality Use of Medicines* (QUM) (Commonwealth of Australia, 2002, p. 1) establishes the following definition:

QUM is one of the four objectives outlined in Australia's National Medicines Policy. It refers to the wise selection of management options (including recognising that non-pharmacological management options may be preferable), selecting medicines that are suitable for an individual and their clinical condition, and using medicines safely and effectively to achieve the best possible health outcomes.

QUM recognises that a multidisciplinary approach is needed to optimise the use of medicines. Examples of potential partners include consumers, carers, healthcare practitioners, healthcare facilities, the pharmaceutical industry, media and healthcare funders (Commonwealth of Australia, 2002). Achieving QUM is of major importance to public health. An estimated 250 000 hospitalisations occur each year in Australia, due to the direct or indirect harms associated with medicine use, with up to two-thirds of these hospitalisations considered potentially preventable (Pharmaceutical Society of Australia, 2019). Medicine safety and the quality use of medicines was declared Australia's 10th national health priority area in November 2019.

TRANSLATION TO PRACTICE

Quality use of medicines

Quality use of medicines means:

- Selecting management options wisely by:
  - considering the place of medicines in treating illness and maintaining health, and
  - recognising that there may be better ways than medicine to manage many disorders.
- Choosing suitable medicines if a medicine is considered necessary so that the best available option is selected by taking into account:
  - the individual
  - the clinical condition
  - risks and benefits
  - dosage and length of treatment
  - any co-existing conditions
  - other therapies
  - monitoring considerations
  - costs for the individual, the community and the health system as a whole.
- Using medicines safely and effectively to get the best possible results by:
  - monitoring outcomes
  - minimising misuse, over-use and under-use, and
  - improving people's ability to solve problems related to medication, such as negative effects or managing multiple medications.

Source: Commonwealth of Australia (2002, p. 1).

Role of the pharmacist in QUM

Pharmacists have increasingly important roles in working with consumers, carers and other healthcare practitioners to achieve QUM. Pharmacists now work across a range of healthcare settings, including in community pharmacies, hospitals, aged-care facilities and general practices. Medication errors often occur at the transitions between healthcare settings. This means that there are roles for pharmacists in ensuring QUM as people are admitted and discharged from hospitals or aged-care facilities.

Services provided by pharmacists in Australian hospitals include review of medicine orders, providing patient education, providing medicine information to nurses, medical and other healthcare practitioners, the manufacture of special medicinal products, monitoring and reporting of adverse events, advising which medicines should be included in the hospital formulary and conducting clinical trials (Society of Hospital Pharmacists of Australia, 2016).

Quality use of medicines in mental health

The QUM guiding principles of wise selection of management options, selecting suitable medicines and safe use of medicines have great significance for mental health care. Choosing options leads us to acknowledge the wider therapeutic or recovery context, in which other therapies and practices can have positive effects. It also highlights choice in relation to benefits and costs. Suitability and safety highlight the important roles of monitoring and evaluation regarding dosage levels and poly pharmacy implications.

An example of the need for monitoring and evaluation is in anti-psychotic use. A recent review on the prevalence of poly pharmacy in Australian consumers examined studies that focused on multiple anti-psychotic use, dosage levels and drug-related side-effects. Westaway and colleagues (2016) found that 19 studies reported varying rates of multiple anti-psychotic use, with the range of multiple use being from 5 to 61 per cent of consumers within respective studies. The authors also reviewed the studies for the dosage levels of consumers taking multiple treatments and found that between one-third and one-half of all consumers had received higher doses than recommended.

How can health practitioners promote better health outcomes for consumers using psychotropic medicines?

- Take an interest in the person's experience of medicine use and enquire about regular physical health monitoring. Ask about the things they do to manage their use of medicines.
- Consider how the consumer's psychotropic medicine use affects the area of health care you are assisting them with. For instance, if they have come into hospital for a diabetes-related crisis, is information about their mental health medicines available? How do these medicines interact with others, including CAMs?
- With consumer permission, engage with service providers responsible for the physical health monitoring and care planning. This may be the person's general practitioner, or it could be public mental health services (e.g. for a medicine such as clozapine). Ask about the monitoring and support processes that may be in place.
- Promote and support lifestyle and care practices that may help protect consumers from the effects of longer-term use of antipsychotics – these include having a healthy diet, regular exercise, regular monitoring and consumer self-knowledge.
- If the consumer is worried about the interactions of different medicines, you can recommend that they request a Home Medicines Review from their pharmacist. This is helpful if the consumer is also taking medicines for a range of chronic health conditions. The pharmacist will review the consumer's medicines for suitability and make recommendations to the doctor and consumer.

TRANSLATION TO PRACTICE

QUM has significance when considering the needs of people from diverse cultural and linguistic backgrounds. As Australia is one of the most multicultural societies in the world, there is a great need to ensure the availability of bilingual or multilingual information regarding safe use of medicines and that literacy issues are taken into account. There is a growing range of bilingual resources regarding different types of psychotropic medication (Transcultural Mental Health Centre, 2015).

Use of psychotropics during a pandemic

The social isolation and lockdown recommendations experienced during the COVID-19 pandemic imposed unforeseen challenges to the management of pharmacological treatment for people in in-patient and out-patient care settings. Initiatives to assist consumers to continue to access medicines during the COVID-19 pandemic (Bell et al., 2020) included digital image prescriptions, fast-tracking of electronic prescribing, continued dispensing by pharmacists and telehealth medication review. Withdrawal or reduction of dosages during the pandemic and in its aftermath was needed, as people were potentially vulnerable to the social and economic changes provoked by the pandemic. Possible increased continuation of psychotropic medication over non-pharmacological approaches was anecdotally observed due to social distancing restrictions. In aged-care facilities, the use of antidepressants and benzodiazepines increased to assist consumers to cope with depression, anxiety and reduced social contact.

Another implication of the pandemic is in relation to long-acting injections (LAIs). To avoid COVID-19 contamination, the number of LAIs administered decreased in some settings, with consumers opting for the more manageable and easy-to-obtain oral medicines (Ifteni, Dima & Teodorescu, 2020).

SUMMARY

This chapter has presented stories and information, supplemented with activities designed to deepen your understanding of:

- Community and personal attitudes and their influence on consumers' decision-making when being prescribed a psychotropic medicine. It is important to listen to consumers about their experience of using psychotropic medicines and to engage consumers and carers in effective problem-solving and shared decision-making.
- The main groups of psychotropic medicines used in mental health care, including medicines for anxiety, depression and psychosis-related illness.
- The importance of understanding safety and quality in the use of medicines, including awareness about common side-effects and adverse events associated with psychotropic medicines, and ways of finding reputable information for consumers and health practitioners.
- Shared decision-making as an approach to, or model of, practitioner–consumer decision-making, which is gaining prominence across all of health care. Shared decision-making considers the best evidence for possible forms of treatment and emphasises the importance

of the consumer in terms of contributing their views, needs, preferences and experiences. Decision aids are used to promote health literacy and to empower consumers.

- Roles that build trusting relationships with consumers and encourage leadership in promoting effective health screening, monitoring for adverse events, and care planning that includes healthy diet and lifestyle practices. The chapter promoted a team-based approach to including both physical and mental health care needs across the healthcare system.

CRITICAL THINKING/LEARNING ACTIVITIES

1   Describe some of the benefits and some of the limitations of taking psychotropic medication.
2   Working on your own or in a small group, brainstorm some reasons consumers may feel their lived experience of medicine use is not well recognised or acknowledged by practitioners. What can be done by practitioners to rectify this situation?
3   Describe how shared decision-making and consumer engagement could be achieved in both (a) an in-patient setting and (b) a community setting.
4   How can person-centred recovery care be advanced and supported by practitioners working with consumers who are taking psychotropic medications?
5   What are some of the challenges to psychotropic treatment that can be experienced during an event such as the COVID-19 pandemic? What are some of the strategies to circumvent such challenges?

LEARNING EXTENSION

The resource available from the link below is designed to help practitioners work with consumers for whom 'non-adherence with psychiatric medication is common and is associated with an increase in rehospitalisation and poorer outcomes' (Cavezza, 2013). Working with others, critically review the resource against consumer experience and decisions about medicines discussed in this chapter. Discuss how and where changes could and should be made to advance a person-centred recovery approach.

Cavezza, C. (2013). A consumer centred intervention to enhance antipsychotic medication adherence. *InPsych, 35*(2). Retrieved from https://www.psychology.org.au/publications/inpsych/2013/april/cavezza

FURTHER READING

iphYs (Website). Retrieved from http://www.iphys.org.au
This website has interesting resources about screening and management for young people using anti-psychotic medicines. The 'Right from the Start' resource and early intervention frameworks (algorithms) provide details of recommended interventions.

NPS Medicinewise Learning (Website). Retrieved from http://learn.nps.org.au
This website is very useful for accessing information about specific medicines and evidence about the benefits and risks.

REFERENCES

Agency for Health Care Research and Quality. (2014). *The SHARE Approach Essential Steps of Shared Decision Making: Quick Reference Guide.* Washington, DC: Department of Health and Human Resources.

Aldridge, M. (2012). Addressing non-adherence to antipsychotic medication: A harm-reduction approach. *Journal of Psychiatric and Mental Health Nursing, 19*(1): 85–96.

Alonso-Pedrero, L., Bes-Rastrollo, M. & Marti, A. (2019). Effects of antidepressant and antipsychotic use on weight gain: A systematic review. *Obesity Reviews, 20*(12): 1680–90.

Alvarez-Jimenez, M., Priede, A., Hetrick, S. E., Bendall, S., Killackey, E., Parker, A. G. ... Gleeson, J. F. (2012). Risk factors for relapse following treatment for first episode psychosis: A systematic review and meta-analysis of longitudinal studies. *Schizophrenia Research, 139*(1–3): 116–28.

Angermeyer, M. C., Van Der Auwera, S., Carta, M. G. & Schomerus, G. (2017). Public attitudes towards psychiatry and psychiatric treatment at the beginning of the 21st century: A systematic review and meta-analysis of population surveys. *World Psychiatry, 16*(1), 50–61.

Armytage, P., Cockram, A., Fels, A. & McSherry, B. (2019). *Royal Commission into Victoria's Mental Health System, Interim report.* Retrieved from https://rcvmhs.vic.gov.au/interim-report

Australian Commission on Safety and Quality in Health Care. (2010). *Australian Safety and Quality Framework for Health Care.* Retrieved from http://www.safetyandquality.gov.au/national-priorities/australian-safety-and-quality-framework-for-health-care/

Australian Medicines Handbook Pty Ltd. (2020). *Australian Medicines Handbook.* Adelaide: Australian Medicines Handbook Pty Ltd.

Bell, J. S., Airaksinen, M. S., Lyles, A., Chen, T. F. & Aslani, P. (2007). Concordance is not synonymous with compliance or adherence. *British Journal of Clinical Pharmacology, 64*(5): 710–11.

Bell, J. S., Blacker, N., Leblanc, V. T., Alderman, C. P., Phillips, A., Rowett, D. ... Husband, A. (2013). Prescribing for older people with chronic renal impairment. *Australian Family Physician, 42*(1–2): 24–8.

Bell, J. S., Reynolds, L., Freeman, C. & Jackson, J. K. (2020). Strategies to promotes access to medications during the COVID-19 pandemic. *Australian Journal of General Practice, 49*(8).

Birks, J., Grimley Evans, J., Iakovidou, V., Tsolaki, M. & Holt, F. E. (2009). Rivastigmine for Alzheimer's disease. *Cochrane Database Systematic Review,* (2): Cd001191.

Blanco-Silvente, L., Castells, X., Saez, M., Barceló, M. A., Garre-Olmo, J., Vilalta-Franch, J. & Capellà, D. (2017). Discontinuation, efficacy, and safety of cholinesterase inhibitors for Alzheimer's disease: A meta-analysis and meta-regression of 43 randomized clinical trials enrolling 16 106 patients. *International Journal of Neuropsychopharmacoly, 20*(7): 519–28.

Bola, J. R. & Mosher, L. R. (2003). Treatment of acute psychosis without neuroleptics: Two-year outcomes from the Soteria project. *The Journal of Nervous and Mental Disease, 191*(4): 219–29.

Breggin, P. R. (2016). Rational principles of psychopharmacology for therapists, healthcare providers and clients. *Journal of Contemporary Psychotherapy, 46*(1): 1–13.

Brett, J. & Murnion, B. (2015). Management of benzodiazepine misuse and dependence. *Australian Prescriber, 38*(5): 152–5.

Britten, N., Riley, R. & Morgan, M. (2010). Resisting psychotropic medicines: A synthesis of qualitative studies of medicine-taking. *Advances in Psychiatric Treatment, 16*(3): 207.

Cipriani, A., Furukawa, T. A., Salanti, G., Chaimani, A., Atkinson, L. Z., Ogawa, Y. ... Geddes, J. R. (2018). Comparative efficacy and acceptability of 21 antidepressant drugs for the acute treatment of adults with major depressive disorder: a systematic review and network meta-analysis. *The Lancet, 391*(10128): 1357–66.

Commonwealth of Australia. (2002). *The National Strategy for Quality Use of Medicines – Plain English Edition.* Canberra: Commonwealth of Australia.

Day, R. O. & Snowden, L. (2016). Where to find information about drugs. *Australian Prescriber, 39*(3): 88–95.

Declercq, T., Petrovic, M., Azermai, M., Vander Stichele, R., De Sutter, A. I., van Driel, M. L. & Christiaens, T. (2013). Withdrawal versus continuation of chronic antipsychotic drugs for behavioural and psychological symptoms in older people with dementia. *Cochrane Database Systematic Reviews,* (3): Cd007726.

Deegan, P. E. (2007). The lived experience of using psychiatric medication in the recovery process and a shared decision-making program to support it. *Psychiatric Rehabilitation Journal*, *31*(1): 62–9.

Desplenter, F. A., Simoens, S. & Laekeman, G. (2006). The impact of informing psychiatric patients about their medication: A systematic review. *Pharmacy World and Science*, *28*(6): 329–41.

Dudas, R., Malouf, R., McCleery, J. & Dening, T. (2018). Antidepressants for treating depression in dementia. *Cochrane Database Systematic Review*, *8*(8): CD003944.

Frederiksen K. S., Cooper C., Frisoni G. B., Frölich L., Georges J., Kramberger M. G. ... Waldemar, G. (2020). A European Academy of Neurology guideline on medical management issues in dementia. *European Journal of Neurology*, *27*(10):1805–20.

Galling, B., Calsina Ferrer, A., Abi Zeid Daou, M., Sangroula, D., Hagi, K. & Correll, C.U. (2015). Safety and tolerability of antidepressant co-treatment in acute major depressive disorder: Results from a systematic review and exploratory meta-analysis. *Expert Opinion on Drug Safety*, *14*(10): 1587–608.

Gisev, N., Hartikainen, S., Chen, T. F., Korhonen, M. & Bell, J. S. (2011). Mortality associated with benzodiazepines and benzodiazepine-related drugs among community-dwelling older people in Finland: A population-based retrospective cohort study. *The Canadian Journal of Psychiatry*, *56*(6): 377–81.

Glue, P. & Herbison, P. (2015). Comparative efficacy and acceptability of combined antipsychotics and mood stabilizers versus individual drug classes for acute mania: Network meta-analysis. *Australian and New Zealand Journal of Psychiatry*, *49*(12): 1215–220.

Gordon, C. & Green, M. (2013). Shared decision making in the treatment of psychosis. *Psychiatric Times*, *30*(4): 33–4, 48.

Haddad, P. M. (2001). Antidepressant discontinuation syndromes. *Drug Safe*, *24*(3): 183–97.

Happell, B., Manias, E. & Roper, C. (2004). Wanting to be heard: Mental health consumers' experiences of information about medication. *International Journal of Mental Health Nursing*, *13*(4): 242–8.

Harrow, M., Jobe, T. & Faull, R. (2012). Do all schizophrenia patients need antipsychotic treatment continuously throughout their lifetime? A 20-year longitudinal study. *Psychological Medicine*, *42*(10): 2145–55.

Healthwise. (2015). *Depression: Should I take antidepressants while I am pregnant?* (Fact sheet). Retrieved from http://www.uwhealth.org/health/topic/decisionpoint/depression-should-i-take-antidepressants-while-im-pregnant/zx1763.html

Hirsch, L., Yang, J., Bresee, L., Jette, N., Patten, S. & Pringsheim, T. (2017). Second-generation antipsychotics and metabolic side effects: A systematic review of population-based studies. *Drug Safety*, 40(9): 771–81.

Holbrook, A. M., Crowther, R., Lotter, A., Cheng, C. & King, D. (2000). Meta-analysis of benzodiazepine use in the treatment of insomnia. *Canadian Medical Association Journal*, *162*(2): 225–33.

Huhn, M., Nikolakopoulou, A., Schneider-Thoma, J., Krause, M., Samara, M., Peter, N., Arndt, T., Bäcker, L., Rothe, P., Cipriani, A., Davis, J., Salanti, G. & Leucht, S. (2019). Comparative efficacy and tolerability of 32 oral antipsychotics for the acute treatment of adults with multi-episode schizophrenia: A systematic review and network meta-analysis. *Lancet*, *394*(10202): 939–51.

Husebo, B. S., Ballard, C., Sandvik, R., Nilsen, O. B. & Aarsland, D. (2011). Efficacy of treating pain to reduce behavioural disturbances in residents of nursing homes with dementia: Cluster randomised clinical trial. *British Medical Journal*, *343*: d4065.

Ifteni, P., Dima, L. & Teodorescu, A. (2020). Long-acting injectable antipsychotics treatment during COVID-19 pandemic – A new challenge. *Schizophrenia Research*, *220*: 265–6.

Jakobsen, J. C., Gluud, C. & Kirsch, I. (2020). Should antidepressants be used for major depressive disorder? *BMJ Evidence-Based Medicine*, *25*(4).

Jakubovski, E., Varigonda, A. L., Freemantle, N., Taylor, M. J. & Bloch, M. H. (2016). Systematic review and meta-analysis: Dose-response relationship of selective serotonin reuptake inhibitors in major depressive disorder. *The American Journal of Psychiatry*, *173*(2): 174–83.

James, J. (2016). Dealing with drug-seeking behaviour. *Australian Prescriber*, *39*: 96–100.

Jorm, A. F. & Wright, A. (2007). Beliefs of young people and their parents about the effectiveness of interventions for mental disorders. *Australian and New Zealand Journal of Psychiatry*, *41*(8): 656–66.

Kaplan, P. W. & Fisher, R. S. (2005). *Imitators of Epilepsy*, 2nd edn. New York: Demos Medical Publisher.

Keks, N., Hope, J. & Keough, S. (2016). Switching and stopping antidepressants. *Australian Prescriber*, *39*(3): 76–83.

Khoo, J.-P. (2012). Mood stabilisers. *Australian Prescriber*, *35*(5): 164–8.

Lalic, S., Ilomäki, J., Bell, S., Korhonen, M. J. & Gisev, N. (2019). Prevalence and incidence of prescription opioid analgesic use in Australia. *British Journal of Clinical Pharmacology*, *85*(1): 202–15.

Ma, H., Huang, Y., Cong, Z., Wang, Y., Jiang, W., Gao, S. & Zhu, G. (2014). The efficacy and safety of atypical antipsychotics for the treatment of dementia: A meta-analysis of randomized placebo-controlled trials. *Journal of Alzheimer's Disease*, *42*(3): 915–37.

MacDonald-Wilson, K. L., Deegan, P. E., Hutchison, S. L., Parrotta, N. & Schuster, J. M. (2013). Integrating personal medicine into service delivery: Empowering people in recovery. *Psychiatric Rehabilitation Journal*, *36*(4): 258.

Maguire, M. J., Weston, J., Singh, J. & Marson, A. G. (2015). Antidepressants for people with epilepsy and depression. *Journal of Neurology, Neurosurgery & Psychiatry*, *86*(9): e3.

Maidment, I. D., Brown, P. & Calnan, M. (2011). An exploratory study of the role of trust in medication management within mental health services. *International Journal of Clinical Pharmacology*, *33*(4): 614–20.

Malhi, G. S. & Outhred, T. (2016). Therapeutic mechanisms of lithium in bipolar disorder: Recent advances and current understanding. *CNS Drugs*, *30*(10): 931–49.

Marshall, K. P., Georgievskava, Z. & Georgievsky, I. (2009). Social reactions to Valium and Prozac: A cultural lag perspective of drug diffusion and adoption. *Research in Social and Administrative Pharmacy*, *5*(2): 94–107.

Masuda, T., Misawa, F., Takase, M., Kane, J. M. & Correll, C. U. (2019). Association with hospitalization and all-cause discontinuation among patients with schizophrenia on clozapine vs other oral second-generation antipsychotics: A systematic review and meta-analysis of cohort studies. *JAMA Psychiatry*, *76*(10): 1052–62.

McCormack, J. & Korownyk, C. (2018). Effectiveness of antidepressants. *British Medical Journal*, *360*: k1073.

McKnight, R. F, de La Motte de Broöns de Vauvert, S. J. G. N., Chesney, E., Amit, B. H., Geddes, J. & Cipriani, A. (2019). Lithium for acute mania. *Cochrane Database Systematic Review*, 6(6):CD004048.

Mental Health Commission of New South Wales. (2015). *Medication and Mental Illness: Perspectives*, Sydney: State of New South Wales.

Morken, G., Widen, J. H. & Grawe, R. W. (2008). Non-adherence to antipsychotic medication, relapse and rehospitalisation in recent-onset schizophrenia. *BMC Psychiatry*, *8*: 32.

Morrison, A. P., Hutton, P., Shiers, D. & Turkington, D. (2012).Antipsychotics: Is it time to introduce patient choice? *British Journal of Psychiatry*, *201*: 83–4.

Moses, T. & Kirk, S. A. (2006). Social workers' attitudes about psychotropic drug treatment with youths. *Social Work*, *51*(3): 211–22.

National Health and Medical Research Council Partnership Centre for Dealing with Cognitive and Related Functional Decline in Older People. (2016). *Clinical Practice Guidelines and Principles of Care for People with Dementia*. Retrieved from https://www.dementia.org.au/resources/clinical-practice-guidelines

Neufeld, K. J., Yue, J., Robinson, T. N., Inouye, S. K. & Needham, D. M. (2016). Antipsychotic medication for prevention and treatment of delirium in hospitalized adults: A systematic review and meta-analysis. *Journal of the American Geriatrics Society*, *64*(4): 705–14.

Nguyen, D., Brakoulias, V. & Boyce, P. (2009). An evaluation of monitoring practices in patients on second generation antipsychotics. *Australasian Psychiatry*, *17*(4): 295–9.

NPS MedicineWise. (2020a). *Australian Prescriber*. Retrieved from http://https://www.nps.org.au/australian-prescriber

——— (2020b). Resources. Retrieved from https://www.nps.org.au/resources

Ostuzzi G., Matcham F., Dauchy S., Barbui C. & Hotopf M. (2018). Antidepressants for the treatment of depression in people with cancer. *Cochrane Database Systematic Review*, *4*(4):CD011006.

Parsaik, A. K., Mascarenhas, S. S., Khosh-Chashm, D., Hashmi, A., John, V., Okusaga, O. & Singh, B. (2016). Mortality associated with anxiolytic and hypnotic drugs: A systematic review and meta-analysis. *Australian and New Zealand Journal of Psychiatry*, *50*(6): 520–33.

Pharmaceutical Society of Australia. (2019). *Medicine Safety: Take care*. Canberra: Pharmaceutical Society of Australia.

Ralph, S. J. & Espinet, A. J. (2018). Increased all-cause mortality by antipsychotic drugs: Updated review and meta-analysis in dementia and general mental health care. *Journal of Alzheimer's Disease Reports*, *2*(1): 1–26.

Reavley, N. J. & Jorm, A. F. (2011). Recognition of mental disorders and beliefs about treatment and outcome: Findings from an Australian national survey of mental health literacy and stigma. *Australian and New Zealand Journal of Psychiatry*, *45*(11): 947–56.

Reeve, E., Farrell, B., Thompson, W., Herrmann, N., Sketris, I., Magin, P. J., Chenoweth, L., Gorman, M., Quirke, L., Bethune, G. & Hilmer, S. N. (2019). Deprescribing cholinesterase inhibitors and memantine in dementia: guideline summary. *Medical Journal of Australia*, *210*(4): 174–9.

Reeve, E., Ong, M., Wu, A., Jansen, J., Petrovic, M. & Gnjidic, D. (2017). A systematic review of interventions to deprescribe benzodiazepines and other hypnotics among older people. *European Journal of Clinical Pharmacology*, *73*(8): 927–35.

Rosenbaum, J. F. (2005). Attitudes toward benzodiazepines over the years. *Journal of Clinical Psychiatry*, *66*(Suppl 2): 4–8.

Royal Commission into Aged Care Quality and Safety. (2019). *Interim Report: Neglect*. Retrieved from https://agedcare.royalcommission.gov.au/publications/interim-report-volume-1

Russ, T. C. & Morling, J. R. (2012). Cholinesterase inhibitors for mild cognitive impairment. *Cochrane Database Systematic Review*, (9): Cd009132.

Sajatovic, M. & Jenkins, J. H. (2007). Is antipsychotic medication stigmatizing for people with mental illness? *International Review of Psychiatry*, *19*(2): 107–112.

Salomon, C., Hamilton, B. & Elsom, S. (2014). Experiencing antipsychotic discontinuation: Results from a survey of Australian consumers. *Journal of Psychiatric Mental Health Nursing*, *21*(10): 917–23.

Siskind, D., McCartney, L., Goldschlager, R. & Kisely, S. (2016). Clozapine v. first and second-generation antipsychotics in treatment-refractory schizophrenia: Systematic review and meta-analysis. *The British Journal of Psychiatry*, *209*(5): 385–92.

Smardon, R. (2008). 'I'd rather not take Prozac': Stigma and commodification in antidepressant consumer narratives. *Health*, *12*(1): 67–86.

Society of Hospital Pharmacists of Australia. (2016). Standards of Practice for Clinical Pharmacy Services. Retrieved from https://www.shpa.org.au/resources/standards-of-practice-for-clinical-pharmacy-services

Starcevic, V. (2014). The reappraisal of benzodiazepines in the treatment of anxiety and related disorders. *Expert Review of Neurotherapeutics*, *14*(11): 1275–86.

Tan, E. C., Hilmer, S. N., Garcia-Ptacek, S. & Bell, S. J. (2018). Current approaches to the pharmacological treatment of Alzheimer's disease. *Australian Journal of General Practice*, 47(9).

Tan, E. C., Jokanovic, N., Koponen, M. P., Thomas, D., Hilmer, S. N. & Bell, J. S. (2015). Prevalence of analgesic use and pain in people with and without dementia or cognitive impairment in aged care facilities: A systematic review and meta-analysis. *Current Clinical Pharmacology*, *10*(3): 194–203.

Therapeutic Guidelines. (2020). About eTG Complete. Retrieved from https://tgldcdp.tg.org.au/etgcomplete

Thompson, W., Quay, T. A., Rojas-Fernandez, C., Farrell, B. & Bjerre, L. M. (2016). Atypical antipsychotics for insomnia: A systematic review. *Sleep Medicine*, *22*: 13–17.

Tiihonen, J., Lönnqvist, J., Wahlbeck, K., Klaukka, T., Niskanen, L., Tanskanen, A. & Haukka, J. (2009). 11-year follow-up of mortality in patients with schizophrenia: A population-based cohort study (FIN11 study). *The Lancet*, *374*(9690): 620–7.

Tiihonen, J., Tanskanen, A. & Taipale, H. (2018). 20-Year nationwide follow-up study on discontinuation of antipsychotic treatment in first-episode schizophrenia. *American Journal of Psychiatry*, *175*(8): 765–73.

Transcultural Mental Health Centre. (2015). Consumer medication brochures. Retrieved from http://www.dhi.health.nsw.gov.au/Transcultural-Mental-Health-Centre/Resources/Translations-/Consumer-Medication-Brochures/default.aspx

US Department of Health & Human Services. (2015). *Shared Decision Making in Mental Health. Decision Aids: Considering the role of antipsychotic medications in my recovery plan.* Retrieved from http://media.samhsa.gov/consumersurvivor/sdm/DA_files/index.html

Westaway, K., Sluggett, J. K., Alderman, C., Procter, N. & Roughead, E. (2016). Prevalence of multiple antipsychotic use and associated adverse effects in Australians with mental illness. *International Journal of Evidence Based Healthcare, 14*(3): 104–12.

Xing, D., Ma, X. L., Ma, J. X., Wang, J., Yang, Y. & Chen, Y. (2014). Association between use of benzodiazepines and risk of fractures: A meta-analysis. *Osteoporosis International, 25*(1): 105–20.

Zhou, X., Teng, T., Zhang, Y., Del Giovane, C., Furukawa, T. A., Weisz, J. R. ... Xie, P. (2020). Comparative efficacy and acceptability of antidepressants, psychotherapies, and their combination for acute treatment of children and adolescents with depressive disorder: a systematic review and network meta-analysis. *Lancet Psychiatry, 7*(7): 581–601.

Legal and ethical aspects in mental health care

Helen P. Hamer and Debra Lampshire
With acknowledgement to Terry Froggatt
for the second edition

LEARNING OBJECTIVES

At the completion of this chapter, you should be able to:

1 Describe a legal and ethical framework for practice.
2 Understand the effects of compulsion or coercion on people with mental health conditions and their families.
3 Describe the tension between the therapeutic relationship and compulsory treatment.
4 Understand a procedural justice framework to underpin human connectedness.
5 Explain the role of the practitioner in implementing mental health legislation.
6 Incorporate alternative approaches to compulsory treatment.

Introduction

This chapter explores the legal and ethical factors that inform mental health nursing, from multiple perspectives. The chapter proposes a legal and ethical framework that promotes human connectedness between the practitioner and people with mental health conditions, and their families and **whānau**. The chapter includes theoretical and practical aspects of working within a legal framework and provides several narratives to bring to life what it means to experience compulsory treatment. It concludes by discussing proposed alternatives to compulsory treatment and a potential future legal framework that embraces a person's autonomy and human rights. Aotearoa New Zealand – and each Australian state and territory – has its own mental health legislation. Although there are differences between them, they share the essential features of providing for treatment without consent, applying criteria of danger or risk to self and others, and certain procedural protections. Throughout this chapter we use the term 'mental health legislation' to refer to common aspects of the legislation in different jurisdictions.

whānau – (Māori) extended family, family group; a familiar term of address to a number of people

An ethical and legal framework for practice

Practitioners encounter many challenges in caring for people with mental health conditions, such as the multifaceted explanations for the origins of mental distress and the requirement to uphold people's well-being and safety though the use of mental health legislation. Such challenges can create moral and ethical dilemmas in practice.

Ethical framework

An ethical framework for nursing practice (Australian Nursing and Midwifery Council, 2008; Nursing Council of New Zealand, 2012) is based on four sound ethical principles: autonomy, beneficence, non-maleficence and justice. Autonomy refers to the respect that is shown by practitioners towards people's decisions and choices. Beneficence requires the nurse to prevent harm to people and non-maleficence obliges the practitioner to avoid inflicting harm. Ethics is a necessary part of nursing practice and concerned with doing the right thing and doing our best to serve the person in our care, their families and the community. When nurses act ethically, demonstrate the values of compassion, kindness and dignity, and are confident to raise concerns when they witness unethical practices, they maintain the trust that members of the public place in health and social systems (Chadwick & Gallagher, 2016). Ventura and colleagues (2020), however, suggest that mental health nurses may find difficulty in engaging with the ethical issues in mental health, such as paternalistic acts. By applying the skills of critical thinking, nurses can protect service users from paternalism and discrimination, and when they place the individual at the centre of a just and ethical discourse, can maintain respect for consumers' **human rights** and autonomy.

human rights – an expression of dignity, respect and equality; regardless of a person's religious, cultural or linguistic background, where the person lives or what the person thinks or believes, human rights are about being treated fairly, treating others fairly and having the ability to make real and genuine choices in our daily lives

Examples of ethical dilemmas in practice

The legal term **conscientious objection** provides health professionals with the power to decline to perform a particular procedure or treatment, based on the perceived threat to their moral integrity. Most jurisdictions have professional regulation authorities that support

conscientious objection – 'an appeal to conscience to refuse to perform acts that threaten a person's sense of moral integrity' (Hallagan, 2013)

the professional to exempt themselves from these situations, and in turn the employer should not discriminate against them. The rule of conscientious objection has been evident in the termination of pregnancy for many decades, and recently there are potentially new moral challenges to health professionals such as voluntary assisted dying (VAD), or euthanasia.

In both Australia and Aotearoa New Zealand, debates about VAD or euthanasia have led to some states enacting these laws and regulations. White, Willmott and Close (2019), however, argue that these laws are yet to be fully translated into clinical practice, and will have major implications for all health professionals, including those who choose *not* to support these laws through conscientious objection. Demedts and colleagues (2018) further argue that attention must be paid to how mental health nurses can be involved in the process of VAD, and ensure adequate cooperation between physicians, nurses and service users (Demedts et al., 2018). Both Pesut and colleagues (2019) and Demedts and colleagues (2018) stress that the need for ethical reflection, adequate training and knowledge of the remaining treatment options; a legal framework; transdisciplinary and multicultural approaches; and evidence of how nurses handle their own emotions will be vital for future practice in this area.

Morley and colleagues (2020) suggest that the COVID-19 pandemic has highlighted many novel ethical issues and, likewise, Sheridan Rains and colleagues (2021) report that the pandemic has had, and continues to have, many potential effects on people with pre-existing mental health conditions and on service delivery, including direct consequences of infection and subsequent societal changes. Mental health nurses may be faced with moral and ethical dilemmas. For example, restrictions on the movement of the public imposed in the COVID-19 'lockdowns' have likely proved difficult for consumers who were unable to access their usual supports, such as attending community groups. Nurses have to be prepared to respond to these ethical dilemmas, to critically reflect on the potential for coercion through these restrictions, and the extent to which the mental health legislation could be invoked to further restrict people's autonomy during this public health crisis (discussed further in this chapter).

REFLECTIVE QUESTION

Think about a nurse or other practitioner you work with: how do they demonstrate the ethical and legal aspects of practice in their behaviour and communication style?

Introduction to a legal framework

The legal framework for health practitioners is underpinned by principles within the United Nations charter (United Nations High Commissioner for Human Rights (UNHCHR), 1991), which describes the rights of people with mental health conditions who are subject to **compulsory treatment**. The charter declares that all people with mental health conditions have the right to voluntary treatment, wherever possible. However, if involuntary treatment is required this must be authorised by a qualified mental health professional; a second medical opinion must be sought; capacity and competence to make such informed decisions must be assessed (see Chapter 18); and treatment must occur within an approved mental health facility.

Maintaining human connectedness within a legal framework and establishing collaborative partnerships with consumers requires practitioners to be cognisant of rights-based

compulsory treatment – the Mental Health Acts in Australia and Aotearoa New Zealand provide specific criteria for compulsory treatment and treatment orders that operate for a fixed duration and that are overseen by an independent legal process, such as an appointed lawyer and Mental Health (Review) Tribunal

approaches to assessment and treatment. Rather than providing a practical, step-by-step guide to the various legislation throughout Australia and Aotearoa New Zealand, we now focus on social and political aspects of mental health law and the tensions that may arise in the art and science of mental health practice.

A background to mental health law

Mental health nursing as a specialty is unique in health care, in that it provides a specific legislative framework for treatment without consent. Mental health legislation sets out the criteria for the compulsory treatment of consumers by the mental health service and, in addition, sets out the rights of consumers, procedures to be followed in conducting assessments, and relevant appeal and review processes. The legislation varies internationally and between jurisdictions, and almost every developed country has some form of mental health legislation.

Several iterations of mental health legislation internationally have occurred over the decades and typically provide for detention and treatment in hospital and compulsory treatment in the community in the form of a community treatment order (CTO). Having a mental health condition is not a sufficient criterion for someone to be made subject to detention and/or compulsory treatment. In addition, as well as being assessed as 'mentally disordered', the person must also present a risk to self or to others because of the mental disorder or illness. Risk may include a substantial threat of self-neglect, in the case of someone who is unable adequately to attend to activities of daily living (Braye, Orr & Preston-Shoot, 2017).

CTOs are used to provide compulsory treatment in the community. Most commonly, the person will have been in hospital under compulsory care, and the CTO is a condition of their discharge from the hospital. CTOs are considered by those who use them as providing for the least-restrictive treatment, with the idea being that treatment in the community, even under legislation, is less restrictive than treatment in a hospital setting. A person subject to a CTO is obliged by the order to accept treatment, which will usually consist of medication, some form of case management and periodic review. A nurse, in the role of case manager, must provide contact in the form of home visits or attendance at a community clinic, and must broker other services such as employment, housing and income support, and therapeutic programs. A person who does not accept compulsory community-based treatment may be returned to hospital, sometimes with the assistance of police and ambulance services.

Despite their widespread adoption internationally, there is limited evidence for the effectiveness of CTOs in achieving their main goal of reduced hospital admissions. Light and colleagues (2017) argue strongly that service deficiencies determine the increased use of CTOs and that practitioners and policymakers need to factor in their clinical and legal justifications for using CTOs for involuntary treatment. They also assert that nurses need to adequately inform consumers about the meaning of the CTO, their legal rights and choices to reduce further constraints on the consumer's full rights as citizens (Banks, Stroud & Doughty, 2016; Hamer & Finlayson, 2015).

As Braye and colleagues (2017) report, ethical dilemmas arise from tensions between respect for autonomy, on the one hand, and the exercise of a protective duty of care, on the other hand. This common-law principle provides the rationale for the police to take responsibility for persons with a mental health condition, and authority to protect the safety and welfare of the community, as well as their obligations to protect individuals who are 'mentally disordered'. However, as first responders, this places the police in a role as the **gatekeeper**, and risks increasing the use of force when attending crises (Blais et al., 2020). Thomas and Watson (2017), however, have suggested that, given police do have a community guardianship role, they would benefit from hands-on training to respond to mental health emergencies, and some mental health services are already offering training for police officers (McKenna et al., 2015).

Mental health legislation sets out the rights of those subject to committal, and the processes available to support those rights and to seek review of their committed status. Rights include the right to information, access to a lawyer, to receive treatment, to receive visitors and other rights. A person may seek the opportunity to have their compulsory status reviewed by a judge who has the power to release the person from compulsory status.

Safeguards for the use of the Act include the role of the Mental Health Review Tribunal (Taylor-Sands & Nicholson, 2020), which hears appeals about the treatment orders that have been put in place and is able to confirm or revoke an order under the legislation. Each person who is subject to the legislation is also supported by a legal representative (a lawyer) free of charge.

Mental health legislation establishes specific statutory roles for practitioners. For example, in New South Wales an accredited person may sign a mental health certificate as part of the process of committal. The accredited person must be a health professional. In Aotearoa New Zealand, the duly authorised officer (DAO) is an accredited role instrumental in providing advice and arranging compulsory assessment, and that role is held by a registered nurse. In addition to these roles, practitioners may be involved in providing opinions to a court about a consumer's compulsory status under mental health legislation. Legislated roles such as these present practitioners with the dilemma that they have dual responsibilities: those created by legislation and those arising from their commitment as practitioners to developing therapeutic relationships with consumers. However, there remains a need for mental health nurses to build their skills in the role of second mental health professional, to better assist in judicial decisions that affect the lives of consumers (McKenna, O'Brien & O'Shea, 2011).

gatekeeper – usually a healthcare practitioner who is the consumer's first contact with the healthcare system and who uses their expertise to facilitate the consumer's access to the appropriate care

INTERPROFESSIONAL PERSPECTIVES

A joint assessment

I work as a clinical nurse specialist and my specialty practice is in primary care mental health consultation–liaison. I am also a DAO, which is an accredited role within the Mental Health Act. I attend the weekly patient review meeting in a general practitioner's clinic. Recently, a practice nurse presented a person who was seated in the waiting room. The practice nurse had recently completed the NZ College of Mental Health Nurses credentialling program, so was confident in her mental state assessments. Her preliminary assessment was that the person met the second limb of the Mental Health Act, therefore was deemed mentally disordered and posed a risk to themselves. We completed a joint assessment with the person and, indeed, compulsory treatment was indicated. As the DAO, I was able to invoke the process of the Act in collaboration with the person's GP, while at the same time demonstrating the process of procedural justice to both the GP and the practice nurse. By working collaboratively with the person and their attending family member, and with the existing rapport the person had with their GP and practice nurse, this created a trusting, respectful and collaborative decision to invoke the Act. I arranged for the person to have further compulsory assessment by a psychiatrist in one of the supervised community respite houses, with the likely option that the person would be released under the Act within a five-day period, and then receive continuing follow-up from the home-based treatment team, as an alternative to acute in-patient care.

Mental health law and human rights

The human rights of people with mental health conditions in Aotearoa New Zealand and Australia have received increasing attention in the past two decades, more recently prompted, in part, by new obligations under the United Nations Convention on the Rights of Persons with Disabilities (UNCRPD) (UNHCHR, 2006). Enshrined in these instruments is the human right of individuals to not be subjected to medical treatment without full, free and **informed consent.**

The UNCRPD defines persons with disabilities as 'those who have long-term physical, mental, intellectual, or sensory impairments which in interaction with various barriers may hinder their full and effective participation in society on an equal basis with others' (UNHCHR, 2006). Though these declarations, principles and guidelines have no binding legal effect, they provide the moral force and practical guidance to governments to domesticate these within their statutes and protocols.

Mental Health Acts in Australia and Aotearoa New Zealand

The UNCRPD has been instrumental in initiating and shaping the reform of mental health legislation within the eight Australian jurisdictions, and in Aotearoa New Zealand (Gill et al., 2020; Gordon & O'Brien, 2014; Ministry of Health, 2020), each primarily replacing the dangerousness standard with a competency and capacity standard (see Chapter 18). The Mental Health Act (hereafter MH Act) in each jurisdiction is intended, in the main, to balance consumer rights and the need for treatment, while recognising the important role of recovery-focused care and the vital role played by the family members and carers of consumers. The legislation is usually designed to enable 'individuals with capacity to make their own choices, while facilitating treatment for individuals who lack decision-making capacity and who need treatment for their own health or safety, or for the safety of others' (Department of Social Services, 2014).

For brevity in describing each jurisdiction's MH Act here, we direct you to the Royal Australian and New Zealand College of Psychiatrists (n.d.), a valuable resource that provides

informed consent – 'a person's decision, given voluntarily, to agree to a healthcare treatment, procedure or other intervention' (ACSQHC, 2020, p. 1). The person must be provided with accurate information regarding the proposed treatment and alternative options available, and must have sufficient knowledge and understanding of the treatment's possible benefits and risks (ACSQHC, 2020).

extensive tables summarising in detail the MH Acts across Australia and Aotearoa New Zealand, including references to Aboriginal and Torres Strait Islander peoples and Māori within each Act. Though each jurisdiction has its own MH Act, each also attempts to balance civil liberties with the need to prevent serious harm and provide care. Gill and colleagues (2020), however, caution that success of the legislative reform may be hampered by a lack of systematised voluntary alternatives to compulsory treatment, the continuation of a paternalistic and restrictive culture in mental health services and risk aversion in clinicians and society. They further recommend that momentum in the reforms in mental health policy and legislation needs to continue, so as to realise the goals in the human rights framework of the UNCRPD (Australian Law Reform Commission, 2014; McCarthy & Duff, 2019; Douglas & Bigby, 2020).

The law, reciprocity and recovery

The potentially conflicting processes of reciprocity and authority represent a challenge in clinical practice. Community mental health professionals are often challenged by consumers who do not wish to receive services or do not follow mutually agreed treatment plans. Rugkåsa and colleagues (2014) report that asserting professional authority is sometimes necessary; however, it can pose a threat to therapeutic relationships. Working in a community setting means that nurses are often involved in many aspects of consumers' personal lives; nurses may, however, take on roles that are both empowering and controlling, and which consumers may perceive as the nurse's way of influencing their behaviour – either helpful and caring, or as pressurising or coercive (Rugkåsa et al., 2014). Therefore, balancing authority and reciprocity is a critical skill of ethical comportment in nursing practice.

Nurses face many ethical dilemmas in practice that require them to balance authority and reciprocity. For example, the COVID-19 pandemic had a major effect on some consumers who were isolated from their usual supports, including community groups, which were curtailed in the strict rules of 'lockdown', leaving some feeling isolated and distressed when confined to their homes. It may be that some consumers refuse to follow the rules; in this situation the nurse faces the therapeutic task of caring for, and at the same time placing controls on, the consumer in order to reduce their physical health risk.

In a public health emergency, such as the COVID-19 pandemic, this ethical dilemma requires the nurse to draw on their legal knowledge to act in good faith, preserve the therapeutic alliance and employ the least-restrictive use of the public health and mental health laws available. In New South Wales, people can be detained under the Mental Health Act for not complying with lockdown restrictions (section 18.2). In Aotearoa New Zealand, once determined that the consumer has full capacity, the Pandemic Health Act (Ministry of Health, 2019) is the relevant legislation in the event that any person fails to comply with appropriate COVID-19 pandemic health requirements. In Aotearoa New Zealand, the MH Act does not allow for people to be compulsory detained on physical health grounds. The person is then likely be held in a managed isolation facility or, if they test positive for the coronavirus, may be held in a quarantine facility for 14 days, with physical and mental health staff in attendance.

The effects of involuntary treatment

Suzy Stevens (2003) gave a compelling account of her experience of involuntary containment and treatment. She suggested that psychiatry understood 'mental illness' as a 'disease of the brain' and completely separate from the human being. Suzy's initial and subsequent involuntary treatment in hospital, therefore, was more about suppressing her distress – by heavily medicating her – than bringing relief and calm to the turmoil she was experiencing at that time. Decisions about involuntary treatment led to irreparable breakdowns in her family relationships.

Considering the ethical framework outlined earlier in this chapter, Stevens experienced significant limitations to her autonomy, and did not experience her care and treatment as beneficent. Her account also suggests that the ethical principle of non-maleficence was breached in her case, leading to her experience of care and treatment as harmful. A greater focus on human connectedness during Stevens's episode of care may have reduced her level of distress and led to better outcomes in terms of her family relationships.

PERSONAL NARRATIVE

Leigh's story

clan – in Australia, an important unit in Indigenous societies, having its own name and territory, and is the land-owning unit; a clan consists of groups of extended families of about 40–50 people with a common territory and totems, each having its own group name

In my role as a family advisor for the district health board, I would urge practitioners to maintain the human connectedness with the person and their loved ones during the legal process of compulsory assessment and treatment, and to help mitigate the effects on all concerned. As a family, *whānau* or **clan** member, I have at times felt in conflict about whether to seek help for my loved one. Encouraging my family member to access help is always the first thing I do. However, when this does not happen, I have in the past been concerned enough to seek assistance on my family member's behalf. One experiences feelings of guilt about calling for assistance and then the person ends up under compulsion to enter the system. Sometimes the process takes on a life of its own, with the person being processed very quickly becoming involved with police and crisis staff. As a family *whānau* we have experienced trauma because of the process. When a family member ends up under compulsion to enter the system and is processed very quickly with police involvement and crisis staff, it is natural to wonder if you have done the right thing. Being involved in and witnessing your family member being taken away by the police is very distressing and potentially traumatic, especially for children. Often, the loved one being placed under the Act blames the family, as the system is too big to blame, and then the family is alienated from the person they care about, left with feelings of guilt and regret which negatively affect their future relationship.

REFLECTIVE QUESTIONS

- Many family members feel excluded from discussions about the processes within the MH Act, and do not understand what their role might be to support their loved one. How would you respond?
- What resources are available in your area for the support of families?

What the family member needs

I would like practitioners to support and strengthen the relationship that the family *whānau* or clan has with their family member. My relationship is not strengthened by being reduced to the role of 'the monitor' or 'the watcher' of my family member or being asked to 'make sure they take their pills'. I would like some skills and knowledge to support my family member who is experiencing mental distress, and not to be afraid of the 'symptoms', so that together we can hopefully reduce the need for compulsory care under the MH Act. With the knowledge I have gained over the years, I no longer have fears about my family member hearing voices. I can talk about what is happening for my family member, normalise the situation and decide more accurately (with my family member) if there is a need to call for help. I would like practitioners to encourage the use of advance directives that enable us as a family, *whānau* or clan member to discuss ahead of time what help and support is needed when things are not going well. The system needs to also model the recovery process and support family, *whānau* and clan members to understand how they can do that, too.

Suzy Stevens (2003) described how the longer-term effects of being subjected to involuntary treatment dehumanised her as a statistic. She had the label and stigma of psychiatric patient, and as she was removed from society she could no longer participate as she had no place within it. Stevens explained that people who are detained by law in a psychiatric hospital have very few rights. One cannot, for example, claim the right to refuse or change one's mind about the treatment on offer (Health and Disability Commission, 1996). Bhugra (2016) and Bhugra and colleagues (2016) report that people admitted to some psychiatric institutions may also miss out on their right to vote when staff do not comply with the UNCRPD. Practitioners must ensure that they provide support for people in hospital settings to make available documentation described in both Australian and Aotearoa New Zealand electoral law. Stevens further explained that when compulsorily detained, it is difficult for consumers to assert their rights, and thus they need the advocacy of others, including nurses.

Compulsion and coercion through legislation represents an intrusion on the rights and liberties of an individual (Bhugra, 2016), and is a form of social control and regulation of the lifestyle of citizens. Boardman (2011) further argues that people with long-term psychoses are the most socially excluded group; if governments promote social policies that attend to economic inequalities and the social exclusion of people with mental health conditions, rather than containing risk and rationing resources for mental health care, they may reduce the need for compulsory admissions (Johnson, 2013). The following section outlines the concept of procedural justice, a framework that acknowledges the experience of coercion when consumers are subject to compulsory treatment, and which provides guidance for practitioners in maintaining human connectedness when practising within mental health legislation.

Procedural justice

In keeping with the spirit of human connectedness promoted within this book, people who face the requirement of compulsory treatment will, more than ever at this time, require practitioners to work within a legal and ethical framework that provides dignity and respect for them during the process of civil commitment. The process of being compulsorily detained can be highly traumatising when the person's liberty, autonomy and personal power are curtailed, and when the use of physical restraint and seclusion (O'Hagan, Divis & Long, 2008) are applied during this process. Leigh's story reminds us of the risk of traumatising the person's loved ones; equally, it can be traumatic for nurses working within acute in-patient settings during the process of compulsory detention, especially the use of physical restraint and seclusion.

In order to reduce the risk of re-traumatising the people we serve, it is recommended that nurses demonstrate the approach of 'universal precautions' (see Chapter 2 for more details), and assume and respond 'as if' the person has a history of trauma, minimising further trauma and for their loved ones, during the process of compulsory detention.

Contemporary mental health law considers moving from substituted decision-making to enabling nurses to provide supported decision-making in clinical practice, and supported by policy in their services (Kokanović et al., 2018; McSherry & Wilson, 2011). Substitute decision-making in mental health settings is prohibited by the UNCRPD under article 12 of the Convention. Therefore, Kokanović and colleagues (2018) argue that this practice relies on nurses having good communication skills and attitudes, adapting practices and removing barriers to providing best practice by introducing these legally supported decision-making mechanisms.

procedural justice – the legal decision-making processes that incorporate the principles of fairness, justice and distribution of resources

The concept of **procedural justice** (Kopelovich et al., 2013) provides a framework for supported decision-making and ensures the practitioner's obligation to include consumers in fair decision-making processes that incorporate the principles of fairness and justice, and that provide an opportunity for any erroneous decisions to be corrected.

The procedural justice framework incorporates the legitimacy of dialogue (Martin & Bradford, 2019) and inclusivity with consumers and their families, and fosters human connectedness by adhering to the following principles:

- *Fairness:* the person believes that the process of commitment is free from bias and self-interest on the part of the practitioner, even when the person has no control over the decision itself.
- *Voice:* the person is able to voice their opinions, choices and wishes about treatment options at that time, even though this may not influence the outcome of the process.
- *Validation:* the person experiences that their views and opinions are taken seriously and their distress is validated.
- *Respect:* the person feels that they have been treated in a respectful and dignified way.
- *Motivation:* the practitioner has conveyed that they are admitting the person into a hospital out of their concern for their well-being.
- *Information:* the person believes that they have had the opportunity to discuss all the relevant information and the goals for this procedure.

insight – in psychiatry, the person's awareness and understanding of theor own attitudes, feelings, behaviours, disturbing symptoms and self-understanding

Such frank discussion may not determine the outcome that the person desires, though. However, the therapeutic alliance is enhanced when the practitioner bears witness to the person's often-traumatic experience of compulsory assessment and treatment.

Here, we turn to the idea of **insight**, a term that is frequently used but poorly defined within mental health law, and its role in compulsory assessment and treatment (Radovic, Eriksson & Dahlin, 2020). Insight forms a critical component of practitioners' assessments of the mental health of consumers, and lack of insight is frequently cited in the clinical reasoning that leads to a practitioner's decision to use mental health legislation. The notion of insight can be 'troubling' (Hamilton & Roper, 2006, p. 416); however, when a person's explanation of their distress does not accord with the professionals' biomedical explanatory framework of illness. Hamilton and Roper (2006) argue further that this often results in any further commentary or decision-making input that consumers have in their care to be considered invalid or mistrusted. However, as the following example illustrates, attending to the individual's account of distress is experienced as validating and respectful.

Longden (2010, p. 256) expressed how the attention to her story changed the relationship with her psychiatrist when she felt 'heard' and able to begin to give her own story or explanation for her mental distress:

> When the psychiatrist said 'I don't want to know what other people have told you about yourself, I want to know about you', it was the first time I had been given the chance to see myself as a life story, not as a genetically determined schizophrenic with aberrant brain chemicals and biological flaws and deficiencies that were beyond my power to heal.

In this case, if the psychiatrist had insisted that their own view of Longden's mental distress was the only correct view, she would have been assessed as lacking insight. In terms of the concept of procedural justice outlined above, Longden would have been denied a voice, would not have felt respected and would not have had her experience validated by the psychiatrist.

REFLECTIVE QUESTIONS

- In pairs, discuss your understanding of the term 'insight'.
- Having read the stories of consumers' lived experiences in this chapter, how might these change your understanding of insight?

The mandate of the state in the MH Act

The use of the MH Act creates a disconnect between the mandate of the state to safeguard the greater public and the autonomy of the individual. Restrictions on the person's autonomy will almost inevitably cause great alarm and distress for the individual. The parameters of the MH Act dictate the responsibilities and role of mental health practitioners toward the person; they then, in turn, determine the restrictions that are to be put in place. However, the individual's focus is on the effect of the restrictions and how this will impede their ability to function and live in the manner in which the person chooses for themself. This tension remains generally intact until the Act is lifted. It is not unusual for people with mental health conditions to feel significantly oppressed by service providers, which can lead to an adversarial relationship with the services and, in particular, the mental health practitioners. It seems a natural response that people will 'push back' when constraints are placed on their liberty and autonomy, particularly if they see the restrictions as unjustified. People then run the risk of being labelled as 'oppositional', 'non-compliant' or 'in-sightless', thereby

TRANSLATION TO PRACTICE

reinforcing the notion that the person is unwell, incompetent and even untrustworthy. The person may perceive that they are being punished for being honest. Yet, by endeavouring to keep their integrity and stay true to their beliefs, people forfeit their freedom. This will add to their sense of persecution. It also raises the question: 'If the person acquiesces to the compulsory treatment and just tells clinicians what they want to hear, is this not an attack on their self-esteem and their honour?'

In Aotearoa New Zealand, and in some parts of Australia, it is a requirement for mental health clinicians to consult with families during the legal process of making an application to place a person under compulsory treatment. Leigh Murray (2013) contends that relationships form the cornerstone of recovery from mental health conditions and the often-traumatic effects that the process of being compulsorily detained has on both the person and their loved ones. She provides a useful acronym, RELATIONSHIP, that can be applied to practitioners' practice of procedural justice:

- **r**espect – build trust and rapport
- **e**nhance – the family's ability to be with the loved one
- **l**isten – in an empathic way
- **a**ddress – the needs of children when a parent is compulsorily detained
- **t**hink – about the implications for the person's relationship with a loved one when you make requests of the family
- **i**nformation – about the process of the MH Act and the service to be provided
- **o**utcome tools – that track progress and improvement in the mental distress of the loved one
- **n**ormalise – the way the family views the situation can determine their response to the event
- **s**trength – keep the door of communication open to help families to learn, grow and change
- **h**elp – the family to hold hope
- **i**nform – the family about available support services
- **p**rotect – families entrust practitioners with their most precious and vulnerable family members, so it is important to protect the relationship between the person with a mental health condition and his or her family.

PERSONAL NARRATIVE

Debra's story

It is hard to speak of the time when I am seated in that room with a group of strangers, all of whom seem to have an excessive amount of influence on my future and how I will live my life, especially when they only know the vulnerable and confused me, not the capable, competent me. To be judged by any person is an uncomfortable and difficult position to be in, and when it is by people who appear to have no understanding or appreciation of your circumstances it appears quite unjust. To speak with any authority on another's life and know their history, one must be witness to all facets of a person's life, surely, not just this snapshot, and this moment in time when things are hard for me. I hardly know these people and, more importantly, they know almost nothing about me, so how can it be fair that they can exert such power over my existence? This cannot be right; it most certainly can't be an honest assessment of me. They speak around me as if I don't exist. It all seems so predetermined. I don't understand why I'm here and no one seems to be listening to me, no one has told me what to expect and what to do. I feel betrayed and assaulted by those very people who profess to help me. If these are the very people who can condemn me, they can also free me. How do I navigate that relationship, knowing I have no choice but to do so? What will this mean for my present and for my future?

REFLECTIVE QUESTIONS

- Reflect on Debra's account, and imagine you are 'in her shoes'; make a list of the thoughts and feelings that she is expressing.
- Now, imagine you are the nurse working with Debra over the next few weeks. What strategies would you use to strengthen the therapeutic relationship with her?

The role of crisis plans and consumer preferences

Since mental health legislation overrides the usually accepted principle of autonomy in health care, it is important that we limit the use of legislation and develop alternative written plans and preferences for consumers experiencing acute episodes of distress. As discussed in Chapter 18, these written plans are usually described as psychiatric advance directives (Lenagh-Glue et al., 2020; Ouliaris & Kealy-Bateman, 2017); or advance preferences statements (Lenagh-Glue et al., 2020). Though terminologies vary, the emphasis of these plans is to support the practitioner to record and have a stronger recognition of the person's autonomy when they cannot account for themselves. However, there is no law that specifically protects someone's advance directive, which can be overridden if the person is subject to MH Acts.

Williams, Smith and Lumbus (2014) report that joint crisis planning enhances the therapeutic relationship and empowers consumers. Typically, the joint crisis plan documents a person's early warning signs of mental health deterioration; specifies responses, such as the consumer initiating contact if they feel a crisis is imminent; and specifies options such as intensive support at home, respite care or voluntary hospital admission, medication and other measures. Williams and colleagues (2014) assert that the plans are more successful if all agencies have been involved and collaborate to support the consumers wishes. Thom and colleagues (2015) further argue that providing intensive coaching for practitioners will support joint crisis plans to be more effectively implemented.

The law and intellectual disability

Intellectual disability is an irreversible genetic or congenital disorder developed at birth and is characterised by the person's limitations in intellectual functioning, such as reasoning and learning, and the person's difficulty in exercising their full autonomy to carry out the functions of daily life. The term 'intellectual disability' has superseded such pejorative labels such as 'mentally retarded', and contemporary practice is now underpinned by the **social model of disability**.

social model of disability – proposes that a person's disablement is caused by the ways in which society is organised, rather than by a person's impairment or difference; the social model looks at ways of removing barriers that restrict life choices for disabled people, and increasing their access to the same rights and responsibilities enjoyed by all citizens

Early work by Prebble and colleagues (2013) argues that, historically, people with intellectual disability or dual disability – having a psychiatric diagnosis and intellectual disability – who required compulsory treatment due to a perceived risk to self or others were disadvantaged in having their specific needs met through mental health legislation. To uphold their rights, both Aotearoa New Zealand and Australia have developed specific legislation, such as the *Intellectual Disability (Compulsory Care and Rehabilitation) Act 2003* (NZ) (ID (CC&R) Act) and the *Disability Amendment Act 2012* (Vic.).

Prebble and colleagues (2013) further suggest that the unique ID (CC&R) Act values the social model of disability and the philosophy of autonomy, choice and normalisation. Similar to mental health legislation, there are specific statutory roles designed to protect the rights of people subject to the ID (CC&R) Act. These roles are care coordinators, care managers (both roles held by registered health practitioners), specialist assessors (usually a psychologist) and medical consultants. The role of the district inspector also applies to this legislation.

The role of the care manager is central in the processing of applications, liaising with the courts and ensuring that assessments, plans and reports are implemented and that regular clinical reviews take place. Care managers also have considerable powers: to seclude and restrain, to grant leave and 'retake' (Ministry of Health, 2001, p. 22) the person when absent without leave (AWOL), and can restrict certain human rights such as communication through letter-writing and phone calls.

The Australian Law Reform Commission (2014) continues to enshrine the principles of equality, capacity and disability in Commonwealth laws. Though these are encouraging legal changes, particularly for people with disabilities in the criminal justice system, McCarthy and Duff (2019) warn that most health professional training schemes have little focus on issues for this population who use mental health and forensic settings. Encouragingly, Douglas and Bigby (2020) have developed the La Trobe practice framework to meet these professional gaps; it offers an evidence-based guide for engaging in effective support for decision-making with people with cognitive disability.

Chapter 16 discusses intellectual and developmental disabilities in more detail.

Mental health legislation in the year 2042

In this concluding section of the chapter, we ask the reader to suspend judgement and consider the future of mental health law if the principles of least-restrictive approaches to mental health care were to be firmly embedded within the legislation, mental health delivery and practice. In the following we have chosen to summarise the innovative ideas of Mary O'Hagan, a consumer activist who has offered many visionary approaches to mental health care within Aotearoa New Zealand and Australia.

In the first instance, we are reminded that mental health legislation is underpinned by the principles of harm to self and harm to others. O'Hagan and colleagues (2008) argue that the harm-to-self principle is unfair in that it does not apply to people who have physical illnesses; for example, people with diabetes are free to refuse treatment. Therefore, she suggests that people who are vulnerable and at risk because of a mental health condition are required to have advanced advocacy and support rather than deprivation of their liberty.

According to O'Hagan, even though the risk of harm to self and others can result in death, this is likely to happen only in extreme circumstances, and need not be a driver of the mental health systems in Australia and Aotearoa New Zealand, which are dominated by risk management.

O'Hagan offers a visionary set of mental health laws to honour the rights of those who experience mental health conditions. She suggests that future legislation will embody the principles of a 'Care without Coercion' law and a 'Health Consumer Treatment Act' (HCT Act), which will support decision-making that recognises the best interests of the person and their family, places least restrictions on the person's autonomy and sustains the person's equal access to the rights accorded to other citizens.

O'Hagan suggests that the in-patient or CTO would be superseded by a 'right to treatment order' (RTO), which will require mental health services to provide specified treatment, support and advocacy for people with cognitive challenges to make their own decisions.

In addition, she recommends a single capacity test that assesses the person's ability to communicate their wishes, facilitated by professional assessors. However, this will be overridden in the case of a medical emergency.

Here, we remind the reader of the importance of advance directives. O'Hagan's idea that the law needs to focus on adequate treatment, rather than containment, means that within a new HCT Act the person or their loved ones can apply to the court for an RTO rather than a CTO.

In conclusion, Mary O'Hagan proposes that such legislation will change the care of people with mental health conditions; for example, all hospitals will be replaced by community-based crisis houses and in-home options for treatment and care. Open access to suicide prevention houses will be established and forensic services will be absorbed into a humanistic criminal justice system.

We urge practitioners working with consumers subject to mental health legislation to familiarise themselves with the ethical framework outlined above, and with the concept of procedural justice. While these measures alone will not resolve all professional and ethical issues arising from the use of compulsion in mental health care, we believe that if they are applied with concern for maintaining human connectedness in clinical practice, they will assist practitioners in providing humanistic interpersonal care, and will promote respectful care for consumers.

SUMMARY

This chapter has presented stories, information and activities designed to deepen your understanding of:

- How Australia and Aotearoa New Zealand enact mental health legislation to protect individuals and communities.
- The effects of coercion and compulsory treatment, which require nurses to be aware of their roles and responsibilities within the legislation and the ethical and moral dilemmas within practice.

- The complexity of the relationship between the law and human connectedness. Developing trust within therapeutic relationships can mitigate against the trauma of compulsory treatment when the principles of procedural justice are enacted.
- Adopting the least restrictive and person-centered approach to care as the goal of every nurse: exploring evidenced-based alternatives is not only a professional responsibility but is also enshrined in much of the contemporary legislation.

CRITICAL THINKING/LEARNING ACTIVITIES

1   Review the acronym RELATIONSHIPS. Are these principles currently being modelled in clinical practice by other practitioners, or by you?
2   Consider the aspects of the procedural justice framework; does it seem easy to implement this framework into your current practice? If not, discuss what may hinder you from doing so.
3   Consider the process of developing your advanced preferences plan; if you became physically or mentally unwell, discuss what wishes you would record for your care.
4   Imagine a world with new mental health legislation as described by Mary O'Hagan. How might this affect your current understanding of the role of the mental health practitioner?
5   Discuss the advantages and disadvantages of having alternative treatment facilities such as community-based crisis houses, in-home options for treatment and care, suicide prevention houses, and the role of peer support workers in these facilities.

LEARNING EXTENSION

1   Mary O'Hagan's description of potential future mental health legislation is strongly linked to a human and citizenship rights-based platform. In small groups, discuss how other marginalised groups, such as people living with a physical and intellectual disability, have claimed their right to fair and just health care.
2   Watch the video 'Recovery is … voting' by the CMCH Foundation on YouTube (https://www.youtube.com/watch?v=PMiqnjkyRqA), which demonstrates how a group of peer support workers in New Haven, Connecticut (United States) set out to improve access to the right to vote for people with mental health disorders. Discuss how nurses can ensure the rights of consumers to vote while in residential care during an election.
3   The following list is from the *Mental Health Act 2015* (ACT) and provides the questions that need to be asked to determine whether the person has the capacity to make a decision. Think of a consumer you have worked with whose capacity was questionable. Imagine that you are using these questions to assess capacity and reflect on your confidence to ask and then respond to the consumer:
    Can the person …
    - Understand that a decision about treatment, care or support needs to be made?
    - Understand the facts related to that decision?
    - Understand the main choices available in relation to the decision?
    - Weigh up the consequences of the main choices?
    - Understand how the consequences of the main choices affect them?
    - Based on the above elements, make the decision?
    - Communicate to you the decision they make in whatever way they can?

FURTHER READING

Department of Health, Western Australia. (2015). *New Mental Health Act for WA*. Retrieved from: https://ww2.health.wa.gov.au/News/New-Mental-Health-Act-for-WA
The *Mental Health Act 2014* (WA) is one example of a jurisdiction that embeds many of the topics discussed in this chapter. The Chief Psychiatrist, Dr Nathan Gibson, talks about the need for the new Act, how it came about and the effect it will have on patients, their families, carers and particularly Indigenous people. (6.55 mins)

Hamilton, B. & Roper, C. (2006). Troubling 'insight': Power and possibilities in mental health care. *Journal of Psychiatric and Mental Health Nursing*, *13*(4): 416–22.
This paper offers both the practitioner's and consumer's view of the concept of insight.

O'Brien, A. J. & Kar, A. (2006). The role of second health professionals under New Zealand mental health legislation. *Journal of Psychiatric and Mental Health Nursing*, *13*(3): 356–63.
This seminal paper discusses the tensions and conflicts practitioners may be confronted with when a person is subjected to compulsory assessment and treatment.

Royal Australian and New Zealand College of Psychiatrists (n.d.). Mental health legislation – Australia and New Zealand (Website). Retrieved from https://www.ranzcp.org/practice-education/guidelines-and-resources-for-practice/mental-health-legislation-australia-and-new-zealan
The Royal Australian and New Zealand College of Psychiatrists provides a comprehensive overview of several sets of mental health legislation related to the topics in this chapter. Read the details that relate to your jurisdiction and assess your own level of knowledge in this area of practice

Stevens, S. (2003). Where is the asylum? In K. Diesfeld & I. R. Freckelton (eds), *Involuntary Detention and Therapeutic Jurisprudence: International perspectives on civil commitment* (pp. 95–112). Aldershot, UK: Ashgate.
This chapter is a first-person account of the effects of compulsory assessment and treatment.

REFERENCES

Australian Commission on Safety and Quality in Health Care (ACSQHC). (2020). Informed consent in health care (Fact sheet). Retrieved from https://www.safetyandquality.gov.au/sites/default/files/2020-09/sq20-030_-_fact_sheet_-_informed_consent_-_nsqhs-8.9a.pdf
Australian Law Reform Commission. (2014). *Equality, Capacity and Disability in Commonwealth Laws: Summary report*. Retrieved from https://www.alrc.gov.au/publication/equality-capacity-and-disability-in-commonwealth-laws-dp-81/
Australian Nursing and Midwifery Council. (2008). Code of Ethics for Practitioners in Australia. Retrieved from www.nursingmidwiferyboard.gov.au/Search.aspx?q=code%20of%20ethics.
Banks, L. C., Stroud, J. & Doughty, K. (2016). Community treatment orders: Exploring the paradox of personalisation under compulsion. *Health & Social Care in the Community*, *24*(6): e181–e190.
Bhugra, D. (2016). Bill of rights for persons with mental illness. *International Review of Psychiatry*, *28*(4): 335.
Bhugra, D., Pathare, S., Gosavi, C., Ventriglio, A., Torales, J., Castaldelli-Maia, J. … Ng, R. (2016). Mental illness and the right to vote: A review of legislation across the world. *International Review of Psychiatry*, *28*(4), 395–9.

Blais, E., Landry, M., Elazhary, N., Carrier, S. & Savard, A.-M. (2020). Assessing the capability of a co-responding police-mental health program to connect emotionally disturbed people with community resources and decrease police use-of-force. *Journal of Experimental Criminology*.

Boardman, J. (2011). Social exclusion and mental health – how people with mental health problems are disadvantaged: An overview. *Mental Health and Social Inclusion, 15*(3): 112–21.

Braye, S., Orr, D. & Preston-Shoot, M. (2017). Autonomy and protection in self-neglect work: The ethical complexity of decision-making. *Ethics and Social Welfare, 11*(4), 320–35.

Chadwick, R. & Gallagher, A. (2016). *Ethics and Nursing Practice*, 2nd edn. London: Palgrave.

Demedts, D., Roelands, M., Libbrecht, J. & Bilsen, J. (2018). The attitudes, role & knowledge of mental health nurses towards euthanasia because of unbearable mental suffering in Belgium: A pilot study. *Journal of Psychiatric and Mental Health Nursing, 25*(7): 400–10.

Department of Social Services. (2014). *National Disability Strategy 2010–2020*. Progress Report to the Council of Australian Governments. Retrieved from https://www.dss.gov.au/sites/default/files/documents/12_2015/nds_progress_report_2014.pdf

Douglas, J. & Bigby, C. (2020). Development of an evidence-based practice framework to guide decision making support for people with cognitive impairment due to acquired brain injury or intellectual disability. *Disability and Rehabilitation, 42*(3): 434–41.

Gill, N. S., Amos, A., Muhsen, H., Hatton, J., Ekanayake, C. & Kisely, S. (2020). Measuring the impact of revised mental health legislation on human rights in Queensland, Australia. *International Journal of Law and Psychiatry, 73*: 101634.

Gordon, S. E. & O'Brien, A. (2014). New Zealand's mental health legislation needs reform to avoid discrimination. *The New Zealand Medical Journal, 127*(1403): 55–65.

Hallagan, C. (2013). *Conscientious Objection in New Zealand: Its Legal Status and Significance*. Retrieved from https://www.nzhpa.org/conscientious-objection-in-new-zealand-its-legal-status-and-significance/

Hamer, H. P. & Finlayson, M. (2015). The rights and responsibilities of citizenship for service users: Some terms and conditions apply. *Journal of Psychiatric and Mental Health Nursing, 22*(9): 698–705.

Hamilton, B. & Roper, C. (2006). Troubling 'insight': Power and possibilities in mental health care. *Journal of Psychiatric and Mental Health Nursing, 13*(4): 416–22.

Health and Disability Commission. (1996). *Health and Disability Commissioner (Code of Health and Disability Services Consumers' Rights) Regulations 1996*. Retrieved from www.legislation.govt.nz/regulation/public/1996/0078/latest/DLM209080.html

Johnson, S. (2013). Can we reverse the rising tide of compulsory admissions? *The Lancet, 381*(9878): 1603–4.

Kokanović, R., Brophy, L., McSherry, B., Flore, J., Moeller-Saxone, K. & Herrman, H. (2018). Supported decision-making from the perspectives of mental health service users, family members supporting them and mental health practitioners. *Australian & New Zealand Journal of Psychiatry, 52*(9): 826–33.

Kopelovich, S., Yanos, P., Pratt, C. & Koerner, J. (2013). Procedural justice in mental health courts: Judicial practices, participant perceptions, and outcomes related to mental health recovery. *International Journal of Law and Psychiatry, 36*(2): 113–20.

Lenagh-Glue, J., Potiki, J., O'Brien, A., Dawson, J., Thom K., Casey, H. & Glue, P. (2020). Help and hindrances to completion of psychiatric advance directives. *Psychiatric Services in Advance*: 1–3.

Lenagh-Glue, J., Thom K., O'Brien, A., Potiki, J., Casey, H., Dawson, J. & Glue, P. (2020). The content of Mental Health Advance Preference statements (MAPs): An assessment of completed advance directives in one New Zealand health board. *International Journal of Law and Psychiatry, 68*: 101537.

Light, E. M., Robertson, M. D., Boyce, P., Carney, T., Rosen, A., Cleary, M. … Kerridge, I. H. (2017). How shortcomings in the mental health system affect the use of involuntary community treatment orders. *Australian Health Review, 41*(3): 351–6.

Longden, E. (2010). Making sense of voices: A personal story of recovery. *Psychosis: Psychological, Social & Integrative Approaches, 2*(3): 255–9.

Martin, R. & Bradford, B. (2019). The anatomy of police legitimacy: Dialogue, power and procedural justice. *Theoretical Criminology*. https://doi.org/10.1177/1362480619890605

McCarthy, J. & Duff, M. (2019). Services for adults with intellectual disability in Aotearoa New Zealand. *British Journal of Psychiatry International, 16*(3): 71–3.

McKenna, B., Furness, T., Oakes, J. & Brown, S. (2015). Police and mental health clinician partnership in response to mental health crisis: A qualitative study. *International Journal of Mental Health Nursing*, *24*(5): 386–93.

McKenna, B., O'Brien, A. J. & O'Shea, M. (2011). Improving the ability of mental health nurses to give second opinion in judicial reviews: An evaluation study. *Journal of Psychiatric and Mental Health Nursing*, *18*(6): 550–7.

McSherry, B. & Wilson, K. (2011). Detention and treatment down under: Human rights and mental health laws in Australia and New Zealand. *Medical Law Review*, *19*(4): 548–80.

Ministry of Health. (2001). *The New Zealand Disability Strategy: Making a world of difference: Whakanui Oranga.* Wellington: Ministry of health.

——— (2019). *Pandemic legislation*. Retrieved from https://www.health.govt.nz/your-health/healthy-living/emergency-management/pandemic-planning-and-response/pandemic-legislation

——— (2020). *Draft revisions to the Guidelines to the Mental Health (Compulsory Assessment and Treatment) Act 1992*. Retrieved from https://consult.health.govt.nz/mental-health/draft-revisions-to-the-guidelines-to-the-mental-he/

Morley, G., Grady, C., McCarthy, J. & Ulrich, C. M. (2020). Covid-19: Ethical challenges for nurses. *Hastings Center Report*, *50*(3): 35–9.

Murray, L. (2013). Ko te whānau te kī mo te oranga o te tangata: The family is the key to the wellbeing of the person. *Handover*, *23*(23): 12–13. Retrieved from www.tepou.co.nz/library/tepou/handover-issue-23–autumn-2013

Nursing Council of New Zealand. (2012). Code of Conduct for Practitioners. Retrieved from http://nursingcouncil.org.nz

O'Hagan, M., Divis, M. & Long, J. (2008). *Best practice in the reduction and elimination of seclusion and restraint. Seclusion: Time for a change?*: Te Pou O Te Whakaaro Nui: The National Centre of Mental Health Research and Workforce Development. Retrieved from https://www.mentalhealth.org.nz/assets/ResourceFinder/FINAL-SECLUSION-REDUCTION-BEST-PRACTICE-Research-Report.pdf

Ouliaris, C. & Kealy-Bateman, W. (2017). Psychiatric advance directives in Australian mental-health legislation. *Australasian Psychiatry*, *25*(6): 574–7.

Pesut, B., Greig, M., Thorne, S., Storch, J., Burgess, M., Tishelman, C. … Janke, R. (2019). Nursing and euthanasia: A narrative review of the nursing ethics literature. *Nursing Ethics*, *27*(1): 152–67.

Prebble, K., Diesfeld, K., Frey, R., Sutton, D., Honey, M., Vickery, R. & McKenna, B. (2013). The care manager's dilemma: Balancing human rights with risk management under the *Intellectual Disability (Compulsory Care and Rehabilitation) Act 2003. Disability & Society*, *28*(1): 110–24.

Radovic, S., Eriksson, L. & Dahlin, M. K. (2020). Absence of insight as a catch-all extra-legislative factor in Swedish mental health law proceedings. *Psychiatry, Psychology and Law*, 27(4): 601–19.

Royal Australian and New Zealand College of Psychiatrists. (n.d.). *Mental Health Legislation – Australia and New Zealand*. Retrieved from https://www.ranzcp.org/practice-education/guidelines-and-resources-for-practice/mental-health-legislation-australia-and-new-zealan

Rugkåsa, J., Canvin, K., Sinclair, J., Sulman, A. & Burns, T. (2014). Trust, deals and authority: Community mental health professionals' experiences of influencing reluctant patients. *Community Mental Health Journal*, *50*(8): 886–95.

Sheridan Rains, L., Johnson, S., Barnett, P., Steare, T., Needle, J. J., Carr, S. … COVID-19 Mental Health Policy Research Unit Group. (2021). Early impacts of the COVID-19 pandemic on mental health care and on people with mental health conditions: A framework synthesis of international experiences and responses. *Social Psychiatry and Psychiatric Epidemiology*, *56*(1): 13–24.

Stevens, S. (2003). Where is the asylum? In K. Diesfeld & I. R. Freckelton (eds), *Involuntary Detention and Therapeutic Jurisprudence: International perspectives on civil commitment* (pp. 95–112). Aldershot, UK: Ashgate.

Taylor-Sands, M. & Nicholson, Z. (2020). The role of the mental health tribunal in setting duration of compulsory treatment in Victoria. *Psychiatry, Psychology and Law*. https://doi.org/10.1080/13218719.2020.1775153

Thom, K., O'Brien, A. J. & Tellez, J. J. (2015). Service user and clinical perspectives of psychiatric advance directives in New Zealand. *International Journal of Mental Health Nursing, 24*(6): 554–60.

Thomas, S. & Watson, A. (2017). A focus for mental health training for police. *Journal of Criminological Research, Policy and Practice, 3*(2): 93–104.

United Nations High Commissioner for Human Rights (UNHCHR). (1991). *United Nations Principles of Care and the Improvement of Mental Health Care.* http://www.un-documents.net/pppmi.htm

——— (2006). *Convention on the Rights of Persons with Disabilities and Optional Protocol.* Retrieved from www.un.org/disabilities/documents/convention/convoptprot-e.pdf

Ventura, C. A. A., Austin, W., Carrara, B. S. & de Brito, E. S. (2020). Nursing care in mental health: Human rights and ethical issues. *Nursing Ethics, 28*(4): 463–80.

White, B. P., Willmott, L. & Close, E. (2019). Victoria's voluntary assisted dying law: Clinical implementation as the next challenge. *The Medical Journal of Australia 210*(5): 207–9.

Williams, T. M., Smith, G. P. & Lumbus, A. M. (2014). Evaluating the introduction of joint crisis plans into routine clinical practice in four community mental health services. *Australasian Psychiatry, 22*(5): 476–80.

e-Mental health

Rhonda L. Wilson

Twitter handle: @rhondawilsonmhn

Facebook: E Mental Health Nurse: Connecting the Region

(https://www.facebook.com/EMentalHealthNurse/)

11

LEARNING OBJECTIVES

At the completion of this chapter, you should be able to:

1 Consider implications for a growing domain of e-mental health.
2 Identify and discuss digital interventions and practice with regard to mental health and well-being.
3 Consider the implications of digital health with regard to health service providers and e-mental health services.
4 Recognise the practicalities of giving and receiving e-mental health care within the online community, and how these relate to health promotion and recovery.
5 Identify some of the ways in which contemporary e-mental health services are delivered and understand how e-mental health professionals interact with others.

Introduction

This chapter introduces students in the health professions to a new and developing area of mental health practice: e-mental health. It describes a range of digital interventions and explores how digital and mobile technologies are providing additional avenues to help people with mental health problems in densely populated and hard-to-reach communities. It is important for practitioners to acquire and develop proficient **digital literacy** skills in the e-mental health service sector. Some types of digital and mobile interventions are considered, along with some of the benefits and limitations that relate to e-mental health in general. As emerging healthcare professionals, students increasingly are expected to utilise e-health interventions and strategies in the delivery of health care. The chapter introduces the e-mental health environment in general and aims to help students to develop the knowledge and skills needed to implement person-centred e-mental health care to individuals and populations.

Readers will have noticed that the start of this chapter includes the author's professional social media handles (names) and identities, because they are relevant to the content of the chapter and the evolving nature of conversations among mental health professionals on social media sites. Readers are invited to visit these sites to learn more about how mental health professionals are using social media within the context of the Web 2.0 environment, which includes social media.

digital literacy – the basic information technology skills and literacy required to be able to interact with others using digital technologies; these include communicating (voice/sound, text, video, image) and navigating by using the internet and online platforms, computers, digital telephones and email

What is digital health?

The World Health Organization (WHO) has a wide interpretation of digital health, which is broadly used to refer to a classification framework for digital and mobile health interventions that are used to support health system needs (WHO, 2018).

The WHO taxonomy of digital health interventions is designed for a primary health context, to support health planners using a common language about the implementation of digital health within the health sector, and is suitable for use within the contexts of developing and developed countries. Digital health interventions, in this sense, are considered as helpful strategies to respond to challenges faced by health service providers, such as information and communication, and availability, quality, acceptability, utilisation, efficiency, cost and accountability of services (WHO, 2018). Health professionals need to be mindful of these health challenges in any clinical setting, and must adhere to the systems in standardised institutional health service information and communication technologies that promote best clinical practice. In particular, it is noted that digital health systems are ideal for maintaining the functionality of electronic medical records, registries and directories for patients and populations, and to enhance client communications. Clinical interventions are supported through telemedicine consultations, and in the use of decisional support systems such as the development of standardised care plans and clinical procedures, as well as enabling the early detection of deterioration (WHO, 2018).

In the clinical setting, the terms used to describe digital health interventions can be confusing due to some ambiguity of terminology. 'Therapeutic digital interventions' has a more directly clinical connotation, inferring the use of technology to enhance the recovery of individuals or to promote the health and well-being of individuals and populations. Digital therapeutics can be delivered using any type of software or digital hardware device that can support patient assessment, monitoring and treatment (Natanson, 2017). Digital therapeutics is especially suited to health care that targets behavioural or lifestyle modifications, or remote monitoring to improve chronic disease outcomes. For example, telehealth (by voice call or video call) has been shown to be acceptable for use by mental health nurses who provide clinical care to support older people with depression (Christensen et al., 2020).

Other terms that are used in the clinical context are e-mental health, telehealth, digital health and videoconferencing. A range of platforms (e.g. open and closed or secure websites), software (e.g. smartphone applications – apps – providing cognitive behavioural therapy (CBT) treatment programs) and hardware (e.g., smartphones and smartwatches, virtual reality devices, personal computers, notebooks/tablets) can be used to deliver therapeutic digital interventions (Wilson, 2018). A growing number of platforms, software and devices make it possible to conduct health interventions in new, timely, innovative and effective ways.

Some priority communities remain underserved in terms of access to the internet; First Nations populations are one example, with only 43 per cent of Indigenous households having access to the internet, compared to 64 per cent of other households in Australia (Hunter & Radoll, 2020). Thus, there are clinical solutions to health problems but there are also health problems that arise from the use of digital technology. Health professionals will need to be competent in the digital therapeutics, and also be prepared to assist a small number of people who become unwell as a result of their personal use of digital technologies. This circumstance illustrates the importance of health professionals using sound clinical decision-making to ensure the right digital therapy is applied to the right circumstance, to support health promotion and recovery each time it is prescribed or administered (Ferguson, Jackson & Hickman, 2018; Wilson, 2018).

Digital health disorder

Conversely, while there are interesting new digital therapeutics to treat health problems, there are new health problems emerging for people arising from their interaction with digital environments. Gaming disorder is one such example described in this chapter.

Gaming disorder: An example of a digital health disorder

Society is increasingly interacting at the social, commercial, vocational and educational levels in online environments. It is inevitable that ill health will occur as a consequence of this shift in social behaviour. Recently, gaming disorder was added to the WHO's International Classification of Diseases (ICD-11) (WHO, 2020). It stands to reason that mental health professionals can anticipate caring for people with a range of digital health disorders in the future. Care planning for such disorders will require a new and evolving set of clinical interventions, and mental health professionals can expect to deliver many of these types of treatments in the future. Selecting, administering and assessing the clinical effectiveness of appropriate interventions for these types of problems will be required. In essence, the clinical decision-making process health professionals use to do so remains unchanged but is applied to a new clinical problem.

TRANSLATION TO PRACTICE

What is e-mental health?

e-Mental health, and the use if communications technologies in healthcare service delivery more broadly, is not a new idea. e-Mental health has been around for the past 50 years, in a more rudimentary sense through the use of two-way UHF (ultra-high frequency) radio and landline telephones. The idea of supporting people in need of health care advice and/or treatment, and their families, by using communications technologies is well established. Telephone services in mental health have been routinely used for many years, but in recent times the use of e-mental health has snowballed and now includes a wide range of electronic and digital technologies that enable mental health promotion, support for people and carers, early intervention and longer-term digital treatments in both standalone and **blended care** formats. For example, *This Way Up* (https://thiswayup.org.au/courses/the-depression-course/) is a scientifically validated internet-delivered cognitive behavioural therapy (iCBT) program available in Australia and suitable for use in the treatment of anxiety and depression disorders. SPARX is a scientifically validated, interactive gamification strategy to support young people with depression and anxiety in Aotearoa New Zealand (https://www.sparx.org.nz/home).

Increasingly, digital health care is seen as a viable and cost-effective strategy for integration as a blended-care modality within a comprehensive suite of mental health service delivery options, making it possible to assist more people at a time and place of convenience to them (Free et al., 2013; Wilson & Usher, 2015). A wide range of **digital interventions** is emerging, although not all of them have been subjected to the rigour of clinical trials that is required to validate their efficacy and qualify them as safe for therapeutic use in the clinical context.

Digital interventions can be described as 'programs that provide information and support – emotional, decisional and/or behavioural – for physical and/or mental health problems via a digital platform' (Alkhaldi et al., 2016). Research and development are required to engineer suitable software and technologies into the future, and to ensure that digital interventions are designed to treat mental health problems and illnesses, effectively and safely. It is recognised that positive engagement of clients using mental health interventions, especially where behavioural change is required, can be improved when technology based strategies are included in the therapeutic context (Alkhaldi et al., 2016). It is apparent that digital interventions are increasing in their appeal to clients and health practitioners, and that health services such as public hospitals and clinics will need to develop expertise appropriate to the delivery of e-mental health care; however, end users of the interventions should be consulted in the co-design and development of digital therapeutic interventions, so as to improve implementation and adherence of interventions in the real world (Cronin, Hungerford & Wilson, 2020; see Table 11.1).

blended care – a strategy that combines traditional face-to-face or centre-based services with digital or mobile technology strategies

digital interventions – programs or resources that provide information and/or emotional, decisional or behavioural support for health problems, using a digital platform for delivery, such as a website

Table 11.1   Benefits and limitations of digital interventions

Benefits	Limitations
Convenient access, 24 hours a day	Internet timing-out can influence drop-out rates in treatment programs
Accessible wherever an internet or telephone connection exists	The cost of access to the internet using a personal device
Free Wifi accessibility in most major cities and many smaller communities	Poorly designed software programs influence drop-out rates Privacy in public settings

Table 11.1   (cont.)

Benefits	Limitations
Enhances face-to-face therapy – especially in blended-care formats	Lack of face-to-face human contact
Universal distribution of service to large geographical regions	Limited digital literacy of some service users and/or practitioners Limited accessibility to some priority populations (e.g. rural or minority populations)
Many people prefer the convenience and privacy of the online environment to address their mental healthcare needs, including engaging in therapy – e.g. iCBT	Variability in the quality and availability of hardware and operating systems Expensive new hardware versus older hardware and slower operating systems Dependent on reliable electricity or battery power supply

Implications of mental health care using the phone in your pocket

e-Mental health is expanding into new and exciting areas of practice; for practitioners and health researchers, this is a particularly dynamic time. The general community has been engaged and ready to use e-mental health innovation for some time (Fox & Duggan, 2012). People now expect to find and gain access to useful mental health information, support and even treatment in digital formats (Free et al., 2013; Fraser et al., 2016). In particular, they expect to be able to do this conveniently by harnessing their personal digital technologies, such as smartphones and other mobile devices (Fraser et al., 2016). Conversely, this now means that the client population itself is now much more accessible to practitioners in terms of reaching them with health promotion messages or implementing targeted digital interventions designed to address specific health problems (Fraser et al., 2016). Today, at least two-thirds of the world's population has a mobile phone in their pocket; in many high-income countries there are more mobile phone subscriptions than there are people, and therefore many people are able to engage with a potentially lifesaving digital intervention close to them, at any time of day (Free et al., 2013).

For example, clinical intervention, risk reduction monitoring and management, and the engagement of health promotion with mental health interventions or services using text messages or short message services (SMS), or digital intervention in the form of smartphones or tablet applications (apps), may provide relief from distress, or access to protective or preventative health information. It is now feasible to administer mental health assistance to a vast population of people, using cost-effective and clinically efficacious communications technologies (Free et al., 2013). Self-care and information-seeking using e-mental health resources are gaining widespread popularity among people with mental health conditions and their families, carers and colleagues (Alkhaldi et al., 2016). Many people prefer to receive information, guidance and even treatment in the privacy and comfort of their own homes, where they remain connected to their familiar personal spaces and are able to best maintain the activities of daily living that underpin their optimal well-being (Bissell, 2015; Christensen et al., 2020).

The 21st-century reality is that healthcare professionals can now deploy a virtual e-mental health clinic to people anywhere, anytime and in any location by connecting via the technology contained within the pockets, handbags or backpacks of the majority of people in the developed world, and, for many people in developing countries also (Brusse et al., 2014; Wilson et al., 2013; Free et al., 2013; ICT Data and Statistics Division, Telecommunication Development Bureau & International Telecommunications Union, 2012; Proudfoot et al., 2014). These are exciting times to work in mental health clinical settings; however, to be successful in this environment, the mental health workforce will need to adapt to the changing dynamics of consumer expectations, and need to develop their own digital literacy skills for enhanced therapeutic effectiveness (Christensen et al., 2020). The pivot to telehealth services as a response to the COVID-19 pandemic, and a need for physical distancing in that context, has accelerated the need for mental health services to adapt rapidly to provide flexible service delivery (Christensen et al., 2020; Wilson et al., 2020). To achieve widespread outcomes, it will be necessary to find ways to improve equity of access and connectivity, as Hunter and Radoll (2020) remind us with a particular note to priorititise First Nations peoples.

REFLECTIVE QUESTIONS

- As you read this chapter right now, at this moment, where is your smartphone located?
- How many hours each day are you within one or two metres of your smartphone?
- How convenient is it to pick up your phone at any time of the day or night?
- If your answers to these questions reveal that you have your smartphone near you most of the time, consider the implications for access to health information at any time you may require it.
- Is it convenient? Desirable? Does it have any limitations? Discuss with your student peers.

Five modes of communications technologies to deliver e-mental health interventions

1 *Voice or text/SMS*
2 *Video* such as YouTube channels and telehealth video consultations
3 *Smart device applications* (apps)
4 *Web 1.* Static, internet-based health information provided by the website owner. For example, fact sheets and password-protected treatment platforms such as iCBT.
5 *Web 2.* Interactive health information or digital treatments using social media platforms or communities of common interest in the worldwide web environment. Web 2 incorporates user-generated content, and this is the key difference between Web 1 and 2.

The nature of Web 2.0 technologies and platforms aligns particularly well with a person-centred approach to mental health care because it incorporates, values and privileges web users using a non-hierarchical approach to communication: in many cases, all users have equal status and power to contribute. This type of real-time collaborative communication lends itself to advances in mental healthcare delivery in the future.

While there are five modes of communication for delivery of e-mental health interventions at present, it should be noted that these are typically accessible across two hardware technology types: mobile devices and computers. **Mobile devices** include mobile telephones, smartphones, tablets and notebooks, while computer-based technologies include laptop and/or desktop internet-connected computer hardware. Current research and innovation in the e-mental health field will see expansions in the hardware communication technologies over time, including new technologies such as wearable monitors or tools, robotics and even drone technology. A diverse array of technologies is available, with the following examples being the most common at this time.

mobile devices – mobile or cell phones, smartphones, tablets, notebooks, wearables and other devices designed to be used in the mobile environment

Examples of voice and text/SMS communications technologies in use in mental health services

- Two-way radio UHF services in locations where mobile phone coverage is poor. For example, the Royal Flying Doctor Service (https://www.flyingdoctor.org.au/what-we-do/tele-health/) in remote regions of Australia.
- Call centre-based services designed for triage purposes and to arrange intake or referral for people who seek entry into mental health services for themselves or others. For example, public health freecall assistance telephone numbers in Australia (https://www.health.nsw.gov.au/mentalhealth/services/Pages/support-contact-list.aspx) (Elsom et al., 2013).
- Call centre-based services providing mental health crisis and support helplines. For example, Australian services Lifeline (https://www.lifeline.org.au/), Suicide Call Back Service (https://www.suicidecallbackservice.org.au/) and Kids Helpline (https://kidshelpline.com.au/). Similar services are available in most countries in which free public mental healthcare services or insurances also exist.
- Many countries have an emergency service freecall telephone number, such as 000 in Australia, 111 in New Zealand, 911 in the United States, 112 in Europe and 999 (or 112) in the United Kingdom.
- Mobile phone, SMS or text-based services provide an opportunity to administer lifesaving assistance to people who are thinking about suicide. In her TED Talk, Nancy Lublin (2012) advocated that mental health practitioners use technology for this purpose.

Examples of video use in the e-mental health context

- **Telepsychiatry** is frequently referred to as a video-linked service between health services and consumers or patients and/or carers in separate locations. A suitable time is arranged between parties for a private consultation by videoconference (e.g. Zoom, Skype and other secure online video platforms). This enables people to receive specialist care without needing to travel to attend an appointment (e.g. see Christensen et al., 2020; Statewide Telehealth Services, 2013).
- More recently, platforms enabling flexible, video-based consultation are available through providers such as Skype, Apple's FaceTime and Zoom, and this has added an element of convenience and simplified technology, together with patient convenience (Shore, 2013; Christensen et al., 2020).
- Video recordings can be incorporated into web-based services and intervention modules to enhance the user experience, or to demonstrate techniques or examples. For example, some computer or internet-delivered CBT modules integrate video recordings and interactions. For some examples, see the Australian-based Mental Health Online (https://www.mentalhealthonline.org.au) and in the United Kingdom, FearFighter CBT app for anxiety, panic and phobias.

telepsychiatry – frequently referred to as video-linked services between health services, whereby the consumer or patient and/or carer in one location is able to communicate with the specialist mental health practitioner/s in a different location

Examples of smart device applications for digital mental health interventions

Social media platforms are useful applications for teaching the public, student health professionals and experienced practitioners about mental health information and clinical skills development. We know that many students in the health professions prefer to gain their discipline-specific information from social media platforms such as Facebook (Usher et al., 2014). We also know that a growing number of health professionals are using social media platforms and apps to create virtual communities for research, practice, knowledge exchange and mentoring purposes.

Examples of Web 1.0 e-mental health services

- Email use and web browser literacy are now generally considered to be basic life skills for adults in developed countries, including older people who were not digital natives. As web literacy develops, people are able to explore, build and connect relevant information that is useful to them for solving a range of problems from a self-help perspective (Alkhaldi et al., 2016). For example, browser search engines such as Google provide free email host services such as gmail and provide a virtual and digital context in which many people have relatively easy access and capacity to search for health information aligned with their health needs and specific health questions.

Web 1.0 – the first iteration of the internet; website content was written and managed by its owners; access was provided to users who chose to go to the site and receive information, and passwords could be used to restrict access to a selected target group

- **Web 1.0** is defined as website-based information generated by the owner or provider of the website. Web 1.0 provides a platform for healthcare professionals to develop static information, education and computer-based therapy resources for the general public. Web 1.0 is a platform for service owners to give information to customers. For example, therapy (see https://assist.ehubhealth.com/), community information and crisis support organisations such as beyondblue (https://www.beyondblue.org.au/) and the Black Dog Institute (https://www.blackdoginstitute.org.au/resources-support/fact-sheets/). Web-based intervention tools include iCBT and mindfulness-based therapies (see https://www.mycompass.org.au/).
- e-Mental health electronic patient records. Safety and confidentiality are high priorities for healthcare services, and this includes the management and storage of data about the health and private information of the people who receive care. In addition, the timely access to patient records by health care providers includes an integrated pathway for a range of services to access relevant health-related data such as pathology reports, communications from general practitioners (GPs) and patient health files. All of these activities are broadly considered components of an e-health strategy for holistic mental health care (Australian Commission on Safety and Quality in Health Care, 2015).
- Call centre-based services have been able to add value to their telephone services by providing additional information of a general nature on websites connected to their services so that they can support callers further (see Lifeline).

Web 2.0 strategies to enhance mental health

Web 2.0 – an internet-based application for user-generated content that is an interactive component of web-based communication platforms; social media channels are an example of Web 2.0

- **Web 2.0**, which is designed for user-generated content that has an interactive component on a web-based communication platform (Kaplan & Haenlein, 2010; Kirmayer, Raikhel & Rahimi, 2013; Leavy et al., 2013; Wilson et al., 2013), has expanded the options for other types of communications technologies in real time, conveniently timed asynchrony and social media-enhanced interactive experiences that are particularly convenient for use by the general population. Social media channels harnessed for e-mental health purposes offer promise for mainstream mental healthcare services as new services and innovative interventions are developed and introduced.

- Smart devices, especially smartphones, enable the use of apps to enhance e-mental health service offerings, with many apps currently available in information or treatment service formats (e.g. see https://www.hopkinsmedicine.org/apps/all-apps/madap).

- Personal electronic devices such as fitness wearable monitoring devices (e.g. Fitbit and Apple Watch) synchronise the monitoring of, for instance, heart rate and calorie consumption, with diary tools to collect personal data on health characteristics and behavioural activities. Fitness wearable technologies have been demonstrated to be effective in monitoring activity to enhance engagement in self-care and to promote health and well-being in general (Paul et al., 2015). The integration of physical and mental health care is an important aspect of holistic care, and over time technologies such as these personal monitors are being integrated as tools in healthcare service provision.

- Gamification in e-mental health enhances engagement in mental health self-care. Gaming-based intervention is an area of particular growth in the development of e-mental health digital intervention. Gamification introduces a fun and engaging way to interact with digital interventions to foster behavioural change. It adds incentives and motivation by stimulating the gamer's sense of satisfaction and giving positive feedback through reward strategies that reinforce healthy behavioural change. Some gamification apps are brief and simple, such as relaxation graphics interchange format (GIF) files (see https://mic.com/articles/127062/looking-at-this-viral-gif-could-be-the-perfect-way-to-cope-with-an-anxiety-attack#.tbkqOmLj9) that prompt and guide the user through breathing exercises, to assist in reducing the experience of panic or anxiety.

- More complex digital interventions using gamification strategies help to connect with target populations, such as with young people, as used in this ReachOut example: https://au.reachout.com/tools-and-apps/superbetter. Integrating gamification software strategies into mental health promotion can be tailored for at-risk populations.

- Gamification within a digital intervention is also amenable to addressing complex comorbid health problems such as severe mental illness and metabolic syndrome, with research conducted to trial a MetaMood app on smart devices (Shaw et al., 2016).

- Many organisations providing mental health promotion and prevention services now include a social media presence as a component of their service structure, including Facebook, Twitter, Pinterest and Instagram (see https://www.facebook.com/LifelineAustralia as an example).

REFLECTIVE QUESTIONS

- Imagine for a moment that you are concerned about your partner, spouse or child, who you think may have depression. Using the web browser of your choice, search for the Black Dog Institute and look for general information that describes depression and its treatment. What resources did you find? How suitable were they for providing basic information? Were they easy to find? What digital skills and hardware types did you need to access this information?

- As a future healthcare professional, how will you support people to gather useful information to help them and the people for whom they care? Discuss your experience of this exercise with your student peers.

INTERPROFESSIONAL PERSPECTIVES

Collaboration in e-mental health

e-Mental health is not aligned to a particular traditional health discipline. As a developing era of practice, e-mental health is emerging as a new interprofessional space within the health professions as a discrete field of expertise. New disciplinary partners are entering the interprofessional environment. For example, collaborators in e-mental health include mental health professionals from a range of disciplines, namely nursing, social work, medicine, psychology, occupational therapy and arts and culture, including Indigenous health, linguistics and human geography, computer sciences, technology, gamification software development and network engineering. The complexity of these interprofessional collaborations stretches the traditional paradigms of healthcare collaborative teams. These non-traditional disciplines are increasingly vital partners in enabling the process, ensuring that digital interventions are developed and delivered with relevant expertise that will translate into convenient use and promotion of high-quality, safe mental health service delivery to people and populations everywhere. The landscape of mental health care is changing and adapting to the needs of the 21st century, and the health disciplines are adapting accordingly.

Digital resources to address clinical problems

Diverse technologies are in use, and are under development for future use, in the clinical setting for the delivery of digital therapy interventions. SMS are useful in prompting people to adhere to treatment plans (Alkhaldi et al., 2016). Health promotion campaigns have long been shown to be effective, such as smoking cessation using internet and phone technologies (Brendryen, Drozd & Kraft, 2008). Monitoring and assessment can be achieved using ecological monitoring technologies that facilitate the collection of health data using personal smart devices (phones/ watches/ notebooks), which can be used to detect changes in health status or adherence to lifestyle modification, particularly useful for use with patients with chronic physical and mental health conditions (Helweg-Joergensen et al., 2019; Heron & Smyth, 2010). While online treatment programs are commonly used to treat anxiety and or depression conditions (Cuijpers, Riper & Andersson, 2015), additional digital techniques are useful to enhance adherence to treatment programs, such as through SMS reminder functions (Zarski et al., 2016). There are many ways that digital interventions can be incorporated in the routine care of people with a diverse range of physical and mental health conditions. Examples include pre-clinical and at-risk health promotion campaigns, self-help or guided health care for people with mild to moderate conditions through to people with moderate to severe and/or chronic conditions, and people who require aged-care support or care in independent home settings or in residential care settings.

Table 11.2   Examples of clinical use of technology for health issues

Technology type	Health issue
Robotics	Personal care and supported independent living (Moyle, Jones, Pu, & Chen, 2018)
Smart watch/ smartphone apps: Bring Your Own Technology (BYO)	Apps for monitoring heart rate and rhythm / cardiac health SMS for cardiac health promotion messaging Apps for medication, mood and weight monitoring (Byambasuren et al., 2018)
Smart devices (phone, watch and notebooks) and gamification.	Diabetes management (Kerfoot et al., 2017) Metabolic syndrome management and mood monitoring (Shaw et al., 2017).
Videoconferencing	Specialist health consultations (Greenhalgh et al., 2018)
Social media	Self management support of hypertension (Ghezeljeh et al., 2018)
Mobile phones	Real-time mobile phone messages targeting reduction of high-risk drinking (Kazemi et al., 2012).
iPad video	Promoting comfort for dementia patients using recorded video techniques (Hung et al., 2018)

PERSONAL NARRATIVE

Paul – meta4RN

Paul McNamara is a mental health nurse who is actively engaged in building a social media-based mental health conversation among mental health nurses. This is his meta4RN story.

There is a famous quote attributed to author, speaker and Harvard Business School graduate Charlene Li: 'Twitter is not a technology. It's a conversation. And it's happening with or without you.' This idea is not unique to Twitter – the same notion applies to all social media.

Over the years there has been a great deal of talk about healthcare matters and nursing, and much of that has occurred without nurses. Since the emergence of social media, nurses do not have to wait to be invited to join in these conversations. We can share our experiences, knowledge and values with the world, whether the world wants to hear from us or not. To paraphrase author, feminist and media expert Jane Caro, social media allows nurses and midwives unmediated access to public conversations for the first time in history.

We would be foolish to let that opportunity slip by.

I'm a mental health nurse working in consultation liaison psychiatry, located in a busy general hospital in a regional city of Australia. People like me often go unheard in the 'big picture' discussions. As a busy clinician, I'm not ever likely to pump out dozens of journal articles or to write books about my role.

Clinical nurses like me are likely to share 'war stories' with each other. Many interesting, funny, sad and (sometimes) scary things happen on the front line. There's a strong oral tradition of storytelling among nurses, and we learn a lot from each other. Social media enables us to share our stories beyond our workplace and beyond our immediate workmates. We can share our stories with nurses, and anyone else who is interested, all over the world.

As our circles of communication and connection become wider and more diverse, our minds expand, we learn more, we have more opportunity to reflect on our work. It's a fun way to do professional development.

Some of your patients, some of your colleagues and some of your current or future employers will use a search engine such as Google to find out more about you. They probably won't be malicious or creepy. They'll probably just be idly curious. Either way – no matter their intention – don't you want to be in charge of what they find?

I think it's important to be clear and intentional when using social media. Nurses already know about boundaries and confidentiality, and are nearly always good at this in the flesh. Sometimes, nurses blur the boundaries online between their social life and professional life. That's where it gets tricky. I suggest having two distinctly different social media identities: a personal one for family and friends, and a professional one for patients, colleagues and employers.

Personal use of social media is where you share photos of holidays and parties with family and friends on platforms such as Facebook and Instagram. Relax. Have fun with it. Don't bother naming your employer or talking too much about work. It's a place to enjoy yourself. Do you have to use your actual name? A nickname will increase your privacy.

Professional use of social media is based on your area of expertise and interests. This use of social media enables you to share information and interact with other people and organisations with similar interests. Here, you don't want to hide your light under a bushel: use your real name.

I have a blog that I usually update every month or so with posts that are of interest to me: have a look at meta4RN.com if you're interested in what a nursing blog looks like. It's not the only nursing blog out there – in fact, there are many nursing blogs that are much fancier and updated more regularly than mine.

Twitter is a fantastic way to connect with people all over the world. The best way to learn about Twitter is to follow people who are already using it – feel free to follow me via my Twitter handle: @meta4RN. By way of explanation, 'meta4RN' is a homophone: read it as either 'metaphor RN' or 'meta for RN'.

I also use the meta4RN handle on Facebook, YouTube, Instagram, Prezi and other online apps. Nearly all of the things I share on these social media platforms relate to my professional life, but there's room for a bit of playfulness and fun too. Professionalism doesn't have to be boring. Just check on yourself as you go, and ask, 'Is this something I want my patients, colleagues and managers to see?' If not, it either belongs on your personal social media accounts, or shouldn't be posted at all.

So, why on earth would a mental health nurse use social media? The answer is to connect and collaborate with others for professional development; to make sure that ordinary clinical nurses have a voice online; and to expand my horizons. Also, it doesn't hurt that when people do search for me online I am in control of what they see.

REFLECTIVE QUESTION

As you reflect on Paul's use of social media, can you think of ways you can draw forward something relevant that you can apply to your own emerging professional experience in mental healthcare development?

Social media policy and guidelines

As meta4RN (aka Paul McNamara) indicates in his story, we need to be sensible and professional about our approach to social media. There are some guides to assist you to stay in the safe zone when using social media:

- The Nursing and Midwifery Board of Australia has developed some guidance for health professionals on using social media (Nursing and Midwifery Board of Australia, 2019).
- A wide range of authors from the health professions has published literature on the usefulness of social media in the context of health – see some of these authors' papers to learn more about how social media is being used to advance health conversations and to transform practice: Arrigoni et al., 2016; Australian Medical Association Council of Doctors-in-Training et al., 2012; Brusse et al., 2014; West & Verran, 2013; Wilson et al., 2013.

Cost-effectiveness and quality of e-mental health digital services

People in society expect that health information and interventions will increasingly be available online. The integrity and efficacy of e-mental health is an emerging field of endeavour, and while some studies have concluded that e-mental health is indeed a cost-effective and a viable delivery mechanism, there is still much to be done to demonstrate the benefits and limitations of e-mental health care, in general. Governments propose telehealth and e-mental health as mechanisms to reduce the inequity inherent in face-to-face mental health service delivery, particularly for hard-to-reach populations such as rural and regional communities (Department of Health and Ageing, 2012). Internet-based services are cheaper to provide than hospital or ambulatory based services. Using digital technologies, it is possible to reach large populations and deliver services while practitioners and technicians are based in a singular location with specialist technologies. These measures are recommended as an adjunct to face-to-face services, or within a blended-care format, rather than as a replacement (Wilson & Usher, 2015).

Telephone triage services

Mental health telephone triage services are gaining increasing popularity in state and territory health services, as part of a telehealth and e-mental health response to managing mental health triage and providing timely support for people with mental health problems or who are in crisis (Elsom et al., 2013). Increasingly, nurses and other health professionals are engaged in the delivery of these types of services and, as a result, it is important that practitioners learn to use online and telehealth modes of service delivery so that they can contribute to the collaborative health workforce. Telephone triage services often serve as the intake point for service users seeking to initiate a first mental health appointment, or a referral to a mental health practitioner, to commence mental health care. The Translation to Practice box highlights some of the clinical characteristics needed to support people using telephone triage services.

TRANSLATION TO PRACTICE

Supporting people using telephone triage services

Hello, my name is ... my role is ... what can I help you with?

Always introduce yourself and identify your delegation. Invite the caller to tell you their preferred name and pronouns, and how you might be able contact them later if you need to. Ask the person what has occurred today or recently to trigger this call.

Remember that the caller already has had to select from a number-based menu of service options and has listened to several automated voice instructions prior to speaking with you. Familiarise yourself with the automated functions of your triage phone service.

Build rapport and trust by demonstrating care through active listening. Maintain a calm and even tone and volume, using a friendly voice that conveys kindness.

Let the caller know that you have heard them by providing regular and frequent verbal feedback. For example: 'Uh-huh' and 'I am hearing you tell me that ... have I understood correctly what you wanted to tell me?' In doing so you will be able to check whether you have missed any non-verbal cues that help to make meaning of the words, and clarify any nuances in communication relating to cultural or linguistic diversity.

Use the health service's usual triage assessment tool to guide your questions and to ascertain what has prompted the caller to phone, and to assess the nature and urgency of response required. In particular, make sure you assess the caller for any thinking or actions that may lead to harm to self or others, suicide, homicide or arson. Every triage call centre has standardised tools and policies to guide this process: apply the concepts to your telehealth practice.

An empathetic attitude and kind verbal demeanour towards the caller is especially important because it is likely that some level of emotional discomfort has preceded their call on this occasion.

Attempt to ascertain the caller's contact details, location and the names of relevant people within the context of the call.

If at any point in during the call you are concerned for the immediate welfare and safety of the caller, you should discuss this immediately with the clinical team leader in the centre and request a police or ambulance attendance to ensure the situation is safe.

End the phone call by establishing and planning what will happen next for the caller. For example, if a moderately urgent response is required, ensure that a practitioner will phone the caller in the next 24 hours to invite them to attend an appointment. Or, if immediate help is required, you may need to advise the caller to attend the accident and emergency department of their nearest hospital. Always end the call by thanking the person for their call, assure them of your authentic interest in their mental health and your desire to ensure their personal capacity for strength and resilience in the midst of their current or apparent vulnerability or distress.

Digital platforms

The health professions, including nursing, have been using online education platforms for some time. Health professional students are increasingly familiar with online learning models and platforms because they are regularly exposed to them during their undergraduate study. Public health services also use digital platforms for professional development and clinical documentation purposes (Paliadelis et al., 2015). In addition, many practitioners and students use the internet and social media in their personal lives as well as for professional development (Wilson et al., 2013). Some students indicate that they prefer to access information about health education in social media environments such as Facebook (Usher et al., 2014). e-Health learning experiences have been integrated into health and nursing curricula with a range of augmented reality, virtual reality, **gamification** and simulation, and these are now regular components of higher education teaching (Ferguson et al., 2015; Wilson, 2010).

Healthcare professionals have been slow, in general, to take up Web 2.0 application of social media for professional use, despite a growing trend worldwide for acquisition of internet-connected smartphones, tablets and computers (Usher, 2010). Mid to late-career health professionals in Australia have demonstrated limited interest in engaging with their clients through the use of digital resources. Early career health professionals are more likely to have previously developed strong digital literacy and are comfortable using online or social media communications, and they are able to translate these generic digital skills into the professional health service delivery context. It is important for new graduates to contribute professionally to the development of clinical digital interventions and, in doing so, they will guide their senior colleagues to adapt to systems that providing safe and effective e-mental health care into the future.

> **gamification (or gaming)** – the process of incorporating games and gaming technology into e-learning or e-health interventions for the purpose of engagement and motivation, and to contribute to learning or changes in health behaviours

Designing health information for digital environments

Ensuring that the design of e-mental health information matches the targeted audience is a priority for successful promotion of health education learning, memory and recall experiences within the client population (Bol et al., 2016). A wide variety of online health information is available to the general population, but little is known as yet about how people process and recall the online health information to which they are exposed.

One Dutch study explored the use of eye tracking of health information on health websites to assess the duration of attention (eye fixation) of older (65 years and older) and younger study participants (Bol et al., 2016). The researchers in this case wanted to know about how people in the two age groups recalled information across three different online learning experiences: text-only, text and cognitive images (e.g. diagrams), and text and affective images (e.g. warm and friendly images). They found that older people could recall information better if they had enough time to read the text, and most of their eye fixation was on the text, while younger people tended to remember what they had learnt from the text and cognitive image scenarios.

There may be several reasons for these findings, and these include evidence that health literacy is generally lower among older people and that older people tend to take longer to process textual information (Bol et al., 2016). However, given sufficient time in the online environment, older people are able to recall the health information equally as well as younger people. Older people generally experience age-related deterioration in eye health, and this may also explain a longer reading time in the online environment. Younger people are usually more fluent with online literacy skills, and so it is more likely that they will be more familiar with the layout of websites, and this may be why they spend less time looking at textual information and integrate their learning with cognitive imagery. The researchers in this study also suggested that while less time was spent by the participants in looking at the affective images supporting the textual information, it is possible that the warmth of the image motivated and engaged people to concentrate on the textual information presented to them (Bol et al., 2016).

e-Mental health literacy

Bol and colleagues' (2016) research is particularly interesting when applied to e-mental health interventions, because the experience of online learning is relevant to mental health literacy and the desired uptake of behavioural changes as the outcomes of successful e-mental health education. Designing an e-mental health intervention should take into consideration the most useful components of information exchange for the target population, while the duration of exposure to textual and/or imaging content will also be relevant. The effective use of diagrams and warm, engaging images has the capacity to enhance, motivate and assist in the learning, memory and recall of health information. In contrast to face-to-face health education interventions, it is not possible to ask the client to 'teach back' the information to the practitioner, to check that a message has been understood and retained, and thus it is important that e-mental health practitioners use evidence to support online interventions and to improve their efficacy in general.

REFLECTIVE QUESTIONS

- Think back to a time when you have used websites or apps to find health-related information for your personal use. What was your experience of gathering web-based information?
- Were you satisfied that you located good-quality information? How did you know you could trust the information? Or, were you suspicious about the quality of information you found? Did you find conflicting advice and, if so, how did you decide which advice was appropriate?
- If you were successful in your online search for health information, what digital literacy skills did you need to be successful? How did you develop those personal skills? How would you assist others who do not have these skills to find quality health information? As a future health professional, what codes of practice will you need to be mindful of to ensure that you provide safe advice about health to people seeking your professional assistance?

The safe administration of digital interventions

It is difficult for consumers and carers to determine the credibility, usefulness and effectiveness of the more than 350 000 health apps currently available in app stores (Research2Guidance, n.d.). Increasingly, they will need to rely on nurses and other health professionals to provide expert professional advice regarding the selection of suitable self-care and blended-health care digital resources. To do this, health professionals will need to be able to determine the validity, effectiveness and suitability of digital therapeutics for safe healthcare advice, based on best practice standards (Ferguson, Jackson & Hickman, 2018).

Health professionals should consider the factors in Table 11.3 when determining the suitability of digital therapeutics for consumers and carers.

Table 11.3 The 'rights' in administration of digital therapeutic intervention

Right digital therapeutic intervention	Clinical reasoning guide
Right digital therapy	Prescription and administration of digital therapy should be guided by the strength of the clinical evidence-base, matched with the digital treatment design and its suitability to effectively treat the clinical or subclinical problem experienced by the patient at that time and place, and for the purpose intended.
Right person	Does the person possess the digital literacy skills required to engage with the digital intervention? Does the person agree to adhere to a digital intervention? Has this intervention been beneficial for others in similar biological, psychosocial, social, developmental, cultural, spiritual and ecological circumstances? Does the digital design align with the person's capacity to engage, their availability and ability to adhere, and their age, gender identity and health beliefs?
Right condition	Has the digital intervention been shown to be useful, effective and safe for the condition?
Right dose	How many exposures to the digital therapy are ideal to produce a clinical effect? Is the duration of exposure, or treatment, a factor? Should the treatment be administered in conjunction with any other activity, location or intervention? Is it a standalone intervention, blended with other face-to-face or located therapies, medications or physical therapies?
Right time	Is there a specific time for administration? Is a reminder message desirable to prompt adherence? Is there a specific sequence that should be followed (e.g. module one should precede module two?) What would occur if a treatment exposure or module is missed or taken out of sequence? What are the risks? Or advantages of maintaining adherence? Is real time intervention critical to effect?
Right (route) platform or device	Which device is best suited to delivery of the intervention? Does the patient have access to a suitable device? What are the threats to success (e.g. loss of internet connection? Data privacy?). How can these be best managed? Do the screen experience and design align with the patient's age, digital literacy, vision, motivation, lifestyle etc.?

(cont.)

Table 11.3 (cont.)

Right digital therapeutic intervention	Clinical reasoning guide
Right agreement and *right* security settings. *Right* to refuse digital engagement.	Does the patient agree to accept the terms and conditions of use? What are the 'side-effects' or consequences of use? Do the institution, health professional and patient all adhere to adequate data security arrangements? Have 'settings' been checked to reduce adverse outcomes and risks through unintended data sharing or security breaches, third-party access to data, paywall or other barriers, password protection, encryption, or access blocks? What alternatives are available to patients if they exercise a right to refuse digital treatment? Are the answers to these questions available in 'plain language' for ease of comprehension by all?
Right evidence	Is there evidence to ensure the conduct of evidence-based digital intervention nursing practice? How can we be certain that there are no adverse side-effects, or unintended harms?
Right effect has been achieved after administration.	How will the effectiveness of the treatment be monitored and assessed? Under what circumstances will it be discontinued? Have there been any adverse reactions? Have there been any unintended benefits or consequences for the patient?

Source: Adapted from Wilson (2018).

Human–computer interaction (HCI) design elements should be considered carefully to enhance the safe administration of digital health interventions (Søgaard Nielsen & Wilson, 2019). It is important to match the technological platforms and devices so they are best suited for an optimal clinical effect for the particular health conditions, age groups, developmental stages, digital literacy abilities and preferences of the patient/s who utilise the digital interventions (Shaw et al., 2017; Morrison et al., 2012). Some of the design features that are likely to influence the clinical effectiveness may include font (type) design and size, colours, text, image, animation, voice, accent, tone and volume (Bol et al., 2016). The screen experience for the patient is important because it is the mechanism that delivers the dose and strength of the intervention, and as such, affects whether sufficient engagement, exposure and adherence to the intervention will lead to a therapeutic result (Kobak, Mundt & Kennard, 2015). While these factors markedly shape users' experiences, most digital therapeutic trials do not provide the details necessary to assess the HCI components of the interventions that they test (Søgaard & Wilson, 2019). Health professionals should be equipped with the competence and skills needed to sufficiently critique the quality of the evidence that supports and validates the digital therapies they administer. They are also responsible for monitoring the quality, safety and effectiveness of the interventions they administer. Health professionals are responsible for advocating for their patients, in pursuit of the most appropriate, fair and reasonable access to health care that best suits the health promotion, well-being and recovery needs of their patients.

Digital interventions and blended care

The common usage of smartphones and access to personal computers and other smart devices has driven a level of integration in which voice, video and web-based resources are widely available, and often in blended formats so that all three can be used simultaneously and in synchronous or asynchronous formats. This provides service users and service providers with a level of flexibility and convenience not seen previously. For example, Mathiasen and colleagues (2016) have conducted a study to examine the experiences of people with anxiety and panic disorders who are waiting for a place in a face-to-face clinical treatment program. In this study, a treatment group was randomly selected from the waiting-list group to receive iCBT (fearfighters.com), while others remained on the waiting list with no additional treatment. This research has shown that people who were supported with the iCBT program reported experiencing a significantly better quality of life while waiting for the face-to-face program to commence (Mathiasen et al., 2016). This is significant because optimism and hope for the future positively influences mental health and assists with recovery overall (Thompson, 2015).

Commercial and social enterprise innovation in e-mental health

Much innovation in the field of e-mental health is occurring, and at a rapid pace, with commercial and social enterprises being quick to respond to a growing global appetite for mental health care in general. There are many apps and websites to choose from, many free of charge. This dynamic has associated benefits and risks.

Benefits

- A general, population-wide awareness and expectation of the availability of mental health information and support in an online environment
- Populations are skilled and literate in the use of electronic devices and digital technologies such as apps, website navigation, email and social media.

Risks and limitations

- The trustworthiness, reliability, dependability and credibility of many e-mental health activities in the commercial and social zones are not known because e-mental health research and development occur at a slower pace than in the commercial and social environments, and often without a rigorous process to demonstrate efficacy and patient safety. Thus, health service providers and practitioners are reluctant to engage in e-mental health initiatives without best-practice guidelines to support their practice.
- Clinical trials take a significant amount of time, planning, design and testing to underpin evidence that supports safe practice. In the context of the rapid pace of change in the digital environment, this poses a challenge.

- Not all practitioners are keen adopters of social media. Thus, a digital literacy and skills base has not dominated the health environment in general to date. The mental health workforce is ageing and, as younger and more digitally literate workers enter the mental health professions they bring with them the ease and comfort of existing and operating in the various digital environments (Wilson et al., 2013).

Opportunities for safe e-mental health development

e-Mental health holds great promise for mental health care now and into the future. There are some gaps at present, and there is a significant need for research to develop practice-ready tools to contribute to a blended-care delivery system (Fraser et al., 2016). Blended care includes elements of face-to-face and online or electronic components of clinical mental health care.

Mental health practitioners and researchers need to develop and refine their skills in the use of e-health care technologies, especially with regard to web-based tools, apps and social media (Wilson et al., 2013). It is encouraging that students in the health professions indicate their likeliness of having a strong grasp of electronic health care and information transfer because they bring pre-existing, web-savvy skills to their pre-qualification studies (Usher et al., 2014).

Governments and funding bodies increasingly anticipate the incorporation of strategic e-mental health care into health service delivery systems, because it aligns with their business plans and population distribution plans (Department of Health, 2015; Department of Health and Ageing, 2012; European Commission, 2012; Shaw et al., 2016). Thus, new mental health professional graduates should anticipate a future requirement to operate safely and proficiently in the e-health environment.

TRANSLATION TO PRACTICE

As a new graduate, you may have more experience in using digital platforms than your health professional peers and senior colleagues. How will you familiarise yourself with the digital platforms to support e-mental health, and to teach your colleagues the digital skills they will need as well? Have you thought of yourself as competent in digital literacy? How do you feel about supporting your senior colleagues as they learn from you as a beginning health practitioner? How will you conduct yourself respectfully while sharing your knowledge with your health professional peers? Practise guiding a friend or relative in the use of a new app or game on their smartphone or computer. Reflect on the experience and draw forward what you learn about yourself as a teacher and guide.

SUMMARY

This chapter has presented stories and information, supplemented with activities designed to deepen your understanding of:

- The growth and community expectations of the use of new technologies to deliver mental health care. People are increasingly embracing new technologies, including hardware, software and interactive social media in their personal and professional lives. A growth of population-level digital literacy provides an opportunity for health service providers to use these technologies to meaningfully provide timely and efficacious mental health services for people everywhere, regardless of their geographic location, and suggests that accessibility is achievable.

- A broad range of digital interventions have been presented, with particular focus on interventions that can be provided across five technology modes: voice and text messaging; video; smart device apps; Web 1.0; and Web 2.0. Mental health promotion, prevention, support and treatment are all suitable for e-mental health delivery; for example, through online support communities, online mental health information and education using static resources to download games that enhance motivation and treatment adherence, and treatments such as iCBT. The continuing adaptation of traditional therapies to the e-mental health environment is changing rapidly, with evidence to support practice growing in volume.

- The important role that exists for new graduates to participate actively with their senior colleagues, to assist them to acquire knowledge and proficiency in digital literacy within the health workforce, thus assisting in a transition towards the successful uptake of e-mental health care, in general. Digital health service delivery is a cost-effective method of distributing health care across populations, and governments are keen to support health initiatives that utilise e-mental health care solutions to meet service delivery needs.

- Digital interpersonal and wider communication skills, which are necessary for the mental health practitioner to develop a therapeutic rapport with consumers, using e-mental health techniques. This chapter has outlined some ways that traditional rapport-building skills can be adapted for e-mental health service delivery, especially in voice, video and textual formats. Particular attention has been given to voice-based service delivery such as telehealth and telephone-based triage services. Additionally, this chapter has presented some of the ways in which health promotion and recovery can be enhanced with the addition of stand-alone or blended e-mental health care.

- Examples of contemporary e-mental health practice, from telephone triage to complex internet-based treatments. The e-mental health practitioner is a relatively new addition to the mental health interdisciplinary team, bringing with them a growing multitude of new interdisciplinary practitioners such as software engineers, gamification technicians, communication professionals, human geographers and more. These new e-mental health care collaborators bring new knowledge and skills to solving the complex problems of mental illness. Interacting with these new professionals will challenge the traditional paradigms of mental health care delivery in the immediate future. In doing so, we will discover innovative, cost-effective and safe ways to assist people with mental health problems, both now and into the future.

CRITICAL THINKING/LEARNING ACTIVITIES

1 Describe some benefits and limitations for delivering e-mental health care that might be experienced by health care professions and their clients.
2 How important is the development and acquisition of digital literacy skills in the healthcare sector, now and into the future?
3 Is e-mental health an opportunity or a threat to the mental health and well-being of people in society in general? Why? Or, why not?
4 What are some of the strengths and limitations of mental health triage call centres?
5 Describe how using e-mental health, telephone interaction or digital intervention enhances person-centred mental health recovery.

LEARNING EXTENSION

Reflective activity

Think back to the last time you called a service provider or company and were greeted by an automated phone service and menu (such as a telecommunications company, perhaps). How did you feel as you listened and made your way through the selections available? Did you want to ask a question, but couldn't? Did you want to talk about something slightly different to the categories offered? Did you feel like your enquiry was going to fit with the options available? Or would you have liked a different option that was not suggested? Did your enquiry fit into the menu available to you? Did you mind having to select numbers and follow instructions? Was it convenient? (And, if so, for whom?) What emotions did you experience? Ambivalence? Frustration? Anger? Confusion? Happiness? Satisfaction? Contented? Reflect on your experiences and feelings about your experiences.

Drawing on your learning from your own reflection on this type of experience, how do you think you would be able to assist a person with a mental health problem (or their carer) in this context? How would you engage with them positively? Can you see any barriers or enablers to the use of telephone triage services in a mental health context? Discuss with your peers.

Planning activity

With a small group of student peers, plan a brief e-mental health education intervention for a carer or a person experiencing an episode of depression, using resources from the websites of beyond blue and/or the Black Dog Institute, using mobile technology such as a smartphone. What preparation will you need to do beforehand? How will you convey the information and resources you have found to your clients? How will you select appropriate information? What education goals will you set? How will you know your intervention has been effective and helpful? How will you guide and facilitate the health learning experience?

ACKNOWLEDGEMENTS

Thanks to Mr Paul McNamara BN MMHN FACMHN for contributing his perspective to this chapter. Thanks to Dr Janene Carey for editorial assistance.

FURTHER READING

Arrigoni, C., Alvaro, R., Vellone, E. & Vanzetta, M. (2016). Social media and nurse education: An integrative review of the literature. *Journal of Mass Communication & Journalism*, *6*(1): 1–8.
This paper discusses social media in the context of nurse education. In particular, the ethical and professional use of social media is discussed.

Australian Medical Association Council of Doctors-in-Training, Australian Medical Students' Association, New Zealand Medical Association Council of Doctors-in-Training & New Zealand Medical Students' Association. (2012). *Social Media and the Medical Profession: A guide to online professionalism for medical practitioners and medical students*. Retrieved from https://ama.com.au/article/social-media-and-medical-profession
This guide provides practical advice about the safe use of social media for health care professionals.

Brusse, C., Gardner, K., McAullay, D. & Dowden, M. (2014). Social media and mobile apps for health promotion in Australian Indigenous populations: Scoping review. *Journal of Medical Internet Research*, *16*(12): e280.
This article describes how social media and smart device apps can be used in the context of specific health conditions and for specific populations.

West, C. & Verran, D. (2013). Something to tweet about: Incorporating social media into your nursing practice. *Transplant Journal of Australasia*, *22*(1): 10–12.
This paper provides insights on how to integrate social media use in professional practice.

Wilson, R. L., Ranse, J., Cashin, A. & McNamara, P. (2014). Nurses and Twitter: The good, the bad, and the reluctant. *Collegian: The Australian Journal of Nursing Practice, Scholarship and Research*, *21*(2): 111–19.
This paper describes how to get started as a health professional in the social media environment.

REFERENCES

Alkhaldi, G., Hamilton, F. L., Lau, R., Webster, R., Michie, S. & Murray, E. (2016). The effectiveness of prompts to promote engagement with digital interventions: A systematic review. *Journal of Medical Internet Research*, *18*(1): e6.

Arrigoni, C., Alvaro, R., Vellone, E. & Vanzetta, M. (2016). Social media and nurse education: An integrative review of the literature. *Journal of Mass Communication & Journalism*, *6*(1): 1–8.

Australian Commission on Safety and Quality in Health Care. (2015). *Australian Commission on Safety* and Quality in Health Care *Annual Report 2014/15*. Retrieved from http://www.safetyandquality.gov.au/wp-content/uploads/2015/10/Annual-Report-2014–15.pdf

Australian Medical Association Council of Doctors-in-Training, Australian Medical Students' Association, New Zealand Medical Association Council of Doctors-in-Training & New Zealand Medical Students' Association. (2012). *Social Media and the Medical Profession: A guide to online professionalism for medical practitioners and medical students*. Retrieved from https://ama.com.au/article/social-media-and-medical-profession

Bissell, D. (2015). Virtual infrastructures of habit; the changing intensities of habit through gracefulness, restlessness and clumsiness. *Cultural Geographies*, *22*(1): 127–46.

Bol, N., van Weert, J. C. M., Loos, E. F., Romano Bergstrom, J. C., Bolle, S. & Smets, E. M. A. (2016). How are online health messages processed? Using eye tracking to predict recall of information in younger and older adults. *Journal of Health Communication*, *21*(4): 387–96.

Brendryen, H., Drozd, F. & Kraft, P. (2008). A digital smoking cessation program delivered through internet and cell phone without nicotine replacement (Happy Ending): Randomized controlled trial. *Journal of Medical Internet Research*, *10*(5): e51.

Brusse, C., Gardner, K., McAullay, D. & Dowden, M. (2014). Social media and mobile apps for health promotion in Australian Indigenous populations: Scoping review. *Journal of Medical Internet Research*, *16*(12): e280.

Byambasuren, O., Sanders, S., Beller, E. & Glasziou, P. (2018). Prescribable mHealth apps identified from an overview of systematic reviews. *npj Digital Medicine*, *1*(12): 814.

Christensen, L. F., Wilson, R., Hansen, J. P., Nielsen, C. T. & Gildberg, F. A. (2020). A qualitative study of patients' and providers' experiences with the use of videoconferences by older adults with depression. *International Journal of Mental Health Nursing*, 30(2): 427–39.

Cronin, C., Hungerford, C. & Wilson, R. L. (2020). Using digital health technologies to manage the psychosocial symptoms of menopause in the workplace: A narrative literature review. *Issues in Mental Health Nursing*, *42*(6): 541–8.

Cuijpers, P., Riper, H. & Andersson, G. (2015). Internet-based treatment of depression. *Current Opinion in Psychology*, (4): 131–5.

Department of Health. (2015). Digital Health (Website). Retrieved from http://www.health.gov.au/internet/main/publishing.nsf/Content/eHealth

Department of Health and Ageing. (2012). *e-Mental Health Strategy for Australia*. Canberra: Commonwealth of Australia. Retrieved from https://www.health.gov.au/internet/main/publishing.nsf/content/7C7B0BFEB985D0EBCA257BF0001BB0A6/$File/emstrat.pdf

Elsom, S., Sands, N., Roper, C., Hoppner, C. & Gerdtz, M. (2013). Telephone survey of service-user experiences of a telephone-based mental health triage service. *International Journal of Mental Health Nursing*, *22*: 437–43.

European Commission. (2012). eHealth Action Plan 2012–2020: Innovative health care for the 21st century (Webpage). Retrieved from https://ec.europa.eu/digital-single-market/en/news/ehealth-action-plan-2012-2020-innovative-healthcare-21st-century

Ferguson, C., Davidson, P. M., Scott, P. J., Jackson, D. & Hickman, L. D. (2015). Augmented reality, virtual reality and gaming: An integral part of nursing. *Contemporary Nurse*, *51*(1): 1–4.

Ferguson, C., Jackson, D. & Hickman, L. D. (2018). 'Use this app twice daily': How digital tools are revolutionizing patient care. *The Conversation*, 24 July. Retrieved from https://theconversation.com/use-this-app-twice-daily-how-digital-tools-are-revolutionising-patient-care-99456

Fox, S. & Duggan, M. (2012). *Mobile Health 2012: Half of smartphone owners use their devices to get health information and one-fifth of smartphone owners have health apps*. Retrieved from http://www.pewinternet.org/files/old-media/Files/Reports/2012/PIP_MobileHealth2012_FINAL.pdf

Fraser, S., Randell, A., DeSilva, S. & Parker, A. (2016). *Research Bulletin: e-Mental health: the future of youth mental health?* Retrieved https://www.orygen.org.au/Training/Resources/digital-technology/Research-bulletins/E-mental-health-the-future-of-youth-mental-health/orygen-e-mental-health-rb?ext=

Free, C., Phillips, G., Galli, L., Watson, L., Felix, L., Edwards, P. … Haines, A. (2013). The effectiveness of mobile-health technology-based health behaviour change or disease management interventions for health care consumers: A systematic review. *PLoS Medicine*, *10*(1): e1001362.

Ghezeljeh, T. N., Sharifian, S., Isfahani, M. N. & Haghani, H. (2018). Comparing the effects of education using telephone follow-up and smartphone-based social networking follow-up on self-management behaviors among patients with hypertension. *Contemporary Nurse*, *54*(4–5): 362–73.

Greenhalgh, T., Shaw, S., Wherton, J., Vijayaraghavan, S., Morris, J., Bhattacharya, S. … Hodkinson, I. (2018). Real-world implementation of video outpatient consultations at macro, meso, and micro levels: mixed-method study. *Journal of Medical Internet Research*, *20*(4): e150. Retrieved from http://europepmc.org/abstract/MED/29625956,http://europepmc.org/articles/PMC5930173,https://doi.org/10.2196/jmir.9897

Helweg-Joergensen, S., Schmidt, T., Lichtenstein, M. B. & Pedersen, S. S. (2019). Using a mobile diary app in the treatment of borderline personality disorder: Mixed methods feasibility study. *JMIR Formative Research*, *3*(3): e12852.

Heron, K. E. & Smyth, J. M. (2010). Ecological momentary interventions: Incorporating mobile technology into psychosocial and health behaviour treatments. *British Journal of Health Psychology*, *15*(1): 1–39.

Hung, L., Au-Yeung, A., Helmer, C., Ip, A., Elijah, L., Wilkins-Ho, M. & Chaudhury, H. (2018). Feasibility and acceptability of an iPad intervention to support dementia care in the hospital setting. *Contemporary Nurse*, 54(4–5): 350–61.

Hunter, B. H. & Radoll, P. J. (2020). Dynamics of digital diffusion and disadoption: A longitudinal analysis of Indigenous and other Australians. *Australasian Journal of Information Systems*, *24*: 1–21.

ICT Data and Statistics Division, Telecommunication Development Bureau & Switzerland International Telecommunications Union. (2012). Mobile cellular subscriptions per 100 inhabitants, 2001–2011 (Excel spreadsheet). Retrieved from http://www.indexmundi.com/facts/switzerland/indicator/IT.CEL.SETS.P2

Kaplan, A. M. & Haenlein, M. (2010). Users of the world, unite! The challenges and opportunities of social media. *Business Horizons*, *53*(1): 59–68.

Kazemi, D. M., Cochran, A. R., Kelly, J. F., Cornelius, J. B. & Belk, C. (2012). Integrating mHealth mobile applications to reduce high risk drinking among underage students. *Health Education Journal*, *73*(3), 262–73.

Kerfoot, B. P., Gagnon, D. R., McMahon, G. T., Orlander, J. D., Kurgansky, K. E. & Conlin, P. R. (2017). A team-based online game improves blood glucose control in veterans with type 2 diabetes: A randomized controlled trial. *Diabetes Care*, *40*(9): 1218–25.

Kirmayer, L. J., Raikhel, E. & Rahimi, S. (2013). Cultures of the internet: Identity, community and mental health. *Transcultural Psychiatry*, *50*(2), 165–91.

Kobak, K. A., Mundt, J. C. & Kennard, B. (2015). Integrating technology into cognitive behavior therapy for adolescent depression: A pilot study. *Annals of General Psychiatry*, *14*(37): 1–10.

Leavy, J. E., Rosenburg, M., Barnes, R., Bauman, A. & Bull, F. C. (2013). Would you find thirty online? Website use in a Western Australian physical activity campaign. *Health Promotion Journal of Australia*, *24*(2): 118–25.

Lublin, N. (2012). Texting That Saves Lives. TED Talk. Retrieved from https://www.youtube.com/watch?v=LiUClSItcy0

Mathiasen, K., Riper, H., Ehlers, L. H., Valentin, J. B. & Rosenberg, N. K. (2016). Internet-based CBT for social phobia and panic disorder in a specialised anxiety clinic in routine care: Results of a pilot randomised controlled trial. *Internet Interventions*, *4*: 92–8.

Morrison, L. G., Yardley, L., Powell, J. & Michie, S. (2012). What design features are used in effective e-health interventions? A review using techniques from critical interpretive synthesis. *Telemedicine Journal and e-Health*, *18*: 137–44.

Moyle, W., Jones, C., Pu, L. & Chen, S. (2018) Applying user-centred research design and evidence to develop and guide the use of technologies, including robots, in aged care, *Contemporary Nurse*, *54*(1): 1–3.

Natanson, E. (2017). Digital therapeutics: The future of health care will be app-based. *Forbes*, 24 July. Retrieved from https://www.forbes.com/sites/eladnatanson/2017/07/24/digital-therapeutics-the-future-of-health-care-will-be-app-based/?sh=169535007637

Nursing and Midwifery Board of Australia. (2019). Social media: How to meet your obligations under the National Law (Webpage). Retrieved from https://www.nursingmidwiferyboard.gov.au/Codes-Guidelines-Statements/Codes-Guidelines/Social-media-guidance.aspx

Paliadelis, P. S., Stupens, I., Parker, V., Piper, D., Gillan, P., Lea, J. … Fagan, A. (2015). The development and evaluation of online stories to enhance clinical learning experiences across health professions in rural Australia. *Collegian*, *22*(4): 397–403.

Paul, S. S., Tiedemann, A., Hassett, L. M., Ramsay, E., Kirkham, C., Chagpar, S. & Sherrington, C. (2015). Validity of the Fitbit activity tracker for measuring steps in community-dwelling older adults. *BMJ Open Exercise and Sport Medicine*, *1*: e000013.

Proudfoot, J., Clarke, J., Birch, M.-R. , Whitton, A. E., Parker, G., Manicavasagar, V. … Hadzi-Pavlovic, D. (2014). Impact of mobile phone and web program on symptom and functional outcomes for people with mild-to-moderate depression, anxiety and stress: A randomised controlled trial. *BMC Psychiatry*, *13*: 312.

Research2Guidance. (n.d.). 325,000 mobile health apps available in 2017 (Webpage). Retrieved from https://research2guidance.com/325000-mobile-health-apps-available-in-2017/)

Shaw, A., Paul, D., Billingsley, W., Kwan, P. & Wilson, R. L. (2017). Gamification in E-mental health: Development of a digital intervention addressing severe mental illness and metabolic syndrome. Paper presented to the International Conference on Internet Technologies & Society, Sydney, Australia.

Shaw, A., Paul, D., Wilson, R. L., Billingsley, W. & Kwan, P. (2016). Gamification in E-Mental Health: Development of a digital intervention addressing severe mental illness and metabolic syndrome. Paper presented to the OzCHI2016 Connected Futures conference, Launceston, Tasmania. Retrieved from http://www.ozchi.org/2016/

Shore, J. H. (2013). Telepsychiatry: Videoconferencing in the delivery of psychiatric care. *American Journal of Psychiatry, 170*: 256–62.

Søgaard Neilsen, A. & Wilson, R. L. (2019). Combining e-mental health intervention development with human computer interaction (HCI) design to enhance technology-facilitated recovery for people with depression and/or anxiety conditions: An integrative literature review. *International Journal of Mental Health Nursing, 28*(1): 22–39.

Statewide Telehealth Services. (2013). *Extending the reach of clinical health services throughout Queensland* (Video). Brisbane: Queensland Health.

Thompson, N. (2015). Responding to trauma: Promoting healing and recovery. *People Skills*, 4th edn (pp. 256–62). London: Palgrave.

Usher, K., Woods, C., Casellac, E., Glass, N., Wilson R. L., Mayner, L. … Irwin, P. (2014). Australian health professions student use of social media. *Collegian, 21*(2): 95–101.

Usher, W. (2010). Australian health professionals' social media (Web 2.0) adoption trends: Early 21st century health care delivery and practice promotion. *Australian Journal of Primary Health, 18*: 31–41.

West, C. & Verran, D. (2013). Something to tweet about: Incorporating social media into your nursing practice. *Transplant Journal of Australasia, 22*(1): 10–12.

Wilson, R. L. (2010). Mental Health Case-Based Simulation and Virtual Learning Environments (VLE) in Mental Health Pre-Registration Nursing Education. Paper presented to the Australian College of Mental Health Nurses 36th International Conference, Hobart, Tasmania.

—— (2018). The right way for nurses to prescribe, administer and critique digital therapies. *Contemporary Nurse, 54*(4–5): 543–5.

Wilson, R. L., Carryer, J., Dewing, J., Rosado, S., Gildberg, F., Hutton, A., Johnson, A., Kaunonen, M. & Sheridan, N. (2020). The state of the nursing profession in the International Year of the Nurse and Midwife 2020 during COVID-19: A nursing standpoint. *Nursing Philosophy, 21*(3): e12314.

Wilson, R. L., Ranse, J., Cashin, A. & McNamara, P. (2013). Nurses and Twitter: The good, the bad, and the reluctant. *Collegian: The Australian Journal of Nursing Practice, Scholarship and Research, 21*(2): 111–19.

Wilson R. L. & Usher, K. (2015). Rural nurses: A convenient co-location strategy for rural mental health care of young people. *Journal of Clinical Nursing, 24*(17–18): 2638–48.

World Health Organization (WHO). (2018). *Classification of digital health interventions v1.0.* (WHO/RHR/18.06). Retrieved from https://apps.who.int/iris/bitstream/handle/10665/260480/WHO-RHR-18.06-eng.pdf

—— (2020). *ICD-11 mortality and morbidity statistics. Mental, behavioural or neurodevelopmental disorders.* Retrieved from https://icd.who.int/browse11/l-m/en#/http%3a%2f%2fid.who.int%2ficd%2fentity%2f1448597234

Zarski, A. C., Lehr, D., Berking, M., Riper, H., Cuijpers, P. & Ebert, D. D. (2016). Adherence to internet-based mobile-supported stress management: A pooled analysis of individual participant data from three randomized controlled trials. *Journal of Medical Internet Research, 18*(6): e146.

Mental health and substance use

12

Rhonda L. Wilson, Andrea E. Donaldson
and Bernadette Solomon

LEARNING OBJECTIVES

At the completion of this chapter, you should be able to:

1 Consider how harm minimisation can be implemented to improve mental health outcomes for individuals and communities.
2 Recognise the effects of legal and illegal drugs which, when misused, can adversely affect mental health and well-being.
3 Consider the ways in which person-centred care can promote the recovery of people with combined drug, alcohol and mental health conditions.
4 Identify holistic care opportunities related to professional care of mental health conditions and drug and alcohol problems.
5 Recognise the physical and mental healthcare needs of people affected by drug misuse.

Introduction

This chapter introduces the intersections between mental health care and drug and alcohol care. It addresses the implications for holistic healthcare needs related to dual drug and alcohol use, and concurrent mental health conditions. It tells the contemporary, real-life story of a person who developed an episode of psychosis following consumption of premixed alcohol and caffeine drinks. The chapter also describes change models applied to substance use and recovery, such as motivational interviewing and stages of change readiness. Both common and less common drugs and their misuse affect the physical, social, cognitive and mental health dimensions of people with mental health conditions. Reflective exercises guide you to consider how you will be able to promote mental health and well-being, and minimise drug-related harm, to individuals and communities in practice context.

Prevalence of co-occurring disorders

The terms 'comorbidity', 'coexisting' or 'co-occurring' refer to 'the co-occurrence of two or more mental disorders within the one individual, either at the same time or within a specified period such as 12 months or over the lifetime' (Oakley Browne, Wells & Scott, 2006).

The issue of comorbidity or co-occurring mental illness and alcohol and drug addiction has become a focus of mental health and alcohol and other drug services in Aotearoa New Zealand and Australia due to the prevalence of these disorders. In Aotearoa New Zealand, *Te Rau Hinengaro: The New Zealand Mental Health Survey* (Oakley Browne et al., 2006) found that 9.4 per cent of people with anxiety disorders also had a substance-use disorder. Only 7.9 per cent of the population experiences a mood disorder, but that figure rises to 29 per cent in people with a 12-month substance-abuse disorder. Comorbidity among substance-use disorders was common: 'Around a quarter of those with alcohol dependence also met criteria for drug dependence (23.5 per cent) or drug abuse (28.1 per cent)' (Oakley Browne et al., 2006, p. 76). Among those with drug-use disorders, even greater proportions had alcohol use disorder comorbidity: 'About half (49.9 per cent) of those with drug dependence also reported alcohol abuse symptoms in the past 12 months, and 43.1 per cent of those with drug dependence were also alcohol dependent' (Oakley Browne et al., 2006, p. 76).

A national survey on mental health and well-being in Australia (ABS, 2007) found that, across a 12-month period, 8.7 per cent of people diagnosed with a mental disorder also had a diagnosis of substance use and one or more other mental disorders (anxiety disorder, affective disorder or both) (AIHW, 2018). The 2016 National Drug Strategy Household Survey (NDSHS; AIHW, 2017) found that '26 per cent of recent illicit drug users had been diagnosed or treated for a mental illness in the previous 12 months' and '22 per cent of recent illicit drug users reported high or very high levels of psychological distress in the previous four weeks' (AIHW, 2018, p. 218). The AIHW states that:

> the 2016 NDSHS showed that self-reported rates of mental illness were higher among people who reported the use of illicit drugs in the previous 12 months than among people who had not used over this period. Specifically, mental illness was reported by 26 per cent of people who had used any illicit drug in the previous 12 months, compared with 14 per cent of people who had not used an illicit drug in the previous 12 months. (AIHW, 2018, p. 218)

Harm minimisation

Australian and Aotearoa New Zealand drug policies have been underpinned by a **harm-minimisation** philosophy, which has a 'three pillars' approach to implementation: supply reduction, demand reduction and harm reduction. This collaborative approach includes stakeholder partnerships across government agencies, including those responsible for health, education and law enforcement (Department of Health and Ageing, 2011; Ritter, King & Hamilton, 2013; He Ara Oranga, 2018). Supply reduction is largely a role for policymakers, legislators and justice systems, while reducing demand and reducing harm to individuals, groups and communities are areas of focus for health and education service providers. Health services aim to provide enough information to assist people to make healthy lifestyle choices and thereby deter the harmful uptake of drug and alcohol use, and/or to help people reduce or cease the use of harmful drugs and alcohol if this has occurred.

harm-minimisation – a multi-agency drug policy approach, aimed at achieving supply reduction, demand reduction and harm reduction

Harm prevention

Any type of substance misuse has the potential to harm people's physical and mental health, social relationships, finances and academic and career prospects. Therefore, as health professionals we need to examine how to support and promote harm-prevention strategies (Dick et al., 2019).

Table 12.1 Harm prevention

Substance	Risk patterns	Prevalence of harm	Recommended harm prevention/reduction
Alcohol	Intoxication Regular use	High: leading cause of harm	Promotion of recommendations for standard drinks (how much alcohol consumed in an hour) Advertising about appropriate alcohol consumption Random breath-testing Thiamine fortification of drinks and flour Increased resources and services
Tobacco	Regular use	Toxicity High risk of lung disease	Early education Cognitive behavioural therapy (CBT) to reduce use Medicinal nicotine Smokeless tobacco e-cigarettes
Cannabis	Regular use Dependence	Low for health- related harms, high for criminal justice costs Low/reduced capacity for productive functioning Low motivation and interest in daily activities (Palmer et al. 2012)	Use of civil penalties rather than criminal penalties Online and mobile platforms to deliver interventions with instant availability and at relatively low cost. Emphasis on elements of social cognitive theory, including self-efficacy, outcome expectation, observational learning, facilitation and self-regulation, which were used to develop text messages focused on substance misuse resistance skills (Haug et al., 2017).
Other illicit substances	Overdose Intoxication Dependence	Lower than legal drugs for health and social costs High for law enforcement costs, social harm (Toumbourou et al., 2007).	Needle-exchange programs Hepatitis B vaccinations for service users and safe injecting areas (Toumbourou et al., 2007). Hepatitis B and hepatitis C health information/ education and early treatment

REFLECTIVE QUESTIONS

Alcohol and tobacco are drugs that are available for purchase in Australia and Aotearoa New Zealand under legally regulated conditions of sale and consumption. Take some time to consider the pros and cons of legalisation and regulation of supply.

- What are the health and social influences and the consequences of alcohol and cigarette smoking in your community?
- Have our laws and regulations achieved a balanced approach to management of these two legal drugs?

List some changes you would like to see in the future and explain why.

An overview of substance-use problems

drugs – in the context of this chapter, legal or illegal substances that have a psychoactive effect on the central nervous system and are taken for the purpose of achieving pleasurable or normative personal experiences

The use of **drugs** can be considered a problem or 'non-problem', based on the health, social, behavioural and cognitive outcomes related to that use. The chemical nature of a particular substance (drug) as well as its availability, including its legality, determines the potential for harm. It is how these substances are used that determines the behavioural patterns and whether it results in harm. There are three main groups of drugs that are used or misused for non-therapeutic purposes, described in Table 12.2. It should be noted that there is a range of subjective variability, related to the experiences people may have with drugs within these categories (Ritter et al., 2013). For instance, alcohol is a depressant but, when used in small quantities, some people experience behavioural stimulation promoting a sense of social disinhibition, which may be considered a desirable outcome by the person consuming the alcohol (Ritter et al., 2013). In addition to these broad categories, it is important to consider poly drug use, which may include the use of drugs across categories, thereby further complicating the effects of the drug. The setting or context in which the drug is taken (Bullock, Ranse & Hutton, 2018), along with the mood in which the drug is consumed, are both important considerations (Zinberg, 1984). Thus, if alcohol is consumed in a context in which the mood is low, and the person is alone, the alcohol effects will most likely reinforce a state of depression. However, if the alcohol is consumed when the person's mood is happy, and in a social and celebratory setting, the alcohol effects more likely will stimulate the drinker's behaviour. An assessment of the drug type, along with the context and mood, will be required in order to understand the dynamics related to an individual's drug experiences. For example, substance use associated with outdoor music festivals has been identified as a context in which high increased substance use and related intoxication may occur, placing higher demands on health services located at the event, or nearby (Bullock et al., 2018).

Table 12.2   Drug categories

Drug category	Description	Examples
Depressants	Drugs that cause the central nervous system to be inhibited or depressed. Symptoms include decreased respiration and heart rate.	Alcohol, benzodiazepines (e.g. Valium), opioids (heroin, pethidine, morphine, methadone, Endone, OxyContin) and cannabis
Stimulants	Drugs that cause an increase in central nervous system activity and arousal. Symptoms include increased heart rate, respirations and blood pressure; increased temperature, especially with amphetamine-based drugs; and some increase in agitation and aggression.	Methylenedioxymethamphetamine (MDMA, or ecstasy), amphetamines, methamphetamine ('ice'), cocaine, caffeine, nicotine and synthetic, cocaine-like 'bath salts'
Hallucinogens	Drugs that alter the central nervous system so that perceptions, thinking or cognition, feelings or emotions and sense of time or place are distorted. Symptoms include the sometimes-frightening experiences of delusions and paranoia.	LSD (acid), mescaline (peyote cactus), psilocybin (magic mushrooms), cannabis, kronic/spice (synthetic cannabis) and *Daytura stramonium* leaf)

An overview of drugs and their effects

Alcohol

Alcohol is a depressant drug, and it acts to slow heart and respiratory rates. Alcohol is often associated with mood-related conditions, and especially so in people who experience depression (Attenborough, 2010; Crum et al., 2013). Alcohol is a legal drug that is the most likely of all drugs to be misused in Australia, and it is sometimes misused by people who attempt to regulate their distress by modifying both low and elevated moods (Attenborough, 2010; AIHW, 2011). Alcohol is frequently associated with death by suicide (Attenborough, 2010; Darvishi et al., 2015; Cobiac & Wilson, 2018). Suicide is the most significant problem caused by alcohol misuse in Aboriginal men and represents the most common cause of death for this group, while alcohol misuse related to suicide is the fourth-most common cause of deaths among Aboriginal women in Australia (Wilkes et al., 2010). Similarly, in Aotearoa New Zealand, there is also a significant link between alcohol misuse and suicide completion (Cobiac & Wilson, 2018). In particular, Māori (who make up 15 per cent of the Aotearoa New Zealand population) have a suicide rate that is 84 per cent higher than non-Māori individuals (Hatcher et al., 2016). Longer-term, risky alcohol consumption is particularly harmful, with implications for decline in physical and mental health (e.g. liver failure and cirrhosis;

gastrointestinal haemorrhage and ulceration; depression; alcohol-related dementia). Withdrawal from alcohol dependence should be monitored and managed carefully because abrupt alcohol withdrawal can trigger seizures resulting in death. A carefully managed, gradual withdrawal is required to support a person who has planned to reduce or cease their use of alcohol (MHDAO, 2008). In addition, social and psychological support will be needed to provide holistic support for a comprehensive withdrawal (MHDAO, 2008).

Low-risk alcohol consumption consists of no more than two standard drinks per day and should include some alcohol-free days each week (National Health and Medical Research Council (NHMRC), 2009). A standard drink is equivalent to 10 grams of alcohol. The percentage by volume of alcohol in any drink will differ depending on the type of beverage consumed; for example, a 'pot' or 'middy' (285 mL) of strong beer (7% alcohol) is equal to 1.4 standard drinks, whereas a 'nip' or 'shot' (30 mL) of spirits (40% alcohol) is equal to 1.0 standard drink (Department of Health and Ageing, 2013; AIHW, 2014). Alcohol is metabolised by the liver, and for a healthy adult it typically takes approximately one hour for the liver to process one standard drink. For a healthy adult, no more than four standard drinks should be consumed in one sitting, as the risk of alcohol-related injury increases considerably for that episode (NHMRC, 2009; Edward & Alderman, 2013).

binge drinking –
drinking alcohol with the
intention of becoming
drunk

Binge drinking is described as drinking alcohol with the intention of drinking to become drunk. Young people are more likely to binge drink, with 20 per cent of young people reporting this behaviour (AIHW, 2011). There is some evidence to suggest that SMS messaging of health promotion and/or brief information is one example of a strategy to reduce alcohol consumption rates among young people, including during episodes of social interaction, thus a real time e-health strategy might be useful in addressing the adverse effects of binge drinking for young people (Hutton et al., 2020).

Caffeine

Caffeine is a stimulant found in products like tea, coffee, chocolate and cola soft drinks. Increasingly, it is found in premixed alcoholic and non-alcoholic energy drinks. In small doses, caffeine has effects that include increased heart rate, energy and stimulation. This is a pleasant sensation for many people; however, even at low doses withdrawal can result in discomfort such as headaches and agitation. At higher doses and in combination with other drugs, caffeine can contribute to the experiences such as those that Mark reports in his story (see p. 261). And, as Mark's story demonstrates, not all people are aware that they are consuming both alcohol and caffeine in premixed alcoholic beverages.

Cannabis

Cannabis (delta-9 tetrahydrocannabinol, or THC) is a drug that is often associated with both depression and psychosis. Attempts to understand causal relationships between the use of cannabis and the experience of these mental health conditions have been the subject of much research; however, empirical evidence of a causal relationship in either direction – that is, that cannabis causes psychosis, or that psychosis predisposes people to decisions to consume cannabis – remains elusive, despite the efforts of many researchers (DiForti et al., 2015; Dubertret et al., 2006; Ferdinand et al., 2005; Fergerson, Horwood & Ridder, 2005; Green, Young & Kavanagh, 2005; Mental Health Council of Australia, 2006; Ritter et al., 2013; Solowij & Michie, 2007; Volkow et al., 2016).

Cannabis is most commonly used by smoking the dried leaves or heads of the cannabis plant, either as a paper-rolled cigarette – sometimes combined with tobacco – or with the use of a water pipe ('bong'). It is also consumed in baked products such as 'hash cookies'. Inhalation provides a fast effect, and for this reason it is most likely to be smoked. A 2015 Aotearoa New Zealand study indicated that Māori men were 2.1 times more likely and Māori women were 2.3 times more likely to use cannabis, in comparison with non-Māori individuals (Ministry of Health, 2015).

Synthetic drugs

Some synthetic copies of cannabis and other drugs have become prominent in recent times. They are frequently marketed as 'herbal cigarettes', or as incense, to connect with customers who are curious and looking for a legal and safe alternative to illegal drugs such as cannabis, amphetamines and cocaine. It is difficult for regulators to keep up with the rapid pace with which these types of drugs are varied and manufactured, and so legislation through therapeutic goods administration and regulation of their sale lag behind in listing new products as illegal substances (Barratt, Cakic & Lenton, 2013). Synthetic cannabinoids are sprayed onto inert plant matter, which is then smoked using the methods typical of cannabis inhalation. Some common names for these substances are 'kronic' and 'spice' (Ritter et al., 2013). These substances should not be considered safe, or a lesser risk, than other known drugs, because it is impossible to accurately know their ingredients and concentration. In the case of kronic, there are known cases of debilitating psychosis and other mental and physical health conditions that have been triggered by the use of these drugs (Barratt et al., 2013; Solomon et al., 2014). Synthetic drugs are best avoided because so little is known about them, and the adverse consequences are thought to be significant. Furthermore, people who use synthetic drugs tend not to seek help (Barratt et al., 2013).

Amphetamines

Amphetamines (sometimes referred to as 'speed') were discovered about 100 years ago, and have been used in the clinical context for much of that time (Heal et al., 2013). However, misuse of amphetamines in its various forms is problematic. Amphetamines act to stimulate the central nervous system. They are consumed in various forms, such as in oral tablets or wafers, inhaled nasally, or injected intravenously. People misuse amphetamines in search of pleasurable, alert and energetic effects. This experience usually lasts for several hours, while with continued heavy misuse paranoid, perceptual, cognitive and delusional problems can occur. The resulting behaviours and sensations can be frightening, and they can place individuals in risky circumstances (e.g. thinking they are safe to drive at high speeds). The physiological risks include increases to blood pressure, heart rate, respiration and body temperature, with increased body temperature placing individuals at high risk of serious and life-threatening neurological damage, in particular. Amphetamine-style drugs are sometimes considered 'party' drugs (e.g. MDMA/ecstasy), and in a party setting where it is hot, there is poor air circulation and cooling, perhaps some dancing and alcohol consumption, the risk of dehydration and elevation in temperature is high.

Methamphetamine

Methamphetamine (sometimes known as 'ice' or 'crystal') is one type of amphetamine that has become popular among people who use stimulant drugs. The prevalence of use has increased significantly over the past 10 years (Degenhardt et al., 2017) with three-quarters of all stimulant use now attributed to methamphetamine use (Peacock et al. 2018). However, it has some particularly challenging side-effects, which include violence, anger and aggression in combination with psychosis, and these have complicated the care of many people presenting to accident and emergency departments in recent years (Cloutier et al., 2013; Jones et al., 2019). Increasingly, many methamphetamine-triggered adverse events requiring pre-hospital care also needs the support of police to ensure safety of the patient and the staff administering health care (Redona et al., 2019). The recent acceleration of methamphetamine use and misuse has highlighted the need for mental health professionals to consider carefully the substance use and misuse history of people in mental health, and other healthcare settings, and to incorporate assessment, de-escalation strategies and safety planning within their professional practice skill development portfolio.

Cocaine

Cocaine is a stimulant drug that is usually injected or inhaled and has many of the same problems and effects as amphetamine drugs. However, the immediate euphoric effects and arousal experienced following consumption of cocaine is short-lived and dissipates within a short time – around half an hour. Despite the reduced sensations, the brain continues to be affected, and often with racing thoughts, irritability, depression and insomnia. People sometimes attempt to modify these symptoms with further doses of cocaine, but while the brain remains saturated with the drug, the pleasurable effects are minimal, and a downward neuro-chemical and behavioural spiral occurs.

Opioids

Opioids are used therapeutically to manage strong pain in the form of injectable (intravenous or intramuscular) morphine or pethidine, or oxycodone in tablet form for pain such as cancer-related pain. Opioids are important clinical medications for the management of both acute and chronic physical pain. However, they are also drugs that are often misused, in the illegal form of heroin, in particular. Fentanyl is a potent synthetic opioid that is an effective analgesic but illegal diversion and use of this drug, when combined with other depressant drugs, has seen an increase in deaths among younger men who have a history of using injectable drugs (Roxburgh et al., 2013).

Heroin is usually injected intravenously and has an immediate euphoric effect; however, less commonly it is smoked, which also has a very quick effect. A sensation of relaxation and calm follows use of this drug, and this can last several hours. Heroin is a depressant drug and its side-effects include respiratory depression, reduced heart rate and low blood pressure. Combining heroin with other depressant drugs such as alcohol can amplify the physiological responses, and this can lead to unconsciousness and death.

Tolerance builds exponentially with continued misuse of opioids, including heroin, which means that people require more of the drug to achieve the desirable effects; however, over time the pleasurable effects are reduced and depression develops. People feel compelled to continue to use this drug to achieve a normal effect, and thus a dependency develops. It is very difficult to break this cycle once it has developed, and the social consequences are complicated because the escalating rates and amounts of use are extremely expensive to maintain, and frequently people become involved in crime, selling their goods, or providing services (e.g. sexual services) to others to pay for their supply of drugs. This circumstance is detrimental to the basic requirements of a healthy life, such as the procurement of quality food, housing, clothing, health care and training. The health, social and economic risks are significant for individuals who misuse heroin, and include the risk of infectious diseases such as HIV/AIDS and hepatitis C if needles, syringes or other drug-using paraphernalia are shared between injecting drug users to reduce costs or enhance convenience.

Benzodiazapines

Benzodiazapines (some common trade names include Diazepam/Valium, Temazepam, Lorazepam and Rohypnol) are among a group of drugs that are legal to use but require a medical prescription to obtain. They can be misused and are sometimes obtained illegally through illicit marketplaces. They are used in a therapeutic form to address the short-term distress of people experiencing anxiety or stress and, sometimes, to assist in enhancing sleep. Benzodiazepines are only effective in the short-term treatment of acute conditions; however, once they are introduced for longer-term use, or misuse, they are extremely difficult to withdraw from. The side-effects are very uncomfortable and include depression, anxiety, panic attacks, psychosis, hallucinations, insomnia and nightmares. People who choose to withdraw from benzodiazepines usually need a great deal of clinical support, which might include cognitive behavioural therapy (CBT), motivational interviewing and change management to achieve withdrawal or reduction in their drug use.

Benzodiazapines are extremely effective depressive drugs, and they will dampen the person's mood; this sometimes makes people think that they are lacking any feeling or emotion at all. To counteract this, some people combine benzodiazapines with other drugs, such as alcohol, to enhance a sense of sociability and confidence. However, the risks associated with this include a bolstered sense of being indestructible, and it is in this condition that coordination is impaired, and sense of self-confidence is high, when risks are taken that can have consequences such as compromising the safety of the person misusing the drugs or other people, and damage to property.

Nicotine

Nicotine is found in tobacco cigarettes. It is a drug that is associated with harm, both to physical and mental health. Nicotine stimulates dopamine neuro-chemical responses and promotes a sense of calm and well-being; however, during withdrawal, anxiety, stress and depression are likely to be experienced (Edward & Alderman, 2013). People with mental health conditions are twice as likely as the general population to smoke cigarettes (Smith, Mazure & McKee, 2014). Smoking increases the risk of respiratory and cardiac diseases, and these are major contributors to the total burden of disease for Australia and Aotearoa New Zealand. Nicotine influences the metabolism of caffeine and some medications for mental health conditions; any reduction or cessation of smoking may also reduce the effective dosage rate of some medications, thereby reducing the effects of high doses and related side-effects (Edward & Alderman, 2013).

Solvents

Solvents are volatile substances. They either vaporise or evaporate when they come in contact with air. People who inhale or sniff these substances are at immediate risk of neurological and/or cardiac and/or respiratory risk, which can include irreparable damage to the brain and cardiac systems. There is no way to assess which episode of use will cause irreversible damage, and the risk is exceedingly high. Solvents are found in products such as aerosol cans, glues, petrol and other fuels, nail polish and correction fluids. People who inhale these solvents experience an immediate effect of the gaseous toxins, which enter the blood stream and central nervous system extremely quickly, followed by a momentary sensation of euphoria that dissipates quickly. Regular use increases tolerance, and this promotes the use of increased doses and increased frequency of use to achieve the desired outcomes, which in turn amplifies the risks. Solvents are relatively cheap to purchase, and they can be easily obtained from a range of common household products, and this availability has an influence on use and access.

Communities in central Australia have identified a particular problem with a high number of young people inhaling petrol, and government, community and retail stakeholders are working together to explore ways to minimise the risks to the population in regard to petrol sniffing. One intervention has reduced the availability of normal petrol and has increased the availability of petrol modified to remove harmful volatile solvents, such as opal fuel, and thereby has minimised the supply of a substance known to cause harm to people (Schwartzkoff et al., 2008).

Paracetamol

Paracetamol and other over-the-counter medications are sometimes used in suicide attempts, or as a method of self-harm. In Aotearoa New Zealand, 'a five-year audit of data (2007–2012) from the Wellington Hospital Emergency Department revealed paracetamol was the most common medication used for overdose (23 per cent)' (Freeman & Quigley, 2015). In 2012, aminophenol derivatives accounted for 22.4 per cent of hospitalisations for poisonings in Aotearoa New Zealand (Freeman & Quigley, 2015). Since 2007, paracetamol toxicity has been implicated in 31 deaths in Aotearoa New Zealand, and the Coroner has often found the overdose was accidental (Schumacher, 2018). Many of the deaths resulted from liver failure due to a combination of excessive alcohol and paracetamol use (Freeman & Quigley, 2015). Some people who overdose on products such as paracetamol report that they do so in an attempt to ease emotional discomfort, and sometimes with a view that they would like to 'go to sleep and not have to wake up'. Frequently, people are not aware of the serious consequences of paracetamol toxicity. Paracetamol toxicity can cause life-threatening liver failure and sometimes requires admission to a critical care unit in a hospital so that liver function can be carefully monitored (Bateman et al. 2014; Daly et al., 2008). Nausea, vomiting and abdominal pain (right upper-quadrant) may signify excessive use of paracetamol. If a person is receiving care in a critical care unit, then consideration should be given to the physical environment, in which there may be many accessible and lethal means of suicide available. Close monitoring in regard to mental health safety and continuing mental health assessment, in conjunction with building a therapeutic rapport, are equally as important as management for prevention of liver failure.

Understanding the time delay between the taking of excess paracetamol and admission to health care will influence the selection of treatment protocols. If within one hour, an orally administered, activated charcoal may be a sufficient response. Up to 8 hours following ingestion and based on the extent of liver function, obtained through a blood test, a decision needs to be made about the level of toxicity and whether intravenous infusion of N-acetylcysteine may need to be commenced, measured against the paracetamol toxicity nomograph tool (Daly et al., 2008). If ingestion is known to have occurred longer than 8 hours prior to receiving health care, then an N-acetylcysteine infusion is likely to be commenced immediately, and liver function monitoring commenced (Daly et al., 2008). If other drugs such as alcohol are also present, this adds further clinical complexity and risk, especially as alcohol is metabolised largely in the liver (Daly et al., 2008). It may be difficult to ascertain a clear history of ingestion of tablets and alcohol if the person is intoxicated, sedated or cognitively compromised. There are no pleasurable effects following use of paracetamol. A vulnerability for repeating overdose of paracetamol has been identified at four weeks following the initial episode, and therefore mental health follow-up is warranted during this period to the reduce risk (Ayonrinde et al., 2005). The safe use of paracetamol is described by New South Wales health polices and clinical guidelines (NSW Health, 2009).

Reasons people use drugs and alcohol

There are some common explanations for drug use. For some people, the pleasure and reward sensations derived from drug use influence and reinforce their drug use or misuse (Heal et al., 2013). For others, drug use creates a normative environment in which people consider they can think, behave or socialise effectively (Ritter et al., 2013). The use of drugs and alcohol for some is a complex matter. Some consideration must be given to the person's environment, social and genetic disposition. In particular, young people may turn to drugs and alcohol in reaction to peer pressure, isolation, family challenges or even just curiosity (Substance Abuse and Mental Health Services Administration (SAMHSA), 2019). Still others might choose to use drugs (e.g. steroids, peptides) to enhance their performance; for example, in sports. The use of drugs to enhance performance is beyond the scope of this chapter. Readers who are interested to know more about this topic should explore the Sport Integrity Australia website (n.d.), and also the Sport and Recreation New Zealand guidelines (2017) to learn more.

TRANSLATION TO PRACTICE

REFLECTIVE QUESTIONS

- Do you, or does anyone close to you, drink wine, beer or other types of alcohol? Why? Reflect on when either you, or others you know well, drink alcohol. How does it make you, or them, feel? Is there any pleasure associated with alcohol consumption? Does it help you/them to 'fit in' with others in a social context? Could you/they manage without alcohol? Does it matter?
- Write a short, reflective paragraph about your experiences with alcohol. How have your experiences shaped your views and beliefs about alcohol consumption, and how will this influence your health care of others?

A holistic framework for understanding people who use drugs and those who misuse drugs

Mental health professionals are often in the position to provide care for people who have both a mental health condition and a drug and/or alcohol problem, and the combination of these conditions can result in increasingly complex situations for people. Both mental health conditions and drug and alcohol problems often need to be managed simultaneously to produce a good health outcome. This is difficult to achieve for a range of reasons, not the least of which is that some health services designate these problems to different streams of care, or service providers, and therefore the coordination and transition of meaningful, comprehensive health care is difficult to achieve for people with a dual diagnosis. Healthcare professionals should consider how they might achieve a seamless and coordinated approach to the care of people with mental health conditions and drug and alcohol problems, and they should work towards an holistic model of care, despite the challenges of service delivery structures and classification systems.

Holistic care models value an approach that is person-centred and recognises that people and their health and well-being are affected by a variety of life circumstances. Health and well-being cannot be fully understood without taking into consideration the *biological*, *psychological*, *social*, *cultural*, *spiritual*, *developmental* and *ecological* elements of human life experiences. Practitioners should take active leadership roles in further developing meaningful, combined mental health and drug and alcohol care. Nursing models of care are central to minimising the harm and promoting health related to these types of problems. A framework is pivotal to understanding how to deliver holistic care to people who have combined mental health conditions and drug and alcohol problems. Central to practice is the concept that health and well-being, health promotion and recovery are critical for individuals, families and communities.

Biological influences on the experiences of mental health and substance use

A broad understanding of the biological explanations of brain functioning is important if we are to understand the mental health and drug and alcohol implications, and if we are to reduce the burden of related health problems in our society. The brain contains around 100 billion neurons (brain cells), each with multiple dendrites that receive incoming information and an axon that sends information outwards; together these neurons, dendrites and axon culminate in about 1000 synapses for each neuron. That translates into about 100 trillion connections within the brain. The synaptic gap between neurons is where messages transfer along the nervous system to achieve actions. Simply stated, the synapses are activated by electrical impulses and neuro-chemicals, and these trigger the transfer of messages along the neural pathways (Blows, 2011).

Some neuro-chemicals of particular interest to the study of drug and alcohol dependence and mental health conditions include serotonin (because it influences a sense of contentment), dopamine (because it influences motivation levels) and adrenaline (because of its capacity to trigger stimulation and alertness) (Blows, 2011). These neuro-chemicals are also described as neuro-transmitters. When triggered, a neuro-transmitter (imagine the shape of a key) travels across the synaptic gap to locate a neuro-receptor (imagine a keyhole to match the key), and a chemical message is transferred along a neural pathway. For example, to achieve the sensation of contentment, sufficient levels of serotonin need to be available to adequately saturate the synaptic gap, and at the same time there needs to be an equally sufficient quantity of serotonin receptors ready to receive the transmission of the serotonin. Too few, too many or unequal supplies of receptor and transmitter chemicals, and a vulnerability exists for mental health conditions or drug and alcohol problems to develop (Blows, 2011). This physiological process goes some way to explaining the influence chemicals have on our mood and cognitive functions and is amplified further during various developmental life stages. For example, during adolescence, the brain goes through significant changes, which can lead to increases in susceptibility to stress, anxiety and high risk behaviours, and has also been linked to hereditary influences (Boisvert et al., 2019; Waaktaar, Kan & Torgersen, 2018). Later in the life spectrum, perhaps when older adults retire or experience the loss of partner, for example, research is increasingly detecting increases in the prevalence of harmful use of alcohol among some people and increased dependence on benzodiazepines related to coping with stress and chronic pain (Lehmann & Fingerhood, 2018).

Chocolate and its biological effects on the brain

Any drugs (and sometimes foods) that alter the chemical balance in our brains will have consequences for our mood and cognition (Cornah & Van De Weyer, n.d.; Van De Weyer, 2005). Chocolate consumption provides a useful way to describe this process. Most people have some experience of eating chocolate and can attest to a temporary enhancement of their mood after consumption. Chocolate gives us a boost of a neuro-chemicals called noradrenalin, oxytocin and dopamine. These chemicals boost our sense of pleasure in, and enthusiasm for, life and they have an immediate effect. The brain is stimulated and begins to down-regulate in an effort to get back to a state of homeostasis. With the flood of chocolate or noradrenalin, the brain receptors start to close down to noradrenalin until the excess can be metabolised, which in turn prompts the person consuming the chocolate to increase their intake (that is, the person eats more chocolate) in order to achieve a release of noradrenalin that the brain now senses it is missing. This results in an imbalance, with more neuro-transmitters and fewer neuro-receptors. To stop this cycle, the brain needs to use up the oversupply of neuro-chemicals and return to homeostasis, but to do so the person needs to stop eating chocolate. Thus, a period of depressed mood will follow, before homeostasis can be achieved again. It is a vicious cycle in some respects, but it is this general process that, in part, describes some of the science behind the craving sensations that can be experienced in relation to chocolate, and the general idea can be extrapolated towards an understanding of the neuro-dynamics related to other drugs. Despite this, people usually repeat the experience of eating chocolate. This analogy mirrors experiences of other drugs by some people.

TRANSLATION TO PRACTICE

Cognitive brain activities, such as learning and memory, are triggered by the repetitive firing of synapses (Blows, 2011; Geake, 2009). The more frequently a synaptic pathway is accessed for cognitive activity the more that pathway is thickened and reinforced, and the easier it is to retrieve the information or memory that is needed; thus the phrase 'neurons that fire together, wire together' (Bennett, 2008a; Blows, 2011; Geake, 2009). People need to have cognitive functionality that is adaptive so that logical decisions can be formulated, problems solved and appropriate behaviours selected (Geake, 2009). Where thinking is slowed, or delays in cognitive processing occur, the capacity for risk taking is accentuated. For example, cannabis is known to impede cognitive functioning, and this is problematic in a practical setting in which perceptual skill is required and decisions need to be made quickly and accurately, such as when driving a motor vehicle.

Long-term use of drugs such as cannabis alters the wiring structure and firing capacity of neural pathways, and this can result in perceptual changes that can in part explain some of the symptoms of mental health conditions such as psychosis (Blows, 2011). However, there is evidence to suggest that the brain has some limited capacity to recover and learn new pathways, in a process known as plasticity, and it can best do this if cannabis is eliminated from the neuro-chemical environment (Early Psychosis Writing Group, 2010).

Psychological influences on the experiences of mental health and substance use

Psychological explanations for drug use and misuse also contribute to an holistic understanding of this topic. Exploring patterns of behaviours displayed by people who use drugs, and the cause-and-effect relationships in connection to human behaviours and experiences, is relevant to the general mental health and well-being of people. A psychological perspective of holistic mental health care seeks to describe and classify behaviours and to look for normal and abnormal parameters for a range of behaviours and experiences. Understanding why people use drugs will help to identify ways in which drug misuse can be reduced. Some people choose to use drugs because they experience satisfying sensations of pleasure in doing so, and generally pleasurable experiences are ones that people choose to replicate in the future (Ritter et al., 2013). Thus, interventions that acknowledge the satisfying experiences of pleasure related to experience of drug use can assist people to identify new and safe ways in which to experience satisfying life experiences and reduce their drug use, which will in turn promote mental health and reduce the risk of harm.

Some people use drugs because they consider that it will assist them by bolstering their confidence in stressful situations (Ritter et al., 2013). Their experiences form a basis from which they have learned to cope in response to stress or anticipated stress, and this then is the underlying mechanism that reinforces future behaviours. Drug use represents a very limited repertoire from which to draw coping skills, and unless other skills are developed, and as tolerance to drugs increases, the only avenue available to solve stress-related problems is to increase drug use. As drug use increases, so, too, does the risk of harm associated with drug misuse, and perhaps, drug dependence. This escalating spiral is a very uncomfortable human experience, and interventions that aim to build a healthy range of coping strategies related to stress management will alleviate the distress that accumulates for people and will also reduce the harm associated with their continued harmful drug use. It is of particular importance to recognise the human distress that accompanies harmful drug use, and for mental healthcare delivery to work towards supporting a person towards recovery.

For some people, the experience of psychological trauma or adversity precipitates vulnerability in regard to the uptake and use of drugs or alcohol. For example, complex mental health and drug and alcohol problems sometimes develop following an experience of child sexual abuse, or other childhood abuses. It is not the aim of this chapter to explore the consequences of abusive circumstances in any depth, but rather to note that frequently the combination of mental health conditions and drug and alcohol problems are linked to early life trauma.

Social influences on the experiences of mental health conditions and substance use

Social interactions are powerful components of human experience. Social connectedness is a critical aspect of a developed sense of self-esteem and confidence. Social interactions also carry a degree of vulnerability, as relationships between people can be sensitive to change, and sometimes flexibility and adaption are difficult to achieve when perspectives or circumstances differ. Some social anxiety is useful because it helps to self-moderate behaviour; however, when anxiety becomes disabling or distressing people often explore ways to deal with this tension. Some choose to isolate themselves from certain social settings, while others choose to utilise drugs to assist in overcoming, or dampening, a sense of anxiety. Alcohol is often used and misused in this way, to achieve a normalising and sociable affect in Australian and Aotearoa New Zealand communities. In rural settings, the local public bar (pub) might be a location for social meetings (and in some communities might be the only avenue for social exchange), thus the setting, and the context, are both linked to the consumption of alcohol. This is by no means problematic for all people; however, for a vulnerable few, the combination of social setting, context and alcohol can pose some risks, and these risks need to be considered in terms of the health and well-being (and the minimisation of harm) for individuals and their communities. Mark's story provides an example of social setting and context in relation to alcohol consumption.

PERSONAL NARRATIVE

Mark – social setting and context

Having a few days of leave from work, I went into the city to catch up with a couple of mates I went to university with about 10 years ago.

It was nearing midnight when I arrived at the club. The music was loud and it was very warm. I usually drink vodka and soda with fresh lime. I went to order one and was told they did not serve anything in a glass after midnight. The bar staff said they had a similar drink but would need to decant it into a plastic cup. I assumed all was fine and didn't think to ask what it was.

REFLECTIVE QUESTION

Have you ever been in a similar circumstance to Mark? Take a moment to reflect on what you might have done in a similar circumstance. Discuss your response with a student peer and compare your responses.

Cultural influences on experiences of mental health conditions and substance use

People are inherently cultural creatures (Kellert, 2012). We are influenced by the culture in which we are immersed in our day-to-day lives. Culture influences our attitudes and our practices in relation to drugs and alcohol. The following examples highlight the diversity of culture and drug or alcohol interactions.

Kava is an active ingredient in the root of a pepper plant (*Piper methysticum*). It is used in Pacific Islander communities and in the northern parts of Australia and Aotearoa New Zealand as a part of cultural ceremonies and social interactions. The effects of kava include sedation and relaxation and, on occasion, psychosis in some individuals (Ritter et al., 2013). The use of kava is intertwined with ceremony and culture, and therefore the social value of this drug is relevant to note. However, there are detrimental consequences in relation to frequent consumption of kava that need to be considered carefully. Legislation exists to minimise the health, social and economic harms associated with use of kava (Northern Territory Government, 2011).

Historically in Aotearoa New Zealand, alcohol has been strongly associated with male culture, mateship and work (James, 2010). These days, people with different gender identities regard drinking as integral to recreation, celebrations and events, and there also seems to be high tolerance of risky behaviours such as drinking to excess and binge drinking. A national survey of people aged 12 years and over conducted by the Alcohol Advisory Council of New Zealand (ALAC) 'found that one-third disagreed with the statement "it's never OK to get drunk", and one-quarter agreed with the statement "it's OK to get drunk as long as it's not every day"' (ALAC, 2006; James, 2010). Furthermore, Māori adults were 1.8 times as likely as non-Māori adults to be hazardous drinkers, after adjusting for age and gender (Ministry of Health, 2020).

Another example is the prevalence of cigarette smoking among Aboriginal and Torres Strait Islander adults and Māori adults (Ministry of Social Development, 2016), which occurs at a much higher incidence than among non-Indigenous people. By way of contrast, the interventions offered in Australia to promote smoking cessation are predominantly targeted towards non-Indigenous people. It has been identified that the cultural basis of interventions such as those offered by Quitline may need to be developed in order to better target health promotion and prevention campaigns that align with Aboriginal and Torres Strait Islander cultures so that healthy outcomes are improved for this section of the community (Cosh et al., 2013).

Spiritual/meaning-making influences on experiences of mental health conditions and substance use

Making meaning from life experiences and circumstances is very important for people. We strive to understand how and why our experiences influence our views of the world, and these experiences have a depth of personal influence that develops our character. Our ability to find some experiences deeply satisfying or meaningful, and to develop a hopefulness for the future, are important aspects of a rich personal inner life, and for some people these experiences have a religious dimension. However, for all people it could be considered that these matters are deeply spiritual. In the real-life story of Mark, which is interwoven in this chapter, Mark expresses something of what it is like to reflect on his life circumstances and to make sense of what happened to him.

Developmental influences on experiences of mental health conditions and substance use

We know that long-term and risky use of drugs such as alcohol and cannabis adversely affect cognitive brain function (MHDAO, 2009; Mental Health Council of Australia, 2006), and this is especially relevant when we consider that the human brain does not complete its developmental growth phrase until about the age of 22 years (Blows, 2011; Lebel & Beaulieu, 2011). Cognitive flexibility is important so that people can learn and remember information and can then select appropriate information to solve problems and make decisions. This process is used in every developmental stage of life; however, the brain structure that has not completed developmental maturation is vulnerable to damage occurring during the developmental phase (Bennett, 2008b; Blows, 2011). Alcohol and drug use pose risks to the developing brain and can compromise, or slow, both the availability of neuro-chemicals and the synaptic actions.

Ecological influences on experiences of mental health conditions and substance use

Family systems and social systems place significant influences on the people within those groups (Kellert, 2012). It is necessary for people to have an environment that fosters thriving and surviving, otherwise mental health will be compromised. Drug and alcohol exposure and misuse can represent a toxic environment, and unless these influences can be minimised, vulnerabilities and risks to mental health will occur.

So – what is it like experience a drug-related mental health condition? Mark's story gives us a real-life example to learn from, and to recognise aspects for both the consumer and the practitioner that influence a respectful and holistic recovery journey.

PERSONAL NARRATIVE

Mark – recognising that something is not quite right and trying to get some help

A few hours later I left the club. I recall catching a taxi to a suburb about 10 minutes away from the city. I then purchased a ticket to go on a train to an outlying suburb, about 30 minutes further out of town. When I left the train, I felt an urge that I needed help. I felt incredibly drunk and was in a very unfamiliar location.

I made my way out of the train station and towards the sound of music. I recall seeing a payphone and decided to call a taxi to take me to the nearest hospital. When I arrived at the hospital, I made my way to the triage nurse. She looked at me and said I looked fine.

I tried to explain that I didn't feel right, but I didn't know what was wrong with me and I couldn't really explain why I felt something was wrong with me. I said I thought my drink had been spiked. She was about to dismiss me for a second time, then decided to allow me to lie down on an emergency room bed. I couldn't articulate what was wrong with me, but I just knew I didn't feel right. I noticed a group of police officers talking to her after I was allowed onto the bed.

It is a very confusing and unsettling situation for people who experience perceptual and cognitive changes as a consequence of drug or alcohol use, especially if they have not experienced these types of situations before. In the next part of Mark's story, he gives a vivid account of his experiences of perceptual changes and paranoid thought processes.

PERSONAL NARRATIVE

Mark – acute psychosis

The accident and emergency department experience during an acute episode of drug and alcohol-induced psychosis

I recall my thoughts starting to become more paranoid. This was because no doctor had seen me and I felt I was not being taken seriously. I recall the sounds of the nurses' voices becoming distorted. They were some 20 metres away, but I could hear, crystal clear, what they were saying; or, at least, what I think was them. Time didn't really seem to have any boundaries.

One of the nurses approached and tried to make me admit what I had taken to make me feel the way I was. I tried to explain my evening, but she was adamant that I must have taken something; that it was not normal to feel the way I did. I tried to explain that I have never consumed any drugs in my life, not even a cigarette. Her questioning kept making me feel more paranoid.

The doctor came over to see me. He asked if I would like to have some tests done to see what was causing me to feel the way I was. I consented and was escorted to a toilet, where I gave a urine sample. I recall returning with it and hesitating to hand it over, fearing that if my drink was spiked and drugs were detected, what would happen to my reputation? Would the police be involved?

The next period became very intense. I started to feel my body tense up and my thoughts become more paranoid. At the time, they just appeared to be what I thought was reality. The examination light overhead turned into a lie detector. It was used by the nurse and police (who I thought were in the bed next to me) to read my thoughts. They would talk or ask questions, and whatever my first thought or opinion was, would be used to determine whether I was telling the truth. If I lied, a particular sound would be heard.

If I told the truth a different sound would be heard. The curtains were drawn around my cubicle so I could not see anyone. All I could focus on was this object above my bed.

The voices and questions started off from the nursing and medical staff. Sometimes, I could hear the voices of the police, who I thought were investigating me. As time went by, I thought I was being set up for something I had not done, so I had to prove them wrong.

I worked out that if I used my mental powers to disarm the lie detector they would not be able to read my thoughts. I felt violated by the interrogation of the hospital staff. I became less trusting of anyone who made an approach to me. I thought they were on the 'other side'.

I learned at times to overcome the power of the machine by focusing on saying 'I love my mum and dad'. Both my parents had passed away – one in 2002 and the other in 2010. I can never recall ever saying to them in my life that I loved them, but somehow, if I focused on my love for them, it stopped the machine from reading my thoughts. This went on for what felt like hours.

The questions became more personal and the intensity of the experience increased tenfold. The voices changed from the medical staff to people from my past, some former students I have taught, current and former colleagues and my extended family. They asked many personal questions, for which only I would have known the answers. Many of the questions were mistakes or oversights I had made in my life. Not remembering to mark a particular question in the detail that I should have, relying on third-hand information about a particular incident are examples. Normally small issues, but with this 'machine' everyone was asking questions.

The voices increased even more in intensity. Rather than the machine having one person speak, all of a sudden more voices appeared and people were in groups, asking questions. At one stage, there were at least four groups asking questions at the same time, often with competing responses from me. If I heard one question, but thought of a response for a different question, it meant I was lying and a sound would indicate that.

I never actually saw any of the people. I could recall very clearly their questions and their voices, but I never saw them. At one stage, I remember thinking it would have been impossible to fly everyone there in time to ask the questions. This sense of reason quickly disappeared under the onslaught of questions

There came a point when I realised I was about to go to gaol. I don't know why I thought that, but it was at this point I felt incredibly fatigued and unable to fight the power of all these questions. I recall believing that a bedside court hearing for bail was being conducted. Again, all of this was behind the curtains. I didn't actually see anything.

Mark goes on to tell us how he began to lose hope, he felt tired and worn out and was no longer able to communicate effectively. Eventually, he was subjected to the relevant section of the Mental Health Act and was required to be transported to an involuntary mental health unit because he was experiencing a psychotic episode. Read on to gain some insights into his experiences.

PERSONAL NARRATIVE

Mark – ideas about dying, losing hope and safety

I thought about just being dead. I knew somehow I couldn't kill myself – I was in a hospital – but if I willed myself to die, that would make this all end. I felt a need to admit defeat as I could no longer keep up. I just lost focus on trying to fight them, and just let them ask the questions. I lost a sense of wanting to prove I was not lying in my thoughts.

There came a point when a doctor, a psychiatrist, came to ask me some questions. I had incredible difficulty focusing on his questions, as I could hear all of these sounds taking place and all these questions being asked of me from all these voices. I would try my hardest to focus on him, but I just couldn't answer sometimes because I was looking at him but hearing all these other questions. I couldn't keep up.

There came a point when I just remember falling asleep. I was so fatigued and I couldn't put up with this anymore.

I woke and the voices had stopped. I was unsure what had happened. Had they left, had they got what they wanted? It was surreal. I didn't know what was happening, but the voices and the sounds had stopped.

The psychiatrist explained that I was being 'scheduled' and that I had elevated levels of alcohol and caffeine in my system. He explained that I had a psychosis and that I needed to get help. I knew what he was saying, but the question in my mind was, 'How'?

REFLECTIVE QUESTION

Mark describes that he was fatigued and extremely tired because of the disturbing thoughts he had encountered. After some sleep, he felt somewhat better. How might you be able to modify the environment to reduce stimulation and support sleep for people such as in Mark's circumstance?

The people Mark met along the way each had an influence on his recovery experience. Some (but not all) of the health services staff members were able to convey respect, care and helpfulness, and where this was achieved Mark felt supported. The unfamiliar environment and people in an involuntary mental health unit, combined with a sense of personal embarrassment and uncertainty, is both a confronting and uncomfortable personal experience. Mark shares some of this discomfort.

PERSONAL NARRATIVE

Mark – experience as an involuntary client

Fear and the experiences of being cared for as an involuntary client in an acute bed-based mental health setting

I was prepared for transport. Security staff came to my bed and assisted me out of the emergency room and into a patient transport vehicle. I recall feeling very embarrassed, as by this stage I thought I looked a wreck. I recall getting into the transport vehicle and being told they were taking me to Inverness. I became concerned as I had driven to Sydney, and what would happen to my car? The nurse, who was with me, became concerned and tried to explain that I had no choice. I understood that, but why Inverness? The hospital there is much smaller. I was settling into what I thought was a six-hour drive. Within about 10 minutes, I arrived at this facility and was told we had arrived. I was hesitant to question why it took so little time. I thought my sense of time was still distorted. Upon walking out of the van, I discovered that Inverness was actually the name of facility, not the name of the country hospital I had thought I was being transferred to. I was relieved.

Once inside, I met the nurse in charge. He was rather large, but very polite. He started a conversation about what I did for work, where I lived etc. He seemed friendly. When I explained to him these details, he looked at me as though he didn't believe me. My belongings – wallet keys etc. – were handed over and I was escorted to a room. I walked through the doors. I could hear screams, voices and noises. I hesitated for a moment, questioning in my own mind if they were real or not. I walked past one room where a large, bearish man was banging and screaming on the door. I could see faeces down the glass panel.

I was shown to my room and my door was opened. I was told that if I heard voices or needed anyone, to press a button in my room. I was assured that only staff could get into my room. I was given some paperwork to read over – my rights and what would happen during this process.

I lay on the bed and could hear the screams and yelling through the air-conditioning ducts. I knew they were real and I looked for logical explanations. I was still trying to understand what I had just been through. I was cautious not to rely on my thoughts because I couldn't be sure that this was not just another trick being played on me.

REFLECTIVE QUESTIONS

Can you imagine what it would be like to have no choice about an admission to hospital? To be transported by security guards? How would it feel to have your liberty removed, and to be detained for medical treatment? Would you have some questions you would like answered? How would you like to be dealt with in such circumstances?

Mental healthcare services are offered in somewhat public settings, and often people receiving care are in close social proximity with each other. Safety is a high priority, and practitioners are responsible for regularly monitoring the safety of the people they are helping. Consideration also needs to be given to the privacy and reputation of people within such a setting. In Mark's excerpt below he describes how he found the care environment to be challenging.

PERSONAL NARRATIVE

Mark – experiencing person-centred and respectful care

Morning came. I was asked to shower. I went into a cubical, where there were cameras. I'm a rather private person, so knowing that I needed a shower but had to shower with others watching made me rather uncomfortable. After the shower, it was time to make my way to breakfast. It was at this point I could see the other people I had heard earlier. I felt they were strange. I sensed they were heavily medicated. We sat to eat breakfast with plastic knives and forks. The staff members were nice and friendly and did whatever they could to ensure I felt comfortable at breakfast.

After breakfast I watched the news on TV. The other people were pacing around the rooms. One gentleman was exceptional with poetry. Staff would give him a topic or word and he would recite or give a poem that lasted hours. His language was sophisticated and he appeared to be very knowledgeable. I recall another person who called herself Miss Monica. She had difficulty keeping her clothes on and would spit at other people. Several times she was excluded to a separate area. Time and time again, staff treated her with respect.

REFLECTIVE QUESTIONS

How do you know when another person shows respect towards you? What are the characteristics of 'respect'? Write down a list of attributes that demonstrate a respectful interaction. Share your list with your student peers and together generate a collaborative understanding of the concept of respectful interactions that might apply in a mental health context.

PERSONAL NARRATIVE

Mark – the importance of therapeutic rapport

At 11.00 a.m. I was due for a meeting with a team of psychiatrists who would make the assessment about whether I needed to be scheduled for 72 hours or if I could be released. There were two. One, a younger woman who took notes and did not speak, and an older woman, who asked all the questions. I felt this older lady was particularly rude. She was the only person who I can recall who didn't show any respect. She attempted to lecture me about drinking and putting myself in a vulnerable state. She said I should be ashamed of myself. What was I thinking? No matter how I attempted to reason with her, she would not accept my position. I was fearful that if I challenged her too much, she would be offended and would schedule me for longer. I didn't want to stay. I needed to play her game. Rather than verbally denigrate her and her 'professional conduct', I just copped it on the chin.

I was released. I was allowed out the back door. I thanked the staff and congratulated them on a good job. They had shown compassion to the patients and I felt assured they cared for them. There was never any treatment of those vulnerable people that made me feel uncomfortable.

REFLECTIVE QUESTIONS

Have you ever experienced shame? If so, do you think it was useful or counter-productive in promoting helpful change in your life? Which would you prefer – a shameful interaction or a respectful interaction with a health professional? Discuss with your peers.

It is important that the interprofessional connections between practitioners and ancillary staff occur respectfully and seamlessly. Building a therapeutic rapport with people enhances communication and supports recovery. Mark was able to identify practitioners with whom he could develop a rapport, and other practitioners with whom there were significant barriers.

INTERPROFESSIONAL PERSPECTIVES

The interprofessional community across mental health and substance use and misuse is broad. You have read about some of the professionals that Mark encountered in his story. Nurses and psychologists make up the largest segment of the mental health workforce. Other professionals you might encounter include occupational therapists, social workers, psychiatrists, medical officers, Indigenous health workers, peer workers, recreational therapists, art therapists, magistrates, guardianship tribunal members, security personnel, police, paramedics and even firefighters. For example, police, paramedic, justice health nurses and firefighters are often engaged in mental health welfare checks in the community setting. Registered health professionals working collaboratively with such a diverse set of professionals creates a unique working environment and recovery environment.

In the next section of Mark's story, he relays how he felt and coped with the various types of communication he was exposed to during his stay in hospital. On reflection, Mark started the process of making meaning of his life experiences. He shares some of the conclusions that he has drawn about his experiences, and what this will mean for his future.

PERSONAL NARRATIVE

Mark – meaning-making and recovery

I spent the next few days with family, trying to overcome and piece together what really had happened. I was trying to figure out how I could move forward. This was a time of deep personal reflection. This event had changed my life.

I made the decision to sell many of my personal assets in the months that followed this experience. I left the job I was in and returned to teaching. I felt comfortable that this experience was an act of God. I obviously had many unresolved matters in my life that I needed to finalise or set to order, and the time was right. I felt a sense of inner peace.

Today, I get worried sometimes when I hear sounds or have strange thoughts. I have to check to make sure they are not foreign thoughts. I never want to experience this again.

So, what was in my system to cause this episode? I had been drinking an alcoholic beverage that was heavily laden with caffeine and alcohol. Each single serve (250 millilitres) contained 1.9 standard drinks and significant amounts of caffeine. I'm a not a coffee drinker (and I don't consume energy drinks), so any caffeine in my system, no matter how much, is significant. I've only ever had about two coffees in my life, and prior to this experience my last coffee had been in 2006, and then I stayed awake for 12 hours after consuming the single cup of coffee (at about 5.00 p.m). I had consumed in the space of three hours the equivalent to 28 standard alcoholic drinks and the equivalent of approximately 30 cups of coffee. That's what they believed caused the episode. My blood tests returned no other traces of drugs.

How could this happen to a well-educated, 30-year-old professional who has spent much of his life working with young people and warning them of these types of problems? How could I have allowed this to happen? Being naïve. Had I just questioned the staff about the alcoholic beverage at the club, this could have been avoided. Had the sweetness of the drink not masked the strong alcohol and caffeine content, this could have been avoided. Had the club served the alcohol beverage in its original packaging, this may have been avoided.

Was this an act of God? I'm not sure. I carry my faith with me and I hold strongly to the power of the experience. It has made me humbler and wiser. It has taught me that even the most innocent people can have such experiences, all because of one foolish mistake.

I have to live with this experience for the rest of my life. The memories and voices have faded over time, but the conviction of the experience is still very strong in my mind.

REFLECTIVE QUESTIONS

Sometimes life course does not go according to plan or our wishes. How do you make meaning of adverse life moments? Do you think that meaning-making can help to making sense of, and draw lessons to apply later in life? Can meaning-making promote mental health in any way, in your view?

Mental health conditions and substance-use problems in combination with each other

Mark's story demonstrates some characteristics of the mental health problems that can occur with drug and alcohol use. This real-life event also demonstrates how easily and rapidly such problems can develop, how frightening the experiences can be and how important it is for health professionals from all disciplines to work together in a collaborative and respectful manner. Drug and alcohol use have implications for the mental health and well-being of people, with studies indicating significant links between drug and alcohol use and comorbid depression, anxiety, bipolar and conduct disorder, and attempted suicide in Aotearoa New Zealand (Cobiac & Wilson, 2018), and the inverse is true, too; personal experiences of mental health and well-being can influence the type, extent and experiences of drug and alcohol consumption. It can be seen from Mark's story that judgement, blame, invoking embarrassment and reinforcing stigma are not useful positions for the people being helped or the health professionals responsible for helping, and that these positions serve to promote discomfort rather than recovery. A more helpful approach is one that is respectful of the person and is both polite and caring, and these characteristics promote hope for the future. Mark's story is a very powerful one; he is a well-educated young man and someone who is able to reflect on his own experiences and convey the meaning of those experiences to others very clearly. But not all people are as skilled as Mark in this regard. Many people may not be able to describe their feelings and experiences in such a clear way.

REFLECTIVE QUESTIONS

Think about what it would be like to be in Mark's shoes.

- How do you think it might feel?
- What if you thought no one believed you?
- How would you act?
- What would you choose to say, or not say?

Mental health and drug and alcohol models of care

Traditionally, mental health services and drug and alcohol services have operated as 'silos' of care; occasionally, health services have been able to integrate care so that people with both mental health conditions and substance use problems can receive simultaneous care. Withdrawal experiences from drugs and alcohol can be very uncomfortable for many people, and many people will benefit from the support of interprofessional mental health and drug and alcohol support during this time. Most public health services have clinical guidelines to promote recovery experiences (MHDAO, 2008).

Motivational interviewing

Motivational interviewing may be a useful strategy to start a conversation with a person experiencing a drug and alcohol problem (Miller & Rollnick, 2002). The aim of motivational interviewing is to engage people to move towards a future in which they are less ambivalent and more engaged and motivated to work towards the changes they will need to make in their lives, so as to minimise the risk of drug-related harm. Initiating and instilling hope for the future is also a useful mental health intervention, and so the same model is useful across both clinical problems.

Stages of change

Understanding the dynamics related to **readiness to change** is a useful framework for drug and alcohol care, and can also apply to mental health care. Distinct phases are evident, and they are precontemplation (no recognition that a change in behaviour is warranted), contemplation (recognition of a need to change, marked with some ambivalence), preparation (engaged in planning for a sustainable life change), action (change behaviour has commenced, including cessation or reduction in drug or alcohol use), maintenance (the desired change has become embedded in a lifestyle for a substantial period of time) and exit/relapse (an exit from the cycle occurs where no relapse has occurred for a long period of time, or a trigger event occurs and the person returns to the original behaviour) (Prochaska, DiClemente & Norcross, 1992; see Figure 12.1). A skilled practitioner is able to apply an understanding of these phases and to assist and motivate people towards phases of action to reduce the harmful effects of drugs and alcohol, to promote health and well-being in a maintenance phase and to assist

readiness to change – a multi-dimensional state concerned with a change in health behaviour; readiness to change is marked by both cognitive and behavioural phases, including precontemplation, contemplation, preparation, action, maintenance and exit/relapse. In later stages of readiness to change, people are actively doing things to change or maintain the changes they have been able to make.

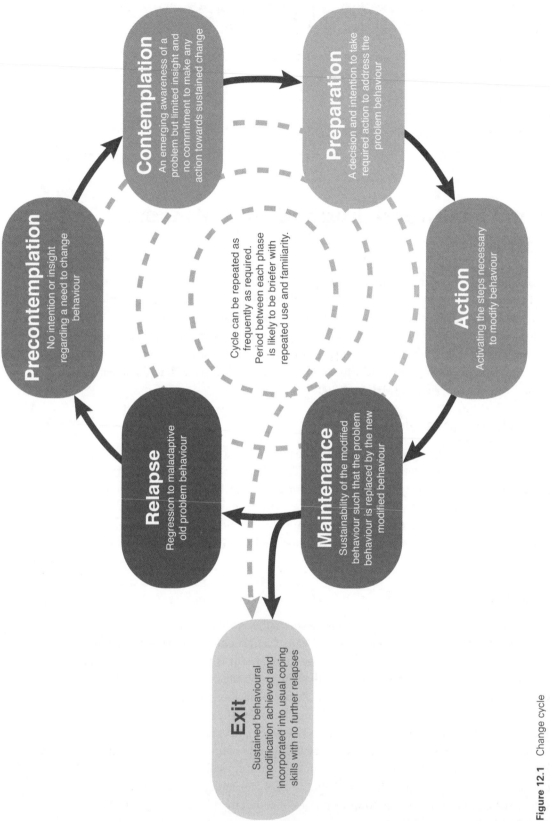

Figure 12.1 Change cycle

Source: Yee Mon Oo (2021) (adapted from Prochaska et al. (1992, p. 1104)).

people to recognise triggers that may result in relapse, with a view to intervention so as to prevent relapse. This process may need to be followed several times before an exit is achieved; however, there are health gains when periods of action and maintenance become longer, and relapses become shorter.

Solution-focused therapy

Solution-focused therapy is a person-centred approach towards helping people with drug and alcohol problems and with mental health conditions, which explores personal strengths, resources for coping and a vision for a healthy future (Wand, 2010). The practitioner aims to help the person to explore and elaborate on what is going well at the moment – rather than confining the discussion to a traditional problem focus – and to help or guide the person to identify for themselves what it is that they are currently doing to survive, and what they might like to be different in the future, so that the person is able to refocus and improve their health and well-being in a supported context (Wand, 2010). Change is seen as a normal dynamic in everyday life and an activity that most people will have a history of success in negotiating in their lives. Adapting to change is something that all people have to do frequently, and so this current problem is an opportunity to adapt normally. The practitioner guides the person towards recovery, helps the person find a way to imagine a future without drug and/or alcohol problems, and to explore ways to create small achievable goals, rather than setting unrealistic, big goals at an early phase. As people see that small things can be changed, and are able to reflect on their success, they are able to take further, constructive steps to achieving more positive changes in their lives. Solution-focused interventions include structuring a scaling process so that people learn to evaluate change within their lives (e.g. on a scale of 0 to 10 rate 'I feel I can make X change in my life'). In this way, outcomes can be recognised and complemented, while new motivation for future changes can be encouraged and nurtured (Wand, 2010). Solution-focused interventions are positively framed and they align usefully with other interventions such as motivational interviewing, change readiness, cognitive behavioural therapy, and withdrawal planning and interventions.

What needs to change in the future?

Remember Mark's story? He has some ideas about improvements that could be made so that others are less likely to experience the distress he did.

PERSONAL NARRATIVE

Mark – reflections and recommendations for change

I wouldn't change the nurses working at the coal-face. Perhaps I was fortunate with the nurses I encountered at the facility, but their care and compassion were very deep and I felt safe with them nearby. I felt human and that I had rights. I felt they were making the best decisions for me.

The experience with the psychiatrist in the facility is one I never want repeated. She thought she had all the answers. I felt that she was annoyed that I didn't have traces of other drugs in my system. I didn't feel a sense of compassion or warmth from her. I felt she was very focused on the power she had in decision-making. Several times, she referred to her authority to make the decision to extend my stay.

Alcohol venues need to be more responsible. While their policy may have stopped me from being 'glassed', it may have contributed to me experiencing this episode. I can never be sure if I would have read the label – I would like to think I would have. At the very least, I would have made an informed decision if I had the chance to read the label. I feel a sense of being personally violated because I could not.

My work, colleagues and extended network were very supportive. I thought they would think I was mad, but they didn't. The support was overwhelming and that was reassuring.

It is interesting that Mark identified that he felt safe, human and that his rights were maintained, and that he could sense the care and compassion of the nurses. These qualities are not tangible; they are not interventions that can be administered from the medication trolley. You cannot get compassion from the treatment room, as you might a dressing; you cannot measure it as if it were a vital sign such as blood pressure, but these characteristics are the invisible hallmarks of excellent nursing care. Safety, care and compassion are noticeable, both in their presence and in their absence; they do require some emotional intelligence and investment by nurses and they are especially vital skills needed for the expert delivery of care towards people with mental health conditions and/or substance-use problems.

SUMMARY

This chapter has presented stories, information and activities designed to deepen your understanding of:

- The three main types of drugs that can be misused for non-therapeutic purposes, as outlined in Table 12.2. Depressants (e.g. alcohol) lower central nervous system activity, leading to lower heart rate and respiration. Stimulants (e.g. amphetamines) increase nervous system activity and can lead to increased heart rate and irritability, among other effects. Hallucinogens alter central nervous system activity and can lead to changed perceptions and thinking. It should be noted that there is a range of subjective variability related to the experiences people may have with drugs within these categories.
- The usefulness of person-centred care approaches in promoting the recovery of people with combined drug, alcohol and mental health problems. Motivational interviewing can start a conversation and instil hope in consumers. Practitioners must understand the dynamics related to readiness to change and acknowledge that consumers may move between stages several times before exiting. Solution-focused therapy explores personal strengths, resources for coping and a vision for a healthy future. Many health services have been able to integrate care and treat mental health conditions and drug and alcohol problems simultaneously. Many people will benefit from the support of interprofessional mental health and drug and alcohol support during this time.

- Holistic care models that value an approach that is person-centred and recognises that people and their health and well-being are affected by a variety of life circumstances, including biological, psychological, social, cultural, spiritual, developmental and ecological circumstances. A framework is pivotal to understanding how to deliver holistic care to people with combined mental health conditions and drug or alcohol problems.
- The effects of drug and alcohol misuse on the physical and mental health of consumers. Both mental health conditions and drug and alcohol problems often need to be managed simultaneously to produce a good health outcome. This is difficult to achieve for a range of reasons, not the least of which is that some health services designate these problems to different streams of care, or service providers, and therefore the coordination and transition of meaningful, comprehensive health care is difficult to achieve for people with a dual diagnosis.
- The harm-minimisation policy consisting of three 'pillars': reduction of supply, reduction of demand and reduction of harm. Implementation of the three pillars into practice is a collaborative effort from governments, health services, education services and law enforcement. Supply reduction is largely the work of policymakers, legislators, justice systems and law enforcement. Health and education services may implement demand reduction through educating consumers to make healthy choices. Harm reduction may involve assisting people to reduce or cease use.

CRITICAL THINKING/LEARNING ACTIVITIES

1 List some ways in which the brain is affected by drug use.
2 List some ways in which you as a new graduate health practitioner could support a person in their decision to reduce or cease consumption of drugs.
3 List the holistic domains that might apply to the care of a person with drug or alcohol problems.
4 What are some of the physical and mental care needs of a person who has ingested excessive quantities of paracetamol?
5 In what ways do harm-minimisation policies affect mental health outcomes for individuals and communities?

LEARNING EXTENSION

Samson and Delilah (directed by Warwick Thornton in 2009) is a film that portrays the experience of a young couple in central Australia who are affected by solvent sniffing. View a trailer by the film's director to find out more about this informative film and to explore some of the complex drug, mental health and social issues that relate to solvent misuse.

ACKNOWLEDGEMENT

Thanks to Mark for sharing his story and for his contribution to this chapter in providing a real-life account of the mental health conditions related to alcohol and caffeine use. Thanks to Dr Janene Carey for editorial support.

FURTHER READING

Department of Health (n.d.) *Ministerial Drug and Alcohol Forum*. Retrieved from
    https://www.nationaldrugstrategy.gov.au
The National Drug Strategy is a cooperative, bipartisan venture between the Australian and state/
territory governments, as well as the non-government sector, to prevent the uptake of harmful
drug use and reduce the harmful effects of illicit drugs in society.

Mental Health Foundation. (2006). *Feeding Minds: The impact of food on mental health*.
    Retrieved from https://www.mentalhealth.org.uk/sites/default/files/Feeding-Minds.pdf
This report summarises the evidence on the role of diet in the care and treatment of people with
mental health problems.

Van de Weyer, C. (2005). *Changing Diets, Changing Minds: How food affects mental well being
    and behaviour*. London: Sustain: The Alliance for Better Food and Farming. Retrieved
    from https://www.mentalhealth.org.uk/sites/default/files/changing_diets.pdf
This is a companion report to *Feeding Minds*, *Changing Diets, Changing Minds*.

Victorian Alcohol and Drug Association (Website). Retrieved from http://www.vaada.org.au/
The Victorian Alcohol and Drug Association aims to reduce the harms associated with alcohol and
other drug use within the Victorian community.

REFERENCES

Alcohol Advisory Council of New Zealand (ALAC). (2006). *The Way We Drink 2005 – Executive
    Summary*. ALAC Occasional Publication No. 27. Wellington: Alcohol Advisory Council of New
    Zealand. Retrieved from https://www.hpa.org.nz/research-library/research-publications/way-
    we-drink-2005-executive-summary
Attenborough, J. (2010). Alcohol and mood disorders. In P. Phillips, O. McKeown & T. Sandford (eds),
    Dual Diagnosis. Practice in context. (pp. 76–88). Oxford, UK: Wiley-Blackwell.
Australian Bureau of Statistics (ABS). (2007). *National Survey on Mental Health and Wellbeing:
    Summary of results, 2007*. ABS cat. no. 4326.0. Canberra: ABS.
Australian Institute of Health and Welfare (AIHW). (2011). *2010 National Drug Strategy Household
    Survey Report*. Drug statistics series no.25. Cat. no. PHE 145. Canberra: AIHW.
—— (2014). *National Drug Strategy Household Survey Detailed Report 2013*. Drug statistics series
    no.28. Cat. no. PHE 145. Canberra: AIWH.
—— (2017). *National Drug Strategy Household Survey 2016: Detailed findings*. Drug statistics
    series no. 31. Cat. no. PHE 214. Canberra: AIHW.
—— (2018). *Australia's Health 2018*. Australia's health series no. 16. AUS 221. Canberra: AIHW.
    Retrieved from https://www.aihw.gov.au/getmedia/7c42913d-295f-4bc9-9c24-4e44eff4a04a/
    aihw-aus-
Ayonrinde, O. T., Phelps, G. J., Hurley, J. C. & Ayonrinde, O. A. (2005). Paracetamol overdose and
    hepatotoxicity at a regional Australian hospital: A 4-year experience. *Internal Medicine Journal*,
    35: 655–60.
Barratt, M. J., Cakic, V. & Lenton, S. (2013). Patterns of synthetic cannabinoid use in Australia. *Drug
    and Alcohol Review*, *32*: 141–6.
Bateman, D. N., Dear, J. W., Thanacoody, H. K. R., Thomas, S. H. L., Eddleston, M., Sandilands,
    E. A., Coyle, J., Cooper, J. G., Rodriguez, A., Butcher, I., Lewis, S. C., Vliegenthart, A. D. B.,
    Veiraiah, A., Webb, D. J. & Gray, A. (2014). Reduction of adverse effects from intravenous
    acetylcysteine treatment for paracetamol poisoning: a randomised controlled trial. *The Lancet*,
    383(9918): 697–704.

Bennett, M. R. (2008a). Dual constraints on synapse formation and regression in schizophrenia: Neuregulin, Neuroligin, dysbindin, DISC1, MuSK and agrin. *Australian and New Zealand Journal of Psychiatry*, *42*: 662–77.

—— (2008b). Stress and anxiety in schizophrenia and depression: Glucocorticoids, corticotrophin-releasing hormone and synapse regression. *Australian and New Zealand Journal of Psychiatry*, *42*: 995–1002.

Blows, W. T. (2011). *The Biological Basis for Mental Health Nursing*, 2nd edn. New York: Routledge.

Boisvert, D. L., Connolly, E. J., Vaske, J. C., Armstrong, T. A. & Boutwell, B. B. (2019). Genetic and environmental overlap between substance use and delinquency in adolescence: An analysis by same-sex twins. *Youth Violence and Juvenile Justice*, *17*(2): 154–73.

Bullock, M., Ranse, J. & Hutton, A. (2018). Impact of patients presenting with alcohol and/or drug intoxication on in-event health care services at mass-gathering events: An integrative literature review. *Prehospital and Disaster Medicine*, *33*(5): 539–42.

Cloutier, R. L., Hendrickson, R. G., Fu, R. R. & Blake, B. (2013). Methamphetamine-related psychiatric visits to an urban academic emergency department: An observational study. *The Journal of Emergency Medicine*, *45*(1): 136–42.

Cobiac, L. & Wilson, N. (2018). *Alcohol and Mental Health: A review of evidence, with a particular focus on New Zealand – Report prepared to inform the Mental Health and Addiction Inquiry.* Retrieved from http://www.ahw.org.nz/Portals/5/Resources/Submissions/2018/Alcohol%20 Healthwatch%20Alcohol%20and%20mental%20health%202018.pdf

Cornah, D. & Van De Weyer, C. (n.d.). *Feeding Minds. The impact of food on mental health.* London: Mental Health Foundation. Retrieved from https://www.mentalhealth.org.nz/assets/ ResourceFinder/Feeding-Minds.pdf

Cosh, S., Maksimovic, A. L., Ettridge, K., Copley, D. & Bowden, J. (2013). Aboriginal and Torres Strait Islander utilisation of the Quitline service for smoking cessation in South Australia. *Australian Journal of Primary Health*, *19*: 113–18.

Crum, R. M., Mojtabai, R., Lazareck, S., Bolton, J. M., Robinson, J., Sareen, J., Green, K. M., Stuart, E. A., La FlairL. , Alvanzo, A. A. H. & StorrC. L. A. (2013). Prospective assessment of reports of drinking to self-medicate mood symptoms with the incidence and persistence of alcohol dependence. *JAMA Psychiatry*, *70*(7):718–26.

Daly, F., Fountain, J. S., Murray, L., Graudins, A. & Buckley, N. A. (2008). Guidelines for the management of paracetamol poisoning in Australia and New Zealand – Explanation and elaboration. A consensus statement from clinical toxicologists consulting to the Australasian poisons information centres. *Medical Journal of Australia*, *188*: 296–301.

Darvishi, N., Farhadi, M., Haghtalab, T. & Poorolajal, J. (2015). Alcohol-related risk of suicidal ideation, suicide attempt, and completed suicide: A meta-analysis. *PLOS One*, *10*(5): e0126870.

Degenhardt, L., Sara, G., McKetin, R., Roxburgh, A., Dobbins, T., Farrell, M., Burns, L. & Hall, W. D. (2017). Crystalline methamphetamine use and methamphetamine-related harms in Australia. *Drug and Alcohol Review*, *36*(2): 160–70.

Department of Health and Ageing. (2011). *National Drug Strategy 2010–2015.* (D0224). Retrieved from www.nationaldrugstrategy.gov.au/internet/drugstrategy/publishing.nsf/Content/nds20102015

—— (2013). *Standard Drinks Guide.* Retrieved from www.health.gov.au/internet/alcohol/publishing .nsf/Content/drinksguide-cnt

Dick, S., Whelan, E., Davoren, M. P., Dockray, S., Heavin, C., Linehan, C. & Byrne, M. (2019). A systematic review of the effectiveness of digital interventions for illicit substance misuse harm reduction in third-level students. *BMC Public Health*, *19*(1244).

DiForti, M., Marconi, A., Carra, E., Fraietta, S., Trotta, A., Bonomo, M., Bianconi, F., Gardner-Sood, P., O'Connor, J., Russo, M., Stilo, S. A., Marques, T. R., Mondelli, V., Dazzan, P., Pariante, C., David, A. S., Gaughran, F., Atakan, Z., Iyegbe, C., Powell, J., Morgan, C., Lynskey, M. & Murray, R. M. (2015). Proportion of patients in south London with first-episode psychosis attributable to use of high potency cannabis: A case-control study. *Lancet Psychiatry*, *2*(3):233–8.

Dubertret, C., Bidard, I., Ades, J. & Gorwood, P. (2006). Lifetime positive symptoms in patients with schizophrenia and cannabis abuse are partially explained by comorbid addiction. *Schizophrenia Research*, *86*: 284–90.

Early Psychosis Writing Group. (2010). *Australian Clinical Guidelines for Early Psychosis*, 2nd edn. Melbourne: ORYGEN Youth Health.

Edward, K. & Alderman, C. (2013). *Psychopharmocology: Practice and contexts*. South Melbourne: Oxford University Press.

Ferdinand, R. F., Sondeijker, F., van der Ende, J., Selten, J.-P. & Huizink, A. (2005). Cannabis use predicts future psychotic symptoms, and vice versa. *Society for the Study of Addiction, 100*: 612–18.

Fergerson, D. M., Horwood, L. J. & Ridder, E. M. (2005). Tests of causal linkages between cannabis use and psychotic symptoms. *Society for the Study of Addiction, 100*: 354–66.

Freeman, N. & Quigley, P. (2015). Care versus convenience: Examining paracetamol overdose in New Zealand and harm reduction strategies through sale and supply. *The New Zealand Medical Journal, 128*(424).

Geake, J. G. (2009). *The Brain at School. Educational neuroscience in the classroom*. Berkshire: Open University Press.

Green, B., Young, R. & Kavanagh, D. (2005). Cannabis use and misuse prevalence among people with psychosis. *British Journal of Psychiatry, 187*: 306–13.

Hatcher, S., Coupe, N., Wikiriwhi, K., Durie, M. & Pillai, A. (2016). Te Ira Tangata: a Zelen randomised controlled trial of a culturally informed treatment compared to treatment as usual in Māori who present to hospital after self-harm. *Social Psychiatry and Psychiatric Epidemiology, 51*: 885–94.

Haug, S., Paz Castro, R., Meyer, C., Filler, A., Kowatsch, T. & Schaub, M. (2017). A mobile phone-based life skills training program for substance use prevention among adolescents: Pre-post study on the acceptance and potential effectiveness of the program, Ready4life. *JMIR mHealth and uHealth, 5*(10):e143.

He Ara Oranga. (2018). *Report of the Governmental Inquiry into Mental Health and Addiction*. Wellington: Ministry of Health. Retrieved from https://mentalhealth.inquiry.govt.nz/inquiry-report/he-ara-oranga/

Heal, D. J., Smith, S. L., Gosden, J. & Nutt, D. J. (2013). Amphetamine, past and present – a pharmacological and clinical perspective. *Journal of Psychopharmacology, 27*(6): 479–96.

Hutton, A., Prichard, I., Whitehead, D., Thomas, S., Rubin, M., Sloand, E., Powell, T. W., Frisch, K., Newman, P. & Goodwin Veenema, T. (2020). mHealth interventions to reduce alcohol use in young people: A systematic review of the literature. *Comprehensive Child and Adolescent Nursing, 43*(3): 171–202.

James, B. (2010). *Under the influence: Reshaping New Zealand's drinking culture*. The Salvation Army Social Policy and Parliamentary Unit. Retrieved from https://www.parliament.nz/resource/0000170714

Jones, R., Woods, C., Barker, R. & Usher, K. (2019). Patterns and features of methamphetamine-related presentations to emergency departments in QLD from 2005 to 2017. *International Journal of Mental Health Nursing, 28*(4): 833–44.

Kellert, S. (2012). *Birthright. People and nature in the modern world*. New Haven, CT: Yale University Press.

Lebel, C. & Beaulieu, C. (2011). Longitudinal development of human brain wiring continues from childhood into adulthood. *The Journal of Neuroscience, 31*(30): 10937–47.

Lehmann, S. W. & Fingerhood, M. (2018). Substance-use disorders in later life. *The New England Journal of Medicine, 379*(24): 2351–60.

Mental Health and Drug and Alcohol Office (MHDAO). (2008). *Drug and Alcohol Withdrawal: Clinical practice guidelines – NSW. (GL2008_011)*. Sydney: NSW Health.

——— (2009). *NSW Clinical Guidelines for the Care of Persons with Comorbid Mental Illness and Substance Use Disorders in Acute Care Settings*. Sydney: NSW Health.

Mental Health Council of Australia. (2006). *Where There's Smoke … Cannabis and Mental Health*. Melbourne: ORYGEN Youth Mental Health Service.

Miller, W. R. & Rollnick, S. (2002). *Motivational Interviewing. Preparing people for change*, 2nd edn. New York: The Guilford Press.

Ministry of Health. (2015). *Cannabis Use 2012/13: New Zealand Health Survey*. Wellington: Ministry of Health. Retrieved from https://www.health.govt.nz/system/files/documents/publications/cannabis-use-2012-13-nzhs-may15-v2.pdf

——— (2020). *Annual Update of Key Results 2019/20: New Zealand Health Survey*. Retrieved from https://www.health.govt.nz/publication/annual-update-key-results-2019-20-new-zealand-health-survey

Ministry of Social Development. (2016). *The Social Report 2016 Te pūrongo oranga tangata*. Wellington: Ministry of Social Development. Retrieved from https://socialreport.msd.govt.nz/documents/2016/msd-the-social-report-2016.pdf

National Health and Medical Research Council (NHMRC). (2009). *Australian Guidelines to Reduce Health Risks from Drinking Alcohol*. Canberra: Australian Government.

Northern Territory Government. (2011). *Kava Management Act*. Darwin: Northern Territory Government.

NSW Health. (2009). *Paracetamol Use*. Clinical Policy PD2009_009). Sydney: Department of Health, NSW. Retrieved from www0.health.nsw.gov.au/policies/pd/2009/pdf/PD2009_009.pdf

Oakley Browne, M. A, Wells, J. E. & Scott K. M. (eds). (2006). *Te Rau Hinengaro: The New Zealand Mental Health Survey*. Wellington: Ministry of Health. Retrieved from https://www.health.govt.nz/system/files/documents/publications/mental-health-survey.pdf

Palmer, R. S., McMahon, T. J., Moreggi, D. I., Rounsaville, B. J. & Ball, S. A. (2012). College student drug use: Patterns, concerns, consequences, and interest in interventions. *Journal of College Student Development*, *53*(1): 123–32.

Peacock, A., Gibbs, D., Sutherland, R., Uporova, J., Karlsson, A., Bruno, R., Dietze, P., Lenton, S., Alati, R., Degenhardt, L. & Farrell, M. (2018). *Australian Drug Trends 2018: Key findings from the National Illicit Drug Reporting System Interviews*. Sydney: National Drug and Alcohol Research Centre, University of New South Wales. Retrieved from https://ndarc.med.unsw.edu.au/resource/australian-drug-trends-2018-key-findings-national-illicit-drug-reporting-system-idrs

Prochaska, J. O., DiClemente, C. C. & Norcross, J. C. (1992). In search of how people change: Applications to addictive behaviours. *American Psychologist*, *47*(9): 1102–14.

Redona, P., Jackson, D., Woods, C., Usher, K., 2019. Increasing use of stimulants in Australia: *Cause for health services concern. International Journal of Mental Health Nursing*, *28*: 795–7.

Ritter, A., King, T. & Hamilton, M. (eds). (2013). *Drug Use in Australian Society*. South Melbourne: Oxford University Press.

Roxburgh, A., Burns, L., Drummer, O. H., Pilgram, J., Farrell, M. & Degenhardt, L. (2013). Trends in fentanyl prescriptions and fentanyl-related mortality in Australia. *Drug and Alcohol Review*, *32*: 269–75.

Schumacher, F.-R. (2018). Fransplaining science: Is paracetamol doing more harm than good? *Radio NZ*, 11 June. Retrieved from https://www.rnz.co.nz/news/the-wireless/375268/fransplaining-science-is-paracetamol-doing-more-harm-than-good

Schwartzkoff, J., Wilczynski, A., Reed-Gilbert, K. & Jones, L. (2008). *Review of the First Phase of the Petrol Sniffing Strategy*. Canberra: Department of Families, Housing, Community Services and Indigenous Affairs.

Smith, P. H., Mazure, C. M. & McKee, S. A. (2014). Smoking and mental illness in the US population. *Tobacco Control*, *23*(e2): e147–53.

Solomon, D., Grewal, P., Taylor, C. & Solomon, B. (2014). Managing misuse of novel psychoactive substances. *Nursing Times*, *110*(22): 12–15.

Solowij, N. & Michie, P. T. (2007). Cannabis and cognitive dysfunction: Parallels with endophenotypes of schizophrenia. *Journal Psychiatry Neuroscience*, *32*(1): 30–52.

Sport and Recreation New Zealand. (2017). *Briefing to the Incoming Minister for Sport and Recreation*. Retrieved from https://www.beehive.govt.nz/sites/default/files/2017-12/Sport%20and%20Recreation%20-%20Sport%20NZ.pdf

Sport Integrity Australia. (n.d.). *Sport Integrity Australia*. Canberra: Sport Integrity Australia. Retrieved from https://www.asada.gov.au/

Substance Abuse and Mental Health Services Administration (SAMHSA). (2019). *Substance Misuse Prevention for Young Adults*. Publication No. PEP19-PL-Guide-1. Rockville, MD: National Mental Health and Substance Use Policy Laboratory.

Toumbourou, J. W., Stockwell, T., Neighbors, C., Marlatt, G. A., Sturge, J. & Rehm, J. (2007). Interventions to reduce harm associated with adolescent substance use. *The Lancet*, *369*(9570): 1391–401.

Van de Weyer, C. (2005). *Changing Diets, Changing Minds: How food affects mental well being and behaviour*. London: Sustain: The Alliance for Better Food and Farming. Retrieved from www.mentalhealth.org.uk/content/assets/PDF/publications/changing_diets.pdf

Volkow, N. D., Swanson, J. M., Evins, A. E., DeLisi, L. E., Meier, M. H., Gonzalez, R., Bloomfield, M. A. P., Curran, H. V. & Baler, R. (2016). Effects of cannabis use on human behavior, including cognition, motivation, and psychosis: A review. *JAMA Psychiatry*, *73*(3): 292–7.

Waaktaar, T., Kan, K. J. & Torgersen, S. (2018). The genetic and environmental architecture of substance use development from early adolescence into young adulthood: A longitudinal twin study of comorbidity of alcohol, tobacco and illicit drug use. *Addiction, 113*(4): 740–8.

Wand, T. (2010). Mental health nursing from a solution focused perspective. *International Journal of Mental Health Nursing, 19*: 210–19.

Wilkes, E., Gray, D., Saggers, S., Casey, W. & Stearne, A. (2010). Substance misuse and mental health among Aboriginal Australians. In N. Purdie, P. Dudgeon & R. Walker (eds), *Working Together: Aboriginal and Torres Strait Islander mental health and wellbeing principles and practice* (pp. 117–33). Canberra: Australian Government, Department of Health and Ageing.

Zinberg, N. (1984). *Drug, Set and Setting: The basis for controlled intoxicant use.* New Haven, CT: Yale University Press.

Nutrition, physical health and behavioural change

13

Anne Storey and Denise McGarry

LEARNING OBJECTIVES

At the completion of this chapter, you should be able to:

1 Understand the interrelationship of care for mental health and physical health.
2 Recognise the common physical health problems of people who experience mental health problems.
3 Incorporate preventative strategies and monitoring approaches into future practice.
4 Acknowledge physical health care as a human rights issue for people with mental ill-health.
5 Approach physical health care as a collaborative endeavour undertaken with the person experiencing mental ill-health and their carers and other members of the health team.

Introduction

The experience of mental ill-health has long been recognised as associated with a range of physical conditions that shorten life or impose limitations on physical well-being. Although the causes of this association are unresolved, it is absolutely clear that the experience of enduring mental ill-health (referred to as **serious mental illness (SMI)** in the research literature) in both Australia and Aotearoa New Zealand are associated with a shorter life span (Firth et al., 2019; Cunningham et al., 2014).

The chapter addresses the more commonly experienced and co-occurring physical conditions (also known as **comorbidities**), looking at the **prevalence** and specific characteristics of each among people experiencing recurring mental ill-health. The effects of medication on physical health and well-being are explored. Complementary approaches to augmenting well-being

serious mental illness (SMI) – also known as 'significant or severe mental illness'; ordinarily, it is used in reference to psychotic illnesses including schizophrenia and affective conditions and may also include anxiety conditions. This chapter uses the expression 'enduring mental ill-health' to avoid possible stigmatising characteristics of the term SMI.

comorbidity – a concomitant or co-occurring but unrelated pathological or disease condition

prevalence – the proportion of a population that experiences a certain condition

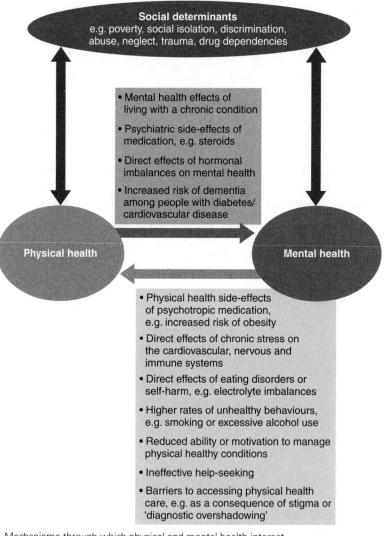

Figure 13.1   Mechanisms through which physical and mental health interact

Source: Naylor et al. (2016).

are addressed. This includes exercise, diet and stress-reduction strategies as well as the use of **over-the-counter (OTC) medications** and **complementary and alternative medicines (CAMs)**.

The final part of the chapter looks at approaches that are useful in preventing or limiting the effects of co-occurring physical ill-health. Physical health care is often overlooked in the presence of enduring mental ill-health or is given a lesser priority. The right to physical health care is independent of a person's mental health status, as described in the United Nations *Convention on the Rights of Persons with Disabilities* (United Nations Office of the High Commissioner for Human Rights, 2007). Article 25 states that 'persons with disabilities have the right to the enjoyment of the highest attainable standard of health without discrimination on the basis of disability' (United Nations Office of the High Commissioner for Human Rights, 2007). Reference in this context is to government policies directing the approaches of mental health services (NSW Ministry of Health, 2017; Te Pou o Te Whakaaro Nui, 2014).

over-the-counter (OTC) medications – drugs that are available for purchase without a medical prescription; these are generally considered to be safe, but this is a misconception as they may be toxic when taken in combination with other drugs, in certain physical conditions or when taken in large amounts

complementary and alternative medicines (CAMs) – medicines not usually prescribed in Western scientific medicine; 'complementary' refers to those approaches that do have some emerging scientific validity, and include diet and exercise. 'Alternative' medicines are those taken instead of Western biomedical treatments and may include Chinese traditional medicines and some herbal remedies. The term 'complementary' broadly refers to approaches that are 'in addition to', whereas 'alternative' refers to those used 'instead of' (see NIH National Cancer Institute, 2021).

REFLECTIVE QUESTIONS

Consider your knowledge of the physical health status of people with mental health problems prior to reading this chapter.

- Were you aware of the differences between the health of people with mental ill-health and the physical health of the general populations in Australia and Aotearoa New Zealand?
- What factors may limit this understanding of the poor physical health experienced by people with mental ill-health?

List a few points in response to these questions.

INTERPROFESSIONAL PERSPECTIVES

The context of mental health care

Any care in the field of mental health services is defined by its collaborative and interprofessional nature (Happell et al., 2019). The primary relationship is the collaborative relationship with the person experiencing mental ill-health, who wherever possible must lead the relationship. In this context, the professional disciplines involved are dictated by need and the expertise they contribute to care. In practice, restrictions exist, as dictated by the legal context of care but the ideal position is to support the person in determining their own care needs. A recent scoping review (Richardson et al., 2020) found mixed results in provision of integrated physical health care for those experiencing mental health problems and/or substance use disorders.

Prevalence

Determining the cause of death among of people with mental ill-health is problematic. It is often difficult to determine the cause of death for someone who may have had a co-existing mental health diagnosis. Consequently, many reports of premature death are derived from examination of people with a diagnosis or reported experience of schizophrenia and mood disorders rather than other diagnoses of mental ill-health.

People experiencing recurring mental ill-health have a life expectancy in Australia of 15–20 years less than the general population (Australian Bureau of Statistics, 2008, 2012; Firth et al., 2019). This range is conservative, and there have been suggestions that life expectancy may be as much as 25 years less than the general population (World Health Organization (WHO), 2014).

In Australia, Indigenous communities experience significantly earlier mortality and greater prevalence of physical diseases overall than the general population (Australian Institute for Health and Welfare (AIHW), 2020a; Parker, 2010; Vos et al., 2009). A review of available studies has confirmed that there is a greater prevalence of mental ill-health in Aboriginal and Torres Strait communities and that this is evident from a younger age (AIHW, 2020a; Jorm et al., 2012). More than 30 per cent of Indigenous young people were reported as experiencing high levels of psychological distress in 2014–2015, compared with one in eight non-Indigenous young people (AIHW, 2020a). Analysis of the physical health of Indigenous people who experience mental health problems is not readily available.

In Aotearoa New Zealand, studies report similar prevalence of physical ill-health in people experiencing mental ill-health (Lockett et al., 2018). Māori who had used mental health services were reported to have 'had more than twice the mortality rate of the general population' (Te Pou o Te Whakaaro, 2014), and those with a diagnosis of a psychotic illness had a rate of three times the general population (Cunningham et al., 2014). The New Zealand Health Survey of 2015/16, found that people who self-reported an internalising disorder (anxiety, depression and bipolar diagnoses) had increased experience of 'stroke (adjusted OR = 2.26, $p < 0.001$); cardiovascular disease (adjusted OR = 1.79, $p < 0.001$); chronic pain (adjusted OR = 2.03, $p < 0.001$); arthritis (adjusted OR = 1.72, $p < 0.001$); asthma (adjusted OR = 1.63, $p < 0.001$); and high cholesterol (adjusted OR = 1.50, $p < 0.001$)' (Lockett et al., 2018, p. 5).

The reduction in lifespan for people diagnosed with mental health problems is also reported in other countries. For example, a Finnish study (Tiihonen et al., 2009) reported a life expectancy of 22.5 years less than the general population in 2006. A later study provided more detailed information. It showed that route of administration of long-acting anti-psychotic made a difference: injections have an approximately 30 per cent lower risk of death compared with equivalent oral preparations (Taipale et al., 2018).

Studies from the United Kingdom report a life expectancy of 16–25 years less for those experiencing mental ill-health than for the general population (Blythe & White, 2012; Department of Health, 2011). This figure was reported to have improved to 15–20 years by 2018 (Public Health England, 2018). Studies from the United States report deaths among people experiencing mental health diagnoses as 25–30 years earlier than in the general population (Newcomer, 2007). The World Health Organization (WHO) reports that the life expectancy of people with severe mental illness is decreased by 10–25 years (WHO, 2014).

The Australian national study, People Living with Psychotic Illness 2010 (Morgan et al., 2011), was primarily concerned with gathering detailed information about the lives of people with psychotic illness who received publicly funded, specialised mental health services. The survey's method randomly sampled 1825 people, most of whom had a diagnosis of schizophrenia, for interview. Topics covered included socio-economic and demographic characteristics, activities of daily life, social participation, family contact, physical conditions, nutrition and exercise. Scales were also included to understand the effects of psychotic illness on a number of different factors, including a person's quality of life, general functioning, alcohol and drug use, smoking, cognitive functioning and their perceived need for mental health and other support services (Morgan et al., 2011). Figure 13.2 is based on participant reports from the study. It describes physical health morbidity as something that is diagnosed or assessed by their doctors at any time in the past and covers a range of conditions. In comparison to the general population, rates for every condition except cancers were higher in people with psychosis (Morgan et al., 2011).

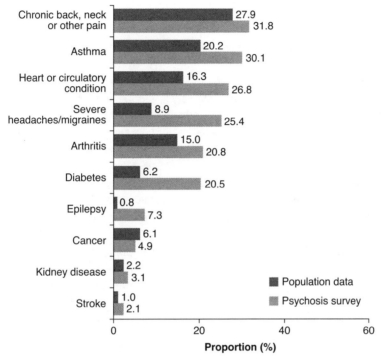

Figure 13.2 Lifetime physical morbidity of people with mental illness compared with the general population

Source: Morgan et al. (2011, p. 42).

Diagnostic overshadowing

The phenomenon of **diagnostic overshadowing** (Jones, Howard & Thornicroft, 2008) is important in understanding the greater rates of ill-health and premature mortality experienced by people diagnosed with mental ill-health and the difficulty in accessing physical health care that underlies this. Diagnostic overshadowing was first proposed as occurring among people with an intellectual disability. It recognised the tendency for physical ailments to be ascribed to the individual's cognitive disability (Reiss, Levitan & Szyszko, 1982). It has also been observed as occurring in other people who experience an enduring health (or other) condition such as mental ill-health. Diagnostic overshadowing is thought to occur because of three factors: the severity of the other (co-occurring) condition and its symptoms; cognitive or communication difficulties the person may also experience; and the understanding of the attending practitioners (Shefer et al., 2014). It is possible to speculate about the contribution of time pressures, and the failure of interprofessional practice evidenced by demarcation of specialties, to diagnostic overshadowing. In the field of mental health, delirium, substance misuse or toxicity may be particularly relevant to the effects of diagnostic overshadowing.

diagnostic overshadowing – the tendency for co-occurring conditions to be ascribed to the individual's initial presenting problem

PERSONAL NARRATIVE

Bree's story – transplantation services

It is often difficult to distinguish between the presentation of mental illness and the effects of liver disease such as hepatic encephalopathy. This creates challenges when nursing patients with both liver disease and mental illness who present for a potential liver transplant, as medical findings and treatment can unfortunately be complicated by diagnostic overshadowing.

Mental illness is a common occurrence in the transplant population. It is not seen as a contradiction to transplantation; however, it can be deemed an obstacle if issues of non-compliance relating to a mental health disorder are identified (Corbett et al., 2013). When supported by friends and family, patients with mental health disorders who undergo transplantation experience outcomes similar to those of the general population (Corbett et al., 2013).

One example is of a patient diagnosed with hepatitis C virus and schizophrenia who was referred to the transplant unit of a tertiary facility for consideration of a liver transplantation. The patient presented with symptoms of confusion, disorganised behaviour and memory loss, as well as other common manifestations of liver disease. Initially, the nursing staff found it difficult to converse with the patient and noticed issues of poor insight and lack of compliance. At times the patient refused regular care and medications, which is usually seen as a barrier to approval for transplantation. Acknowledging that this behaviour could potentially be caused by schizophrenia, hepatic encephalopathy, or a combination of both, it was imperative for further assessment to be initiated to determine the cause. A comprehensive psychiatric assessment was performed to determine the cause of behaviour. It was recognised that the patient was suffering from symptoms of hepatic encephalopathy, and therefore their mental health diagnosis was not the cause of concern. The patient was subsequently approved for liver transplantation on the understanding that the behaviours would resolve following transplantation.

REFLECTIVE QUESTION

While waiting for definitive results from testing, what considerations should be taken for safety and the engagement of the person?

PERSONAL NARRATIVE

Michelle's story – part one

I was first diagnosed in 2003 with schizophrenia. At this stage of my life it was devastating and distressing. I am now 40 years old and have some life experience behind me.

My life before schizophrenia was relatively normal. I went to a selective high school in New South Wales and went on to study a health science degree at university. My degree was actually in acupuncture, so I came from a background of complementary medicine. I was not anti-medicine; I just found from experience that Western medicine did not always have a cure. In Chinese medicine also, there is an ethos of treating people while they are well, in order to prevent disease in the first place. This background made it difficult for me to accept that I could not heal myself and that I, indeed, needed to take anti-psychotic medication.

It was a huge leap for me. I spent years going in and out of hospital, always thinking that I would be fine without medication. After about five years of relapse after relapse, I made a promise to myself that I would take the medication and work with the doctors to find the right treatment for me. I now take olanzapine every night without fail, as I have too much to lose, including a job and a relationship.

Relationships can be challenging. I do a lot of online dating as it is better to meet people that way rather than, for example, at a club or a pub. I tell potential partners about my mental distress on the third or fourth date and most people are okay with it. It is more likely that I end the relationship than the other way around!

I also want to tell you about my experience with physical health and mental health. When I was first diagnosed, I weighed 50 kilograms and was a size 6. Over the years and with different medications and their side-effects, I slowly gained 40 kilograms.

After I was divorced, I ballooned out to my heaviest, at 90 kilograms. I was taking clozapine and had the unusual side-effect of feeling nauseous and sometimes vomiting, particularly in the morning. Despite me knowing that the nausea was due to the clozapine, my psychiatrist ignored my pleas to change me to a different medication as my mental health was great on the clozapine.

After a couple of years of daily nausea, I finally got a referral to a gastroenterologist who, after hearing my story and conducting a gastroscopy, concluded that the nausea was due to the clozapine. I asked her to write a letter to my psychiatrist and she did this for me. I finally was switched to olanzapine.

I was then able to work on my physical health. I went to see the community dietitian, who introduced me to the Australian Guide to Healthy Eating, the new food pyramid. It was hard to change my diet and I was also on the pension so unable to afford the best food. Over a 12-month period, I started walking, first to the shops and back, and then further, working my way up to hour-long walks at least times three times a week. I did change my diet to include more fruit and vegetables and less carbohydrates, and I ended up losing about 15 kilograms.

I was also given a TheraBand™ by the exercise physiologist and she explained how important it was to include strength exercises in my regimen.

I still monitor my diet and make sure I exercise but I am in a much better position physically than I was before.

Side-effects of the medication is probably the biggest obstacle I find to keeping my weight at a respectable level. I get hungry at night and often indulge in carbs and sugar, and have to pull myself out of this mindset and return to healthy eating, which means having a couple of carrots at night when I'm hungry. Exercise is also important.

Consumers often say that you can't lose weight on anti-psychotics. I am proof that you can; it just takes a concerted effort.

Good physical health makes a space for good mental health. I strongly believe this.

REFLECTIVE QUESTIONS

Michelle's story highlights the importance of collaboration with the consumer for holistic, person-centred health care.

- Did Michelle experience barriers to accessing physical health care during periods of mental ill-health?
- How may her physical health have been best maintained alongside her mental health care?

- Whose responsibility is it to ensure Michelle, or any other person in her situation, has her physical health needs addressed?
- How can the risks to mental health and to physical health be best reconciled? Can they always be reconciled? If treatment for mental health results in effects on physical health, should mental health outcomes be compromised? In your answer, take into account the potential effects of enduring or recurrent episodes of mental ill-health for physical health, and recovery principles.

Common co-occurring physical conditions

Physical health concerns in those experiencing serious mental illness are varied. The discussion of co-occurring physical conditions includes:

- metabolic syndrome
- diabetes
- hyperlipideamia
- cardiovascular diseases
- obesity.

Metabolic syndrome

The metabolic syndrome is a cluster of factors that significantly increase the risk of developing and dying from cardiovascular disease. There is a variety of definitions, and the definition endorsed by the International Diabetes Federation (IDF, 2006, updated 2020) requires central obesity (abdominal girth) and at least a further two of the following factors be present. These are summarised in Table 13.1.

Table 13.1 Metabolic syndrome risk factors

According to the new IDF definition, for a person to be defined as having the metabolic syndrome they must have: **Central obesity** (defined as waist circumference* with ethnicity specific values) **plus any two of the following four factors:**	
Raised triglycerides	≥ 150 mg/dL (1.7 mmol/L) **or specific treatment for this lipid abnormality**
Reduced HDL cholesterol	< 40 mg/dL (1.03 mmol/L) in males < 50 mg/dL (1.29 mmol/L) in females **or specific treatment for this lipid abnormality**
Raised blood pressure	systolic BP ≥ 130 of diastolic BP ≥ 85 mm Hg **or treatment of previously diagnosed hypertension**
Raised fasting plasma glucose	(FPG) ≥ 100 mg/dL (5.6 mmol/L) **or previously diagnosed type 2 diabetes** If above 5.6 mmol/L or 100 mg/dL, OGTT is strong recommended but is not necessary to define presence of the syndrome.

*If BMI is > 30 kg/m², central obesity can be assumed, and waist circumference does not need to be measured.

Source: IDF (2006, updated 2020, p. 10).

Lambert and Chapman (2004) attributed the premature age at death in people experiencing mental ill-health to an increased prevalence of the metabolic syndrome and its components, which are risk factors for cardiovascular diseases and type 2 diabetes. These factors have to be assessed against the general population, in which rates of metabolic syndrome have increased (Moodie et al., 2013). But evidence strongly suggests that the prevalence of metabolic syndrome is much greater among people experiencing mental ill-health (Newcomer, 2007; Zuko et al., 2020). It has been reported that 32 per cent of men and 51 per cent of women diagnosed with schizophrenia meet criteria for metabolic syndrome (John et al., 2009; Scott et al., 2019); the prevalence is higher in women than in men (Lopuszanska et al., 2014; Narasimhan & Raynor, 2010). Overweight and obesity, hyperglycaemia, dyslipidaemia and hypertension are all risk factors of this syndrome that have higher prevalence among people with mental ill-health (Lambert, 2009; Lambert et al., 2017).

The reasons metabolic syndrome rates are high are complex and contested. Social factors such as poverty and reduced access to medical services are recognised contributors (Wheeler, McKenna & Madell, 2014). So, too, is the use of psychotropic medications (Hammoudeh et al., 2020; Van Winkel et al., 2008). Understanding these factors may help consumers of mental health services make informed decisions about their treatment options. However, reversal of increased risk is not simple for those experiencing mental ill-health, as it also is not for the general population. Risk factors may be screened for and recognised. Reversing or countering such factors as overweight, obesity, hyperlipidaemia and hyperglycaemia is difficult as these are stubborn issues. There are no simple responses, as shown by the achievement of only modest improvements over the past decade (Lambert & Newcomer, 2009; Rødevand et al., 2019).

Diabetes

The prevalence of diabetes has increased rapidly in the developed world over the past several decades. The IDF has reported that 'the number of people around the world suffering from diabetes has skyrocketed in the two decades 1990–2010, from 30 million to 230 million' (World Federation for Mental Health, 2010, p. 12). The association of depression with diabetes has been recognised for some time. The World Federation for Mental Health has reported that 25 per cent of people with diabetes experience depression, and that the risk of developing depression and the prevalence of depression is twice that of the general population (World Federation for Mental Health, 2010). Further, the risk of mortality in people with diabetes is increased by 30 per cent when they also experience depression (World Federation for Mental Health, 2010).

The occurrence of diabetes among people with mental ill-health has been observed for a long time. Maudsley, the famous British psychiatrist, observed in 1897 that 'diabetes is a disease which often shows itself in families in which insanity prevails' (cited in Koran, 2004, p. 65). While the rate of diabetes among the general population is thought to be around 5–7 per cent (Busche & Holt, 2004; Robson & Gray, 2007; Shaw, Sicree & Zimmet, 2010), the prevalence among those diagnosed with enduring mental ill-health is 10.2 per cent (Stubbs et al., 2015) and 15 per cent for those diagnosed with schizophrenia (Holt & Peveler, 2005).

Understanding of why diabetes is more widely prevalent among people with enduring mental ill-health is not clear. The best explanations point to the recurrent association with family history, low physical activity, poor diet, smoking and the metabolic effects of some anti-psychotic medications (Mitchell et al., 2013; Nordentoft et al., 2013; Vancampfort et al., 2019; Vancampfort et al., 2017; Vancampfort et al., 2012).

An additional concern observed about diabetes in the general population is an extreme delay in diagnosis. Explanations of this delay are not clear but the delay is estimated at up to 12 years (De Hert et al., 2011; Ronaldson et al., 2020). Moreover, this delay in recognition, diagnosis and treatment has several serious health effects. Eye damage and blindness, kidney impairment that may result in renal failure, and nerve damage are all potential consequences. This is also the case for people with enduring mental ill-health who develop diabetes. Data about delays in diagnosis for people with mental ill-health is not available, but it is possible to speculate that the delay is greater than for the general population. If this is the case, the consequences on health could be serious.

Hyperlipidaemia

Monitoring of lipids is low among people experiencing enduring mental ill-health, despite long-standing position statements by relevant professional bodies (Royal Australian & New Zealand College of Psychiatrists (RANZCP), 2015). Further, the efficacy of statins, the usual pharmacological treatment for hyperlipidaemia, has rarely been studied among people who are also being treated for mental ill-health (Gierisch et al., 2014; Gierisch et al., 2013). This raises concerns that there may be effects other than those intended.

Cardiovascular diseases (hypertension, cardiac arrhythmias)

Cardiovascular disease rates are higher among people experiencing mental ill-health than the general population (Ward, White & Druss, 2015). This is not solely as a result of hyperlipidaemia but arises from the higher prevalence of hypertension and cardiac arrhythmias. Table 13.2 summarises data collected by Morgan and colleagues (2011) in Australia pertaining to consumers living with psychotic illness, most commonly schizophrenia. Nearly one-third of people who were assessed were at absolute risk of experiencing a cardiovascular event in 5 years' time, with 7.2 per cent of the total number of participants at medium risk and 24.0 per cent at high risk (Morgan et al., 2011). Although lifestyle factors such as reduced activity levels, obesity, poor diet and limited medical screening are implicated, medications used to treat mental ill-health are known to contribute (Ronaldson et al., 2020). Drugs such as tricyclic antidepressants and some anti-psychotics are understood to change cardiac function (Gierisch et al., 2014). For example the anti-psychotic clozapine requires monitoring to respond to iatrogenic cardiac effects, including myocarditis (Alawami et al., 2014; Raedler, 2010).

Table 13.2   Absolute 5-year risk of cardiovascular disease

Risk	Proportion (%) of population		
	18–34 years*	35–64 years	Total
Low	87.2	56.3	68.8
Medium	0.0	12.0	7.2
High	12.8	31.7	24.0

*Framingham risk equation 15–16 applied to those with no missing data. The Framingham risk equation is not normally used with people under 35 years of age. However, 12.8 per cent in the younger age group met risk criteria. In all cases, this was due to pre-existing cardiovascular disease or other high-risk medical conditions.

Source: Morgan et al. (2011).

Cardiovascular disease is the primary cause of early mortality reported in people experiencing enduring mental ill-health (De Hert et al., 2011; Hammoudeh et al., 2020).

Obesity

Rates of overweight and obesity have risen markedly over the past 20 years and continue throughout the world (Friedrich, 2017; Sassi et al., 2009). In 2017, Australia ranked fifth in rates of obesity (out of 23 member countries of the Organisation for Economic Co-operation and Development (OECD) for people aged 15 years and over (AIHW, 2020b, p. 5). This is also true of people in Aotearoa New Zealand with enduring mental ill-health. Māori and Pacific Islander peoples living in Aotearoa New Zealand who have enduring mental ill-health have been found to have a higher **body mass index (BMI)** than New Zealanders of European heritage (Wheeler, McKenna & Madell, 2013). All the reasons suggested as significant for the rises in obesity in the general population – a food-rich environment, reduced levels of incidental physical activity and increased consumption of calorie-rich foods – also hold true for those with mental ill-health. However, there are additional factors that make the challenge of maintaining a healthy BMI more difficult.

A useful measurement of obesity, independent of height or musculature is waist circumference. This is a simple measurement that often correlates with BMI, except in athletes, for example. The waist circumference may indicate fat distribution, especially visceral fat that maybe detrimental to health. Waist circumference used in conjunction with BMI gives a more complete understanding of a person's obesity.

Figure 13.3, which presents data from the Morgan and colleagues (2011) study, used the International Physical Activity Questionnaire to measure the level of physical activity of participants in the previous 7 days. The results revealed that 'one-third (33.5 per cent) of participants were classified as sedentary; that is, inactive or with very low levels of activity, while the other two-thirds were classified as having a low level of activity' (Morgan et al., 2011). These patterns have been reported to continue (Vancampfort et al., 2017).

body mass index (BMI) – an index of weight-for-height that is commonly used to classify underweight, overweight and obesity in adults. BMI = kg/m² where kg is a person's weight in kilograms and m² is their height in metres squared. See Heart Foundation (n.d.) for further details.

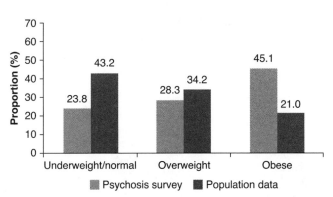

Figure 13.3 Weight status of people with mental illness compared with the general Australian population

Source: Morgan et al. (2011, p. 44).

The reduced income – indeed, poverty – of many people experiencing mental ill-health, especially those enduring mental ill-health, presents the first hurdle. Prepared (fast) foods are often perceived as cheaper as well as more convenient. These foods are often high in calories and include a range of ingredients detrimental to good health, such as saturated fats, low fibre and high levels of sodium and sugar. A range of semi-prepared foods is now more available, but not cheap and not as convenient as fast foods.

Poverty or significantly reduced income also increases the individual's chances of weight gain by yet another means. The capacity to pay for exercise opportunities, whether through gym membership or sporting club registration, is severely limited, if not lost. A common response to activity needs of the general population is often denied to those with enduring mental ill-health before any application of stigma that may reduce social inclusion in such venues.

Psychotropic medications also play a role. Many have sedative qualities. Measures of basal metabolic rates for people taking clozapine are very low, further enhancing weight-gain trajectories. People often experience lethargy when taking many of the anti-psychotics, such as olanzapine (Kishimoto et al., 2019; McEvoy et al., 2007).

There is also an association between anti-psychotic medications and weight gain. Young people experiencing their first episode of psychosis are particularly vulnerable to rapid weight gain (Curtis et al., 2016). This can lead to development of cardio-metabolic changes (Kishimoto et al. 2019). The observation has been made that increased appetite is also experienced in association with anti-psychotic medication use (Deng, Weston-Green & Huang, 2010).

Psychotropic drugs are suspected of interfering with the sensation of satiety. This in-built physiological feedback mechanism does not react to signals that the person has consumed sufficient food or calories. Some people have been known to complain of constant hunger that severely impedes self-restraint and moderation in eating. Histamine neuro-transmitters are suspected to be instrumental in these second-generation, anti-psychotic-induced weight gain effects (Deng, Weston-Green & Huang, 2010), Consider Michelle's comments regarding this problem.

Finally, the nature of most enduring mental ill-health in itself can reduce a person's motivation to participate actively in life – including healthy rates of daily exercise. The study of people living with psychotic illness (Morgan et al., 2011; see Figure 13.4) found that those in the age group 35–64 years were more likely to be in the sedentary category when compared with a younger age group of 18–34 years. According to the results, the most frequently reported barriers to being physically active were lack of motivation (36.4 per cent), tiredness (19.2 per cent) and pain or discomfort (15.2 per cent).

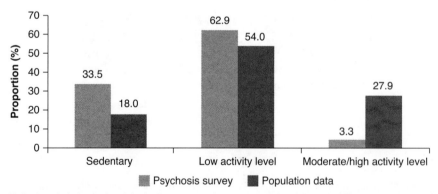

Figure 13.4   Level of physical activity in the past week among people with mental illness compared with the general Australian population

Source: Morgan et al. (2011, p. 44).

Nutritional patterns

Independent of the effects of psychotropic drugs, the nutritional patterns of people experiencing mental ill-health are poor and do not meet healthy eating guidelines (Ministry of Health, 2018; National Health and Medical Research Council (NHMRC), 2013; Teasdale et al., 2019). In a study of 159 people who had been diagnosed with schizophrenia, Simonelli-Muñoz and colleagues (2012) found that that 51 per cent of people reported that their meal times took less than 15 minutes, while 40.8 per cent did not eat fresh food daily and 63.1 per cent did not eat fish. Additionally, portion sizes are critical to weight control. 'Super-sizing' has become commonplace in Westernised societies. These poor dietary habits were associated with increases in BMI and waist circumference – a prime indicator of adipose fat patterns, the development of obesity and metabolic syndrome.

The effects and use of nutrition as treatment are largely unknown. A recent randomised control study of nutrition (Jacka et al., 2017; Opie et al., 2018) has suggested that nutrition may offer fresh approaches in therapeutic interventions for depression; this adds to suggestions in the literature that diet can act as a preventative factor in the development or resolution of the experience of mental ill-health. It is a field of study that suggests approaches that may minimise the experience of side-effects or adverse effects from pharmacological treatment.

Exercise behaviours

The evidence about the efficacy of exercise is tentative and, as yet, a comprehensive understanding of its contribution across the full diversity of mental ill-health is unclear. Adjunctive rather than first-line treatment is considered a safe and conservative option until further study clarifies the contribution of exercise (Stanton et al., 2015).

A range of studies support the clinical observation that exercise interventions have a place in the treatment of several different mental health problems. This may be as an adjunct to traditional psychotherapy and psychopharmaceuticals such as antidepressants; for example, in the treatment of depression (Stanton et al., 2015). The Royal Australian & New Zealand College of Psychiatrists (RANZCP) guidelines for the treatment of depression suggest that 'adequate exercise may be of benefit' (RANZCP, 2015). Critically, an explanation of what constitutes 'adequate exercise' is lacking.

The efficacy of yoga and general stretching exercises are also gaining some traction within the mental health field (Snaith et al., 2020). It has been postulated that the mindfulness aspects of yoga and gentle stretching can help with anxiety and depression by assisting in emotional regulation (Snaith et al., 2020). However, accessing yoga classes in the community due to cost, perceived stigma and access is not always feasible.

Nursing staff are well placed to explore exercise patterns and preferences with consumers. Their position within and across mental health services, coupled with their unique and privileged therapeutic relationship with consumers, can facilitate examination of the possible contribution exercise can make to an individual's well-being (Stanton, Raeburn & Happell, 2015). Exercise physiologists and physiotherapists are among the allied health disciplines with whom consultative interventions could be developed.

PERSONAL NARRATIVE

Michelle's story – part two

After taking the anti-psychotics, clozapine and olanzapine, I gained 40 kilograms, going from a size 6 to a size 18.

It took a long time to motivate myself to eat healthily, and I was on the pension for a while, so I would only buy fruit and vegetables that were in season. I had pretty much given up on myself and felt that I couldn't afford to eat healthily.

I went to my GP to do annual blood work and the GP diagnosed me with pre-diabetes. This was a great motivator for me as I didn't want to end up diabetic and on another medication. Diabetes was a serious illness for me.

I went to see a community dietitian, who helped me with portion sizes and increasing fruit and vegetable intake. She also helped to keep me accountable, meaning that I had to see her every two weeks and she would weigh me and discuss my progress. I felt that someone checking up on me motivated me to change my habits.

The dietitian also talked about the importance of exercise. I found that by developing a routine it was easier to motivate myself to change. I would get up in the morning, put on my exercise gear and go straight out for a walk. I started off in a small way, walking for 15 minutes and then built this to an hour-long walk.

I ended up losing 15 kilograms and was in a much healthier place and out of the risk of developing diabetes.

Maintenance is important too, and it is easy to fall back into old habits. I still count the amount of carbs that I have during the day and often (though not always) have a couple of carrots at night when I feel the need to eat. I find it harder to deal with cravings, especially at night, and I think this is a side-effect of the medication. I have cheat days, too.

REFLECTIVE QUESTION
How could you support Michelle to maintain a healthy diet and weight?

REFLECTIVE QUESTIONS

Keep a diary for one week, detailing your exercise and eating. Note your emotional state as the context of your exercise and eating.

- Write a critique on your eating and exercise behaviours, compared to national guidelines for your age group.
- Reflect on any variation in your behaviours, relative to those recommendations. Do you perceived any relationship between these and your emotional state?
- How difficult was it to accurately undertake this activity?
- What insights may be relevant for people experiencing mental ill-health for whom you may be recommending dietary and exercise interventions?

Cancers

The prevalence of cancers among people with mental health problems shows contradictory patterns. On the one hand, some cancers appear more frequently while others are less frequently experienced. This apparently confusing pattern has been explained by a closer analysis of individual cancers, suggesting that some cancers that may be expected to be common causes of mortality, such as lung cancer, are not represented as expected because people experiencing enduring mental ill-health have died earlier from other causes, such as cardiovascular diseases. Lung cancer typically occurs at a later age than death from cardiovascular disease, providing a possible explanation for its lower representation, and given the high levels of smoking among people with enduring mental ill-health (Robson & Gray, 2007; Solmi et al., 2020).

Digestive and breast cancers, however, are well recognised as having higher rates of mortality than in the general population (Iglay et al., 2017). Several possible explanations are offered for this situation in relation to breast cancers. Among these includes lower participation by people experiencing mental ill-health in screening activities: routine self-examination, examination by GPs and breast scans. In addition to reduced screening participation, increased prevalence of digestive cancers among people with mental ill-health is associated with poor diet and increased alcohol consumption.

Overall, people experiencing enduring mental ill-health and cancer have worse outcomes (Davis et al., 2020). This can be attributed, in part, to poorer access and quality of healthcare treatment (Ronaldson et al., 2020).

Hepatitis and HIV/AIDS

Hepatitis and HIV/AIDS are over-represented in people with a diagnosois of mental ill-health. A recent meta-analysis by Hughes and colleagues (2016) demonstrated that people with enduring mental ill-health had high rates of hepatitis B and C. Many studies have reported an increased HIV seroprevalence among people diagnosed with mental ill-health, compared to the general population (Bauer-Staeb et al., 2017; Hughes & et al., 2016). Although the number of newly diagnosed cases of HIV in Australia has declined by 7 per cent over the past 5 years, to a total of 963 new notifications of HIV in 2017 (Kirkby Institute, 2018), the vulnerability of people diagnosed with mental ill-health remains a concern.

Behaviours that expose people with mental ill-health, in particular, to increased risk include sexual disinhibition and disorganisation. Sex may be considered a currency in a population living in poverty. Coexisting substance misuse is common, along with an increase in at-risk partners in sexual networks and difficulty in accessing medical care.

Mental ill-health, especially depression and psychosis, have been associated with poor adherence to antiretroviral treatment. Consequently, the progression of the disease may be unimpeded (Corr, 2012, p. 333).

Sexual health

Access to sexual health resources and the ability to experience a safe expression of sexuality is a fundamental human right (WHO, 2006, 2015). Sexual health concerns carry with them a certain stigma. They are not easy problems to discuss, both for the consumer and the health professional. Most mental health assessments do not include sexual health.

Therefore, in order to understand how best to guide consumers, we need to also be able to discuss sexual health along with sexual dysfunction (Bartlett et al., 2010; Pacitti & Thornicroft, 2009).

Mental ill-health, substance misuse and prescribed psychotropic medication all can cause sexual dysfunction. In first-episode psychosis, up to 82 per cent of men and 96 per cent of women report problems with sexual dysfunction that lead to reduction in quality of life (Taylor, Barnes & Young, 2018, p. 141).

It has been estimated that 50–60 per cent of people diagnosed with schizophrenia report sexual dysfunction, compared to 30 per cent of the general population. One study found that 37 per cent of consumers with psychosis spontaneously reported experiencing sexual dysfunction, whereas 46 per cent reported experiencing sexual difficulties when asked directly (Taylor et al., 2018, p. 141). Therefore, direct questioning is indicated to establish baseline sexual functioning.

Sexual dysfunction has been reported as an adverse effect of anti-psychotic medications. Anti-psychotics decrease dopaminergic transmission, which can lower libido, although a negative feedback loop may also increase prolactin levels. It has been estimated that increases in prolactin levels account for 40 per cent of the sexual dysfunction associated with anti-psychotic medication, (Taylor et al., 2018, p. 142).

Both depression and the treatment of depression can cause sexual dysfunction. The precise nature of the sexual dysfunction can indicate whether the depression itself or the medication causes the sexual dysfunction. Sexual dysfunction has also been reported as an adverse effect of all antidepressants (Taylor et al., 2018, p. 243). It needs to be noted that sexual dysfunction with antidepressants is often dose-related and fully reversible. Sexual dysfunction can be minimised by the careful selection of an antidepressant medication. In some instances, antidepressants are used to assist in sexual dysfunction with medications helping to reduce premature ejaculation and paraphilias (Taylor et al., 2018, p. 243).

The prevalence of high-risk sexual behaviours among people with mental ill-health are difficult to determine, but there is some evidence that sexually transmissible infections are more common than in the general community (Brown & Paxton 2008; Corr, 2012, p. 333; Dyer & McGuinness 2008; Hughes et al. 2018).

Although sexual health seems a major concern for many people experiencing enduring mental ill-health, according to the literature it is rarely spoken about. This could be for many reasons, including health practitioners feeling uncomfortable about discussing these personal concerns, along with the health practitioner not having a clear understanding of how to assist the consumer. According to an Australian study, mental health nurses generally avoid discussing sexual health with patients (Quinn, Happell & Browne, 2011). Reasons postulated were concerns about professional boundaries, sexual health concerns of consumers not being a priority and that it is was not their responsibility (Quinn et al., 2011).

Health practitioners are in a powerful position to discuss sexual health with their consumers. While not all practitioners may be comfortable discussing these issues, a few simple questions could lead to a discussion with a psychiatrist about the possibility of changing the consumer's medication (Quinn & Happell, 2012). In large city hospitals, mental health practitioners can readily refer consumers to sexual health clinics for consultation and treatment. This may not be the case for people in regional, rural and remote areas. It needs to be noted that consumers aspire to have safe and supportive intimate relationships, and that health practitioners can be the agents to ensure this (Hughes et al., 2018; WHO, 2015).

REFLECTIVE QUESTIONS

- How would you talk about sexuality with people who have mental health problems?
- How do your beliefs, both about sexuality and mental ill-health, influence your ability to provide this care?

Back pain, migraine and arthritis

A 2010 survey of people with enduring mental ill-health and their physical health (Morgan et al., 2011) established that back pain, migraine and arthritis were experienced more commonly than among the general Australian population.

Harris and colleagues (2018) suggested that the experience of back pain occurs earlier in people with mental ill-health than in the general population, thereby resulting in a lower quality of life for a longer period. Morgan and colleagues (2011) reported that one in three people with a psychotic illness who participated in their survey reported experiencing back pain. The relationship between pain and mental ill-health is suggested by Harris and colleagues (2018) as potentially bi-dimensional, with each influencing the other.

Arthritis (including osteoarthritis and rheumatoid arthritis) in 959 000 people experiencing mental ill-health was reported by more men (66 per cent) than women (46 per cent) (Morgan et al., 2011). Arthritis is more often experienced by people from lower socio-economic groups, and more in rural and regional areas (Harris et al., 2018). This leaves people with mental ill-health suffering a greater burden of disease as it occurs earlier in life than for the general population, affecting them during their productive working lives. This flows on to reports of limitations in self-care, mobility and employment, and disruption to social interaction.

Smoking

The links between tobacco smoking and heart disease, cancers and other health conditions is well established. In Australia, 12.8 per cent of the population smokes daily, but this is not evenly distributed through all parts of the population (Harris et al., 2018). Morgan and colleagues (2011) found that rates of smoking among people with enduring mental ill-health are significantly higher than in the general population. Of the study participants, males were more likely to smoke than females, with 71.1 per cent reporting that they were current smokers at the time of interview, compared to 58.8 per cent of females (Morgan et al., 2011). Participants in the study smoked on average 21 cigarettes per day.

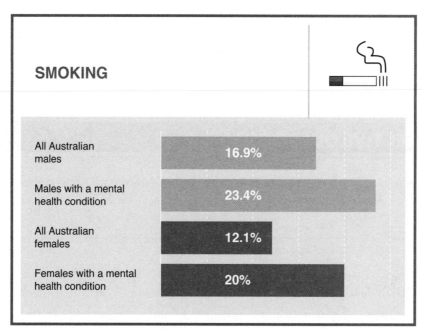

Figure 13.5   Tobacco consumption among people with mental illness and comparison with the general population

Source: Harris et al. (2018, p. 21).

The interest of people experiencing enduring mental ill-health in reducing or quitting smoking tends to be at rates similar to the general public (Prochaska, 2010; Prochaska et al., 2014). However, success is lower in part because ready access to support for quitting is less than in the general community. This indicates that a routine component of all mental health care should include assessment of tobacco use and the person's desire to reduce or cease usage. The most-commonly used measure is the Fagerström Test for Nicotine Dependence. Health promotion has been successful and safe when including harm-reduction measures using nicotine replacement therapy (NRT) in the presence of continued smoking (Bittoun et al., 2015, p. 954). Current 'stop smoking medications' such as varenicline (Champix) have been shown to be helpful for some people (Taylor et al. 2018, p. 434). This suggests that smoking-cessation programs need not take an 'all or nothing' approach. Very low nicotine-content cigarettes may also have a role in supporting harm minimisation related to smoking (Tidey et al., 2019). Electronic cigarettes (vaping, vapes, e-cigarettes) can also assist people to reduce their smoking (Mental Health Smoking Partnership, 2020; Taylor, et al., 2018).

Health professions, especially in primary heathcare settings, are in an excellent position to support smoking reduction and cessation. Schemes exist for subsidised NRT, often through local authorities. Access may require medical prescription and, in some areas, qualified nursing staff are credentialled to prescribe NRT. If a person chooses to stop smoking completely, and especially if this is abruptly, it calls for discussion of available support measures. Adjustments in dosage is required for clozapine as plasma levels can rise significantly (Wagner et al., 2020).

Urinary incontinence

People experiencing enduring mental ill-health have a heightened risk for urinary incontinence. A number of psychotropic medications appear to be implicated, specifically anti-psychotics, benzodiazepines and antidepressants (Harrison-Woolrych et al., 2011; Movig et al., 2002; Tsakiris, Oelke & Michel, 2008). Clozapine is recognised as contributing to increased urinary incontinence, especially nocturnal incontinence (Harrison-Woolrych et al., 2011). Anti-cholinergic and antidepressant medications are associated with urinary retention and overflow.

The effects of urinary incontinence are multiple. Individuals may be less able to advocate for active investigation and treatment of this physical health issue, and so may not have access to expert services. This can cause additional effects to consumers' self-esteem when they are already affected by the incontinence. Incontinence can be experienced at an early age due to the introduction of medications. This can cause additional alienation from peer groups. Additionally, staff may be challenged by urinary incontinence among in-patients and may be rejecting in their attitudes. Stigma and stereotypes can be reinforced by incontinence. When living on a restricted income or in poverty, the cost of seeking treatment and incontinence aids can be prohibitive.

It is important that incontinence screening and treatment be routinely incorporated into the physical health care of people with mental ill-health. Active approaches when clozapine is prescribed should be taken to manage or minimise the development or problems of incontinence. Standard assessment tools, such as 24-hour urine collections and bladder diaries, can prove difficult for some people experiencing mental health problems. Tools may need to be adapted or developed to better serve people with these problems.

Direct questioning of people prescribed psychotropic medication is indicated as the topic is often embarrassing, and many people do not volunteer this information. Privacy and sensitivity are important.

TRANSLATION TO PRACTICE

Dental health

A review of the published literature on oral health advice for people with enduring mental ill-health (Arnaiz et al., 2011; Khokhar et al., 2011) reported that people with mental health problems had worse oral health than the general population. It has been noted that people with enduring mental ill-health experience greater prevalence of oral disease and find accessing care for this difficult (Arnaiz et al., 2011; Khokhar et al., 2011).

For many people with mental health problems, barriers to accessing routine dental care may exist. These include prohibitory costs in private care and complex schemes that differ across services within the public health arena (AIHW, 2020c).

In addition to this financial impediment for good dental care, enduring mental ill-health can result in difficulties with the level of organisation required of the individual for

xerostomia – a condition of dry mouth that may be a result of several different causes, such as the adverse side-effects of medications and salivary gland dysfunction due to a variety of causes, including radiotherapy and fluid balance

preventative dental activities, such as routine cleaning and dental visits. The side-effects of medications (e.g. **xerostomia**) can create a poor oral environment, and poor dietary and nutritional habits may also contribute.

The effects of poor oral health are multiple. Poor oral health can affect a person's everyday functioning, as pain or discomfort from poor dentition can affect the ability to eat. People's diet may be restricted in response to this, and when coupled with low economic resources, may even result in nutritional deficits. Poor oral health has been associated with coronary heart disease. Appearance may also be affected by poor oral health. Missing or discoloured teeth and halitosis can reduce social acceptability. In turn, self-esteem may be reduced (AIHW, 2020c). Good oral health is part of overall good health.

Xerostomia (dry mouth) is a side-effect of many psychotropic medications, including anti-psychotics, antidepressants and mood stabilisers. Reduction in salivation is an uncomfortable experience. It increases the risk of periodontal diseases, such as gingivitis, that can lead to tooth loss (Persson et al., 2009). Xerostomia may also affect the capacity to swallow food. The mechanical ability to chew food and create a bolus for swallowing becomes impaired. Saliva is essential in this process. The bolus produced may be large and dry (Arnaiz et al., 2011). This increases the risk of choking, which is a cause of death among people with enduring mental ill-health that occurs with greater frequency than in the general population.

TRANSLATION TO PRACTICE

A conversation about oral health whenever possible can include discussion on diet, and on pain. The time needed for the conversation needs to be considered. People may have altered their diet in response to pain, so asking about these modifications may require a direct line of questioning, as people may take this for granted or may be embarrassed. Discussing fluid intake is also important, as pain may also be implicated in reduced fluid intake.

Remember to ask about the person's most recent visit to the dentist and why it has or has not been a routine. Frequency of dental visits may by reflected by the long waiting periods for public services, difficulties in receiving reminders, or financial burden. In addition, pain during treatment may be a factor. Consideration should be given to access, especially if the person is located in rural or regional areas.

Dysphagia

Dysphagia is a problem that has been recognised as occurring more commonly among people experiencing mental ill-health problems than among the general population. It is estimated that 9–42 per cent of people with a mental health diagnosis experience dysphagia, compared with 6 per cent of the general population (Aldridge & Taylor, 2012). This seems to be related to behavioural factors and adverse reactions to anti-psychotic medications (Allen, de Nesnera & Robinson, 2012; Ruschena et al., 2003). Fast-eating syndrome is the most common behavioural cause of choking among people with mental ill-health (Kulkarni, Kamath & Stewart, 2017). It is compounded by people taking large mouthfuls of food, gorging and pocketing (saving) food in the cheek (Corcoran & Walsh, 2003; McMannus 2001; Warner, 2004). An Australian study of choking deaths reported that people who had died from choking were 20 times more likely to have had a medical diagnosis of schizophrenia than others who had died from choking (Lu et al., 2017).

Complementary and alternative therapies and mental health care

CAMs encompass various disease-preventing and disease-treating practices. Common therapies in mental health include folate and tryptophan supplements, acupuncture, aromatherapy, Tai Chi, exercise and homeopathy as adjuncts to antidepressants (Bryant & Knights, 2014).

Frequent problems with the use of natural products in mental health is that often the purity and the strength of the product is not known and cannot be guaranteed from product to product. This can be a problem as the active ingredient can vary between products and between batches (Bryant & Knights, 2014).

Perhaps the most common herbal product known in Australia and Aotearoa New Zealand is St John's wort (*Hypericum perforatum*). About 450 products containing St John's wort (SJW) are listed in Australia (Bryant & Knights, 2014). There is significant evidence for the effectiveness of SJW in treating depression. Preparations of SJW are often unregulated, however, which makes the interpretation of clinical trials more complex (Taylor et al., 2018). Some preparations of SJW have gained a traditional herbal registration but needs to be noted that this is based on traditional rather than proven efficacy (Taylor et al., 2018). SJW is licensed in Germany as a treatment for depression (Taylor et al., 2018, p. 355). It can be purchased without prescription, so many health providers may be unaware that a consumer is taking this medication. Various studies have shown that SJW lowers the plasma concentration of many prescription drugs, including warfarin, hormonal contraception, digoxin and some HIV medications. According to case reports, SJW has also lowered the plasma concentrations of clozapine and other drugs (Taylor et al., 2018). Serotonin syndrome has also been reported when SJW is taken with specific SSRI medications (Taylor et al., 2018, p. 356).

SJW should not be taken with any drugs that have a predominantly serotonergic action (Taylor et al., 2018, p. 356), which can lead the health practitioner to assume that an increase in medication is required. This has the potential to lead to various problems. It is essential that practitioners ask and discuss with consumers about all CAMs taken, especially SJW.

Fish oils contain the omega-3 fatty acids, which in some animal studies have suggested a treatment for a variety of mental health problems. According to the *Maudsley Prescribing Guidelines in Psychiatry* (Taylor et al., 2018, p. 88), fish oils are no longer recommended for the treatment of residual symptoms of schizophrenia or for the transition to psychosis in young people considered at high risk.

An emerging trend is the increasing use of melatonin preparations as an aid to sleep. In Australia and Aotearoa New Zealand, this may require a prescription but is available as an over-the-counter preparation in many countries.

Over-the-counter medications

Over-the-counter (OTC) medications are often regarded as safe and effective for the treatment of minor ailments. They are drugs with a variable range of preparations that may include different concentrations of the active ingredients. This makes interchangeability unclear in clinical usage. They are effective for a large proportion of the population when directions are followed. Thousands of different preparations are available, with the most common being analgesics, antacids, laxatives, anti-diarrhoeals, cough-and-cold preparations, antihistamines, vitamins and mineral supplements (Bryant & Knights, 2014). The ubiquitous nature of OTC medications in Australia and Aotearoa New Zealand often leads to them being regarded as unremarkable and therefore omitted in history-taking by both health practitioners and consumers. Further, their use may be increased among people experiencing mental ill-health if they experience traditional health services as expensive, difficult to access or stigmatising.

The best possible medication history (BPMH) (Australian Commission on Safety and Quality in Health Care (ACSQHC), 2019) addresses this by asking about CAMs and herbal preparations. Medication reconciliation includes this aspect and routinely documents consumer usage.

Exercise and well-being strategies

The beneficial effects of lifestyle interventions have an extensive history. It has long been recognised that the ways in which we live our lives have implications for not only our physical health but also our mental health. Restful sleep, regular exercise and healthy diet are valuable to our well-being. Sleep hygiene, gentle stretching exercises such as yoga and Pilates, reductions in caffeine and alcohol consumption are readily accessible and of value.

Interventions

Practitioners and other staff working with people who have mental ill-health recognise that extending care to include physical health interventions is an important part of holistic care (Happell, Davies & Scott, 2012; RANZCP, 2015). However, several factors act as barriers to ready adoption of such interventions into day-to-day practices, including the manner in which work is organised (i.e. models of care). Happell and colleagues (2012), in a study of the adoption of exercise in mental health care, suggested that such barriers may operate at both the individual and systemic levels, and may include factors such as geography, financial and social circumstances, current state of health and stigma. They acknowledged that these factors were significant barriers to most people in changing behaviours to adopt healthier levels of exercise but pointed out that the situation of those with enduring mental ill-health, in particular, can be difficult.

As many people experiencing mental ill-health are known to have experienced trauma, it is essential that approaches to delivery of physical health care is trauma-informed; that is, healthcare practitioners are mindful that people may avoid seeking care due to past unsatisfactory encounters, which may delay or interfere with timely delivery of care.

Increasingly, mental health services are developing so-called 'wellness' or 'lifestyle' clinics to address these challenges. Such clinics take many forms in response to the needs and desires of their recipients. They may be found in in-patient, forensic and community settings, and increasingly in primary healthcare settings, and may take a particular focus on a part of the lifespan, such older people or adolescents (Lundstrom et al., 2020). Interventions for young people experiencing their first episode of psychosis are recognised as critical, as comorbid physical conditions rapidly become evident (Curtis et al., 2016). Some community mental health facilities are embracing physical health and have designated clinical staff, including peer workers, who are responsible for encouraging consumers' attention to physical health care.

A range of screening tools is being introduced in different practice settings, to deliver screening interventions where and when people with mental ill-health are encountered in health or mental health services. These tools include prompts to help practitioners recall the most important physical health tests to administer and questions to ask. Physical health care in New South Wales, for example, has a set of guidelines for practice: the Physical Health Care of Mental Health Consumers Guidelines (NSW Ministry Of Health, 2017; Te Pou o Te Whakaaro Nui, 2014). All of these documents, tools and guidelines share certain characteristics: an annual list of recommended health-screening checks, prompt questions about general lifestyle factors and a symptoms checklist. Private-sector mental health services in Australia also recognise responsibility to integrate physical health care with mental health care (Nadjidai et al., 2020).

The practitioner is well placed to be the agent for these interventions (Harris et al., 2018; Lundstrom et al., 2020). Practitioners are prepared educationally with the knowledge, skills and attitudes to perform these screening interventions and to arrange follow-up if required. In addition, practitioners work in many of the contexts in which people with mental ill-health are to be found. Ensuring that physical screening is a routine component of any intervention should be part of every practitioner's approach. Services redesigned or developed to address the physical health needs of people experiencing mental ill-health must incorporate the opinions, desires and insights of those for whom the services are being developed (Happell et al., 2019).

Figure 13.6 summarises the data collected by Morgan and colleagues (2011), described earlier in the chapter. In the year prior to data being collected in 2010, almost all participants (97.4 per cent) had undergone one or more of eight different types of assessments to monitor the status of their health (Morgan et al., 2011). For most people (85.6 per cent) this was a blood-pressure check or having waist or weight measurements taken (approximately 75 per cent). Approximately two-thirds (67.3 per cent) had had a physical examination in the previous year and 63.3 per cent had had a blood test.

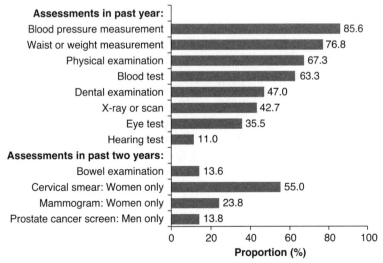

Figure 13.6 Rates of physical health assessment among people with mental illness, Australia

Source: Morgan et al. (2011, p. 44).

INTERPROFESSIONAL PERSPECTIVE

Brendan's story – peer worker

Working in the health clinic in my role as a health peer support worker was a valuable experience. It enabled me to meet many consumers at Camperdown CHC, hear their stories, and listen and respond to their health concerns. The clinic was a place I could use my lived experience of recovery to support consumers to make healthier decisions about diet and exercise. It was also a space where consumers were introduced to several community-based exercise programs, such as Camperdown Walking Group and the Healthy Lifestyles Gym and Swim group. The diet, exercise and lifestyle changes consumers made, with the support of the health clinic and peer-led community groups, have been long lasting and given many a better quality of life.

More broadly, working in the community as a health peer support worker has been rewarding, challenging and, at times, fun! My one-on-one work supporting consumers to recognise their strengths and achieve their health and life goals has been a constant source of inspiration and variety; filling my work day with trips to the gym, the park and, at one point, a music studio. Further, supporting consumers to make GP and clinical appointments, to monitor their physical and mental health, to make friends and engage with their communities, and to maintain links to community services, has been a valuable aspect of the role.

Implications for mental health practice

Mental health practitioners are in the best position to develop long-standing relationships that facilitate the use of their 'clinical lens'. This means that mental health practitioners, particularly mental health nurses and peer workers, may observe changes in physical health prior to direct measurements or routine screening. A conversation is critical, to respectfully explore consumers' physical health prior to any interventions. Direct inquiry is important but is most helpful when it employs a strengths-based approach.

Strengths-based approach

Helping consumers toward recovery has become the fundamental goal for mental health practitioners. A strengths-based approach to treating mental health problems encompasses recovery as a personal journey of gaining an increasingly meaningful life despite the presence of mental ill-health. Recovery does not mean that a consumer will no longer experience symptoms, or will no longer have struggles or require medications, nor does it mean they will be completely independent in meeting all their needs.

The strengths-based approach works on six principles:

1   All people have the capacity to recover, reclaim and transform their lives.
2   Focus on strengths rather than deficits.
3   The relationship between practitioner and consumer is primary and essential.
4   The person receiving services is the director of the helping relationship.
5   The preferred setting is the community.
6   The community has many naturally occurring resources.

INTERPROFESSIONAL PERSPECTIVE

Although the need is well established, achieving interprofessional services for people with mental and physical ill-health remains patchy. People experiencing mental ill-health desire for physical health but may be let down by the dislocation of health services. This can extend to the reticence of health professionals to expand their practices sufficiently to meet the needs of this group of people. Such reticence can include problems related to geographic co-location and the confidence of health practitioners to recognise conditions indicating the consumers' need for specialist services (Harris et al., 2018). Building on the capacity of peer workers and carers may improve health outcomes, but also signals a need to support this workforce to deliver this care. Health promotion is the critical lens that will improve outcomes, leveraging the advantages of the therapeutic alliance.

Emerging physical health challenges

It is clear that the global profile of physical health is changing. The internationalisation of economies worldwide has seen infectious diseases take on pandemic proportions in ways rarely witnessed before. Climate change, as seen in the increasing prevalence and severity of bush-fire activity, is another emerging challenge to physical health. All these changes have mental health dimensions for populations, given the disruption to norms and predictability. For people with pre-existing mental health problems, the challenges may have unique features.

SUMMARY

This chapter has presented stories, information and activities designed to deepen your understanding of:

- The poor physical health experiences of people diagnosed with enduring mental ill-health, and their premature deaths. Physical effects of treatments were explored, as was the clear association of poor physical health with the experience of enduring mental ill-health. Practitioners must include physical health care as a routine component of all care.
- A comprehensive range of commonly encountered physical health problems and their interactions. The chapter focused on the way in which discrete physical health problems manifest and interact with a range of other factors, including mental health issues and social determinants of health.
- Current strategies and preventative approaches that demonstrate challenges to current and future practice. Metabolic monitoring is a clear example of this approach.
- The application of human rights to physical health care, which must inform healthcare provision.
- The contemporary model for healthcare delivery, which is central to mental health services. The need for strengths-based approaches demands collaboration to ensure the attainment of consumer goals and recovery objectives.

CRITICAL THINKING/LEARNING ACTIVITIES

1   Evidence of effective preventative factors for the metabolic syndrome are not clear, and people who are being treated with some common anti-psychotic medications develop the precursors (weight gain, insulin resistance). What approach could be used to promote physical health?

2   Sexuality is an aspect of health that is affected by the experience of mental ill-health. Nominate some of the reasons sexuality may be negatively affected, and some possible remedies.

3   Many psychotropic medications affect the swallowing reflex, suggesting orthodox treatment recommendations such as dietary modification. People with enduring mental ill-health may face an indefinite future with texture-modified diets. Discuss the consequences for consumers and possible responses to support attaining the best possible quality of life.

4   List the factors required to maintain good oral health across the lifespan. What factors impede this for people who experience mental ill-health?

5   People who experience enduring mental ill-health continue to smoke tobacco at higher rates than the general population. What strategies may support people to revise this smoking behaviour and work toward reducing and eliminating smoking?

LEARNING EXTENSION

Design a series of posters addressing the physical health needs of people experiencing mental ill-health. Discuss which services should be targeted and which disciplines this could involve. For example, primary healthcare staff might design posters with GPs as their target audience. Posters may be designed to attract the attention of emergency department staff, to encourage comprehensive health assessment of people presenting with mental health problems, so that physical health is incorporated. Brochures could be produced for consumers of mental health services and their carers about the risks of metabolic syndrome.

FURTHER READING

Australian Commission on Safety and Quality in Health Care. (n.d.). Medical reconciliation – resources for obtaining a best possible medication history. Retrieved from https://www.safetyandquality.gov.au/medical-reconciliation-resources-obtaining-best-possible-medication-history

The Australian Safety and Quality Council provides information about how to take a best possible medication history (BPMH), including an online learning module and videos. Explore this resource and especially consider how to take a history that includes OTC medications and CAMs.

Harris, B., Duggan, M., Batterham, P., Bartlem, K., Clinton-Mcharg, T., Dunbar, J., Fehily, C., Lawrence, D., Morgan, M. & Rosenbaum, S. (2018). *Australia's Mental and Physical Health Tracker*. Melbourne: Australian Health Policy Collaboration. Retrieved from https://www.vu.edu.au/sites/default/files/australias-mental-and-physical-health-tracker-background-paper.pdf

This resource discusses the disparities in physical health that are evident for those experiencing mental ill-health. It suggests some strategies for improvement, including a greater integration of services, improvement in staff attitudes and the separation of mental and physical health services.

Health Education and Training, NSW Government. (n.d.). Positive Cardiometabolic Health.
Retrieved from https://www.heti.nsw.gov.au/resources-and-links/resource-library/
positive-cardiometabolic-health

This algorithm (2011 version) has been adopted for use in New South Wales Health training and is described as ' … provid(ing) trainees and clinicians an opportunity to increase knowledge and skills in the assessment and management of cardiometabolic syndrome and related physical health issues in patients with severe mental illness. Included is a practical algorithm for screening and intervention.'

Mental Health Commission. (2012). *Blueprint II: Improving mental health and wellbeing for all New Zealanders. How things need to be*. Wellington: Mental Health Commission.
Retrieved from https://www.wdhb.org.nz/assets/Uploads/Documents/2f2bc04cb3/
blueprint-ii-how-things-need-to-be.pdf

This document revises the initial Blueprint published in 1998. It reflects the changes since that time and provides a pathway for the next decade for mental health and well-being.

Mental Health Commission of NSW. (2016). *Physical Health and Mental Wellbeing: Evidence guide*. Sydney: Mental Health Commission of NSW. Retrieved from https://www
.nswmentalhealthcommission.com.au/evidence/physical-health-and-mental-wellbeing-
evidence-guide

An evidence guide for physical health and mental well-being. It is clear that a comprehensive and collaborative approach to service reform is needed to improve the physical health of mental health consumers. This guide provides an outline and evidence base for such reform.

National Centre of Mental Health Research Information and Workforce Development. (2014).
The physical health of people with a serious mental illness and/or addiction: An evidence review. Auckland: Te Pou o Te Whakaaro Nui. Retrieved from https://www.tepou.co.nz/
uploads/files/resources/the-physical-health-of-people-with-a-serious-mental-illness-andor-
addiction-an-evidence-review_2021-05-24-233432.pdf

An evidence review of physical health of people with enduring mental ill-health and/or addiction. This review pragmatically reviews evidence-seeking ways to respond to the poorer physical health of those who experience enduring mental ill-health and/or addiction.

National Health and Medical Research Council (NHMRC). (2013). *Australian Dietary Guidelines*.
Canberra: Australian Government. Retrieved from https://www.nhmrc.gov.au/adg

These guidelines were developed by the National Health and Medical Research Council from contemporary best evidence. It is the most authoritative source in this field and should be the basis of understanding, advice and evaluations made of dietary habits.

REFERENCES

Alawami, M., Wasywich, C., Cicovic, A. & Kenedi, C. (2014). A systematic review of clozapine induced cardiomyopathy. *International Journal of Cardiology*, *176*(2): 315–20.

Aldridge, K. J. & Taylor, N. F. (2012). Dysphagia is a common and serious problem for adults with mental illness: a systematic review. *Dysphagia*, *27*(1): 124–37.

Allen, D. E., de Nesnera, A. & Robinson, D. A. (2012). Psychiatric patients are at increased risk of falling and choking. *Journal of the American Psychiatric Nurses Association*, *18*(2): 91–5.

Arnaiz, A., Zumárraga, M., Díez-Altuna, I., Uriarte, J. J., Moro, J. & Pérez-Ansorena, M. A. (2011). Oral health and the symptoms of schizophrenia. *Psychiatry Research*, *188*(1): 24–8.

Australian Bureau of Statistics (ABS). (2008). *National Survey of Mental Health and Wellbeing. Summary of results 2007*. ABS Cat No 4326 0. Canberra: ABS. Retrieved from http://www.abs.gov.au/AUSSTATS

———— (2012). Causes of Death, Australia, 2010, 20 March 2012 edn. Canberra: ABS. Retrieved from http://www.abs.gov.au/AUSSTATS/abs@.nsf/DetailsPage/3303.02010?OpenDocument

Australian Commission on Safety and Quality in Health Care (ACSQHC). (2019). *Medical Reconciliation – resources for obtaining a best possible medication history*. Sydney: ACSQHC. Retrieved from https://www.safetyandquality.gov.au/medical-reconciliation-resources-obtaining-best-possible-medication-history

Australian Institute for Health and Welfare (AIHW). (2020a). *Indigenous Australians*. Canberra: AIHW. Retrieved from https://www.aihw.gov.au/reports-data/population-groups/indigenous-australians/overview

———— (2020b). *Australia's Health 2020: In brief*. Canberra: AIHW.

———— (2020c). *Oral Health and Dental Care in Australia*. Canberra: AIHW. Retrieved from https://www.aihw.gov.au/reports/dental-oral-health/oral-health-and-dental-care-in-australia/contents/introduction

Bartlett, P., Mantovani, N., Cratsley, K., Dillon, C. & Eastman, N. 2010, 'You may kiss the bride, but you may not open your mouth when you do so': Policies concerning sex, marriage and relationships in English forensic psychiatric facilities. *Liverpool Law Review*, *31*(2): 155–76.

Bauer-Staeb, C. B., Jörgensen, L., Lewis, G., Dalman, C., Osborn, D. P. J. & Hayes, J. F. (2017). Prevalence and risk factors for HIV, hepatitis B, and hepatitis C in people with severe mental illness: a total population study of Sweden. *Lancet Psychiatry*, *4*(9): 685–93.

Bittoun, R., Barone, M., Mendelsohn, C. P., Elcombe, E. L. & Glozier, N. (2015). Promoting positive attitudes of tobacco dependent mental health patients towards NRT supported harm reduction and smoking cessation. *Australian & New Zealand Journal of Psychiatry*, *48*(10): 954–6.

Blythe, J. & White, J. (2012). Role of the mental health nurse towards physical health care in serious mental illness: An integrative review of 10 years of UK literature. *International Journal of Mental Health Nursing*, *21*(3): 193–201.

Brown, A. P. & Paxton, S. J. (2008). STIs and blood borne viruses: Risk factors for individuals with mental illness. *Australian Journal of General Practice*, *37*(7): 531.

Bryant, B. & Knights, K. (2014). *Pharmacology for Health Professionals ebook*. Chatswood, NSW: Elsevier Health Sciences.

Busche, B. & Holt, R. (2004). Prevalence of diabetes and impaired glucose tolerance in patients with schizophrenia. *British Journal of Psychiatry*, *184*(Suppl.): s67–s71.

Corbett, C., Armstrong, M. J., Parker, R., Webb, K. & Neuberger, J. M. (2013). Mental health disorders and solid-organ transplant recipients. *Transplantation*, *96*(7): 593–600.

Corcoran, E. & Walsh, D. (2003). Obstructive asphyxia: A cause of excess mortality in psychiatric patients. *Irish journal of Psychological Medicine*, *20*(3): 88–90.

Corr, M. (2012). HIV and Liaison Psychiatry. In E. Guthrie, S. Roa & M. Temple (eds), *Seminars in Liaison Psychiatry*, 2nd edn (pp. 330–44). London: Royal College of Psychiatrists.

Cunningham, R., Peterson, D., Sarfati, D., Stanley, J. & Collings, S. (2014). Premature mortality in adults using New Zealand psychiatric services. *The New Zealand Medical Journal*, *127*(1394): 31–41.

Curtis, J., Watkins, A., Rosenbaum, S., Teasdale, S., Kalucy, M., Samaras, K. & Ward, P. B. (2016). Evaluating an individualized lifestyle and life skills intervention to prevent antipsychotic-induced weight gain in first-episode psychosis. *Early Intervention in Psychiatry*, *10*(3): 267–76.

Davis, L. E., Bogner, E., Coburn, N. G., Hanna, T. P., Kurdyak, P., Groome, P. A. & Mahar, A. L. (2020). Stage at diagnosis and survival in patients with cancer and a pre-existing mental illness: a meta-analysis. *Journal of Epidemiology and Community Health*, *74*(1): 84–94.

De Hert, M., Correll, C. U., Bobes, J., Cetkovich-Bakmas, M., Cohen, D., Asai, I., Detraux, J., Gautam, S., Möller, H.-J., Ndetei, D. M., Newcomer, J. W., Uwakwe, R. & Leucht, S. (2011). Physical illness in patients with severe mental disorders. I. Prevalence, impact of medications and disparities in health care. *World Psychiatry*, *10*(1): 52–77.

Deng, C., Weston-Green, K. & Huang, X.-F. (2010). The role of histaminergic H1 and H3 receptors in food intake: a mechanism for atypical antipsychotic-induced weight gain? *Progress in Neuro-Psychopharmacology & Biological Psychiatry*, *34*(1): 1–4.

Department of Health. (2011). *No Health without Mental Health*. London: Department of Health.

Dyer, J. G. & McGuinness, T. M. (2008). Reducing HIV risk among people with serious mental illness. *Journal of Psychosocial Nursing and Mental Health Services*, *46*(4): 26–34.

Firth, J., Siddiqi, N., Koyanagi, A., Siskind, D., Rosenbaum, S., Galletly, C. … Stubbs, B. (2019). The Lancet Psychiatry Commission: A blueprint for protecting physical health in people with mental illness. *The Lancet Psychiatry*, *6*(8): 675–712.

Friedrich, M. (2017). Global obesity epidemic worsening. *JAMA*, *318*(7): 603.

Gierisch, J. M., Nieuwsma, J. A., Bradford, D. W., Wilder, C. M., Mann-Wrobel, M. C., McBroom, A. J., Hasselblad, V. & Williams, J. W. (2014). Pharmacologic and behavioral interventions to improve cardiovascular risk factors in adults with serious mental illness: A systematic review and meta-analysis. *Journal of Clinical Psychiatry*, *75*(5): e424–e40.

Gierisch, J. M., Nieuwsma, J. A., Bradford, D. W., Wilder, C. M., Mann-Wrobel, M. C., McBroom, A. J., Wing, L., Musty, M. D., Chobot, M .M. & Hasselblad, V. (2013). *Interventions to Improve Cardiovascular Risk Factors in People with Serious Mental illness*. Rockville, MD: Agency for Healthcare Research and Quality.

Hammoudeh, S. I., Al Lawati, H., Ghuloum, S., Iram, H., Yehya, A., Becetti, I., Al-Fakhri, N., Ghabrash, H., Shehata, M. & Ajmal, N. (2020). Risk factors of metabolic syndrome among patients receiving antipsychotics: A retrospective study. *Community Mental Health Journal*, *56*(4): 760–70.

Happell, B., Davies, C. & Scott, D. (2012). Health behaviour interventions to improve physical health in individuals diagnosed with a mental illness: A systematic review. *International Journal of Mental Health Nursing*, *21*(3): 236–47.

Happell, B., Platania-Phung, C., Bocking, J., Ewart, S. B., Scholz, B. & Stanton, R. (2019). Consumers at the centre: interprofessional solutions for meeting mental health consumers' physical health needs. *Journal of Interprofessional Care*, *33*(2): 226–34.

Harris, B., Duggan, M., Batterham, P., Bartlem, K., Clinton-Mcharg, T., Dunbar, J., Fehily, C., Lawrence, D., Morgan, M. & Rosenbaum, S. (2018). *Australia's Mental and Physical Health Tracker: Background Paper*. Australian Health Policy Collaboration issues paper No 2018-2. Melbourne: Australian Health Policy Collaboration.

Harrison-Woolrych, M., Skegg, K., Ashton, J., Herbison, P. & Skegg, D. C. (2011). Nocturnal enuresis in patients taking clozapine, risperidone, olanzapine and quetiapine: comparative cohort study. *The British Journal of Psychiatry*, *199*(2): 140–4.

Heart Foundation. (n.d.). What's your BMI? (Website). Retrieved from https://www.heartfoundation.org.au/bmi-calculator

Holt, R. I. G. & Peveler, R. C. (2005). Association between antipsychotic drugs and diabetes. *Diabetes, Obesity and Metabolism*, *8*(2): 125–35.

Hughes, E., Bassi, S., Gilbody, S., Bland, M. & Martin, F. (2016). Prevalence of HIV, hepatitis B, and hepatitis C in people with severe mental illness: A systematic review and meta-analysis. *Lancet Psychiatry*, *3*(1): 40–8.

Hughes, E., Edmondson, A. J., Onyekwe, I., Quinn, C. & Nolan, F. (2018). Identifying and addressing sexual health in serious mental illness: Views of mental health staff working in two National Health Service organizations in England. *International Journal of Mental Health Nursing*, *27*(3): 966–74.

Iglay, K., Santorelli, M. L., Hirshfield, K. M., Williams, J. M., Rhoads, G. G., Lin, Y. & Demissie, K. (2017). Diagnosis and treatment delays among elderly breast cancer patients with pre-existing mental illness. *Breast Cancer Research and Treatment*, *166*(1): 267–75.

International Diabetes Federation (IDF). (2006, updated 2020). *The IDF Consensus Worldwide Definition of the Metabolic Syndrome*. Belgium: International Diabetes Federation.

Jacka, F. N., O'Neil, A., Opie, R., Itsiopoulos, C., Cotton, S., Mohebbi, M., Castle, D., Dash, S., Mihalopoulos, C., Chatterton, M. L., Brazionis, L., Dean, O. M., Hodge, A. M. & Berk, M. (2017). A randomised controlled trial of dietary improvement for adults with major depression (the 'SMILES' trial). *BMC Medicine*, 15(1): 23.

John, A. P., Koloth, R., Dragovic, M. & Lim, S. C. (2009). Prevalence of metabolic syndrome among Australians with severe mental illness. *Medical Journal of Australia, 190*(4): 176–9.

Jones, S., Howard, L. & Thornicroft, G. (2008). 'Diagnostic overshadowing': Worse physical health care for people with mental illness. *Acta Psychiatrica Scandinavica, 118*(3): 169–71

Jorm, A. F., Bourchier, S. J., Cvetkovski, S. & Stewart, G. (2012). Systematic review: Mental health of Indigenous Australians: A review of findings from community surveys. *Medical Journal of Australia, 196*(2): 118–23.

Khokhar, W. A., Clifton, A., Jones, H. & Tosh, G. (2011). Oral health advice for people with serious mental illness. *Cochrane Database of Systematic Reviews*, (11).

Kirkby Institute. (2018). *HIV in Australia: Annual surveillance short report 2018*. Sydney: Kirkby Institute, UNSW Sydney.

Kishimoto, T., Hagi, K., Nitta, M., Kane, J. M. & Correll, C. U. (2019). Long-term effectiveness of oral second-generation antipsychotics in patients with schizophrenia and related disorders: A systematic review and meta-analysis of direct head-to-head comparisons. *World Psychiatry, 18*(2): 208–24.

Koran, D. (2004). Diabetes mellitus and schizophrenia: historical perspective. *British Journal of Psychiatry, 184*(Suppl 47): s64–s66.

Kulkarni, D. P., Kamath, V. D. & Stewart, J. T. (2017). Swallowing disorders in schizophrenia. *Dysphagia, 32*(4): 467–71.

Lambert, T. J. (2009). Successful implementation of cardiometabolic monitoring of patients treated with antipsychotics. *The Medical Journal of Australia, 191*(9): 516–8.

Lambert, T. J. & Chapman, L. H. (2004). Diabetes, psychotic disorders and antipsychotic therapy: A consensus statement. *The Medical Journal of Australia, 181*(10): 544–8.

Lambert, T. J. & Newcomer, J. W. (2009). Are the cardiometabolic complications of schizophrenia still neglected? Barriers to care. *Medical Journal of Australia, 190*(S4): S39–S42.

Lambert, T. J., Reavley, N. J., Jorm, A. F. & Oakley Browne, M. A. (2017). Royal Australian and New Zealand College of Psychiatrists expert consensus statement for the treatment, management and monitoring of the physical health of people with an enduring psychotic illness. *Australian & New Zealand Journal of Psychiatry, 51*(4): 322–37.

Lockett, H., Jury, A., Tuason, C., Lai, J. & Fergusson, D. (2018). Comorbidities between mental and physical health problems: An analysis of the New Zealand Health Survey data. *New Zealand Journal of Psychology, 47*(3): 5–11.

Lopuszanska, U. J., Skorzynska-Dziduszko, K., Lupa-Zatwarnicka, K. & Makara-Studzinska, M. (2014). Mental illness and metabolic syndrome-a literature review. *Annals of Agricultural and Environmental Medicine, 21*(4).

Lu, Q. F., Ma, Q., Rithwan, S. M. S., Ng, H. C., Lee, S. L., Lee, K. M., Umarani, K. & Xie, H. (2017). Risk factors and nursing strategies to manage choking in adults with mental illness: a systematic review protocol. *JBI Database of Systematic Reviews and Implementation Reports, 15*(8): 1998–2003.

Lundstrom, S., Jormfeldt, H., Hedman Ahlstrom, B. & Skarsater, I. (2020). Mental health nurses' experience of physical health care and health promotion initiatives for people with severe mental illness. *International Journal of Mental Health Nursing, 29*(2): 244–53.

McEvoy, J., Lieberman, J., Perkins, D., Hamer, R., Gu, H., Lazarus, A., Sweitzer, D., Olexy, C., Weiden, P. & Strakowski, S. (2007). Efficacy and tolerability of olanzapine, quetiapine, and risperidone in the treatment of early psychosis: A randomized, double-blind 52-week comparison. *American journal of Psychiatry, 164*(7): 1050–60.

McMannus, M. (2001). Dysphagia in psychiatric patients. *Journal of Psychosocial Nursing, 39*(2): 24–30.

Mental Health Smoking Partnership. (2020). *Use of Electronic Cigarettes by People with Mental Health Problems: A guide for mental health professionals*. UK: Mental Health Smoking Partnership. Retrieved from https://smokefreeaction.org.uk

Ministry of Health. (2018). *Eating and Activity Guidelines: Guideline statements for New Zealand Adults*. Retrieved from https://www.health.govt.nz/our-work/eating-and-activity-guidelines

Mitchell, A. J., Vancampfort, D., Sweers, K., van Winkel, R., Yu, W. & De Hert, M. (2013). Prevalence of metabolic syndrome and metabolic abnormalities in schizophrenia and related disorders – a systematic review and meta-analysis. *Schizophrenia Bulletin, 39*(2): 306–18.

Moodie, R., Stuckler, D., Monteiro, C., Sheron, N., Neal, B., Thamarangsi, T., Lincoln, P. & Casswell, S. (2013). Profits and pandemics: prevention of harmful effects of tobacco, alcohol, and ultra-processed food and drink industries. *The Lancet, 381*(9867): 670–9.

Morgan, V. A., Waterreus, A., Jablensky, A., Mackinnon, A., McGrath, J. J., Carr, V., Bush, R., Castle, D., Cohen, M., Harvey, C., Galletly, C., Stain, H. J., Neil, A., McGorry, P., Hocking, B., Shah, S. & Saw, S. (2011). *People Living with Psychotic Illness 2010. Report on the second Australian national survey.* Canberra: Australian Government.

Movig, K., Leufkens, H., Belitser, S., Lenderink, A. & Egberts, A. (2002). Selective serotonin reuptake inhibitor-induced urinary incontinence. *Pharmacoepidemiology and Drug Safety, 11*(4): 271–9.

Nadjidai, S. E., Kusljic, S., Dowling, N. L., Magennis, J., Stokes, L., Ng, C. H. & Daniel, C. (2020). Physical comorbidities in private psychiatric inpatients: Prevalence and its association with quality of life and functional impairment. *International Journal of Mental Health Nursing, 29*(6): 1253–61.

Narasimhan, M. & Raynor, J. (2010). Evidence-based perspective on metabolic syndrome and use of antipsychotics. *Drug Benefit Trends, 22*: 77–88.

National Health and Medical Research Council (NHMRC). (2013). *Australian Dietary Guidelines (2013).* Canberra: Australian Government. Retrieved from http://www.nhmrc.gov.au/guidelines/publications/n55.

Naylor, C., Das, P., Ross, S., Honeyman, M., Thompson, J. & Gilburt, H. (2016) *Bringing Together Physical and Mental Health: A new frontier for integrated care.* London: King's Fund.

Newcomer, J. W. (2007). Metabolic syndrome and mental illness. *American Journal of Managed Care, 13*: S170–S177.

NIH National Cancer Institute. (2021). Complementary and alternative medicine (Website). Retrieved from https://www.cancer.gov/about-cancer/treatment/cam

Nordentoft, M., Wahlbeck, K., Hällgren, J., Westman, J., Ösby, U., Alinaghizadeh, H., Gissler, M. & Laursen, T. M. (2013). Excess mortality, causes of death and life expectancy in 270,770 patients with recent onset of mental disorders in Denmark, Finland and Sweden. *PloS one, 8*(1): e55176.

NSW Ministry of Health. (2017). *Physical Health Care of Mental Health Consumers Guidelines.* North Sydney: NSW Ministry of Health. Retrieved from https://www1.health.nsw.gov.au/pds/ActivePDSDocuments/GL2017_019.pdf

Opie, R. S., O'Neil, A., Jacka, F. N., Pizzinga, J. & Itsiopoulos, C. (2018). A modified Mediterranean dietary intervention for adults with major depression: Dietary protocol and feasibility data from the SMILES trial. *Nutritional Neuroscience, 21*(7): 487–501.

Pacitti, R. & Thornicroft, G. (2009). Sex, relationships and mental health. *Mental Health and Social Inclusion, 13*(1): 27.

Parker, R. (2010). Australia's Aboriginal population and mental health. *The Journal of Nervous and Mental Disease, 198*(1): 3–7.

Persson, K., Axtelius, B., Söderfeldt, B. & Östman, M. (2009). Monitoring oral health and dental attendance in an outpatient psychiatric population. *Journal of Psychiatric and Mental Health Nursing, 16*(3): 263–71.

Prochaska, J. J. (2010). Failure to treat tobacco use in mental health and addiction treatment settings: A form of harm reduction? *Drug and Alcohol Dependence, 110*(3): 177–82.

Prochaska, J. J., Hall, S. E., Delucchi, K. & Hall, S. M. (2014). Efficacy of initiating tobacco dependence treatment in inpatient psychiatry: A randomized controlled trial. *American Journal of Public Health, 104*(8): 1557–65.

Public Health England (2018). *Severe Mental Illness (SMI) and Physical Health Inequalities: Briefing.* UK: Public Health England. Retrieved from https://www.gov.uk/government/publications/severe-mental-illness-smi-physical-health-inequalities/severe-mental-illness-and-physical-health-inequalities-briefing#fn

Quinn, C. & Happell, B. (2012). Getting BETTER: Breaking the ice and warming to the inclusion of sexuality in mental health nursing care. *International Journal of Mental Health Nursing, 21*(2): 154–62.

Quinn, C., Happell, B. & Browne, G. (2011). Talking or avoiding? Mental health nurses' views about discussing sexual health with consumer. *International Journal of Mental Health Nursing*, *20*: 21–8.

Raedler, T. J. (2010). Cardiovascular aspects of antipsychotics. *Current Opinion in Psychiatry*, *23*(6): 574–81.

Reiss, S., Levitan, G. & Szyszko, J. (1982). Emotional disturbance and mental retardation: Diagnostic overshadowing. *American Journal of Mental Deficiency*, *86*: 567–74.

Richardson, A., Richard, L., Gunter, K., Cunningham, R., Hamer, H., Lockett, H., Wyeth, E., Stokes, T., Burke, M., Green, M., Cox, A. & Derrett, S. (2020). A systematic scoping review of interventions to integrate physical and mental healthcare for people with serious mental illness and substance use disorders. *Journal of Psychiatric Research*, *128*: 52–67.

Robson, D. & Gray, R. (2007). Serious mental illness and physical health problems: A discussion paper. *International Journal of Nursing Studies*, *44*(3): 457–66.

Rødevand, L., Steen, N., Elvsåshagen, T., Quintana, D., Reponen, E., Mørch, R., Lunding, S., Vedal, T., Dieset, I. & Melle, I. (2019). Cardiovascular risk remains high in schizophrenia with modest improvements in bipolar disorder during past decade. *Acta Psychiatrica Scandinavica*, *139*(4): 348–60.

Ronaldson, A., Elton, L., Jayakumar, S., Jieman, A., Halvorsrud, K. & Bhui, K. (2020). Severe mental illness and health service utilisation for nonpsychiatric medical disorders: A systematic review and meta-analysis. *PLoS Medicine*, *17*(9): e1003284.

Royal Australian & New Zealand College of Psychiatrists (RANZCP). (2015), *Keeping Body and Mind Together. Improving the physical health and life expectancy of people with serious mental illness*. Melbourne and Wellington: RANZCP.

Ruschena, D., Mullen, P. E., Palmer, S., Burgess, P., Cordner, S. M., Drummer, O. H., Wallace, C. & Barry-Walsh, J. (2003). Choking deaths: The role of antipsychotic medication. *The British Journal of Psychiatry*, *183*(5): 446–50.

Sassi, F., Devaux, M., Cecchini, M. & Rusticelli, E. (2009). *The Obesity Epidemic: Analysis of past and projected future trends in selected OECD countries*. Paris: OECD Publishing.

Scott, E. M., Carpenter, J. S., Iorfino, F., Cross, S. P., Hermens, D. F., Gehue, J., Wilson, C., White, D., Naismith, S. L. & Guastella, A. J. (2019). What is the prevalence, and what are the clinical correlates, of insulin resistance in young people presenting for mental health care? A cross-sectional study. *BMJ Open*, *9*(5): e025674.

Shaw, J. E., Sicree, R. A. & Zimmet, P. Z. (2010). Global estimates of the prevalence of diabetes for 2010 and 2030. *Diabetes Research and Clinical Practice*, *87*(1): 4–14.

Shefer, G., Henderson, C., Howard, L. M., Murray, J. & Thornicroft, G. (2014). Diagnostic overshadowing and other challenges involved in the diagnostic process of patients with mental illness who present in emergency departments with physical symptoms–a qualitative study. *PLoS One*, *9*(11): e111682.

Simonelli-Muñoz, A. J., Fortea, M. I., Salorio, P., Gallego-Gomez, J. I., Sánchez-Bautista, S. & Balanza, S. (2012). Dietary habits of patients with schizophrenia: A self-reported questionnaire survey. *International Journal of Mental Health Nursing*, *21*(3): 220–8.

Snaith, N., Rasmussen, P., Schultz, T. & Proeve, M. (2020). The practicability and relevance of developing a yoga intervention for mental health consumers: A qualitative study. *International Journal of Mental Health Nursing*, *29*(4): 622–31.

Solmi, M., Firth, J., Miola, A., Fornaro, M., Frison, E., Fusar-Poli, P., Dragioti, E., Shin, J. I., Carvalho, A. F. & Stubbs, B. (2020). Disparities in cancer screening in people with mental illness across the world versus the general population: prevalence and comparative meta-analysis including 4 717 839 people. *The Lancet Psychiatry*, *7*(1): 52–63.

Stanton, R., Franck, C., Reaburn, P. & Happell, B. (2015). A pilot study of the views of general practitioners regarding exercise for the treatment of depression. *Perspectives in Psychiatric Care*, *51*: 253–9.

Stanton, R., Raeburn, P. & Happell, B. (2015). Barriers to exercise prescription and participation in people with mental illness: the perspectives of nurses working in mental health. *Journal of Psychiatric & Mental Health Nursing*, *22*: 440–8.

Stubbs, B., Vancampfort, D., De Hert, M. & Mitchell, A. (2015). The prevalence and predictors of type two diabetes mellitus in people with schizophrenia: a systematic review and comparative meta-analysis. *Acta Psychiatrica Scandinavica*, *132*(2): 144–57.

Taipale, H., Mittendorfer-Rutz, E., Alexanderson, K., Majak, M., Mehtälä, J., Hoti, F., Jedenius, E., Enkusson, D., Leval, A. & Sermon, J. (2018). Antipsychotics and mortality in a nationwide cohort of 29,823 patients with schizophrenia. *Schizophrenia Research*, *197*: 274–80.

Taylor, D. M., Barnes, T. R .E. & Young, A. H. (2018). *The Maudsley Prescribing Guidelines in Psychiatry*, 13th edn. Wiley Blackwell.

Te Pou o Te Whakaaro Nui. (2014). *The Physical Health of People with a Serious Mental Illness and/ or Addiction. An evidence review*. Auckland: The National Centre of Mental Health Research, Information and Workforce Development.

Teasdale, S. B., Ward, P. B., Samaras, K., Firth, J., Stubbs, B., Tripodi, E. & Burrows, T. L. (2019). Dietary intake of people with severe mental illness: Systematic review and meta-analysis. *The British Journal of Psychiatry*, *214*(5): 251–9.

Tidey, J. W., Colby, S. M., Denlinger-Apte, R. L., Goodwin, C., Cioe, P. A., Cassidy, R. N., Swift, R. M., Lindgren, B. R., Rubin, N. & Murphy, S. E. (2019). Effects of 6-week use of very low nicotine content cigarettes in smokers with serious mental illness. *Nicotine and Tobacco Research*, 21(Suppl.1): S38–S45.

Tiihonen, J., Lönnqvist, J., Wahlbeck, K., Klaukka, T., Niskanen, L., Tanskanen, A. & Haukka, J. (2009). 11-year follow-up of mortality in patients with schizophrenia: A population-based cohort study (FIN11 study). *The Lancet*, *374*(9690): 620–7.

Tsakiris, P., Oelke, M. & Michel, M. (2008). Drug induced urinary incontinence. *Drugs and Aging*, *25*(7): 541–9.

United Nations Office of the High Commissioner for Human Rights. (2007). *Convention on the Rights of Persons with Disabilities*. Geneva: Committee on the Rights of People with Disabilities. Retrieved from http://www.ohchr.org/EN/HRBodies/CRPD/Pages/ConventionRightsPersonsWithDisabilities.aspx

Van Winkel, R., De Hert, M., Van Eyck, D., Hanssens, L., Wampers, M., Scheen, A. & Peuskens, J. (2008). Prevalence of diabetes and the metabolic syndrome in a sample of patients with bipolar disorder. *Bipolar Disorders*, *10*(2): 342–8.

Vancampfort, D., Firth, J., Correll, C. U., Solmi, M., Siskind, D., De Hert, M., Carney, R., Koyanagi, A., Carvalho, A. F. & Gaughran, F. (2019). The impact of pharmacological and non-pharmacological interventions to improve physical health outcomes in people with schizophrenia: A meta-review of meta-analyses of randomized controlled trials. *World Psychiatry*, *18*(1): 53–66.

Vancampfort, D., Firth, J., Schuch, F. B., Rosenbaum, S., Mugisha, J., Hallgren, M., Probst, M., Ward, P. B., Gaughran, F. & De Hert, M. (2017). Sedentary behavior and physical activity levels in people with schizophrenia, bipolar disorder and major depressive disorder: A global systematic review and meta-analysis. *World Psychiatry*, *16*(3): 308–15.

Vancampfort, D., Knapen, J., Probst, M., Scheewe, T., Remans, S. & De Hert, M. (2012). A systematic review of correlates of physical activity in patients with schizophrenia. *Acta Psychiatrica Scandinavica*, *125*(5): 352–62.

Vos, T., Barker, B., Begg, S., Stanley, L. & Lopez, A. D. (2009). Burden of disease and injury in Aboriginal and Torres Strait Islander peoples: The Indigenous health gap. *International Journal of Epidemiology*, *38*(2): 470–7.

Wagner, E., McMahon, L., Falkai, P., Hasan, A. & Siskind, D. (2020). Impact of smoking behavior on clozapine blood levels – a systematic review and meta-analysis. *Acta Psychiatrica Scandinavica*, *142*(6): 456–66.

Ward, M. C., White, D. T. & Druss, B. G. (2015). A meta-review of lifestyle interventions for cardiovascular risk factors in the general medical population: Lessons for individuals with serious mental illness. *The Journal of Clinical Psychiatry*, *76*(4): 1478–86.

Warner, J. (2004). Risk of choking in mental illness. *The Lancet*, *363*(9410): 674.

Wheeler, A., McKenna, B. & Madell, D. (2013). Stereotypes do not always apply: Findings from a survey of the health behaviours of mental health consumers compared with the general population in New Zealand. *The New Zealand Medical Journal*, *126*(1385): 35–46.

——— (2014). Access to general health care services by a New Zealand population with serious mental illness. *Journal of Primary Health Care*, *6*(1): 7–16.

World Federation for Mental Health. (2010). *Mental health and chronic physical illnesses. The need for continued and integrated care*. Retrieved from https://www.encontrarse.pt/wp-content/uploads/2016/12/docs_wmfh2010.pdf

World Health Organization (WHO). (2006). *Sexual and Reproductive Health – Laying the foundation for a more just world through research and action: Biennial report 2004–2005*. Geneva: WHO.

———— (2014). Premature death among people with severe mental disorders (Information sheet). Geneva: WHO. Retrieved from http://www.who.int/mental_health/management/info_sheet .pdf

———— (2015). *Brief sexuality-related communication: Recommendations for a public health approach*. Geneva: WHO.

Zuko, M., Fazlić, A., Sokić Begović, E., Halvadžić, E. & Halilović Šuškić, S. (2020). Incidence of unrecognized myocardial infraction in patients with schizophrenia. *Cardiologia Croatica*, *15*(1–2): 9–15.

Mental health of people of immigrant and refugee backgrounds

14

Nicholas Procter, Amy Baker, Mary Anne Kenny,
Davi Macedo and Monika Ferguson

LEARNING OBJECTIVES

At the completion of this chapter, you should be able to:

1 Define the terms refugee, immigrant and asylum seeker, and explain visa
   categories for temporary protection.
2 Describe the mental health problems, needs and risk and protective factors
   for mental health conditions among people from immigrant and refugee
   backgrounds.
3 Identify and discuss the implications of cultural explanatory models in
   mental health.
4 Identify and discuss the implications of mental illness for people of refugee
   and asylum seeker backgrounds as they interact with mainstream health and
   mental health services.
5 Demonstrate awareness of trauma-informed practice when engaging
   with consumers and carers from immigrant, asylum seeker and refugee
   backgrounds, including enablers and barriers to meaningful engagement in
   mental health.
6 Reflect on the experience of older people with immigrant and refugee
   backgrounds and how to support them in mental health distress.
7 Discuss the potential effects of COVID-19 on the mental health and well-
   being of people with immigrant and refugee backgrounds.

Introduction

While the health systems in Australia, Aotearoa New Zealand and other developed countries are regarded as some of the finest in the world, there is an ever-present need to ensure flexibility regarding **cultural competence and responsiveness,** and cultural inclusivity across a range of practice settings. Australia, for example, has one of the most diverse populations in the world, with 33 per cent of its current population being born overseas. More than one-fifth (21 per cent) of Australians speak a language other than English at home, such as Mandarin, Arabic and Vietnamese (Australian Bureau of Statistics (ABS), 2017). If current rates of immigration to Australia continue to grow, it is estimated that by 2050 approximately one-third of Australia's population will be overseas-born (Cully & Pejozki, 2012).

This chapter examines the mental health needs of people from **refugee** and immigrant backgrounds, with emphasis given to **asylum seekers**. Mental health issues that may affect these populations are explored, as is engagement between people of refugee and asylum seeker backgrounds and mainstream mental health services. This chapter seeks to deepen and broaden readers' understanding of the effects of trauma on people of refugee background, and links this to strategies in response, by mainstream mental health practitioners and services.

cultural competence and responsiveness – the ability to recognise different cultural beliefs and patterns, to prevent one's own cultural bias and judgement to influence their interpretation; also requires the person to remain objective when interacting with people from different cultural backgrounds and involves understanding behaviours and intentions in the light of having a different cultural perspective and in the context in which this occurs. The term can also be applied to services, organisations and broader systems that function in interaction with people from culturally and linguistically diverse backgrounds.

refugee – a person who leaves their country of origin or usual residence due to fear of persecution 'for reasons of race, religion, nationality, or membership in a particular group or political opinion and is unable or unwilling to return to it' (Pollard et al., 2014)

asylum seeker – a person who has left their country of origin in search of refuge

PERSONAL NARRATIVE

Hanan's story – part one

My name is Hanan. I am a 51-year-old housewife and mother of two from Iraq, where I worked as a teacher for 10 years. My journey began in 1996, when I left Iraq with my family and spent time living in Jordan, Syria, Iran, Malaysia and Indonesia, then Nauru before eventually, in 2004, being granted refugee protection and permanent residence in Australia.

Traumas to my mental health started during the journey to Australia in a leaky fishing boat, upon which 270 people were squashed, including my young sons. During the boat journey I felt uncertain of my survival from one hour to the next and was in a constant state of high stress for several days. This constant fear was compounded by my children becoming ill, the lack of a bathroom (with only one toilet on board) and the smugglers constantly demanding that all passengers move around to balance the boat and stop it from taking on too much water and sinking. When the boat was no longer safe, I was told to wait for another ship to pick us up. We waited for seven days on the boat while it took on water. I suffered a constant fear of death.

My family spent three-and-a-half years on Nauru, where we lived in tents and, later, in rooms with tin roofs. It was very hot and dirty, and we were constantly harassed by mosquitoes. We had limited access to water, which was particularly difficult as all island inhabitants had a 30-minute window of time to use water each day, with only five bathrooms for over 1000 people. There were regularly quarrels about the use of showers. For the first two years it was very distressing as there were no schools for the children, no activities and no access to health care. It was only after the initial two years that a mental health clinic was provided and two hours of schooling per day for children. This followed repeated hunger strikes, which my husband was a part of, and some asylum seekers sewed their lips or attempted to hang themselves in their tents. It was 10 years ago that this happened, but I still feel the effects today.

During our time on Nauru, I developed anxiety over the status of my family's application for a protection visa. I was anxious and worried about my children's mental health, which was being affected by the suicides and self-mutilation of other asylum seekers. I was also anxious about my vision impairment problems, which I attribute to my constant state of distress. A specialist declared me legally blind and in need of surgery to restore my vision. This advice was ignored for over three years – the time I was held on Nauru. It was only after I arrived in Australia that I managed to get surgery to restore my vision.

REFLECTIVE QUESTIONS

Based on Hanan's story of leaving her home country as a refugee, consider the following questions.

- What is the importance of trauma-informed practice when working with people from immigrant or refugee backgrounds?
- How can neglecting the effects of trauma on Hanan and her family's mental health affect them in the future? What life domains might be compromised if they do not receive appropriate care?
- What services and professionals might be important to involve when working with a person with a similar experience to that of Hanan and her family?

PERSONAL NARRATIVE

Ali's story

My name is Ali. I am 19 years old, from Afghanistan and work in a metal scrap yard in Sydney. My parents were from different ethnicities. My father was killed when I was 12 years old, and I escaped Afghanistan with my mother and two younger siblings to live as refugees in Quetta, Pakistan. At age 16, I left Pakistan to come to Australia to support my family. My uncle in Russia sent $10 000 to pay people smugglers so that I could take the journey from Pakistan to Australia.

I spent six months in the detention centre on Christmas Island, after arriving by boat. Since that dangerous, frightening journey I have been scared of the ocean, and still can't go to the beach with my friends without fear and feeling tense. I refuse to go.

Most of the asylum seekers in the detention centre were Afghan and, because of my young age, the older men took care of me, keeping me company and providing me with reassurance. A few months after being released from detention, I found out that a bomb had exploded near my mother's house in Pakistan. I couldn't contact her for several days and was extremely worried and anxious because I didn't know what was going on. Three days after the bomb-blast report, I found out that my mother had been in the vicinity of the bomb, had seen the blast and was uninjured, but badly shaken from seeing other people die. She was at risk of losing her life and extremely frightened.

I felt helpless and agitated. This caused me to start thinking about life, and my sense of hopelessness grew because my intellectual disability hindered my learning of English. My mother called regularly, telling me to forget about school and to start working to fix my life and get the family to Australia. All this pressure has made me hate my mental incapacity for not being able to learn and study fast enough to save my family.

I felt that no matter what I did I kept hitting barriers. I felt hopeless and helpless to solve my problems. As the eldest son, I had pressure from family responsibility to help my family, who were in danger.

I was having more and more mental issues but refused psychological treatment, which seemed worthless to solve my problems. The pressure to make money became very important so I moved out from foster care into a house with other single refugee men who had come to work to support their families. Now, after much difficulty, I feel like I am doing something worthwhile and successful rather than wasting time at school, where I know I won't learn English.

REFLECTIVE QUESTIONS

- Based on what you have learnt about mental health conditions in previous chapters, what conditions might Ali be at risk of developing? How could you verify whether further assessment for mental illness is needed?
- How would you engage with Ali to discuss his need for psychological treatment (in case your assessment concludes it is necessary)? What are some of the barriers likely to emerge and how could you facilitate his access to the right support?

What is meant by the terms refugee, immigrant and asylum seeker?

The stories of Hanan and Ali are first-person accounts of extremely difficult life circumstances, similar to those faced by many other refugees and asylum seekers. According to the United Nations Convention on the Status of Refugees, a refugee is a person who:

> ... owing to a well-founded fear of being persecuted for reasons of race, religion, national-ity, membership of a particular social group or political opinion, is outside the country of his nationality and is unable or, owing to such fear, is unwilling to avail himself of the protection of that country; or who, not having a nationality and being outside the country of his former habit-ual residence as a result of such events, is unable or, owing to such fear, is unwilling to return to it. (United Nations High Commission for Refugees (UNHCR), 2012)

At some point in time, every person who is a refugee has been an asylum seeker. In countries such as Australia and Aotearoa New Zealand, a person is officially designated a refugee when their claim for asylum has been accepted through the process of refugee status determination.

An asylum seeker is a person seeking protection under the 1951 Refugee Convention (UNHCR, 2012). Typically, an asylum seeker has left their country of origin and formally applied for asylum in another country but the application has not yet been assessed (UNHCR,

2012). By contrast, an economic migrant is someone who has moved to another country to work or to seek work. Refugees and asylum seekers are not economic migrants (UNHCR, 2012).

Each year, the UNHCR publishes reports on the number and location of refugees, asylum seekers and displaced persons around the world. During 2019, the UNHCR (2020) reported that the number of displaced people had exceeded 79.5 million worldwide. 'To put these numbers in perspective, in 2019 on average 37 000 new people were forced to flee their homes every day' (UNHCR, 2020). By 2020, the number of forcibly displaced people had grown to 82.4 million, more than double the level of a decade ago (41 million in 2010) (UNHCR, 2021). More specifically, the 2020 report states that an estimated 765 200 people were granted international protection in 2020, a number significantly lower than that of 2019 (952 800). Most asylum applications originated from Syria (6.6 million), Afghanistan (2.6 million) and South Sudan (2.2 million). While approximately 171 800 are registered as refugees, a further 3.9 million Venezuelans are displaced abroad without a formal refugee status (UNHCR, 2021).

The statistical evidence shows that high-income countries host just 17 per cent of people displaced across borders, while upper-middle income countries such as Turkey, Colombia, the Islamic Republic of Iran, Lebanon and Jordan hosted an estimated 43 per cent of displaced people at the end of 2020. The evidence also shows that nearly three-quarters of people displaced across borders remain in those neighbouring countries (UNHCR, 2021). Of the total number of asylum applications made in the Asia and Pacific regions in 2019, Australia was the second-largest recipient, with 188 600 new asylum claims recorded. Over the past 10 years, Australia welcomed 11 per cent (114 500) of all resettled refugees worldwide. The main nationalities applying for asylum in Australia in 2019 included people from Malaysia, China and India (Refugee Council of Australia, 2021). By comparison, approximately 494 applications were received by Aotearoa New Zealand in 2020, with most recent statistics showing the five most frequent nationalities of those claiming refugee status were Indonesia, China, Malaysia and Sri Lanka (New Zealand Government, 2021).

While the adjusted prevalence of depression in refugee populations has been found to be 30.8 per cent in a meta-analysis of 117 studies, depression in refugee populations is reported to be as high as 85.5 per cent (Steel et al., 2009; Young & Gordon, 2016).

Temporary protection

In some jurisdictions such as Australia, asylum seekers who are found to be refugees may be granted a visa that entitles them to temporary residence. This may be a Temporary Protection Visa (TPV) or a Safe Haven Enterprise Visa (SHEV). These visas are granted to people who arrived in an 'unauthorised way'; that is, without a valid visa. TPVs were granted to people who arrived in Australia by boat between 1990 and 2001. They were abolished and then reintroduced for people who arrived by boat between August 2012 and December 2014. These temporary visas entitle a person to live in Australia for three to five years. For a TPV to be renewed, the applicant's circumstances are re-assessed to determine whether it is safe enough for the person to return to their home country. People granted a SHEV who have lived in a designated 'regional' area may be entitled also to apply for a permanent work visa or a partner visa, in limited circumstances. The impermanent nature of these temporary visas and the processes associated with their renewal – such as the lack of certainty about when interviews to re-assess claims would occur and how the safety of the person's homeland would be assessed, or whether they can apply for another visa – mean that TPV and SHEV holders face considerable anxiety (Procter et al., 2018), mental distress and uncertainty about their continuing personal circumstances (Procter, 2005; Procter et al., 2018). This uncertainty, coupled with strongly held beliefs that it is unsafe to return to their country of origin, can results in substantial psychological and physical effects in some visa holders (Procter, 2005; Procter, 2016).

Studies have suggested that temporary refugee protection contributes substantially to the risk of depression, suicidal intent, post-traumatic stress and problems related to mental illness in refugees (Nickerson et al., 2019; Newnham et al., 2019), including intrusive, anxiety-based symptoms in the form of constant worrying about the possibility of being deported (Coffey et al., 2010). In the study by Coffey and colleagues (2010), asylum seekers' marginalised status arising from TPVs reinforced the sense of insecurity, powerlessness and helplessness that had characterised the experience of detention. In a study investigating the effects of temporary protection on the mental health of Mandaean refugees, temporary protection status was strongly associated with daily stresses related to financial and work difficulties, and problems in accessing health care, language classes and other opportunities (Steel et al., 2006). Since temporary visa holders are unable to sponsor close family members to Australia and to re-enter Australia if they travel overseas, without seeking express permission from the Immigration Department, they are unable to assist family members to flee dangerous situations, thereby reinforcing feelings of guilt and powerlessness (Procter, 2016).

Mental health of people of immigrant and refugee backgrounds

Many studies have been conducted into the mental health experiences of refugees and asylum seekers, detailing the prevalence of serious mental illnesses, particularly in refugees who have relocated to developed countries. Some of the key issues associated with the mental health of refugees relate to previous experiences during their flight to settlement – sometimes temporary and unstable, and in harsh and difficult circumstances. The sense of hopelessness, loss of future aspirations and uncertainty about family and friends left behind (Posselt et al., 2019; Fazel, Reed & Stein, 2015) that accompany such traumatic experiences are risk factors for self-harm, which affect mental health and the recovery process (Commonwealth and Immigration Ombudsman, 2013). A major review of mental health in forcibly displaced children and adolescents settled in low-income and middle-income countries confirmed that exposure to violence is a well-established risk factor for mental illness (Reed et al., 2012). High levels of distress and mental illness were reported in a review of studies investigating the mental health effects of immigration detention (Robjant, Hassam & Katona, 2009). The most common conditions reported in the research focusing on experiences in detention include depression, post-traumatic stress and anxiety, and time spent in detention has emerged as a significant contributing factor to mental deterioration and sense of hopelessness (Newman, Procter & Dudley, 2013). Behavioural responses to distress and inner turmoil expressed as self-harm and suicidal behaviour have also been reported (Commonwealth and Immigration Ombudsman, 2013).

Risk and protective factors

People from refugee and asylum seeker backgrounds are at greater risk of developing mental illness and suicidal behaviours than the general Australian population (Procter et al., 2011). Prolonged periods of being held in immigration detention are associated with diminishing mental health in refugees and asylum seekers, particularly among children and young people, and those with pre-existing vulnerabilities. Typically, there is an initial improvement in mental health upon release from detention, but this tends to be short-lived. In most instances, there is a re-emergence of mental health issues and symptoms of mental illness within six months of release (Procter et al., 2011).

The factors contributing to increased risk of mental health issues and mental illness among people from refugee and immigrant backgrounds include:

- low English-language proficiency
- thwarted cultural, religious and spiritual identity
- loss of close family bonds and confidantes
- racism, discrimination and feeling marginalised and disenfranchised
- limited knowledge of how the health system works
- previous exposure to trauma prior to settlement.

The most significant protective factors for mental health among people from refugee and asylum seeker backgrounds include:

- positive family relationships
- positive peer relationships
- verbalisation ability (self-expression)
- problem-solving and cognitive abilities
- assertiveness
- having confidantes
- clear cultural and linguistic identities
- satisfaction with family success and acculturation.

An overall absence of previous traumatic events, a recognised professional occupation and employment in that occupation are also considered protective of mental health (Procter et al., 2011). Although employment is a **protective factor**, the conditions of employment appear to be most critical, with the occupational setting in which work takes place being particularly important (Bhui, 2008).

protective factor – a personal quality, attribute or characteristic that helps to reduce the likelihood of poor mental health and the development of mental illness

REFLECTIVE QUESTIONS

Imagine you are working with a refugee family. They are seeking information and guidance. Consider the following questions.

- What community contacts or collaborative relationships might the family want to establish with health and community services as a means of helping to manage the transition from refugee to citizen?
- Why might it be important to focus on protective factors? Outline the specific risk and protective factors associated with being from a refugee or asylum seeker background.

Physical illness

People from refugee and asylum seeker backgrounds are not only at increased risk of experiencing mental illness but also physical health conditions. Refugees and asylum seekers often come from countries with poor access to health care. In 2015, over a million refugees and asylum seekers entered Europe (Kupferschmidt, 2016; Clayton & Holland, 2015). Coinciding with this influx of new arrivals, the tuberculosis rates in Germany rose by 30 per cent (Kupferschmidt, 2016). A study that explored child and adolescent refugees of Karen ethnicity from refugee camps situated along the Thai–Burma border, who were settled in outer metropolitan Melbourne, revealed high rates of nutritional deficiencies and infectious diseases (Paxton et al., 2012). The potential for post-arrival health screenings and accessible, funded immunisation among newly arrived refugees has also been described (Rungan et al., 2013). A community-based refugee service in Darwin undertook a retrospective clinical audit of newly arrived refugees attending for general and mental health needs (Johnston, Smith & Roydhouse, 2011). The most common diagnoses confirmed by testing were vitamin D deficiency, hepatitis B carrier status, tuberculosis infection, schistosomiasis and anaemia (Johnston et al., 2011).

Isolation

People from immigrant or refugee backgrounds may experience isolation due to a range of factors. The process of emigration often means leaving behind an established social network, and may involve other losses, such as of language and self-identity. More broadly, emigration may lead to a sense of losing one's cultural identity. Other factors may also create or contribute to a sense of isolation for people from immigrant or refugee backgrounds. Stigma and shame surrounding mental illness can be significant among some cultural groups. A high level of stigma can have a severe effect on a person's or family's desire or ability to seek help, and may further isolate the person or their family from the community. Isolation is particularly relevant to immigrant elders. Immigrant elders who live in cultural enclaves are more likely to have trouble understanding their host country's language, even if they have lived in the host country for an extended period (Procter, 2008). Immigrant elders are also more likely to experience social isolation, due to the disappearance of traditional, intergenerational relationships in Australian culture (Procter, 2008). The increasing urban sprawl characterising Australian cities can result in social dislocation of both young and old people, without adequate social support measures and extended family in place. If the immigrant elder is a refugee or displaced person, they are likely to arrive with only a few family members for support. As time goes on, younger generations may be less willing to provide the kinds of support the immigrant elder expects (Chiriboga, Yee & Jang, 2005). Immigrant elders have described as a profound loss the lack of availability of members in their community of origin with whom to socialise (Giuntoli & Cattan, 2012).

REFLECTIVE QUESTION

Discuss the considerations that should be taken into account when collaborating with older people from immigrant and refugee backgrounds who are reluctant to seek support from others. What skills do mental health practitioners have that enable them to advance collaborative care?

Culture and explanatory models in mental health

The combined elements of social, **cultural** and interpersonal factors in mental health should lead practitioners to consider the deeper meaning of structures held by people from immigrant and refugee backgrounds. Based on the work of Kleinman and Seeman (2000), this means that practitioners must be open to the **explanatory model of mental health and mental illness** used by a person in distress. This will involve challenging taken-for-granted assumptions regarding symptoms and experiences of health and illness, help-seeking, and the way care is evaluated by consumers. The clinical work of any health professional – no matter how willing or keen to help – will be compromised if it does not consider the person's understanding of health difficulties and what practitioners themselves consider to be perceived causes of illness, optimal care and culturally appropriate support and treatment. This is particularly so in the mental health arena (Procter, 2016).

All consumers make interpretations of their health and well-being, the way in which their health is shaped by events and circumstances, and the practical help they need to enable change or improve their situation. Cultural explanatory models attempt to answer these and related questions, such as what something is called, why it started when it did, as well as the severity and potential treatment outcome.

cultural – from the shared and learned systems of beliefs transmitted within a community that shape the social context and set norms and expectations. Culture shapes how individuals interpret the world and how they adjust, behave and attribute meaning to social phenomena. Cultures can vary within subgroups and broader communities, and are subject to continuous development and changes in internal and external circumstances.

How to explore the experience of mental illness in a culturally informed way

The cultural awareness questions listed here are adapted from Procter (2007) and are designed to help practitioners respond to people in the context of their mental health issues or mental illness.

- Can you tell me about what brought you here? What do you call (use the person's words for their problem)?
- When do you think it started, and why did it start then?
- What are the main problems it is causing you?
- What have you done to try and stop/manage to make it go away or make it better?
- How would you usually manage in your own culture to make it go away or make it better?
- How have you been coping so far with it?
- In your culture, is your (person's words for their problem) considered 'severe'? What is the worst problem this could cause you?
- What type of help would you be expecting from me/our service?
- Are there people in your community who are aware that you have this condition? What do they think or believe caused it? Are they doing anything to help you?

TRANSLATION TO PRACTICE

explanatory model of mental health and mental illness – an approach used to explore the way an individual explains, understands or interprets their own or someone else's mental health problems or illness and mental well-being; 'a person's explanatory model will influence the way in which feelings and symptoms are presented, the nature and scope of distress, behaviour, pattern of help seeking, perception of a good outcome as well as adherence or non-adherence to treatment' (Procter, 2016)

In thinking about cultural explanatory models, it is important to be aware that a person's cultural and linguistic backgrounds can significantly affect how they understand concepts such as well-being and illness, and therefore should influence how their health conditions should be treated (Galletly et al., 2016). For example, in some cultures or religions, mental illness may be understood as resulting from reasons as diverse as karma, spiritual possession or mind–body imbalance (Nguyen, Yamanda & Dinh, 2012). The 'mind' may be considered as part of rather than separate from the body, as it tends to be conceptualised within the biomedical model, and this can lead to differences in understanding and explaining a mental illness. Furthermore, in some languages there may not be a word or expression for a particular mental illness such as depression. It is important for health professionals to be aware of such differences and to be prepared to discuss mental health and illness in alternative ways, where necessary. However, in line with the recovery approach in mental health, it is also important to acknowledge that individuals are unique and there can be distinct differences in beliefs, both across and within cultures.

PERSONAL NARRATIVE

Hanan's story – part two

All this experience has made me feel hopeless for myself and my family's future … helpless to escape the prison I was put in without a crime, and worthless. I cannot say strongly enough that we feel like the world has forgotten us and doesn't know we are here. We are humans, not animals. As I tell this story again, I worry about the people coming today and being put into detention centres. My husband and I regret coming to Australia and would not have come if we knew there would be such a high cost to my family's life and health. My husband and I share a great deal of ongoing guilt and self-blame for putting our two sons through this traumatic experience, which has had irreversible and lifelong consequences. I know we chose to come; they were too young to have a say.

In my life now I often go to my room and sit alone with the lights off for hours to cry. Sometimes, I feel agitated and upset with sounds of the TV and conversation, and sometimes I yell at my children or fight with my husband for no reason. My sons often try to calm me down. I respond by telling them to leave me alone and I cope with the situation by removing myself from the room. Afterwards, I feel bad for how I treated my family and sad that I have become like this.

I feel that I have not benefitted from my treatment at the community-based torture and trauma recovery service. They can't solve my problems; they just listen but don't do anything. Talking makes me feel worse. I feel sad for reliving the experiences and exhausted from crying in front of the doctor. It is always so slow. I can't read, speak or write English very well, so I need an interpreter. I also often find that this sadness shows itself physically by making me lethargic and causes pain in my stomach and diarrhoea. I now have limited mobility due to back problems and arthritis, but I don't like to go out anyway, as I feel reluctant and lacking energy to leave the house. My emotions fluctuate from anger to sadness and from fear and worry to hopelessness.

REFLECTIVE QUESTIONS

Imagine you are working with Hanan, who tells you that getting help for her problems is useless, that her life is never going to improve and there is no point talking about the situation as no one really understands her point of view.

- What type of response would be important in this situation?
- What skills or interventions would you use to build a collaborative relationship with Hanan?

A nurse's approach

As a registered nurse working in an acute-care setting and seeing someone like Hanan, my first challenge would be to try and understand her perspective. For this to happen, I would be aware of the need to have an accredited interpreter available for the initial assessment interview. From there, the key would be to try and understand the way in which Hanan's symptoms and experiences are presented, when, how and why help is being sought, and what we both might see as a good outcome. At the same time, I would consciously try to work towards helping to develop and build trust. To my mind, it is critical to look beyond taken-for-granted assumptions when working with people from immigrant and refugee backgrounds, by ensuring that such a human connection is not tokenistic and adds genuine value to the lives of people seeking assistance. Clear communication is the real key. Wherever possible, Hanan should be able to use her preferred language, especially in stressful situations. If Hanan requests an interpreter or expresses a hesitation about her language skills, a professional interpreter should always be used. In general terms, the only exception to this would be in emergency situations. Below are some additional tips (adapted from Procter, 2009) to consider when working collaboratively in determining how well and to what extent a person speaks and understands English.

1   Avoid asking questions that the person can answer with a single word, such as 'yes', 'maybe' or 'no'. Instead, ask open-ended questions that require the person to answer in a sentence. It is preferable to use 'what' or 'why'? 'how'? 'when'? questions, as these help to facilitate an expression of views and ideas, as well as allow for an 'opening-up'. Through this process there may be fewer obstacles for dialogue to occur.
2   Ask the person to repeat the information you have provided, in their own words.
3   Ask for the help of a professional interpreter if the person is struggling to answer any questions or to repeat the information you've provided.
    When working with people in this situation, it is important to remember that:

1   You cannot properly test a person's English-language skills by asking for their name, address, date of birth and other personal information.
2   Being able to have a social conversation with someone else in English does not guarantee that a person will understand complex information presented to them, whether verbally or written down in English.
3   To be culturally competent, practitioners need to be culturally aware and understanding.

Engagement with mainstream mental health services

Health workers supporting people from culturally and linguistically diverse (CALD) backgrounds should take account of cultural idioms of distress and provide care in the person's preferred language. If the person's English proficiency is limited, it is also important to consider what this may mean for their explanation of distress and what the person sees as the problem or areas of concern and their treatment preferences.

Clinical assessment, health and helping strategies for people from immigrant and refugee backgrounds must use personal reflection, therapeutic sensitivity, compassion, patience and understanding. Effective communication, an important basis for building trust, means that health professionals should establish the person's preferred language and whether an interpreter is required. Practitioners should not assume that a lack of proficiency in English is caused by poor language attainment, as it could be associated with dysphasia due to a current or previous stroke or other neuro-muscular disease, or due to the loss of an acquired language resulting from cognitive decline, such as dementia. Care should be tailored to the consumer's customs and beliefs, as well as practices regarding health, illness and death, and people should be asked what *they believe* is the cause of their problem. The practitioner should offer consumers the opportunity to discuss any concerns, needs or problems they may be experiencing in the hospital or community setting. Each consumer should be responsible for deciding the level of family involvement they wish to have and which additional networks may be available for informal support, such as faith-based groups or friends (Procter, 2008). This is a particularly important concern when working with people from collectivist cultures, in which the family and/or wider community is seen as key to achieving well-being and recovery.

With people from refugee and asylum seeker backgrounds presenting distinctive mental illnesses, there is a need for considered and culturally safe ways to engage consumers, **carers** and other key people who may be involved. A monocultural 'business as usual approach' should not be taken, whereby services and individuals adopt a 'one size fits all' approach to service delivery and care planning. There may be a tendency for services to put an assessment and care plan together that suits the needs of the service provider, rather than the CALD consumer. The key issue pertaining to mental health service delivery for people from immigrant and refugee backgrounds is to ensure culturally competent and appropriate care.

carer – a person who offers support, personal care and any type of assistance to someone experiencing a mental health condition. This may include immediate family members, relatives, neighbours, friends, grandparents and foster carers. In transcultural and other contexts, it is important to acknowledge this through use of humanistic language, in line with a recovery approach (e.g. the terms 'support person/ people' and 'support networks' may be preferable to the term 'carer').

Traumatic stress

Personal loss and the loss of loved ones, especially for people who have had to leave their homelands involuntarily (because of social and political unrest), may create a context for trauma (Procter, 2008). The stories of Hanan and Ali highlight how an experience of trauma is a notable risk factor for the development of mental illness among people from immigrant and refugee backgrounds. Certain traumatic experiences (e.g. torture and violence) are very strongly associated with mental illnesses, such as post-traumatic stress and depression (Steel et al., 2009). Recognising the presence of trauma symptoms and acknowledging the role that trauma has played in a person's life is central to the recovery process. When a practitioner (and the wider service system) takes this approach, it is referred to as trauma-informed care.

Trauma-informed care

Trauma-informed care has been applied to address various mental health concerns associated with varying degrees or forms of trauma. It is a relatively recent development, with its aims of accurately identifying trauma and associated symptoms; training practitioners to develop an awareness of how trauma affects the person; minimising re-traumatisation; and an overarching 'do no harm' approach (Miller & Najavits, 2012). Central to trauma-informed care is the goal of ameliorating, rather than exacerbating, the negative effects of trauma (Brown, Baker & Wilcox, 2012). Providing appropriate care requires practitioner education on issues related to trauma and the lived experiences and effects of trauma on the individual (Jennings, 2007). It is essential that systems are informed by and adapted according to available knowledge of the role that trauma plays in the consumer experience of mental illness (Jennings, 2007). Such a system must recognise that trauma can contribute towards a person's vulnerability and has effects on different aspects of a person's life, throughout the lifespan. This understanding is central to designing services that are appropriate to the individual consumer.

Practising trauma-informed care enables practitioners to make decisions about necessary treatments and approaches to an individual's situation. In particular, Blanch (2008) has warned that it cannot be assumed that all refugees have been traumatised and require trauma treatment, even though they have all faced a challenging journey. Having a heightened understanding of the effects of trauma as well as symptoms of trauma enables approaches to be best tailored to individual consumers.

Elliot and colleagues (2005) described 10 principles of trauma-informed services, which are deemed necessary if services are to be both accessible and effective for those who have experienced trauma:

1 Recognise the effects of trauma on the development and coping strategies of the consumer.
2 Set recovery from trauma as a key goal.
3 Employ an empowerment model, to facilitate the person taking control of their life.
4 Work towards maximising the person's choice and control over the recovery process.
5 Strive for therapeutic relationships that develop safety and trust (that is, relationships that are the opposite of traumatising).
6 Create an atmosphere respectful of the person's need for safety, respect and acceptance.
7 Emphasise the person's strengths (focusing on adaptations rather than symptoms, and resilience rather than pathology).
8 Aim to minimise the possibilities of re-traumatisation.
9 Be culturally competent, understanding the person in the context of their cultural background.
10 Encourage consumer input, in designing and evaluating services.

Barriers to talking about trauma with practitioners

The process of telling one's story is central to understanding the trauma experienced by individuals from immigrant and refugee backgrounds and working towards recovery (de Haene et al., 2012). However, there are several barriers that may prevent these individuals from discussing and disclosing their traumatic experiences. In the primary care setting, for example, such barriers have been found to include feeling that it is only appropriate to discuss trauma if the practitioner asks about it first; not considering the effects of trauma upon health; and a desire to not retrieve upsetting memories (Shannon, O'Dougherty & Mehta, 2012). These, and other barriers, need to be addressed to facilitate discussion with consumers and maximise the potential for trauma-informed care.

REFLECTIVE QUESTIONS

Self-assessment of beliefs and attitudes is an important aspect of working across cultures because it can improve the practitioner's clinical care in various situations. Cultural sensitivity should frame how engagement unfolds. Simply asking a question can provide an opportunity for the development of a trusting and effective therapeutic relationship. To achieve these aims and ideals, practitioners working in mental health must also identify their own prejudices and biases, and reflect on how these may influence their clinical practice. The following questions can guide this reflective process. Working in small groups, answer the following questions:

- What are my own views and feelings about immigrants and refugees?
- Am I comfortable working with people who are distressed and non-communicative?
- Do I fear or dislike them? Do they unsettle me? Am I ambivalent towards them and, if so, why?
- How are my ideas, thoughts and feelings about working with refugees and immigrants evident during clinical practice?
- How do media and popular opinions regarding certain immigrant and religious groups shape my views?
- To what extent do I encourage and facilitate consumers from immigrant and refugee backgrounds and their families, where appropriate, to make key decisions about their care?

Source: Adapted from Procter (2008).

Access and engagement when in distress

Perhaps the most challenging aspect of mental healthcare practice is in the emergency context, with people seeking access to the healthcare system at the very point of their distress. From all service access points, practitioners working in mental health are able to assist refugees to 'make sense of an increasingly globalised and at times hostile world, better understand and respond to individual need, develop culturally competent problem-solving abilities and appreciate the factors that can promote health and comfort' (Procter, 2008, p. 439). Having informed knowledge of background issues in the wider world – including the sociopolitical – enables practitioners to collaborate with people from immigrant and refugee backgrounds, their families and significant networks to target strategies and support programs that maximise their capacity to cope on an ongoing basis and to improve their mental health (Procter, 2008).

INTERPROFESSIONAL PERSPECTIVES

Supporting John, a Rwandan refugee

I am a legal professional supporting John, a Rwandan refugee who arrived in Australia more than 12 years ago on a valid passport. He and his wife (and son) were found to be refugees. Both had experienced severely traumatic events in their home country, including surviving the 1993 genocide. John is an intelligent man but has had limited education due to disruptions of war in his home country. He now works as an Uber driver and interpreter. He is in his 40s.

John applied for Australian citizenship in February 2016. He tried to attend the Immigration Department to sit the citizenship test but was refused on the grounds that his identity documents were insufficient (he provided his travel document, driver's licence and Medicare card). The Department gave John a handwritten 'Post-It' note, stating that they needed him to provide a passport or birth certificate. John was also told that he had to contact the Rwandan Embassy. He explained that he is a refugee and therefore cannot contact the Embassy. John also told the Department that he has no birth certificate as he was born in a remote village in Rwanda where births were not registered.

John returned in September to sit the test. Again, he was refused, for the same reason. He was asked for his Rwandan passport and replied that an immigration officer had seized it during the visa application process (as it had had some false visas in it). The immigration officer told John that the Department would locate the file but that 'this could take several months to over a year'. Again, they suggested he contact his home Embassy for a new passport or birth certificate. John asked them to write this down, but they did not. He returned in October, and again he was refused the opportunity to sit the exam, for the same reasons.

Soon afterwards, John came to see me for assistance. I looked online to see how to contact the Immigration Department – there is a general enquiries number. When I called, an automated message informed me that the waiting time would be over an hour and that I would be called back if I choose to leave a number. I left my mobile number, and when the officer called back they told me they were unable to talk to me as John was not with me to give them permission to speak on his behalf (he had left by then).

I arranged to meet John at the Immigration Department. As we walked into the reception area I could see that there were computers for visitors to obtain a ticket for assistance. I ask John if he had a ticket; he said no and so I approached the screen to obtain one. I was stopped by an Immigration Officer in uniform, who bodily stood in front of the screen, preventing me from taking a ticket. There was also a security guard in uniform in the area.

'What are you here for?'

'He has an enquiry about citizenship. I am here to help him.'

'Do you have an appointment?'

'No, he has an application already and we want to arrange to see someone to talk about his case.'

'You cannot see anyone without an appointment – you have to ring the general enquiries number.'

'Yes, I have rung that number but they were not able to assist me, nor would they allow me to make an appointment, so we thought we would come in here to speak to someone.'

'There is no one here who will see you. You have to ring the number.'

'Yes, but I have rung the number. Can't we get a ticket in order to see someone to make an appointment?'

'No, there is no one here for you to see.'

'Do you realise how frustrating this is?'

'You have to ring the number.'

'This is incredibly unhelpful. I have rung the number and told them I would come here! Why did they not tell me that it was not possible to do this, to see anyone?'

There was no answer …

John and I left together. I was furious. John said to me, 'I am glad you saw that; this is how they treat everyone.'

We left the Immigration Department and we rang the number together, waiting for 90 minutes before we were able speak to someone (they rang back). John get on the phone and asked about his case. He was told that 'It is being processed.'

I got on the phone and said, 'No, they wanted his identity documents.'

'Has he provided them?'

'No, he can't and he explained why he can't.'

'Well, they would have given him something in writing about that.'

'No, they haven't.'

'Well, it is being processed and they will contact you when they need anything.'

I composed an email to the citizenship section of the Immigration Department and sent it along with a statutory declaration and specific questions about John's case. I received a standardised email response that the Department does not provide information on the processing of individual cases.

Trust and human connectedness in mental health

Building trust and rapport with consumers from immigrant or refugee backgrounds, their families and/or the wider ethnic community is fundamental. Ambiguity and uncertainty associated with obtaining or maintaining a visa (as in the case of John), or dealing with trauma, war or being held in detention may compromise or threaten a person's ability to trust and reach out for help when needed. Such experiences, which may have been endured by consumers over a long period of time, are quite often the contributing factors to a person's mental illness. As such, it is critical, if and when consumers are ready to share their stories, fears and hopes, that health professionals are ready to listen, be compassionate, sensitive and flexible in their approach and, most of all, have patience and a commitment to their work. These and other qualities are key to building trust and connecting with consumers from immigrant and refugee backgrounds, their families and wider supports.

Older people with immigrant backgrounds

Procter and Baker (2014) described how the cultural and linguistic diversity of older people necessitate the development of an appropriate policy and service response. *The World Health Statistics 2021* highlighted that particular attention must be paid to the difficulties faced by ethnic and migrant groups in accessing health services (World Health Organization (WHO), 2021). In 2019, worldwide there was an estimated 703 million people aged 65 years and older (United Nations, 2019). By 2050, it is estimated there will be approximately 1.5 billion people worldwide aged over 60 years (United Nations, 2019). In addition:

- Between 2019 and 2050, the number of older people in less-developed countries is projected to increase by over 225 per cent, rising from 37 million in 2019 to 120 million persons aged 65 years and older in 2050 (United Nations, 2019).

- Women outlive men in virtually all societies by up to 4.8 years; this global gender gap is expected to narrow over the forthcoming three decades. Projections indicated that in 2050 women will comprise 54 per cent of the global population aged 65 years and over (United Nations, 2019).

In Australia, the population is ageing at a fast rate. In 2019, people aged 65 years and over made up 16 per cent of Australia's population (Australian Bureau of Statistics (ABS), 2019). It is estimated that, by 2057, 22 per cent of the population will be older than 65 years. By 2097, this percentage will correspond to 25 per cent (ABS, 2014). These statistics are similar to those from other developed nations. Future projections of ageing populations in the United States, Canada, Australia and across Europe reveal increasing heterogeneity of immigrant elders, and it is expected that numbers will increase more so than that of non-immigrant elders (Procter, 2008; Wilson et al., 2020).

Older people from immigrant and refugee backgrounds are exposed to unique risk factors for mental health. The *Framework for Mental Health in Multicultural Australia* (Mental Health Australia, 2021a) highlights the following key concerns, including that older people of refugee and immigrant backgrounds:

- have reduced access to mental health services when compared with other Australians
- are over-represented in involuntary admissions and acute in-patient units
- are exposed to more quality and safety risks due to cultural and linguistic barriers (Galletly et al., 2016).

Mental health practitioners working in both health care and human services face two intertwined challenges: how to properly address the mental health concerns of immigrant elders and how to develop the cultural competence skills to be able to meaningfully engage, assess and treat patients, accepting both the challenges and opportunities posed by diversity (Procter & Baker 2014; Mental Health Australia, 2021b).

Consequences of the COVID-19 pandemic for refugees and asylum seekers

The unprecedented conditions observed during the COVID-19 pandemic has had several consequences for refugees and asylum seekers, both in detention centres and in the community. For refugees detained in Australian detention centres and alternative places of detention, for example, reports on failing to comply with safety recommendations were observed (Asylum Seeker Resource Centre (ASRC), 2020a). Concerns were raised due to COVID-19 infections among staff members working in the facilities. Detainees and human rights advocates stated that transparent protocols for physical distancing and use of personal protective equipment (PPE) were non-existent for staff members. Furthermore, no quarantine or testing measures were implemented after staff tested positive, increasing the sense of vulnerability of detention centre residents. Beyond this, despite residents being recommended to wash their hands and maintain social distancing protocols, detainees reported being kept crowded in narrow spaces, sometimes with little sunlight and no fresh air (ASRC, 2020b). This apparent lack of concern could be especially triggering for the detainees, considering the recurrent experience of trauma and lack of control faced by many refugees. Fear of an outbreak spreading, and death, was reported by residents, who were particularly concerned when presenting risk factors for COVID-19 complications, such as respiratory diseases and chronic conditions (ASRC, 2020a, 2020b).

Refugee and asylum seekers were also vulnerable to the socio-economic effects of the COVID-19 pandemic. Unemployment was estimated as affecting many people from refugee backgrounds as they are usually employed in low-income and insecure jobs likely to be affected by lockdowns. At the time of writing, refugee and asylum seekers were not eligible to apply for social welfare funds and government safety net support. Among bridging visa, SHEV and TPV holders, unemployment rates were estimated to rise from 19 per cent to 42 per cent during the COVID-19 pandemic (Kooy, 2020). It was estimated that approximately 19 000 refugees and asylum seekers would lose their jobs. Consequently, rates of homelessness and seeking support networks such as foodbanks, housing and healthcare services were projected to also increase, occasioning increases in expenses for state and territory governments. In this scenario, an extra \$23.4 million per year was estimated as needed to cover increased costs of hospital admissions for mental health conditions, drug overdose, self-harm, injury or heart disease (Kooy, 2020). Health practitioners must be aware of the likely risk factors experienced by people from refugee and asylum-seeking backgrounds. This likely vulnerability reinforces the need for trauma-informed and culturally safe interventions to mobilise available community resources and support people in the recovery process. Trauma-informed responses might include validation of emotional responses (e.g. feeling sad, confused or angry), promotion of engagement with meaningful community based groups and development of a personalised safety plan, including culturally appropriate protective factors (Kenny, Grech & Procter, 2021).

SUMMARY

This chapter has presented stories and information, supplemented with activities designed to deepen your understanding of:

- People of immigrant and refugee backgrounds and their increased risk of developing mental illness and suicidal tendencies when compared to the general population. Some of the factors that may contribute to the manifestation of mental illness among people from immigrant and refugee backgrounds include isolation, pre-migration experiences such as trauma and displacement, and stigma of mental illness in some cultures.
- Risk factors for mental illness among people of immigrant and refugee backgrounds, including low English-language proficiency, loss of support networks and prior trauma. Protective factors for mental health include positive relationships, strong cultural and linguistic identities, and ability to express concerns.
- The need for mainstream health and mental health service providers to consider and enact culturally safe and appropriate ways to engage with consumers from immigrant and refugee backgrounds and their supports. Such care needs to be consumer-focused and recovery focused, and committed to addressing barriers, including language barriers, which prevent or hinder access to good quality care.
- Cultural explanatory models as pathways for discovering a range of issues related to a person's mental health, such as consumers' interpretations of their conditions, their beliefs as to why the problem started and what would help to improve the situation.

- Engaging with consumers and carers from immigrant, asylum-seeker and refugee backgrounds by avoiding a monocultural, 'one size fits all' approach to service provision. To enable engagement, it is important that health professionals take the time to listen to consumers and understand their stories, are flexible and consider the potential involvement of others, such as family and community supports, who may be important to the person's recovery.

CRITICAL THINKING/LEARNING ACTIVITIES

1   On your own, think about a time when you or someone you are close to experienced a mental illness or distress. Brainstorm some reasons you think this occurred. Then, in small groups, share and compare your suggested reasons for the occurrence of mental illness. Discuss any differences and how you developed your individual views about mental illness.
2   In pairs, role-play how you might discuss mental health issues or concerns in a culturally aware manner. To do this, first discuss what you understand by the term 'culturally aware'. Second, imagine that one of you is a practitioner and the other is a person from a refugee or immigrant background.
3   In pairs, role-play how you might go about determining the extent to which a consumer speaks and understands English, and whether the person requires assistance from an interpreter.
4   After reading the stories of Hanan and Ali, brainstorm a list of challenges that may be faced by people from immigrant and refugee backgrounds. In small groups, discuss: (a) possible mental health protective factors to help shift risk associated with mental distress and/or illness, and (b) how protective factors could contribute to an increased ability to cope with adversity and reduce the risk of mental illness.
5   In pairs, take turns to describe an experience you have had at some point in your life that was particularly traumatic or distressing for you. After you have done this, write down how you felt when discussing this experience. Can you identify some factors that were barriers to discussing this experience? Can you identify some factors that made talking about this experience easier?

LEARNING EXTENSION

Consider the following story.

I am a nurse working with Thanh, a 27-year-old single man who arrived from Vietnam to Australia about 10 years ago. He has no family in Australia and moves from one Housing Trust home to another. Thanh was diagnosed with schizophrenia about three years ago. He is currently on oral anti-psychotic medication. Thanh has been seeing me in my capacity as a community nurse for the past 12 months. Last week, he had a dental problem and was required to have follow-up treatment. He requested practical support from the Vietnamese community. In response, a community elder provided transport to attend the appointment that day. However, due to the complexity of the dental work required, the support Thanh needed had to be extended for another two days.

Thanh asked the community elder for two more days of practical support. The elder discussed this with me and together we decided that I would pick up Thanh on the second day only. For the return trip of the second day and on the third day, Thanh and I agreed that he needed to make his own arrangements and take care of himself. The community elder informed Thanh about this decision. However, Thanh did not seem to hear the elder. Thanh was unhappy about this decision and kept ringing the elder several times during the day and night, demanding support. Thanh sounded very worried and confused. He told the elder that he felt he could not make it to treatment on his own on the second day. Thanh also became verbally aggressive and threatened both me and the elder for not helping him.

The following morning, I turned up at Thanh's home. Thanh was disoriented, restless, shaky, confused (e.g. about the time and date) and talking very loudly. He was in a rush, leaving his home without knowing where the keys were. He was concerned that he had lost his keys. He also said things that did not make sense (e.g. words were spoken in a confused and non-logical progression), worried that he was going to be locked up and suspicious others were 'out to get him'. He also mentioned that he had not taken his medication that morning.

I tried to reassure Thanh and attempted to do some practical problem-solving for the situation (I reassured him that it was okay to close the door, see the dentist first then look for the keys later on). I then drove Thanh to the dentist for treatment. Afterwards, Thanh got home by himself. Since this day the elders and I have found it very difficult to work with Thanh. We are reluctant to visit his home and do not want to see him on our own – especially at his home. Thanh continues to be suspicious, accusing and hostile. I am now left feeling unsure about what to do next. I am also unsure about how to engage with him. I am concerned for my safety.

Consider the following questions:

- What questions would you like to ask Thanh and the community elder to be able to understand what everyday life is really like for them?
- List what you consider to be the cultural considerations that have shaped the interaction between Thanh, the nurse and the community elder.
- What are 'culturally safe practices'? What skills should the practitioner use to enhance access and utilisation of healthcare services for immigrant groups?

ACKNOWLEDGEMENT

The authors wish to acknowledge the assistance of Asma Babakarkhil, who assisted with the development of the first edition of this chapter.

FURTHER READING

Conversations Matter. (n.d.). Resources for Culturally and Linguistically Diverse (CALD) communities. Retrieved from https://conversationsmatter.org.au/resources/resources-for-cald-communities/
Forming trusting and meaningful connections with people from diverse backgrounds is essential in person-centred mental health care. This resource is practical and applied, designed to assist practitioners to create engagement that is helping and healing for consumers.

Mares, P. (2016). *Not Quite Australian: How temporary migration is changing the nation*. Melbourne: Text Publishing Company.
This book makes an important contribution as it offers deep societal and historical analyses of immigration policies and the human dimensions of acceptance and belonging. While increasing movement of immigrants and refugees around the globe are political issues for some, the author

of this text links events in Australian society to broader ideas of national identity and cultural diversity.

National Mental Health Commission. (n.d.). Spotlight reports: Multicultural Mental Health and Suicide Prevention (Website). Retrieved from: https://www.mentalhealthcommission .gov.au/monitoring-and-reporting/spotlight-reports/multicultural-mental-health-and-suicide-prevention

This publication provides a rigorous and systematic review and analysis of literature regarding how people from culturally and linguistically diverse backgrounds are identified in mental health care. There is an extensive review of literature on the interconnections between migration and mental health.

Queensland Health. (2007). *Working with Interpreters – Guidelines.* Retrieved from https://www.health.qld.gov.au/multicultural/interpreters/guidelines_int.pdf

Working with translators and interpreters is an essential aspect of health care in a multicultural and multilingual society. This guide is designed to assist practitioners to engage with confidence with accredited interpreters.

Victorian Transcultural Mental Health (Website). Retrieved from https://vtmh.org.au/

This service provides a range of free resources to help understand and interpret mental health across the lifespan in a transcultural context.

REFERENCES

Asylum Seeker Resource Centre (ASRC). (2020a). *They don't care about our lives.* Retrieved from https://www.asrc.org.au/2020/07/23/they-dont-care-about-our-lives/
——— (2020b). *Why asylum seekers are at higher risk of COVID-19.* Retrieved from https://www .asrc.org.au/why-asylum-seekers-are-at-a-higher-risk-of-covid-19/
Australian Bureau of Statistics (ABS). (2014). *Australian Historical Population Statistics, 2014.* ABS cat. No. 3105. 0.65.001. Canberra: ABS.
——— (2017). *Census of Population and Housing: Reflecting Australia – stories from the census, 2016.* Retrieved from https://www.abs.gov.au/ausstats/abs@.nsf/Lookup/by%20 Subject/2071.0~2016~Main%20Features~Cultural%20Diversity%20Data%20Summary~30
——— (2019). *Australian Demographic Statistics, Jun 2019.* Retrieved from https://www.abs.gov.au/ ausstats/abs@.nsf/0/1CD2B1952AFC5E7ACA257298000F2E76?OpenDocument
Bhui, K. (2008). Migration and mental health. In H. Freeman & S Stansfeld (eds), *The Impact of the Environment on Psychiatric Disorder* (pp. 184–209). New York: Routledge.
Blanch, A. (2008). *Transcending Violence: Emerging models for trauma healing in refugee communities.* Alexandria, VA: National Center for Trauma Informed Care.
Brown, S. M., Baker, C. N. & Wilcox, P. (2012). Risking connection trauma training: A pathway toward trauma-informed care in child congregate care settings. *Psychological Trauma: Theory, Research, Practice, and Policy, 4*: 507–15.
Chiriboga, D. A., Yee, B. W. K. & Jang, Y. (2005). Minority and cultural issues in late-life depression. *Clinical Psychology: Science and Practice, 12*: 358–63.
Clayton, J. & Holland, H. (2015). *Over One Million Sea Arrivals Reach Europe in 2015.* Geneva: UNHCR. Retrieved from http://www.unhcr.org/news/latest/2015/12/5683d0b56/million-sea-arrivals-reach-europe-2015.html
Coffey, G. J., Kaplan, I., Sampson, R. C. & Tucci, M. M. (2010). The meaning and mental health consequences of long-term immigration detention for people seeking asylum. *Social Science & Medicine, 70*(12): 2070–9.
Commonwealth and Immigration Ombudsman. (2013). *Suicide and Self-harm in the Immigration Detention Network.* Canberra: Commonwealth of Australia.

Cully, M. & Pejozki, L. (2012). Australia unbound? Migration, openness and population futures. In J. Pincus & G. Hugo (eds), *A Greater Australia: Population, policies and governance* (pp. 60–71). Melbourne: Committee for Economic Development in Australia.

de Haene, L., Rober, P., Adriaenssens, P. & Verschueren, K. (2012). Voices of dialogue and directivity in family therapy with refugees: Evolving ideas about dialogical refugee care. *Family Process*, *51*: 391–404.

Elliot, D. E., Bjelajac, P., Fallot, R. D., Markoff, L. S. & Glover Reed, B. (2005). Trauma-informed or trauma-denied: Principles and implementation of trauma-informed services for women. *Journal of Community Psychology, 33*: 461–77.

Fazel, M., Reed, R. & Stein, A. (2015). Refugee, asylum-seeking and internally displaced children and adolescents. In A. Thapar, D. S. Pine, J. F. Leckman, S. Scott, M. J. Snowling & E. Taylor (eds), *Rutter's Child and Adolescent Psychiatry*, 6th edn (pp. 573–85). John Wiley & Sons.

Galletly, C., Castle, D., Dark, F., Humberstone, V., Jablensky, A., Killackey, E., Kulkarni, J., McGorry, P., Nielssen, O. & Tran, N. (2016). Royal Australian and New Zealand College of Psychiatrists clinical practice guidelines for the management of schizophrenia and related disorders. *Australian and New Zealand Journal of Psychiatry, 50*(5): 1–117.

Giuntoli, G. & Cattan, M. (2012). The experiences and expectations of care and support among older migrants in the UK. *European Journal of Social Work, 15*: 131–47.

Jennings, A. (2007). Blueprint for Action: Building trauma-informed mental health service systems (Draft). Retrieved from www.theannainstitute.org/2007%202008%20Blueprint%20By%20Criteria%202%2015%2008.pdf

Johnston, V., Smith, L. & Roydhouse, H. (2011). The health of newly arrived refugees to the top end of Australia: Results of a clinical audit at the Darwin Refugee Health Service. *Australian Journal of Primary Health, 18*: 242–7.

Kenny, M. A., Grech, C. & Procter, N. (2021). A trauma informed response to COVID 19 and the deteriorating mental health of refugees and asylum seekers with insecure status in Australia. *International Journal of Mental Health Nursing.* https://doi.org/10.1111/inm.12932

Kleinman, A. & Seeman, D. (2000). Personal experience of illness. In G. L. Albrecht, R. Fitzpatrick & S. C. Scrimshaw (eds), *Handbook of Social Studies in Health and Medicine* (pp. 230–43). London: Sage Publications.

Kooy, J. V. (2020). *COVID-19 and humanitarian migrants on temporary visas: Assessing the public costs*. Retrieved from https://www.refugeecouncil.org.au/covid-19-assessing-the-public-costs/

Kupferschmidt, K. (2016). Refugee crisis brings new health challenges, *Science*, 352(6284): 391–2.

Mental Health Australia. (2021a). *Framework for Mental Health in Multicultural Australia: Towards culturally inclusive service delivery*. Retrieved from http://embracementalhealth.org.au/service-providers/framework

——— (2021b). *Rationale: Why is cultural responsiveness important for mental health services?* Retrieved from http://embracementalhealth.org.au/sites/default/files/framework/rationale_factsheet.pdf

Miller, N. A. & Najavits, L. M. (2012). Creating trauma-informed correctional care: A balance of goals and environment. *European Journal of Psychotraumatology, 3*: 17246.

New Zealand Government. (2021). *Refugee and Protection Statistics Pack*. Ministry of Business, Innovation and Employment. Retrieved from https://www.immigration.govt.nz/documents/statistics/statistics-refugee-and-protection.pdf

Newman, L., Procter, N. & Dudley, M. (2013). Seeking asylum in Australia: Immigration detention, human rights and mental health care, *Australasian Psychiatry, 21*: 315–20.

Newnham, E. A., Pearman, A., Olinga-Shannon, S. & Nickerson, A. (2019). The mental health effects of visa insecurity for refugees and people seeking asylum: a latent class analysis. *International Journal of Public Health, 64*(5): 763–72.

Nguyen, H. T., Yamanda, A. M. & Dinh, T. Q. (2012). Religious leaders' assessment and attribution of the causes of mental illness: An in-depth exploration of Vietnamese American Buddhist leaders. *Mental Health Religion & Culture, 15*: 511–27.

Nickerson, A., Byrow, Y., O'Donnell, M., Mau, V., McMahon, T., Pajak, R., Li, S., Hamilton, A., Minihan, S., Liu, C., Bryant, R. A., Berle, D., & Liddell, B. J. (2019). The association between visa insecurity and mental health, disability and social engagement in refugees living in Australia. *European Journal of Psychotraumatology, 10*(1): 1688129.

Paxton, G. A., Sangster, K. J., Maxwell, E. L., McBride, C. R. J. & Drewe, R. H. (2012). Post-arrival screening in Karen refugees in Australia. *PLoS ONE*, 7: e28194.

Pollard, R., Betts, W., Carroll, J., Waxmonsky, J., Barnett, S., de Gruy, F. V., Pickler, L. L. & Kellar-Guenther, Y. (2014). Integrating primary care and behavioral health with four special solutions: Children with special needs, people with serious mental illness, refugees, and deaf people. *American Psychologist, 69*(4): 377–87.

Posselt, M., Deans, C., Baker, A. & Procter, N. (2019). Clinician wellbeing: The impact of supporting refugee and asylum seeker survivors of torture and trauma in the Australian context. *Australian Psychologist, 54*(5): 415–26.

Procter, N. G. (2005). Providing emergency mental health care to asylum seekers at a time when claims for permanent protection have been rejected. *International Journal of Mental Health Nursing, 14*(1): 2–6.

———— (2007). Mental health emergencies. In K. Curtis, C. Ramsden & J. Friendship (eds), *Emergency and Trauma Nursing*. New York: Elsevier Press.

———— (2008). Immigrant elders. In *The Encyclopedia of Elder Care* (pp. 437–9). New York: Springer Publishing Company.

———— (2009). Services for asylum seekers and refugees. In P. Barker (ed.) *Psychiatric and Mental Health Nursing: The craft of caring*. Milton Park: Taylor & Francis.

———— (2016). Person-centred care for people of refugee background. *Journal of Pharmacy Practice and Research, 46*: 103–4.

Procter, N. G. & Baker, A. (2014). Immigrant elders. In A. Capezuti, M. L. Malone, P. R. Katz & M. D. Mezey (eds), *The Encyclopedia of Elder Care: The comprehensive resource on geriatric health and social care*, 3rd edn. New York: Springer.

Procter, N. G., Kenny, M. A., Eaton, H. & Grech, C. (2018). Lethal hopelessness: Understanding and responding to asylum seeker distress and mental deterioration. *International Journal of Mental Health Nursing, 27*(1): 448–54.

Procter, N. G., Williamson, P., Gordon, A. & McDonough, D. (2011). Refugee and asylum seeker self-harm with implications for transition to employment participation: A review. *Suicidologi, 16*: 30–8.

Reed, R. V., Fazel, M., Jones, L., Panter-Brick, C. & Stein, A. (2012). Mental health of displaced and refugee children resettled in low-income and middle-income countries: Risk and protective factors. *Lancet, 379*: 250–65.

Refugee Council of Australia. (2021). *Statistics on People Seeking Asylum in the Community*. Retrieved from https://www.refugeecouncil.org.au/asylum-community/3/

Robjant, K., Hassam, R. & Katona, C. (2009). Mental health implications of detaining asylum seekers: Systematic review. *British Journal of Psychiatry, 194*: 306–12.

Rungan, S., Reeve, A. M., Reed, P. W. & Voss, L. (2013) Health needs of refugee children younger than 5 years arriving in New Zealand. *Pediatric Infectious Diseases Journal, 32*(12): e432–6.

Shannon, P., O'Dougherty, M. & Mehta, E. (2012). Refugees' perspectives on barriers to communication about trauma histories in primary care. *Mental Health in Family Medicine, 9*: 47–55.

Steel, Z., Chey, T., Silove, D., Marnane, C., Bryant, R. A. & van Ommeren, M. (2009). Association of torture and other potentially traumatic events with mental health outcomes among populations exposed to mass conflict and displacement. *Journal of the American Medical Association, 302*: 537–49.

Steel, Z., Silove, D., Brooks, R., Momartin, S., Alzuhairi, B. & Susljik, I. (2006). Impact of immigration detention and temporary protection on the mental health of refugees. *British Journal of Psychiatry, 188*(1): 58–64.

United Nations. (2019). *World Population Ageing 2019*, ST/ESA/SER.A/430. Department of Economic and Social Affairs, Population Division.

United Nations High Commission for Refugees (UNHCR). (2012). *Convention Relating to the Status of Refugees*. Retrieved from www.unhcr.org/pages/49da0e466.html

———— (2020). *Figures at a Glance. Global Trends: Forced displacement in 2019*. Geneva: United Nations. Retrieved from http://www.unhcr.org/figures-at-a-glance.html

———— (2021). *Global Trends: Forced displacement in 2019*. Geneva: United Nations. Retrieved from https://www.unhcr.org/60b638e37/unhcr-global-trends-2020

Wilson, T., McDonald, P., Temple, J., Brijnath, B. & Utomo, A. (2020). Past and projected growth of Australia's older migrant populations. *Genus, 76*(1): 1–21.

World Health Organization (WHO). (2021). *The World Health Statistics 2021 – Monitoring health for the Sustainable Development Goals*. Geneva: WHO. Retrieved from https://reliefweb.int/sites/reliefweb.int/files/resources/whs-2021_20may.pdf

Young, P. & Gordon, M. S. (2016). Mental health screening in immigration detention: A fresh look at Australian government data. *Australasian Psychiatry, 24*(1): 19–22.

Gender, sexuality and mental health

15

Helen P. Hamer, Jane Barrington and Debra Lampshire
With acknowledgement to Joe Macdonald
for the second edition

LEARNING OBJECTIVES

At the completion of this chapter, you should be able to:

1 Understand the continua of sexuality and gender identity.
2 Define the difference between sexual orientation and gender identity.
3 Reflect on how gender and sexual diversity have been pathologised within the mental health system.
4 Develop skills to practise cultural competence and human connectedness.
5 Understand the effects of hetero-sexism and hetero-normativity on people's mental health.
6 Develop skills and confidence in asking and responding to disclosures of interpersonal violence and abuse.

Introduction

As mental health practitioners, we encounter the broad and diverse range of sexual orientations and gender identities in the people we serve. In this chapter we focus on the cultural diversity of gender and sexuality, and the effects of marginalisation and interpersonal and intimate partner violence and abuse on people's mental health (Bosse et al., 2018). We describe the ways in which mental health practitioners can practise empathically and effectively in matters related to gender, diversity and disclosures of violence and abuse. Throughout the chapter, we read Riley's story to help us understand how mental health services can be supportive and accepting of gender and sexual diversity.

Continua of sexuality and gender

sexual orientation – denotes a person's sexuality relative to their biological sex or their sexuality (e.g. homosexual, heterosexual, bisexual, pansexual)

Many people are familiar with the idea that there exists a range of **sexual orientations** within society. One way to conceptualise gender as more than the binary of male and female is to imagine a continuum of gender identity (United Nations High Commissioner for Human Rights, 2012), with heterosexual, or straight, at one end and lesbian or gay at the other end. Many people position themselves at either end, while others place themselves at myriad places in between. Some people move along the continuum over the course of their lifetime. It is less commonly acknowledged that there is also a wide range of gender identities. Some terms that people use include transgender, transsexual, intersex, gender-queer, woman and man.

'Transgender' is a term that encompasses a range of identities for people who do not identify with the sex they were assigned at birth. Some of these people identify as transmen (assigned female at birth, identify as male) or as transwomen (assigned male at birth, identify as female). Some people do not identify with the binary concept of male or female, and therefore may use terms like 'gender-queer' and 'non-binary'. Gender-queer people identify as both male and female, or as neither. This is different to intersex, which is a general term used for a variety of states in which a person is born with a reproductive or sexual anatomy that does not fit the typical biological definitions of female or male.

Some people identify as transsexual, a term often used to refer to a person whose gender identity is opposite to the physical sex they were assigned at birth, and who has changed, or is in the process of changing, their physical sex to conform to this gender identity. Some gender-diverse people identify as 'gender-conforming', as within the binary of male and female, woman and man. Other gender-diverse people identify as gender non-conforming, as outside or beyond the binary of male and female (non-binary), woman and man. People who are transgender, transsexual, intersex, gender-queer, gender diverse and non-binary also

gender identity – an aspect of identity that can be understood as one's psychological sex and may not correspond to one's physical sex

sexuality – how you love and how you express desire romantically or sexually

have sexual orientations, which can be straight, gay, bisexual, lesbian, queer and so on. Some people may describe their sexual orientation as transitory or unfixed. Therefore, the term 'gender fluidity' refers to change over time in a person's gender expression or gender identity, or both. For some people, gender fluidity may be a way to explore their gender expression before settling on a more stable gender identity. For others, gender identity may continue indefinitely as part of their life experience with gender (Harvard Medical School, 2021).

It is important to note the distinction between sexual orientation and **gender identity**. Sexual orientation is about **sexuality**. Gender identity is about your own gender: who you are and how you identify your gender. There are socially determined norms about both sexuality and gender. With regard to sexuality, people are generally expected to be heterosexual; to be attracted to people of the opposite sex. For example, a woman is expected to be attracted exclusively to men. With regard to gender, people are generally expected to identify with the sex they are assigned at birth; for example, an infant who is assigned female at birth is expected to grow up to identify as a woman. However, many people do not follow the patterns of these social expectations.

The social pressure exerted through these expectations about sexuality is called **hetero-normativity** and the equivalent for gender is **cis-normativity**. Cis-normativity assumes that being cis-gendered is superior and more desirable than being transgender, transsexual or intersex.

hetero-normativity – a concept that represents punitive rules (social, familial, and legal) that compel individuals to conform to dominant heterosexual standards of identity

cis-normativity – the assumption that all people are cis-gendered, that people assigned male at birth always grow up to be men and that those assigned female at birth always grow up to be women

Examples of cis-normativity in the clinical context

You are working in an acute mental health unit. Imagine the following scenarios.

- A person who is female assigned at birth walks in wearing masculine clothes. You could assume that this person is a 'butch' lesbian. However, the person may identify as a transman, and not as a woman or as a lesbian. If you have assumed that the person is 'female' and a 'lesbian', then you will probably use female pronouns such as 'she' and 'her'. This is problematic because if the person identifies as a transman they will probably prefer male pronouns such as 'he' and 'him'.
- A person who is male assigned at birth, whom you have assumed to be a man, starts wearing women's clothes in the acute unit. You could assume that this person is a 'cross-dresser' and encourage the person to only wear men's clothes. This person may identify as a woman, or as a transwoman. Inclusive practice would involve asking the person whether they would prefer to be in a women-only room or dormitory. Also, check the person's preferred pronouns – whether they would prefer to be known as 'she', 'he' or 'they', and check whether they use a different name on a day-to-day basis (regardless of whether this is their legal name).

TRANSLATION TO PRACTICE

Most people, regardless of how they identify, experience the pressure of social norms in relation to gender and sexuality. Different cultures frame gender and sexuality in different ways. In the Māori context, there is a less clear distinction between gender identity and sexual orientation, and the Māori term *takatāpui* is used collectively to refer to both men and women. *Takatāpui* can include anyone who has a diverse sexuality and/or gender. The Māori term *Ia* represents the pronouns 'he/him', 'she/her'. In Australia, though there is no similar Aboriginal or Torres Strait Islander term to describe gender and sexually diverse people, some clans use the term 'sister-girls' to describe relationships between women, and the term extends to transgender people. The term 'two-one' expresses Aboriginal views of gender and sexually diverse populations and their view that two spirits (both male and female) live within one person (Global Gayz Australia, 2009). This flexibility is not found in **paradigms** of gender and sexuality that dominate in the non-Indigenous populations of Australia and Aotearoa New Zealand. Regardless of terms used, practitioners need to extend the notion of cultural humility when working with this population group (Bennett & Gates, 2019).

paradigm / paradigm shift – concerned with changing one's perspective and developing new ways of looking at, or thinking about, a standard, a perspective or a set of ideas

There are too many labels for both gender identity and sexual orientation for a comprehensive list to be provided here, and relying on labels, categories or acronyms such as LGBTTIQ (lesbian, gay, bisexual, transgender, *takatāpui*, intersex and queer) risks alienating or excluding people whose terms are not included, or who do not identify with any of the terms offered. In this chapter we prefer to use a more inclusive term, gender and sexual diversity (GSD), which includes the widest possible range of genders and sexualities.

Self-identification

It is crucial to respect the self-identification of any person. With regard to sexual orientation, this means acknowledging how a person experiences and describes their sexuality. Respect the words the person uses to identify themselves, regardless of assumptions you may have made about the person's sexual orientation. Similarly, respecting self-identification in relation to gender means acknowledging how a person experiences and describes their gender. For some people, gender correlates to the sex they were assigned at birth. The term currently used for this is 'cis-gender', which is a companion and contrasting term to transgender, so that people do not talk about 'transgender' and 'normal gender', as this further entrenches cis-normativity.

For some people, the sex they were assigned at birth does not match how they feel, or how they would identify their gender. Sometimes this leads to a gender transition, which is a process of changing one's gender from male to female or from female to male. This process may involve any combination of social, legal and medical elements. It may be purely social: changing one's name and gendered pronouns such as 'he' and 'she', and may include legal changes of name or sex, or may involve medical support such as hormone therapy or surgery. Some gender-diverse people do not transition, or do not identify as part of a binary system of male and female. Gender-diverse people often face barriers when accessing medical services because of the potential disjunction between how they experience and identify their gender and how it is recorded on public documents or medical records.

Intersex

intersex – an umbrella term used to include a range of bodily expressions, identities and conditions

When an infant is born, the medical team assigns a sex that is recorded on the birth certificate. Usually, female or male is recorded on the birth certificate; however, 'indeterminate' or '**intersex**' are terms used to describe a person whose reproductive and sexual anatomy do not fit the typical definitions of male or female (Human Rights Commission of New Zealand, 2020).

When a clinical term is necessary, the most common is Disorders of Sex Development (DSD). There is a continuing negotiation between intersex communities and medical institutions about the medicalisation of intersex identities and embodiments. The most controversial issue is the continued use of invasive genital surgery on intersex infants to enable a clear determination of male or female (for information and resources see Intersex Awareness New Zealand: https://www.gayline.org.nz/intersex-trust-aotearoa-nz). In recent years, some countries have been considering amending their laws regarding the recording of births, deaths and marriages to extend the options under gender and include intersex or indeterminate (Australian Government, 2013).

PERSONAL NARRATIVE

Riley – early gender identity

I was assigned female at birth, but I identify as male. I was a really happy kid, and even a happy girl, until I was about 20 years old. I had come out as a dyke when I was 15 years old and felt really comfortable in my sexuality. But I had some discomfort about the assumptions people made about my gender; when thinking about my body I could honestly say that I felt comfortable in it for the most part, but that socially other people didn't seem to understand what my body meant. I didn't think that having breasts should mean I was female, but when other people saw my chest they assumed I was a girl. The problem was not me; it was the assumptions of the people around me who knew nothing more than the binary of male and female.

REFLECTIVE QUESTION

During your nursing assessment, if the person says: 'I look like a woman, but I feel like a man', how would you respond?

The idea that gender can be fluid, can change over time or move beyond the binary of male and female is increasingly evident in younger populations. The original work by Bornstein and Bergman (2010) is still seminal in the collections of creative work about non-binary gender, and demonstrates the challenge that gender non-conforming people, who may or may not identify as transgender, present to the dominant hetero-normative paradigm.

PERSONAL NARRATIVE

Riley – transition

I explored different ways of 'doing' my gender from when I was about 20 years old, until I was about 25 years old. I found some excellent support from the queer communities I was already part of, where there were lots of different people, some who identified as transgender, some as gender-queer, some as man or woman – it was clear to me that there was a wide range of options.

When I turned 25 years old, I decided it was time to investigate what my options were if I wanted medical support with my transition. I wanted to go on testosterone medication because I wanted to look more masculine; however, I had to see a psychiatrist before the endocrinologist would proceed with treatment.

The psychiatrist at Student Health was someone I knew. I had worked with her doing diversity training workshops for staff and students, so I felt comfortable being honest with her. We talked for almost an hour, about my desire to transition and what that might involve for me. She asked about my childhood, about my relationship with my body, about my sexuality and how I currently identified my gender. We talked about the continuum of gender, and I said that I had started life at the female end of the continuum, and now identified as being more towards the male end. I felt distressed that my boyhood wasn't seen by other people very often, apart from my close friends and in some queer circles.

I mentioned that I liked using words like 'gender-queer', because for me that was about moving beyond a binary understanding of being either male or female. I understand that the binary system works for some people, but it doesn't work for me. And I know there are other cultures that have more expansive understandings of gender, because gender is culturally specific and socially constructed.

REFLECTIVE QUESTION

Many people who are attracted to people of the same sex do not want to attach a label to their sexual orientation. Why might this be so?

Pathologising gender and sexual diversity

Theoretical positions on human sexuality have been historically understood through the dominance of the male/female, masculine/feminine and heterosexual/homosexual binaries. For many years, the diagnosis of gender identity disorder (GID) (American Psychiatric Association (APA), 2000) required the person to identify as heterosexual. GID was renamed 'gender dysphoria' in the *Diagnostic and Statistical Manual of Mental Disorders* (APA, 2013) or DSM-5. Along with these changes was the creation of separate categories for gender dysphoria in children, adolescents and adults. The grouping was given its own category.

The perpetuation of social stigma towards same-sex attracted people resulted in the category of homosexuality being moved from the realm of religious and moral understandings to the realm of pathology (Loue, 2020). Homosexuality was thus perceived as a behaviour rather than an identity, and therefore classified as a mental illness in the DSM-1 (APA, 1952). However, social changes precipitated by equal rights movements led to gay rights activists pressuring the medical establishment to remove homosexuality from the DSM-3 in 1973. Gay and lesbian activism in Aotearoa New Zealand also led to the decriminalisation of homosexuality in 1986, through the *Homosexual Law Reform Act 1986* (NZ). Nonetheless, gender diversity continues to be pathologised, particularly non-binary genders. In order to access health care, especially health care relevant to gender transition, most gender-diverse people have to submit to the pathologising medical paradigm, which regards diversity as something to be treated and fixed. It is proposed that further legislative changes will have a positive effect on the well-being of GSD people. The passing of the *Marriage (Definition of Marriage) Amendment Act 2013* in Aotearoa New Zealand and the *Marriage Equality (Same Sex) Act 2013* in Australia has afforded same-sex couples the same rights as heterosexuals; for example, queer partners are now recognised as next of kin, which means they are able to make healthcare decisions on behalf of their partners in the same way as a spouse in a heterosexual relationship.

Intersex people face a different challenge because medical interventions on intersex bodies often occur when the infant or child is too young to understand the situation. The medicalisation and subsequent surgical interventions upon intersex infants and children remain continuing human rights issues (Carpenter, 2016; Roen, 2019).

Hetero-sexism and hetero-normativity

Hetero-sexism is described as the predisposition to considering heterosexuality as normal, and is biased against people from other sexual orientations within health systems (Vargas, Huey & Miranda, 2020). In their story, Riley uses the word 'queer'; a term that has been regarded as derogatory in the past but has been reclaimed (Barker & Scheele, 2016) to explain that the understandings of normal sexuality lie within a frame of hetero-normativity. Hetero-normativity also shapes how perceptions of otherness are constructed, and who deserves to be accepted in society. Queer analysis therefore highlights that hetero-normative understandings of gender diversity are embedded within the context of power and that such dominant heterosexual and gender roles exist in order to regulate social life (Weeks, 2017).

Gender and health

Gender roles, norms and responsibilities are some of the social determinants of mental health in people. For example, the feeling that one lacks autonomy over one's life increases the risk of developing a depressive disorder, particularly in women. Similarly, the socialisation of men not to show certain emotions also puts them at risk of developing mental and physical health problems when faced with the loss of a partner (World Health Organization (WHO), 2015). Women experience considerably more psychological distress and mental illness associated with reproductive health than men (WHO, 2013).

Maternal mental health

Mental health practitioners have an important role to play in the well-being of mothers and babies, and have developed specialist practices within the area of maternal mental health. Pregnancy and childbirth also place women at greater risk of mental illness; for example in Aotearoa New Zealand, post-natal depression was higher in respondents with Asian ethnicity, lower household income, lower levels of formal education and younger age (Deverick & Guiney, 2017). Practitioners in this specialty offer a broad range of interventions, such as the assessment and support of women who have serious and enduring mental illness, and guidance and advice on medication during the pregnancy trimesters and while breastfeeding. Practitioners are also instrumental in preparing women and their partners in caring for the new baby. Treatments provided by these specialist practitioners are evidence-based talking therapies, such as cognitive behavioural therapy (CBT) for the individual mother or couple, group work and family therapy. Support for both the partner and the wider family is also essential at this stage of human development. The practitioner must also avoid making hetero-normative assumptions about who is the mother's partner and who is the father of the baby. About 11 per cent of Australian gay men and 33 per cent of lesbians have children (Dempsey, 2013); these numbers are increasing, and therefore practitioners need to work in a culturally inclusive way to ensure they do not further marginalise GSD groups (Kelly & Surtees, 2013; O'Neill, Hamer & Dixon, 2013) .

Reducing the risk of mental distress during the perinatal period is achieved when the maternal mental health practitioner works collaboratively with the midwife, a general practitioner (GP) or obstetrician to provide comprehensive care and support to mothers and their significant others. Seng and Taylor (2015) emphasised that as trauma-informed care and interventions increase in mental health and addiction settings, practitioners are required also to address the intergenerational cycles of childhood trauma and psychiatric vulnerability in childbearing women with a history of childhood maltreatment.

For example, one in three women who have a history of sexual violence are likely to experience a post-traumatic stress disorder; therefore, careful consideration must be given to developing a suitable birth plan for the mother, in an approach that is trauma-informed. In so doing, the risk factors are decreased for the mother and promote maternal bonding and overall welfare of the new baby (Erickson, Julian & Muzik, 2019).

Culturally competent human connectedness

Cultural competence within practice ensures that practitioners have the appropriate cultural competencies, knowledge and skills to respond effectively in all cultural encounters (Campinha-Bacote, 2006). For registered health practitioners, cultural competencies are determined by the practitioner's registering body. Increasing one's awareness of the historical, social and political influences on health will foster the development of relationships that engender trust and respect (Jeffreys, 2016).

It is equally important for practitioners to reflect on their own gender and sexual orientation and to consider the inherent assumptions and values derived from their socialisation within a predominantly hetero-normative environment. Essentially, if the practitioner does not use inclusive language then they cannot be regarded as providing safe care (Flemmer et al., 2012). Within a culturally competent human connectedness (CCHC) framework, the practitioner can demonstrate an understanding of the specific needs of the cultural group in question. However, the mental health system is not immune to the power structures that perpetuate heterosexist and homophobic attitudes. Reflections on the practitioner's own cultural safety are paramount, and support from senior practitioners who are also challenging and changing such discriminatory practices will reduce the moral distress that is present in everyday practice.

Exploring the relationship of gender identity and sexual orientation with mental distress is important to the person's recovery journey. However, GSD users of mental health services have reported that most health professionals they encounter do not ask about their sexual orientation within the standard mental health assessment (Semp & Read, 2015). When health professionals do ask and respond positively to disclosures of sexual orientation, it increases the person's sense of safety and acceptance, rather than feelings of invisibility, fear and alienation (Cahill & Makadon, 2014).

Likewise, similar skills are transferrable in response to disclosures of interpersonal violence. Unfortunately, the myth is perpetuated that interpersonal violence does not occur within the GSD population (Human Rights Commission, 2020). Practitioners can demonstrate use of the above CCHC framework to address the specific needs of this cultural group, so as to dispel such myths and provide appropriate support and resources for victims of violence and abuse.

How to talk to people about sexual orientation and gender diversity

Human connectedness is fostered when the practitioner puts the person at ease at the beginning of the assessment process. Some of the following suggestions will help practitioners learn how to ask these important questions:

- An open and safe approach is to tell people that it is 'standard policy' to ask questions about gender and sexuality because they are important topics for many people. You could say: 'Some people want to talk about gender identity or sexual orientation. Is there anything about those topics you would like to discuss?' Or: 'When we are discussing your personal history, this is a safe place to talk about gender or sexuality, if you want to.'
- Check the person's gender identity by asking: 'We have you recorded on the referral form as female/male (as relevant). Is this how you would like me to record your gender?'
- When collecting information about sexual orientation or gender identity, it is always important to respect privacy and check with the person whether they are comfortable with you recording details of the conversation, or disclosing this information to other staff members. Use the person's preferred name and pronouns ('he' or 'she' or 'they'), as requested, in conversation and clinical note-taking.

REFLECTIVE QUESTIONS

- If the person asks why you are asking the above questions, one response could be: 'We ask about sexuality and gender as they can be important yet difficult issues to discuss in our society, and it is important that people know they can discuss these issues here without being judged' (Semp & Read, 2015). What are some other responses you can think of?
- When you ask about relationships, ask: 'Do you have a partner?' and, if so, 'What do they do?', rather than 'What does your husband do?' The former response demonstrates openness and acceptance. What other, similar, inclusive assessment questions might you ask?
- In sum, hetero-normativity and cis-normativity are often perpetuated through language, unintentionally, and perpetuate the person's experience of being treated as 'not normal' or 'lesser than' in some way. Therefore, it is good practice to use gender-neutral language as much as possible, especially about relationships, such as use of the term 'partner' rather than 'husband' or 'wife', which some people find exclusive.

Source: Birkenhead & Rands (2012) and Semp & Read (2015).

PERSONAL NARRATIVE

Riley – gender recognition

I talked about the continuum of gender with my psychiatrist because I wanted her to understand the variety of options that I had seen out in the queer worlds. I wanted to bring that expansiveness into this medical encounter. None of my answers matched the criteria in the DSM.

I told the psychiatrist that I knew that there was a clash between the white, Western medical paradigm, which only acknowledges the existence of binary male and female genders, and my lived experience. My experience, and my own identity, had taught me that gender is a complicated dance of self and body within a wider context of social recognition. There is a vast array of genders, but often people experience violence because they do not fit into either male or female construction, or are considered not 'masculine enough' or 'feminine enough' for either.

I said that I knew that sexuality was more complex than we generally admit, and I knew many people who did not identify as simply gay or straight. When she asked me about my sexuality, I said, 'I am attracted to people'. I specified that gender-diverse or queer people were usually the ones I was more attracted to, but there isn't a label for that, except maybe 'queer'.

In the end, the psychiatrist looked at me, sighed, and said with some resignation: 'I cannot diagnose you with gender identity disorder, or gender dysphoria'.

I agreed, enthusiastically! She asked what we should do. I suggested that she write a letter to the endocrinologist, stating that I was mentally healthy and capable of making this decision. She did so, right there in front of me. I was so impressed by that.

We basically used an 'informed consent' model, instead of a diagnostic model. She still needed to know that I understood all the risks and had realistic expectations about what testosterone injections would do to my body. She needed to know that I also had support from family and friends.

Although the psychiatrist and I composed the letter to send to the endocrinologist, I noticed she was using female pronouns in reference to me in the letter. I asked if she could change them to male pronouns, which was what most of my friends were using for me. She said no, because 'it would only confuse the doctor'. I didn't want to push my luck, so I said okay. Later I reflected on how frustrating it was that I was asking to be recognised as the person that I already knew I was (even if that is somewhat ambiguous, because we're all in the process of 'becoming' all the time). I was being asked to identify as male, in order to access testosterone therapy, but in the same hour I was told I couldn't use male pronouns in a referral letter because other medical professionals would get 'confused'.

I felt powerless in that moment, as if I had offered to show a very vulnerable part of myself, and someone had said, 'No, you do not get to decide who you are'. I got the impression that I could only be 'he' when I looked 'typically male'. It felt to me as though I was 'not allowed' to be 'he' while I still looked, to them, like an androgynous, queer girl. It was sad and frustrating because I had talked about identifying as a boy, and how I felt more comfortable with 'he' rather than 'she', but it was assumed (by a lot of people, my psychiatrist included) that until I had completed some kind of medical transition, I could not legitimately be a boy.

I could only expect to be recognised as myself, and be treated as a boy, when I was no longer 'confusing'. Instead of expanding the understanding of my medical support people (psychiatrist, GP, mental health practitioners, endocrinologist), I felt like I had to shrink myself down to fit into the narrow criteria of acceptable masculinity. I had to wait for them to respect how I identified, wait until I looked male enough that they wouldn't feel too troubled calling me 'he'.

REFLECTIVE QUESTION

Riley's account demonstrates how he helped the psychiatrist understand gender fluidity; reflect on your own confidence and skill in responding, in the same way as Riley did, to one of your colleagues in your clinical setting.

In this encounter with the psychiatrist, Riley knew that there was a tension between the continuing influences of the biomedical view of homosexuality and psychiatric treatment that may still exist for some medical practitioners, particularly that the person can be viewed as a passive recipient of care. In contrast, the informed consent model accepts that Riley has full capacity to make an informed choice, and therefore this represents a rights-based approach to practice. The power of Riley's narrative in the encounter with the psychiatrist helped to change the outcome because the psychiatrist heard and validated Riley's informed opinions. Riley's explanation was accepted as their truth and not translated into the biomedical paradigm. Therefore, when Riley began their hormone treatment they found that the nurse at the endocrinology clinic who was administering Riley's injections was equally supportive and inclusive of their identity, likely because the approach by the psychiatrist was a rights-based approach and Riley was not labelled as 'mentally ill'. That these practitioners worked in tandem to support diversity is an example of culturally competent human connectedness between the psychiatrist, the nurse and Riley. In so doing, their practice sustained Riley's autonomy and ability to take the lead in directing future medical interventions that were appropriate to them.

PERSONAL NARRATIVE

Riley – privileged support

Throughout this process with my psychiatrist, I also reflected on how my privilege, as a well-educated *pākehā* (a non-Māori New Zealander) with white skin, had greatly improved my chances of being understood and being recognised as an expert on my own experience. I got what I needed from this medical encounter, and my endocrinologist accepted the informed consent letter that my psychiatrist had written. I knew that if I hadn't been as confident and articulate, if I hadn't known all the right academic and community terms to use, I would've had a much harder time. I felt grateful that I had successfully negotiated a way to access the treatment I needed, without relying on the DSM. But I was also left with a feeling of frustration about how the medical system failed to recognise my complex, or 'confusing', gender. It was my privilege that enabled me to get the support I needed. I feel worried about a medical system that relies on us having this level of privilege, since many of us are not white or middle-class and do not go to university. What happens then?

REFLECTIVE QUESTION

In pairs, discuss the psychiatrist's decision to use the 'she' pronoun and the possible link to cis-normativity (and to a lesser extent hetero-normativity) within the medical profession. If the psychiatrist had used the 'he' pronoun, do you think it would have confused the endocrinologist?

Effects of homophobia, homonegativity and trans-phobia

homophobia – the fear of, or aversion to, homosexuals

homonegativity – the negative behaviours, attitudes or expressions towards queer people

trans-phobia – a feeling of disgust toward individuals who do not conform to society's gender expectations

Although the Yogyakarta Principles (International Commission of Jurists, 2007) embody the rights of GSD to attain similar standards of physical and mental health as heterosexuals, the effects of **homophobia**, **homonegativity** and **trans-phobia** continue to have a profound effect on the mental health of GSD people (Morandini et al., 2015). For example, people who identify as lesbian or gay have higher rates of mental illness, self-harm and suicide attempts than heterosexuals (Lytle, De Luca & Blosnich, 2014; Rehman, Lopes & Jaspal, 2020). Further, people who identify as lesbian or gay who experience higher levels of homophobia are significantly more likely to use drugs and alcohol (Green & Feinstein, 2012), and four times more likely to develop a substance abuse disorder (McCabe et al., 2010). Given that GSD groups experience higher levels of mental health conditions (Leonard, Lyons & Bariola, 2015; Adams, Dickinson & Asiasiga, 2012) than their heterosexual counterparts, it should be of concern to all practitioners that this vulnerable population continues to avoid seeking health care due to hetero-normative and homophobic attitudes within health settings (Barefoot et al., 2015; Hayman et al., 2013).

REFLECTIVE QUESTION

In pairs, discuss the role of the practitioner in influencing a safe passage through the health system for people who are perceived as not fitting the norm. How will you establish trusting relationships with people who have not had positive experiences with clinical staff in the past?

Genders, sexualities and power

Foucault (1979) argued that, as sexual subjects, humans are the object of power. Communities interpret biological differences between men and women to create a set of social norms and behaviours that are considered appropriate for these genders. These norms determine men's and women's access to their rights, resources, influence and power within society, such as health care. Although the specific nature and degree of these differences vary from one society or ethnicity to the next, they typically favour men, creating an imbalance in power, gender and ethnic inequity that perpetuate; for example, family violence (Pihama et al., 2016). The notion of intimacy within a relationship assumes that there is equal power between partners (Williams, 2008), yet the influence of social norms and gender roles can affect the sharing of equal power. Adams (2012) argues that traditionally men have maintained dominance in many aspects of society, such as work and the home, by sharing a collective masculine identity and central belief that men should be 'in charge' (p. 14). As practitioners, it is important that we are aware of these structural inequities that inform the experiences of consumers, such as how women are socialised, the effects of pathologising difference, stigma, labelling and hetero-normativity. Such hostile and benevolent sexism and misogyny within society affect all people, perpetuate negative stereotypes against men and women, and create an environment that supports and perpetuates interpersonal and intimate partner violence and abuse (World Health Organization (WHO), 2005).

Interpersonal and intimate partner violence and abuse

This final section of the chapter looks at the nature of abusive interpersonal and **intimate partner abuse** (hereafter **interpersonal abuse**) experiences many people have endured and survived, and the ways in which such experiences can manifest as psychological distress and mental illness. Suggestions are made about how practitioners might create safe interpersonal spaces in which to engage with peoples' narratives of interpersonal abuse, helping to avoid re-traumatisation and promoting recovery.

Developing a therapeutic relationship is a fundamental skill or technology in mental health practice. It creates a safe space within which the person can talk about their life, worries, current challenges, and hopes and dreams for the future. The therapeutic relationship creates the place in which the unspeakable may be spoken, and in which the unspoken can be expressed in symbolic language or behaviour and can be recognised and accepted. In listening to accounts of interpersonal abuse, the practitioner helps the person to find understanding, meaning, acceptance and compassion for themselves. It is the profound human connection between the person and the practitioner that enables a sharing and co-construction of a personal narrative that constitutes the work of recovery. For many people, psychological distress often arises from terrible experiences of abuse caused by a known and often loved and trusted person. Our witnessing of these accounts is part of the work of the mental health practitioner.

Interpersonal and intimate partner abuse

Interpersonal abuse occurs in the context of an interpersonal or intimate relationship or situation that is distressing and harmful (Australian Institute of Health and Welfare, 2019). Interpersonal abuse occurs among people who know each other; for example, intimate partners, family members, friends, colleagues, teachers and religious leaders. Most interpersonal abuse is said to be perpetrated by men upon women and children, although women have also been shown to be abusers (Gannon & Alleyne, 2012; McNulty, 2012). Despite the progress of human rights legislation, a male sense of entitlement to power, control and the privilege of access to female bodies for sexual and domestic services remains pervasive. The Duluth model of power and control (Duluth Domestic Abuse Intervention Projects, 2017) (see Figure 15.1) summarises the strategies used to achieve compliance and acquiescence within interpersonal relationships, described as intimate or sexual terrorism (Frye et al., 2006).

intimate partner abuse – any behaviour within an intimate relationship that causes physical, psychological or sexual harm to those in the relationship; such behaviours include acts of physical aggression such as slapping, hitting, kicking and beating (WHO, 2012)

interpersonal abuse – interpersonal abuse and violence include intimate partner abuse, sexual assault, child abuse, bullying and elder abuse. Violence is not just physical: it includes emotional, sexual, economic and social abuse (RACGP 2014).

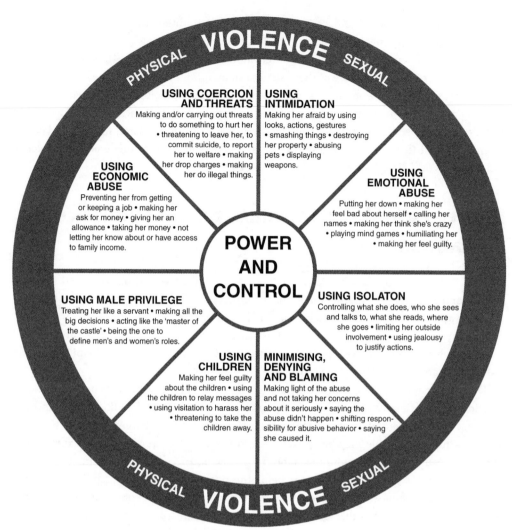

Figure 15.1   The Duluth Power and Control Wheel

Source: Domestic Abuse Intervention Project (2017).

Family and intimate partner violence

Female victims are often held responsible for violent acts of sexual terrorism against them and because these assaults often are not taken seriously by authorities; it has been estimated that 90 per cent of victims do not report these crimes to police (Ministry of Justice, 2009). In Aotearoa New Zealand, one in three women has experienced family or intimate partner violence (Fenrich & Contesse, 2009). Similarly, in Australia, an estimated one in six Australian women (1.6 million or 17 per cent) and one in 16 men (547 600 or 6.1 per cent) aged 18 years and over has experienced partner violence since the age of 15 (Australian Bureau of Statistics, 2017, 2020).

In recognition of this high rate of family and intimate partner violence, a systematic approach to screening (Miller et al., 2015), needs to be the responsibility of all health professionals, particularly in emergency departments (Sprague et al., 2012).

It is of note that family and intimate partner violence are evident in GSD populations; however, barriers to victims seeking help continue to exist (Calton, Cattaneo & Gebhard, 2016). Though this is an area that requires more research, Edwards and Sylaska (2012) have reported that minority-group stress, such as victimisation, stigma and internal homonegativity, may play a part in family and intimate partner violence.

Currently, in Aotearoa New Zealand (New Zealand Ministry of Justice, n.d.), all women aged 16 to 65 years who present to any health service are screened for family or intimate partner physical violence upon arrival. Three standard questions that are perceived as non-threatening and safe are recommended and should be asked in the context of an overall assessment. These are:

1   Have you been hit, kicked, punched or otherwise hurt by someone within the past year? If so, by whom?
2   Do you feel safe in your current relationship?
3   Is there a partner from a previous relationship who is making you feel unsafe now?

The screening focuses on current *physical* abuse and safety rather than historical abuse and its effects. Screening for histories of abuse and trauma in all people who present to mental health and addiction services is discussed further in Chapter 2, including a broader overview of trauma-informed care and how to translate this approach into your everyday practice.

Helen's story – disclosure of interpersonal abuse

Asking people about interpersonal abuse requires confidence and skill in the practitioner. People are waiting to be asked yet are unlikely to spontaneously disclose; if we do not ask then the person will think that their experiences are not relevant to their current situation. It is also important to consider that the person has likely been sworn to secrecy by the perpetrator, hence we need to guide the disclosure safely. To do so, I developed the skills of the following steps, described as the *funnel technique* (see Figure 15.2).

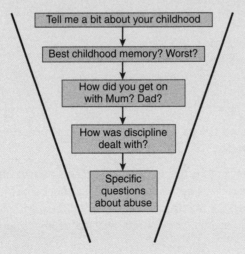

TRANSLATION TO PRACTICE

Figure 15.2   The funnel technique, from general to specific questions

Source: Read, Hammersley & Rudegeair (2007, p. 105).

The funnelling questions begin with gathering information about the person's childhood and upbringing; for example, 'Tell me about your best childhood memories'. Then they lead on to asking about how discipline was dealt with in the family: 'Were you ever chastised, or sent to your room?' This opens a space for the person to talk further about details, such as being hit with a belt etc., as a means of discipline. I can then then respond by introducing the term 'physical abuse'.

At all stages of the interview it is also important that I read the person's body language to be assured that I am progressing the interview safely and with compassion. I can then elicit whether there were any experiences that involved psychological or sexual abuse, and remain aware that the person may describe these experiences as part of the 'norm' in their family. I am also mindful that the perpetrator may have groomed the person as the child, therefore I take the opportunity to link their experiences to the term 'abuse'. Particularly in mental health settings, it is important that we believe the person and not reinforce the stereotype that their experiences are symptoms of a psychiatric disorder, such as a delusion. My role is to normalise the notion that abuse is commonly reported by people seeking help and that they are not alone in these experiences.

At this point, the person may be both relieved and ashamed, upset, or angry about the realisation that they have been betrayed by the abuser. Therefore, I need to express confidence and a non-judgemental approach in developing a collaborative plan to support the person over the next few days. Having revealed the 'secret' about their abuse, I will need to assure the person that they have some control over what happens next.

My role is to consult with other practitioners in the team, develop a plan to keep the person emotionally and physically safe, and to document some details in their clinical notes – while remaining fully collaborative with the person to increase their sense of control. If there are imminent risks to themselves or others, then safety is paramount. My goal is to help the person connect with the appropriate agency to begin their journey of trauma resolution and healing; this may be an external agency rather than my current clinical service. It is also important that I seek support from my team members to address my own responses upon hearing these accounts, which may trigger my own sadness, anger and sense of injustice about what the people I serve have had to endure.

SUMMARY

This chapter has presented stories and information, supplemented by activities designed to deepen your understanding of:

- The mental health needs of the range of gender and sexually diverse identities across the life span. There are many societal assumptions and rules about sexuality and gender; therefore, having an understanding of the gender and sexually diverse communities will assist nurses to actively reduce the stigma, homophobia and the traumatising effects of these on this population.
- The practice of cultural competence and cultural humility to promote human connectedness, and to foster relationships that engender trust and respect. Nurses need to reflect on their

own gender and sexual orientation to consider the inherent assumptions and values derived from their socialisation within a predominantly hetero-normative health system. By adopting inclusive language, nurses can demonstrate safe care as well as challenge and change discriminatory practices in everyday practice.

- The higher rates of interpersonal violence and abuse experienced by gender and sexually diverse people. Nurses can play a role in screening and responding safely to victims of violence and abuse. In so doing, nurses promote the person's mental well-being and their physical health, and increase their personal power

CRITICAL THINKING/LEARNING ACTIVITIES

1   Re-read the definition of hetero-normativity and then make a list of what you perceive to be the traditional gender roles within couple relationships that are perpetuated; for example, by the cinema and print and social media. Compare these roles to the changes, if any, that you are witnessing in society or within your social circle.

2   In the first section of Riley's narrative he told us that the 'problem was not me; it was the assumptions of the people around me who knew nothing more than the binary of male and female'. What may be some of the similar assumptions and actions that practitioners may engage in that could be disrespectful of Riley and his gender identity?

3   Riley also said: 'I feel worried about a medical system that relies on us having this level of privilege, since many of us are not white or middle-class and do not go to university. What happens then?' If you were able to continue this conversation with Riley and respond to his question, what may be some of the key points that you would like to discuss and debate in response to his concerns?

4   The Duluth model of power and control (Figure 15.1) summarised the strategies used to achieve compliance and acquiescence within interpersonal relationships. Either individually or with one of your peers, reflect on these strategies and note any that may apply to people you know, or even to yourself.

5   Review the funnel technique diagram (Figure 15.2) and, in pairs, practise asking the questions to assess the presence of violence and/or abuse. Reflect on your own reactions to asking and responding to the disclosures.

LEARNING EXTENSION

Riley explained that even though there is a vast array of genders, people continue to experience violence because they do not fit into either male or female gender roles or are considered not 'masculine enough' or 'feminine enough'. Make a list of the negative words commonly used to describe people who do not fit the above stereotypes. Write a paragraph answering the following reflective questions:

- How would you feel if these terms were applied to you, your friends or your family?
- How might practitioners assist in challenging and changing this hurtful language in our personal and work lives?

FURTHER READING

Barbara, A. M., Doctor, F. & Chaim, G. (2007). *Asking the Right Questions 2: Talking with clients about sexual orientation and gender identity in mental health, counselling and addiction settings.* Toronto: Centre for Addiction and Mental Health.

This manual is very practical and applicable in both the mental health and substance abuse services, and is relevant to the Australasian setting.

Read, J., Hammersley, P. & Rudegeair, T. (2007). Why, when and how to ask about childhood abuse. *Advances in Psychiatric Treatment, 13*(2): 101–10.

This seminal paper gives an excellent account of the interviewing skills described as the 'funnelling technique', and will complement your further learning in Chapter 2.

Stevens, M. W. (2013). *Rainbow Health: The public health needs of LGBTTI communities in Aotearoa New Zealand with policy recommendations.* Auckland: Affinity Services. Retrieved from http://www.rainbowtick.nz/wp-content/uploads/2019/03/Affinity_Services_Rainbow_Health_Report.pdf

This report discusses the health needs and the marginalising factors that lead to discrimination – both personal and structural – and that affect this marginalised group.

United Nations High Commissioner for Human Rights. (2012). *Born Free and Equal: Sexual orientation and gender identity in international human rights law.* New York: United Nations High Commissioner for Human Rights. Retrieved from http://www.ohchr.org/Documents/Publications/BornFreeAndEqualLowRes.pdf

The United Nations Human Rights Office released this publication on sexual orientation and gender identity in international human rights law. It sets out the source and scope of some of the core legal obligations that nation states have in protecting the human rights of gender and sexually diverse populations.

REFERENCES

Adams, J., Dickinson, P. & Asiasiga, L. (2012). *Mental Health Promotion and Prevention Services to Gay Lesbian, Bisexual, Transgender and Intersex Populations in New Zealand: Needs assessment report.* Retrieved from www.mentalhealth.org.nz/file/downloads/pdf/file_459.pdf

Adams, P. J. (2012). *Masculine Empire: How men use violence to keep women in line.* Auckland: Dunmore Publishing Ltd.

American Psychiatric Association (APA). (1952). *Diagnostic and Statistical Manual of Mental Disorders.* Washington, DC: APA.

——— (2000). *Diagnostic and Statistical Manual of Mental Disorders: DSM-IV-TR,* 4th edn. Washington, DC: APA.

——— (2013). *Diagnostic and Statistical Manual of Mental Disorders: DSM-V,* 5th edn. Washington, DC: APA.

Australian Bureau of Statistics (ABS). (2017). *Personal safety.* Retrieved from http://www.abs.gov.au/ausstats/abs@.nsf/mf/4906.0

——— (2020). *Partner Violence – In focus: Crime and justice statistics.* Retrieved from https://www.abs.gov.au/statistics/people/crime-and-justice/focus-crime-and-justice-statistics/january-2020

Australian Government. (2013). *Australian Government Guidelines on the Recognition of Sex and Gender.* Retrieved from https://www.ag.gov.au/rights-and-protections/publications/australian-government-guidelines-recognition-sex-and-gender

Australian Institute of Health Welfare. (2019). *Family, Domestic and Sexual Violence in Australia: Continuing the national story 2019.* Retrieved from https://www.aihw.gov.au/reports/domestic-violence/family-domestic-sexual-violence-australia-2019/contents/summary

Barefoot, K. N., Rickard, A., Smalley, K. B. & Warren, J. C. (2015). Rural lesbians: Unique challenges and implications for mental health providers. *Journal of Rural Mental Health, 39*(1): 22–33.

Barker, M.-J. & Scheele, J. (2016). *Queer: A graphic history.* London: Icon Books.

Bennett, B. & Gates, T. G. (2019). Teaching cultural humility for social workers serving LGBTQI Aboriginal communities in Australia. *Social Work Education, 38*(5): 604–17.

Birkenhead, A. & Rands, D. (2012). *Let's Talk about Sex (Sexuality and Gender): Improving mental health and addiction services for rainbow communities.* Auckland: District Health Board.

Bornstein, K. & Bergman, S. B. (eds) (2010). *Gender Outlaws: The next generation.* New York: Seal Press.

Bosse, J. D., Leblanc, R. G., Jackman, K. & Bjarnadottir, R. I. (2018). Benefits of implementing and improving collection of sexual orientation and gender identity data in electronic health records. *CIN: Computers, Informatics, Nursing, 36*(6): 267–74.

Cahill, S. & Makadon, H. (2014). Sexual orientation and gender identity data collection in clinical settings and in electronic health records: A key to ending LGBT health disparities. *LGBT Health, 1*(1): 34–41.

Calton, J. M., Cattaneo, L. B. & Gebhard, K. T. (2016). Barriers to help seeking for lesbian, gay, bisexual, transgender, and queer survivors of intimate partner violence. *Trauma, Violence, & Abuse, 17*(5): 585–600.

Campinha-Bacote, J. (2006). Cultural competence in nursing curricula: How are we doing 20 years later? *Journal of Nursing Education, 45*(7): 243–4.

Carpenter, M. (2016). The human rights of intersex people: Addressing harmful practices and rhetoric of change. *Reproductive Health Matters, 24*(47): 74–84.

Dempsey, D. (2013). *Same-sex Parented Families in Australia.* Retrieved from https://www.gaylawnet .com/ezine/family/cfca18.pdf

Deverick, Z. & Guiney, H. (2017). *Findings from the 2015 New Mothers' Mental Health Survey.* Retrieved from www.hpa.org.nz

Domestic Abuse Intervention Project. (2017). *The Duluth Model: Power and Control Wheel.* Retrieved from https://www.theduluthmodel.org/wp-content/uploads/2017/03/PowerandControl.pdf

Edwards, K. M. & Sylaska, K. M. (2012). The perpetration of intimate partner violence among LGBTQ college youth: The role of minority stress. *Journal of Youth and Adolescence, 1*(11): 1721–31.

Erickson, N., Julian, M. & Muzik, M. (2019). Perinatal depression, PTSD, and trauma: Impact on mother–infant attachment and interventions to mitigate the transmission of risk. *International Review of Psychiatry, 31*(3): 245–63.

Fenrich, J. & Contesse, J. (2009). *'It's Not OK': New Zealand's efforts to eliminate violence against women.* New York: Leitner Centre for International Law and Justice.

Flemmer, N., Doutrich, D., Dekker, L. & Rondeau, D. (2012). Creating a safe and caring health care context for women who have sex with women. *Journal for Practitioner Practitioners, 8*(6): 421–96.

Foucault, M. (1979). *The History of Sexuality, Volume 1: An introduction.* New York: Vintage.

Frye, V., Manganello, J., Campbell, J. C., Walton-Moss, B. & Wilt, S. (2006). The distribution of and factors associated with intimate terrorism and situational couple violence among a population-based sample of urban women in the United States. *Journal of Interpersonal Violence, 21*(10): 1286–313.

Gannon, T. A. & Alleyne, E. K. A. (2012). Female sexual abusers' cognition: A systematic review. *Trauma, Violence, & Abuse, 14*(1): 67–79.

Global Gayz Australia. (2009). (Webpage). Retrieved from http://archive.globalgayz.com/oceania/ australia/gay-australia-aborigine-resources/

Green, K. E. & Feinstein, B. A. (2012). Substance use in lesbian, gay, and bisexual populations: An update on empirical research and implications for treatment. *Psychology of Addictive Behaviors, 26*(2): 265–78.

Harvard Medical School. (2021). Gender fluidity: What it means and why support matters (Webpage). Harvard Health Publishing. Retrieved from https://www.health.harvard.edu/blog/gender-fluidity-what-it-means-and-why-support-matters-2020120321544

Hayman, B., Wilkes, L., Halcomb, E. & Jackson, D. (2013). Marginalised mothers: Lesbian women negotiating heteronormative healthcare services. *Contemporary Nurse, 44*(1): 120–7.

Human Rights Commission. (2020). Common Myths about LGBTQ Domestic Violence (News blog). Retrieved from https://www.hrc.org/news/common-myths-about-lgbtq-domestic-violence

Human Rights Commission of New Zealand. (2020). Sexual Orientation and Gender Identity (Website). Retrieved from https://www.hrc.co.nz/our-work/sogiesc/

International Commission of Jurists. (2007). *Yogyakarta Principles: Principles on the application of international human rights law in relation to sexual orientation and gender identity*. Retrieved from www.unhcr.org/refworld/docid/48244e602.html

Jeffreys, M. R. (2016). *Teaching Cultural Competence in Nursing and Healthcare: Inquiry, action and innovation*, 3rd edn. New York: Springer.

Kelly, J. & Surtees, N. (2013). 'We are a family': Legal issues for lesbian and gay parented families in New Zealand. *Plymouth Law and Criminal Justice Review*, *5*: 39–49.

Leonard, W., Lyons, A. & Bariola, E. (2015). A closer look at private lives 2: Addressing the mental health and wellbeing of lesbian, gay, bisexual, and transgender (LGBT) Australians. Australian Policy Online (Website). Retrieved from http://apo.org.au/resource/closer-look-private-lives-2-addressing-mental-health-and-wellbeing-lesbian-gay-bisexual-and

Loue, S. (2020). Homosexuality: Sin, crime, pathology, identity, behavior. In S. Loue (ed.), *Case studies in society, religion, and bioethics* (pp. 13–36). New York: Springer.

Lytle, M. C., De Luca, S. M. & Blosnich, J. R. (2014). The influence of intersecting identities on self-harm, suicidal behaviors, and depression among lesbian, gay, and bisexual individuals. *Suicide and Life-Threatening Behavior*, *44*(4): 384–91.

McCabe S., Bostwick, W., Hughes, T., West, B. & Boyd, D. (2010). The relationship between discrimination and substance use disorders among lesbian, gay, and bisexual adults in the United States. *American Journal of Public Health*, *100*(10): 1946–52.

McNulty, E. A. (2012). Transcription and analysis of qualitative data in a study of women who sexually offended against children. *Qualitative Report*, *17*(47): 1–18.

Miller, E., McCaw, B., Humphreys, B. L. & Mitchell, C. (2015). Integrating intimate partner violence assessment and intervention into healthcare in the United States: A systems approach. *Journal of Women's Health*, *24*(1): 92–9.

Ministry of Justice. (2009). *Te toiora mata tauherenga: Report of the task force for action on sexual violence incorporating the views of Te Ohaakii a Hine* – National network ending sexual violence together – task force for action on sexual violence. Retrieved from www.justice.govt.nz/policy/supporting-victims/taskforce-for-action-on-sexual-violence/policy-and-consultation/taskforce-for-action-on-sexual-violence/documents/tasv-report-full

Morandini, J. S., Blaszczynski, A., Dar-Nimrod, I. & Ross, M. W. (2015). Minority stress and community connectedness among gay, lesbian and bisexual Australians: A comparison of rural and metropolitan localities. *Australia and New Zealand Journal of Public Health*, *39*(3): 260–6.

New Zealand Ministry of Justice. (n.d.). *Risk Assessment Management Framework*. Retrieved from https://www.justice.govt.nz/justice-sector-policy/key-initiatives/addressing-family-violence-and-sexual-violence/work-programme/risk-assessment-management-framework/

O'Neill, K. R., Hamer, H. P. & Dixon, R. (2013). Perspectives from lesbian women: Their experiences with healthcare professionals when transitioning to planned parenthood. *Diversity and Equality in Health and Care*, *10*(4): 213–22. Retrieved from http://www.ingentaconnect.com

Pihama, L., Te Nana, R., Cameron, N., Smith, C., Reid, J. & Southey, K. (2016). Māori cultural definitions of sexual violence. *Sexual Abuse in Australia and New Zealand: An Interdisciplinary Journal*, *7*(1): 43–51.

Read, J., Hammersley, P. & Rudegeair, T. (2007). Why, when and how to ask about childhood abuse. *Advances in Psychiatric Treatment*, *13*(2): 101–10.

Rehman, Z., Lopes, B. & Jaspal, R. (2020). Predicting self-harm in an ethnically diverse sample of lesbian, gay and bisexual people in the United Kingdom. *International Journal of Social Psychiatry*, *66*(4): 349–60.

Roen, K. (2019). Intersex or diverse sex development: Critical review of psychosocial health care research and indications for practice. *The Journal of Sex Research*, *56*(4–5): 511–28.

Royal Australian College of General Practitioners (RACGP). (2014). *Abuse and Violence: Working with our patients in general practice*. East Melbourne: RACGP.

Semp, D. & Read, J. (2015). Queer conversations: Improving access to, and quality of, mental health services for same-sex-attracted clients. *Psychology & Sexuality*, *6*(3): 217–228.

Seng, J. & Taylor, J. (2015). *Trauma Informed Care in the Perinatal Period*. Dunedin: Dunedin Academic Press.

Sprague, S., Madden, K., Simunovic, N., Godin, K., Pham, N. K., Bhandari, M., & Goslings, J. C. (2012). Barriers to screening for intimate partner violence. *Women & Health, 52*(6): 587–605.

United Nations High Commissioner for Human Rights. (2012). *Born Free and Equal: Sexual orientation and gender identity in international human rights law*. Retrieved from www.ohchr.org/Documents/Publications/BornFreeAndEqualLowRes.pdf

Vargas, S. M., Huey Jr, S. J. & Miranda, J. (2020). A critical review of current evidence on multiple types of discrimination and mental health. *American Journal of Orthopsychiatry, 90*(3): 374–90.

Weeks, J. (2017). *Sex, Politics and Society: The regulation of society since 1800*, 4th edn. London and New York: Routledge.

Williams, A. (2008). A literature review on the concept of intimacy in nursing. *Journal of Advanced Nursing, 33*(5): 660–7.

World Health Organization (WHO). (2005). *WHO Multi-country Study on Women's Health and Domestic Violence Against Women: Summary report of initial results on prevalence, health outcomes and women's responses*. Retrieved from www.who.int/gender/violence/who_multicountry_study/en

—— (2012). *Understanding and Addressing Violence Against Women: Intimate partner violence*. Retrieved from http://apps.who.int/iris/bitstream/handle/10665/77432/WHO_RHR_12.36_eng.pdf;jsessionid=45B95A76AF9EEE2C73C6BB96B9D26E6C?sequence=1

—— (2013). *Maternal and Child Mental Health*. Retrieved from http://www.who.int/mental_health/maternal-child/en/

—— (2015). *Sustainable Development Goal 5: Improving mental health*. Retrieved from http://www.who.int/gender-equity-rights/news/gender-health-sdgs/en/

16 Intellectual and developmental disability

Henrietta Trip, Margaret Hughes, Reece Adams
and Isaac Tait

LEARNING OBJECTIVES

On completion of this chapter, you should be able to:

1 Define and explain the nature and scope of learning, intellectual and developmental disability (IDD) and dual diagnosis.

2 Describe philosophical approaches that inform community living for people with IDD in contemporary society, including normalisation, social-role valorisation, the social model of disability, Enabling Good Lives – Aotearoa New Zealand and the National Disability Insurance Scheme – Australia.

3 Discuss and practise key concepts and approaches to inform, support and optimise the potential for meaningful lives for this population, including autonomy, choice and consent to facilitate supported decision-making.

4 Identify and discuss determinants of physical and mental health and illness that affect access, equity and well-being for people with IDD.

5 Explore enablers and barriers to reduce marginalisation and promote equitable engagement between the individual and their family/*whānau* and health and disability professionals, to meet the mental health needs of this population.

Introduction

This chapter provides a brief synopsis of the terminology of learning disability (LD), intellectual disability (ID) and developmental disability (DD). Determinants of physical and mental well-being and associated comorbidities for people living with IDD are explained. The personal narratives of an individual's and parent's perspective illustrate the fundamental principles, interpretations and translations to practice. This will help students to recognise, facilitate and optimise an individual's rights, identity, autonomy, and self-determination in any community or mental health setting.

In previous decades, deinstitutionalisation of people with IDD was informed by philosophical approaches including normalisation (Wolfensberger, 1972; Nirje, 1969), social-role valorisation (Wolfensberger, 1983) and more recently the social model of disability (Oliver, 2013; Race, Boxall & Carson, 2005). These approaches continue to inform mental health assessment and responsiveness through **reasonable adjustments** or accommodations; for example, in employment law (Heslop et al., 2019). Within Aotearoa New Zealand and Australia, these philosophies are exemplified through the principles embedded within Enabling Good Lives – Aotearoa New Zealand (EGL), and the National Disability Insurance Scheme – Australia (NDIS), respectively, and are linked to responsibilities under the *Convention on the Rights of Persons with Disabilities* (UNCRPD; United Nations, 2007) when working with people in mental distress.

> **reasonable adjustment** – this is multifactorial and includes organisational policies, environmental access and interested parties making adjustments or adaptations to the delivery of health and disability care, communication, information and services

Defining the terminology

Historically, LD, ID and DD were considered synonymous with mental illness, and changes in terminology reflect societal influences over time (Roth, Sarawgi & Fodstad, 2019). People with **intellectual and developmental disability (IDD)** were seen as abnormal and defective, were often institutionalised and therefore were excluded from the mainstream. Labels can be both diagnostic and identity-forming (Callard et al., 2012; Scior, Connolly & Williams, 2013), and when they are stigmatising, the focus is often on the deficits framed and perpetuated by society at the time. For example, until the 20th century 'the idiot', 'imbecile' and 'feeble-minded' were people determined unfit to be part of society and thus were subject to the *Mental Defectives Act 1911* (NZ) and similar legislation in the Australian states and territories.

In the United Kingdom, the preferred term for IDD is 'learning disability', whereas in Australasia it is 'intellectual disability' and, until recently, 'mental retardation' in the United States (Luckasson et al., 2002). Today, the purpose of diagnostic labels is to focus on a person's functioning and contextual factors that facilitate their learning and enable application of their abilities. Stigmatising terms and diagnostic labels continue to perpetuate misunderstandings and challenge perceptions about individuals, their *whānau* and their networks of support (Scior et al., 2013). Since population groups are not homogenous, the value and purpose of these labels remain contentious. Labels may identify individual need, can inform the development of responsive health and disability systems, and highlight gaps in service delivery (Scior et al., 2013). ID, DD and LD might be used interchangeably, depending on the jurisdiction, discipline and population. We recommend the term 'IDD' for health professionals, to encompass what this population can teach us. An understanding of these terms as both

> **intellectual and developmental disability (IDD)** – people living with limitations in intellectual, social and adaptive functioning that may include sensory or neurodevelopmental challenges

diagnostic and sociopolitical constructs informs what community access means in the context of a dual diagnosis. There has been a substantial move from perspectives of limitation to those which understand:

> disability as a function of the fit between the person's capacities and the demands of the environment ... Of course, it is not just how the construct is understood that is important; it is how the people so labelled both are perceived and perceive themselves. (Wehmeyer, 2013, p. 124)

Intellectual disability

The three core criteria for a diagnosis of IDD are deficits in intellectual functioning (intelligence quotient (IQ) < 70), challenges in social and adaptive functioning and evidence of onset within the developmental period, which is deemed to be prior to 18 years of age (American Psychiatric Association (APA), 2013). It is important to note that while this appears to be a deficits model, strengths always coexist with deficits and, an understanding of a person's skills and abilities informs the basis of the supports and interventions needed.

Developmental disability

People who live with a DD may, or may not, match the above criteria, as DD represents a lifelong impairment or degenerative condition that may affect the sensory system (e.g. cytomegalovirus), nervous system (e.g. cerebral palsy, fragile X) or metabolism (e.g. phenylketonuria, congenital hypothyroidism). Autism spectrum disorder (ASD), for example, is a neuro-developmental disorder and is defined in the DSM-V as those who present with 'persistent difficulties with social communication and social interaction ... restricted and repetitive patterns of behaviours, activities or interests', which may include hyper-sensory or hypo-sensory reactivity (APA, 2013).

Learning disability

It is important not to confuse LD as used in the United Kingdom with *learning difficulty*, which is used to refer to a specific remediable condition, such as dyslexia, in which the person usually functions without supports beyond this need. While jurisdictions use different terms, People First New Zealand – Ngā Tāngata Tuatahi, (https://www.peoplefirst.org.nz/), a self-advocacy organisation, is seeking to change the preferred term to 'LD', to better reflect a strengths-based approach. In Australia, the term 'ID' is preferred; however, a strengths-based emphasis to increase this population's social participation and community engagement through avenues such as the NDIS.

It is estimated that 1 per cent of the global population has an ID, although the range is considerable, and higher in low-to-middle income countries (Maulik et al., 2011). Establishing the prevalence of ID in Aotearoa New Zealand on the basis of actual diagnostic information is flawed. According to Statistics New Zealand (2013), people with a primary ID comprise 2 per cent of the total population, based upon self-report or proxy reporting on primary disability as part of the census. In Australia, the prevalence of ID is estimated at 1.8 per cent of the total population (Trollor et al., 2017); however, the diagnosis of people with ID also remains inconsistent, and the need for a standardised assessment has been identified (Maulik et al., 2011).

Dual diagnosis or dual disability

Dual diagnosis is a term that has been used historically to refer to people who live with a mental illness and/or a substance use disorder. It is a term that has also been used to refer to people who live with a mental illness and an ID (Tang et al., 2008), and considerations about assessment for mental illness in people with IDD are complex and multifactorial (Britt, Davies & Daffue, 2017).

dual diagnosis/ disability – people who live with a mental illness and an ID

Aetiology

There are more than 450 genetic causes for intellectual, developmental and learning disability, beyond which unknown aetiology accounts for up to 61.4 per cent (Goldfarb & Frankel, 2007). Neuro-developmental disorders (NDD) is a broad term that encompasses disorders that interfere with people's functioning, concentration, decision-making, memory, communication, problem-solving and social interaction. Only a small proportion of people with a NDD, such as ASD or attention deficit and hyperactivity disorder (ADHD) will have an intellectual disability and/or develop a mental illness (Morris-Rosendahl & Crocq, 2020). This section provides a brief introduction to some of the attributable causative factors of IDD.

Common causes

Among others (Yim, 2015), Fragile X is the leading genetic and neuro-developmental cause of ID, followed by Down syndrome. The former is more common in males and the latter, also known as Trisomy 21, means a person has three copies of chromosome 21 (del Hoyo Soriano et al., 2020). Table 16.1 outlines a few non-genetic causes.

Table 16.1 Non-genetic causes of intellectual and developmental disability

Type	Description and examples
Nutritional deficiency	When the body lacks sufficient input or ability to metabolise vitamins and minerals that sustain foetal development – including folic acid, iodine deficiency and malnutrition (Gernand et al., 2016)
Pregnancy and labour issues	Viral infections including rubella or cytomegalovirus, pre-term delivery. Birth complications – hypoxia
Environmental factors	Teratogenic effects include prenatal exposure to drugs, alcohol, radiation or other chemicals, resulting in foetal alcohol syndrome or other neuro-developmental effects.
Medical condition/events	Viral infections such as rubella, cytomegalovirus, meningitis Traumatic brain injury
Sociocultural causes	Abuse, trauma and socio-economic deprivation increase the risk of poor physical and mental health in young people with IDD (Emerson, 2012).

Philosophical approaches to service provision

Deinstitutionalisation saw the transfer of people with IDD from congregate, long-stay settings into the community and, in 2006, Aotearoa New Zealand closed its last long-stay institution. Burrell and Trip (2011) note that while such settings deprived some people of their rights, they also promoted a sense of identity and connectedness. The authors caution that forms of re-institutionalisation may still occur, albeit in smaller community contexts. Similarly, in Australia, deinstitutionalisation began in the 1980s and promoted the inclusion of people with mental health and ID into the wider community. The challenge for health professionals remains how to best support people with IDD to have meaningful lives of their choosing despite changing funding arrangements and systems of service delivery. When working with this population, it is not a single philosophical model that alone informs true citizenship of people with IDD; rather, it is the intercepting and integrated principles embraced by society that will make a difference and avoid history being repeated.

Normalisation, social-role valorisation and the social model of disability

The late 20th century heralded significant changes in thinking about the roles, and rights, of people with IDD to be involved in decisions about their own lives. Normalisation (Wolfensberger 1972; Nirje 1969) and social-role valorisation (Wolfensberger, 1983) were the theoretical drivers for deinstitutionalisation, globally; the former sought to reflect socially normed ways of living and the latter placed emphasis on socially valued roles attached to this achievement.

The social model of disability (SMD) emerged from the Union of the Physically Impaired Against Segregation (UPIAS) which produced the *Fundamental Principles of Disability* in 1976 (Race et al., 2005). Definitions of impairment and disability were respectively distinguished to being of a physical nature and socially constructed phenomena (Carlson, 2010). This refers to intentional or unintentional limitations imposed by society and which *dis-able* others (Goodley, 2001; Oliver, 2013). The UNCRPD (Articles 24, 25, 27) specifically relates to people with disabilities having equitable access to the same resources as others and being able to realise their goals in the education, health and employment sectors (United Nations, 2007), which is in keeping with the SMD. Under this model, disability is defined as:

> Something that happens when people with impairments face barriers in society that limit their movements, senses or activities. (Ministry of Social Development (MSD), 2016, p. 49)

It is also important to note how the person defines disability for themself. The SMD definition differs from the medical model of disability in that the latter implies disability as a deficit that reduces the person's quality of life and needs to be 'fixed' or treated (Shakespeare & Watson, 2001; Walker & Shaw, 2018).

Frameworks and models simply stipulate what is known or understood about how people function in relation to others (Barnes & Mercer, 2004). The philosophy underpinning the social model of health promotes accessible, equitable, fair and safe communities in which people with disabilities have choice and control over their own lives: this can be achieved through professional and clinical leadership by demonstrating respectful and dignified ways of communicating and consulting with people who live with physical, sensory, mental health or other impairments so they can define and articulate their own choices, decisions and needs (Beresford, 2005; MSD, 2016).

Philosophical principles in practice

Enabling Good Lives – New Zealand

Underpinned by the aforementioned philosophical approaches, the EGL principles seek to put the person with IDD in the driver's seat by enabling them to have control over the funding that is identified through a *needs assessment* process. The intention of this is to establish the supports needed to enable a person to access their home and community in a meaningful way. The eight principles informing service provision are: *self-determination; beginning early; person-centred; ordinary life outcomes; mainstream first;* mana-*enhancing or cognition and respect for a persons' abilities and contributions; easy to use;* and *relationship building* (Enabling Good Lives, 2021).

National Disability Insurance Scheme – Australia

Similarly, at its core, the NDIS promotes the social and economic participation of Australians in the community, as the needs of the person with a functional impairment are independently assessed by healthcare professionals. Approximately 70 per cent of NDIS users have a diagnosis of IDD, and just over 9 per cent of NDIS users have a diagnosed psychosocial disability (or mental health diagnosis) (Australian Institute of Health and Welfare (AIHW), 2020). The NDIS provides individuals with dual disability access to essential resources, to support their functioning and well-being. However, it is expected that the health needs of participants under NDIS will still be met by current healthcare systems serviced by state and federal (Medicare) funding. This emphasises the importance of healthcare professionals in Australia understanding the complex interface between health and disability.

O'Brien and Lyle's accomplishments for community living

As the movement of people from institutions into the community was occurring in the 1980s, O'Brien and Lyle (1986) proposed a person-centred approach to working alongside people with IDD. Quite simply, the five accomplishments are as follows and reflect the focus and manner in which all professionals should strive to work with this population:

1 *Respect* – for the person as someone with rights, to be treated with dignity about the expertise they have about themselves
2 *Choice* – is a skill, and people need to be supported to learn how to make their own choices, to identify options and the ability to exercise them
3 *Community presence* – in places within and external to family and natural supports, which provides opportunity to facilitate access physically within a space and to acknowledge the person as an individual with contributions to make. This enables the fourth accomplishment.
4 *Community participation* – meaningful engagement with people, resources and activities of their choosing in mainstream and disability specific settings
5 *Skill acquisition* – may become part of the above processes and/or be the result. This requires continuing vigilance, both in the maintenance and development of functional skills (O'Brien & Lyle, 1986).

What person-centred practice looks like

Fundamentally, if something is not working well for a person, one of the five accomplishments may be missing, so check: Is the person being respected? Are they supported to make a choice? Do they have access to people and places that they value and can truly engage with to draw on their own or others' skills?

PERSONAL NARRATIVE

Mary's story – part one

When my son, Jacob, was offered a job at a local fast-food chain, we had no idea what would unfold. We were happy for him that another one of his life goals would be reached: to be like his big brother, going to live independently and getting a job.

This achievement came at a cost to Jacob's health as he is often targeted by customers and staff because he is different, and he is naïve to the world. I have often wondered if I should step in and make him leave this place. It is a tough call and difficult to watch him make mistakes and become overwhelmed by anxiety.

Jacob feels very lucky to have a job. His job is much more than earning some money, although that is welcome too! It also structures his day, helps him to organise his week, gets him out of the flat and motivates him to shave and catch a bus.

He is the bravest person I know, to still be there after 10 years and to survive the experiences there that he has. Jacob does not give up and, although he might not say it this way, he lives in hope of one day being accepted and included by the staff and customers.

REFLECTIVE QUESTIONS

- When Jacob's day-to-day experiences of living and working with an IDD are viewed through the lens of the social model of disability, what are the barriers and enablers to quality of life for Jacob?
- In your role as a member of a non-government organisation you are asked to attend a seminar titled 'Supporting someone with a disability or impairment: An employer's guide'. What questions will you ask the expert panel on behalf of the people you support?
- Put yourself in the shoes of an employer. What reasonable adjustments would you put in place for people with IDD?

Physical health, mental illness and well-being

Determinants of health are pre-existing, continuing or acquired factors that influence a person's ability to secure timely and equitable access to the right supports that affect their physical and mental well-being (World Health Organization (WHO), 2017). Examples include geographical barriers for people who live in rural or remote areas, financial barriers, socio-economic status, inadequate government support, under-employment and unemployment, limitations in the knowledge of health professionals to understand and engage people living with IDD, and cultural inequity due to stereotypical attitudes. Social disadvantage is also prevalent among people with IDD and includes reduced social capital, which is defined as 'shared norms, values, beliefs, trust, networks, social relations, and institutions that facilitate cooperation and collective action for mutual benefits' (Bhandari & Yasunobu, 2009, p. 480). These are additional risk factors for physical and mental health issues in people with IDD (Emerson & Hatton, 2007).

In keeping with global trends, people with IDD are living longer (MSD, 2016; Janicki, 2009) and may experience higher rates of ill health, mortality and frailty at an earlier age, when compared with the general population (McCarron et al., 2011; Evenhuis et al., 2012; Trip, Whitehead & Crowe, 2020), despite presenting more frequently to emergency and primary care settings (Ministry of Health, 2011). Trollor and colleagues (2017) found that a high prevalence of respiratory and digestive disorders was related to mortality, and the average age of mortality was significantly younger when compared to the general population. It is important to note that as people with IDD age, individuals who have never sought assistance from specialist services can find it a challenge to seek access to supports. Forty years of age is commonly considered an important reference point in the ageing process for this population (Taggart, Coates & Truesdale-Kennedy, 2012) as they are at risk of earlier and/or have a higher likelihood of health and age-related conditions than the general population (Davidson et al., 2008).

The determinants of health are associated with IDD and a greater prevalence of mental illness (Emerson et al., 2012). A systematic review found that in children and adolescents with IDD this could be as high as 30–50 per cent (Einfeld et al., 2011). It is fair to assume that this trend does not diminish altogether when they reach adulthood (Emerson & Hatton, 2014), although maturation may be a factor for young people with ADHD, for example (Tonge, 2007). Mood disorders are not uncommon, and their presentation may be atypical. Understanding a person's usual baseline level of functioning and presentation is important as it is against this that changes may indicate mental distress (Sikabofori & Iyer, 2012). While eating disorders, personality and psychotic disorders are not as common, anxiety disorders are on the rise, alongside substance misuse (Ruedrich, 2010). Links are evident between the presentation of a mental illness and behaviours that challenge. Bowring and colleagues' model (2019) proposes understanding this in the context of known biological and psychosocial vulnerabilities as determinant risk factors. 'Developing communication pathways for adults with communication impairments' (Bowring, Painter & Hastings, 2019, p. 178) will assist in reducing the effects of presenting changes in an individual's behavioural and/or mental health presentation.

Alzheimer's-type dementia is more common in people with Down syndrome (DS), with onset at an earlier age compared to the general population. For people with DS, the incidence is estimated at 50 per cent in those over 50 years and 75 per cent for those 65 years and over (Lott & Head, 2019). Onset of symptoms can be as early as 40 years of age and is due to the amyloid precursor protein, linked to Alzheimer's disease, which is seen on chromosome 21: DS is also known as Trisomy 21 and therefore individuals have three copies, which increases the risk (Lott & Head, 2019). Ageing per se, as well as the diagnosis and management of dementia in people with IDD, is complex and multifaceted.

Aside from physical multi-morbidity, there may be underlying grief associated with both planned and unplanned transitions for all parties involved – be it to a residential setting, or between family members – particularly siblings, as a result of the illness or death of the primary caregiver (Trip et al., 2019). Nurses and other healthcare professionals have long-term relationships with people with IDD and they are often best placed to notice subtle changes in the person's usual cognitive or adaptive functioning (Stanton & Coetzee, 2004); therefore, this presents an opportunity for specialist input by advanced practice nurses.

Table 16.2   Comparison of intellectual disability and mental illness

Domain	Intellectual disability	Mental illness
Age of onset	Evidence prior to age 18	Through the lifespan
Development	Delay in reaching milestones	Usual development Changes in thinking and presentation
Duration	Lifelong	One-off episode or recurring
Main effects	Deficits in adaptive functioning include interpersonal skills, self-care, activities of daily living, communication, access to supports and services, problem-solving, socialisation, decision-making, education, memory, processing, recall	Disturbances in thinking, mood, thought form, judgement, cognition, perception and insight
Examples	Genetics (Down syndrome; Fragile X) Birth complications, infection, toxins, trauma	Mood disorders, schizophrenia, anxiety or eating disorders, dementia and delirium
Management or treatment	Residential, supported living, behavioural intervention Life-skills training, counselling	Assessment/intervention, acute or community based Medication and/or psychosocial intervention
Measurability/ diagnosis	Psychometric assessment of intellectual and adaptive functioning, usually by a clinical psychologist	Diagnosis through assessment of changes in mood, cognition, judgement, perception, decision-making, risk and insight

Diagnostic overshadowing

diagnostic overshadowing – occurs when the healthcare professional assumes that the signs and symptoms they are observing, and the behaviours the person with the IDD is presenting with, are caused by the ID, mental illness or other primary diagnosis

Diagnostic overshadowing occurs when a health professional assumes that the presenting behaviours of the person are caused by an existing condition or diagnosis. Furthermore, assumptions may be made that the person's behaviour is intentional rather than serving the function of communication to indicate an altered sense of being (Blair, 2016). This can result in misdiagnosis or restrictive practices (Deveau, 2012) through dismissive or incorrect assessment and treatment, and a lack of resolution of the presenting concern, which might include physical or mental pain or discomfort and ultimately can result in poor quality of life outcomes. Therefore, the first step in a mental health assessment is to undertake a comprehensive assessment to rule out any physical complaint or, emotional or social distress. If not fully explored, the risk of polypharmacy is heightened as it may be used to address the presenting behaviour. Polypharmacy is commonly understood as taking five or more medications, and can include those accessed over the counter (Cadogan, Ryan & Hughes, 2016).

According to Bigby (2004, cited in Trip et al., 2020), 'age-related conditions also tend to be either under diagnosed or masked by unmet health needs'. Additional factors that contribute to diagnostic overshadowing include, but are not limited to, psychosocial masking, communication challenges, polypharmacy, acquiescence (the person wants to please, or agrees and is not wanting nor able to question content), and the reliability or under-reporting from the person themselves, and/or that by others.

Intersectionality

The theory of intersectionality creates the opportunity to improve healthcare access for people with disabilities by identifying the barriers a person may experience in accessing health care, such as the inability to comprehend the health literature provided to them, and therefore can reduce the inequalities and inequities of healthcare access experienced by people with IDD. Intersectionality has most commonly been associated with gender and racism (King et al., 2019); however, the concept can be expanded to encompass multiple facets that define an individual, including socio-economic status, and ability, as these factors also influence the way the individual accesses health care. The inclusion of intersectionality theory in practice can promote inclusiveness of vulnerable groups in practice and research (Heard et al., 2020).

Similar to intersectionality theory, the World Health Organization's (WHO) *International Classification of Functioning, Disability and Health* encompasses six key elements: health condition (disorder or disease), activity, body structure and function, environmental factors, participation, and personal factors (WHO, 2001). Understanding the interrelationships between these elements enables greater opportunity for positive health outcomes for persons with a disability. For example, the relationship between participation in activities and mental health is well known; however, the individual may rely on the availability of their support network (personal factors) to be able to access the activity in which they usually participate. In the absence of their support network, the individual cannot participate in their meaningful activity, and therefore they may be likely to experience a deterioration in mental well-being.

Reflection: self-in-action

For some healthcare professionals, interacting with people with IDD is an unfamiliar situation. While this may lead to diagnostic overshadowing, it can also create opportunities to learn from family/*whānau* and support networks, and can change the way healthcare professionals communicate, assess and select interventions (Blair, 2016; Gates & Barr, 2009). Fundamentally, diagnostic overshadowing can be attended to when it is acknowledged as a potential challenge, and when the reasons it occurs can be addressed and made visible.

Diagnostic overshadowing occurs for many reasons, and no healthcare worker seeks to intentionally stigmatise or discriminate against people with an IDD and/or mental illness. However, when the experience and non-verbal communication of the individual, and the family/*whānau* or support network voice is dismissed, and privacy and confidentiality within the doctor–patient relationship are privileged over familial concerns, diagnostic overshadowing follows.

TRANSLATION TO PRACTICE

REFLECTIVE QUESTIONS

- You are asked to explain your understanding of diagnostic overshadowing to (a) a newly enrolled group of interprofessional health and disability students, and (b) a family member who has seen the term written in a referral letter by the GP. How will you explain diagnostic overshadowing to this diverse group of potential healthcare professionals, and the family member? Will the approach be the same? *What* will you say? *How* will you say it or present it? What recommendations would you include?
- Explore and reflect on the barriers, challenges and enablers for the person when attending government agencies, services and non-government organisations.

Autonomy, consent and self-determination and strategies to promote healthcare access

Article 3 of the UNCRPD (United Nations, 2007) identifies the principles that apply for the interdependence of all its Articles to be attained. These include respect, non-discrimination, effective participation and inclusion in society, respect for difference and acceptance – as part of human diversity, humanity, accessibility, equality of opportunity between men and woman, and the evolving capacities of children (United Nations, 2007). This is in keeping with the Aotearoa New Zealand Health and Disability Services Code of Consumer's Rights (Health and Disability Commissioner Te Toihau Hauora Hauatanga, 1996). The expectation of services is to uphold a person's right to respect, freedom from discrimination, coercion, harassment and exploitation, and the right to dignity and independence. Services must be of an appropriate standard, effective communication should be provided to ensure consumers are fully informed, able to make an informed choice and to give informed consent, the right to support, to complain and in respect to teaching and research.

There are several core strategies that can support health professionals to put this into practice, and Article 12 of the UNCRPD (United Nations, 2007) requires supported decision-making be integral to this process. The achievement of Article 25 (health) of the UNCRPD (United Nations, 2007) requires application of the tenets of intersectionality, to ensure people with IDD have access to health promotion, mental health assessment, screening and management programs, to optimise health and quality of life. Part of this is ensuring autonomy in health care, which can be adapted and negotiated to optimise the inclusion of the person themself in decisions about their lives (Whitehead et al., 2016).

TRANSLATION TO PRACTICE

Strategies to facilitate healthcare access for people with IDD

- Minimise waiting time, take more time and provide a quiet space.
- Adapt communication:
  - Use simple sentences and avoid medical terms if possible.
  - Use strategies that the person would normally use in communicating, including gesture dictionaries, social scripts, technology and picture boards.

- – Check their understanding by using words or phrases that they know in reference to their body or health. Consistency in responses can be checked by reframing questions to check the person is agreeing to treatment rather than responding as they think you want them to.
- Ask if the person has a health passport and use this to guide care. A health passport provides essential information about the person and how to support them when they use health services.
- Plan appointments to meet the person's needs, and show them any equipment to be used.
- Listen to the person, speak directly to them and include family or support workers, with the person's permission.
- The way in which individuals present or respond to their symptoms might include crying, laughing, repetitive questioning, trying to hurt themselves or others, or becoming withdrawn.

Source: Ministry of Health (2020).

PERSONAL NARRATIVE

For anybody who has a difficulty

A poem by Isaac Tait
Life is tough and there is so much hurt.
Stand beside them and keep trying.
Even though you may think that you're no one.
This is for you. Keep trying
Do not let life get you down. Although it will
Chill out. Pill out. Chill pill it out
Music it, read it or walk it
Be cool. Be you
Talk to someone
Take care. Don't stress it. Beat it
Sleep it. Walk tall
Sniff the roses or coffee at the mall
Paint a painting or drink a fine drink
Kindness and kind re-wind. And unwind

REFLECTIVE QUESTIONS

- The author of this poem has identified several strategies he uses to cope. What are they, and what other strategies can you recommend? Be aware of possible challenges and strengths presenting for this young man.
- Social isolation can negatively affect quality of life and mental health for people living with IDD. How can social involvement and meaningful relationships be supported?
- In groups of three, role-play the approach you would use to promote healthy choices for a person with an IDD and a newly diagnosed mental illness.

Chronic sorrow

chronic sorrow – a long-term sadness experienced by caregivers such as family members of people with disabilities or those with chronic illness, as they redefine and adjust their expectations

Chronic sorrow captures the difference between depression and grief. It is a normal response to ongoing loss experienced by significant people caring for a family member with a disability or chronic illness (Coughlin & Sethares, 2017). This may include the child newly diagnosed with ID, multiple births and mental illness, or learning disability, type 1 diabetes, cancer, epilepsy or cerebral palsy (Bolch et al., 2012; Bowes et al., 2009; Nikfarid et al., 2015). It is described as a natural reaction in response to continuing grief and multiple losses over time, but does not necessarily interfere with daily functioning despite being considered permanent and periodic. There are several specific times or developmental stages across the life span of the person living with IDD or a newly diagnosed health concern, when chronic sorrow can be triggered or predicted for the significant people who care for them. These include when the child is diagnosed, when alternative care is considered, when a younger sibling exceeds the developmental stage of their older sibling, when power of attorney or legal guardianship is explored, and when professional help and support are sought. This can result in sorrow that is never resolved or accepted, as it is continuing for parents, significant others and caregivers as they realise how the young person's life will be affected over the long term (Coughlin & Sethares, 2017).

PERSONAL NARRATIVE

Mary's story – part two

There have been successes and challenges on our journey to support our son, especially as he has grown, faced social milestones and become a man. Throughout this journey the motivating factor has always been, 'how do I keep my son safe while at the same time supporting his independence, decision-making and choices?' While I have been able to accept that failure is not an option, it has been a lonely journey as I watch friends and colleagues celebrate their children's successes at school, when they graduate, leave home to live independently, start jobs, make friends, marry, or have children. As a mother I have to persevere with the teaching and inevitable re-teaching of activities of daily living and everyday executive functioning, and I am kept on task because one day when I'm gone he will have to face these challenges alone. As a nurse I watch him try to cope with newly diagnosed depression and anxiety, and longstanding type 1 diabetes when he has no numeracy and cannot comprehend the fatal or just debilitating consequences of poor blood sugar control, and I have to respect the choices he makes. As a nursing lecturer I try to support his independence while navigating through the medical system and interacting with the government benefits provider that operates by a medical model of disability assessment and intervention, while we are operating from a social model of disability, where he is often *dis-abled* by others' choices.

REFLECTIVE QUESTION

Consider the role of chronic sorrow (Coughlin & Sethares, 2017), as opposed to the grief process and expectation of accepting the loss, for the significant people who care for people living with an IDD. How can knowing about chronic sorrow support or empower *whānau* or family?

INTERPROFESSIONAL PERSPECTIVES

Character of the IDD workforce

Access to clinical placements in IDD services varies significantly. While deinstitutionalisation heralded the de-medicalisation of these populations, many individuals continue to require access to a range of registered health professionals to enable community access and optimise their physical and mental well-being. In many Australasian jurisdictions, people with IDD may be referred to mainstream or disability specific community services to access dietetics, occupational therapy, physiotherapy or music therapy, for example.

Specialist IDD in-patient and out-patient services often sit within mental health settings: people are commonly referred for assessment when there are concerns about changes in their presentation, suspected mental illness and/or cognitive impairment. Additionally, in Aotearoa New Zealand, it is in these settings that people with IDD may also be remanded for assessment under the *Intellectual Disability (Compulsory Care and Rehabilitation) Act 2003* if they have been charged of an imprisonable offence. This legislation was established to provide a pathway for people with IDD to be assessed and for there to be a range of secure and community-based orders within which they would receive ongoing assessment and habilitation over time. These specialist interprofessional teams draw on a range of clinical and therapeutic skills, including clinical psychologists, psychiatrists, occupational therapists, social workers, nurses and specialist teachers in schools.

Within community, primary, secondary or tertiary settings, the focus is on the person themself, their family/*whānau* and their network of support. A key goal is to establish the individual's preferences, strengths and abilities, and to use these to support the habilitation or maintenance of existing skills and, where possible, develop or improve their adaptive functioning.

REFLECTIVE QUESTIONS

- How do members of the interdisciplinary team (IDT) develop and improve the adaptive skills of the person living with a disability?
- What values, skills and attitudes would IDT members need to develop or maintain to communicate well *within* IDT, to benefit and support the person living with IDD and their family?
- You are asked to debate the topic: 'The consumer, client/person living with the IDD is also a member of the IDT'. Write brief, bullet-point notes that capture your arguments.
- List eight constructive practices consistent with your discipline that you would use to support communicating well with a person living with an IDD who has difficulty communicating verbally.

SUMMARY

This chapter has presented stories, information and activities designed to deepen your understanding of:

- The use of labels to define people with an IDD as both a strength and a weakness. Although stigmatising labels persist, the intention is to capture the person's functional abilities and provide resources to meet their needs.
- Meaningful lives and true citizenship, which can be enhanced for people with IDD when the issues and concerns of the people themselves and their families are heard and acted upon.
- The ability to access services as a fundamental right in Australasia, although the experience for people living with IDD varies across populations and jurisdictions. Social disadvantage and diagnostic overshadowing can amplify geographical, financial and cultural inaccessibility.
- People's right to develop and express their autonomy through supported decision-making, regardless of their impairment. It is imperative that society does not disable people through the known and unconscious barriers that exist. 'Kindness must persist' – Isaac Tait.

CRITICAL THINKING/LEARNING ACTIVITIES

1 Now that you have read this chapter, describe the changes you would make to assessment or interview processes for a person living with an IDD. How do you manage risk and maintain safety while enabling the independence of this person? If the person you are interviewing is a family member, how do you support *both* the family and the person living with an IDD when preferred outcomes diverge?

2 You have been asked to facilitate a seminar to a group of healthcare professionals, related to living and working with IDD. List the 10 most important concepts you will communicate.

3 List eight negative terms or phrases used to describe a person living with an IDD. How could these negative labels and words used in the media and popular culture, define their reality (how they see themselves) and contribute to or lessen the potential for stigma and discrimination?

4 Identify and access a film that portrays the life and experiences of a person living with IDD. How are they portrayed and represented?

LEARNING EXTENSION

There may be several people or agencies involved in a person's care and support. How do the roles of the members of the interdisciplinary team responsible for the care and support of the person living with an IDD differ? How is this coordinated? Choose for example, general practitioner, practice nurse, behavioural specialist, family member or support worker. What are the consequences if interprofessional communication is ignored?

FURTHER READING

Matson, J. L. (2019). *Handbook of Intellectual Disabilities: Integrating theory, research and practice*. Switzerland: Springer Nature AG.

This book provides an in-depth collection of evidence-based expertise on a comprehensive range of relevant topics and considerations for working with this population across the lifespan – the extent to which is unable to be captured in this chapter.

Ministry of Social Development. (2016). *New Zealand Disability Strategy 2016–2026*. Wellington: Office for Disability Issues, Ministry of Social Development. Retrieved from https://www .odi.govt.nz/nz-disability-strategy/

This government document supports people living and working with a disability, impairment or chronic illness in Aotearoa New Zealand.

Therapeutic Guidelines Limited. (2012). *Management Guidelines: Developmental disability version 3*. Melbourne: Therapeutic Guidelines Limited.

As an ebook this publication is an accessible reference that covers an informative format with assessment, intervention and monitoring guidelines, with a both lifespan and body systems approach, and applies it to a range of (intellectual) and developmental conditions.

REFERENCES

American Psychiatric Association (APA). (2013). *Diagnostic and Statistical Manual of Mental Disorders*, 5th edn: *DSM-5*. Virginia: APA.

Australian Institute of Health and Welfare (AIHW). (2020). *People with Disability in Australia*. Retrieved from https://www.aihw.gov.au/getmedia/ee5ee3c2-152d-4b5f-9901-71d483b47f03/aihw-dis-72.pdf.aspx?inline=true

Barnes, C. & Mercer, G. (2004). Theorising and researching disability from a social model perspective. In C. Barnes & G. Mercer (eds). *Implementing the Social Model of Disability: Theory and research* (pp. 1–17). Leeds: The Disability Press.

Beresford, P. (2005). Social work and a social model of madness and distress: Developing a viable role for the future. *Social Work and Social Sciences Review*, *12*(2): 59–73.

Bhandari, H. & Yasunobu, K. (2009). What is social capital? A comprehensive review of the concept. *Asian Journal of Social Science*, *37*(3): 480–510.

Bigby, C. (2004). *Ageing with a Lifelong Disability*. London: Jessica Kingsley Publishers.

Blair, J. (2016). Diagnostic overshadowing: See beyond the diagnosis. *British Journal of Family Medicine*, March/April: 37–41.

Bolch, E., Davis, P .G., Umstad, M. P. & Fisher J. R. W. (2012) Multiple birth families with children with special needs: A qualitative investigation of mothers' experiences. *Twin Research and Human Genetics*, *15*(4): 503–15.

Bowes, S., Lowes., L., Warner, J. & Gregory, J. W. (2009). Chronic sorrow in parents of children with type 1 diabetes. *Journal of Advanced Nursing*, *65*(5): 992–1000.

Bowring, D. L., Painter, J. & Hastings, R. P. (2019). Prevalence of challenging behavior in adults in intellectual disabilities, correlates, and association with mental health. *Current Developmental Disorders Reports*, *6*: 173–81.

Britt, E., Davies, K. & Daffue, C. (2017). Context and tension in psychiatric diagnosis in people with intellectual disabilities: Challenges and responses. *Research and Practice in Intellectual and Developmental Disabilities*, *5*(2): 103–13.

Burrell, B. & Trip, H. (2011). Reform and community care: Has de-institutionalisation delivered for people with intellectual disability? *Nursing Inquiry*, *18*(2): 174–83.

Cadogan, C. A., Ryan, C. & Hughes, C. M. (2016). Appropriate polypharmacy and medicine safety: When many is not too many. *Drug Safety*, *39*: 109–16.

Callard, F., Sartorius, N., Arboleda-Florez, J., Bartlett, P., Helmchen, H., Stuart, H.... Thornicroft, G. (2012). *Mental Illness, Discrimination, and the Law: Fighting for social justice*. Chichester, UK: John Wiley & Sons.

Carlson, L. (2010). *The Faces of Intellectual Disability: Philosophical reflections*. Bloomington, Indiana: Indiana University Press.

Coughlin, M. B. & Sethares, K. A. (2017). Chronic sorrow in parents of children with a chronic illness or disability: An integrative literature review. *Journal of Pediatric Nursing*, *37*: 108–16.

Davidson, P. W., Henderson, C. M., Janicki, M. P., Robinson, L. M., Bishop, K. M., Wells, A.… Wexler, O. (2008). Ascertaining health-related information on adults with intellectual disabilities: Development and field testing of the Rochester Health Status Survey. *Journal of Policy and Practice in Intellectual Disabilities*, *5*(1): 12–23.

del Hoyo Soriano, L., Thurman, A. J., Harvey, D., Kover, S. T. & Abbeduto, L. (2020). Expressive language development in adolescents with Down syndrome and fragile X syndrome: change over time and the role of family-related factors. *Journal of Neurodevelopmental Disorders*, *12*(1): 1–18.

Deveau, R. (2012). Reducing the use of restrictive practices with people who have intellectual disabilities: A practical approach. *Tizard Learning Disability Review*, *17*(1): 49–51.

Einfeld, S. L., Ellis, L. A. & Emerson, E. (2011). Comorbidity of intellectual disability and mental disorder in children and adolescents: A systematic review. *Journal of Intellectual & Developmental Disability*, *36*(2): 137–43.

Emerson, E. (2012). Deprivation, ethnicity and the prevalence of intellectual and developmental disabilities. *Journal of Epidemiology and Community Health*, *66*(3): 218–24.

Emerson, E., Baines, S., Allerton, L., & Welch, V. (2012). *Health Inequalities & People with Learning Disabilities in the UK: 2012*. England: Improving Health and Lives -Learning Disability Observatory. Retrieved from https://www.basw.co.uk/system/files/resources/basw_14846-4_0.pdf

Emerson, E. & Hatton, C. (2007). Poverty, socio-economic position, social capital and the health of children and adolescents with intellectual disabilities in Britain: A replication. *Journal of Intellectual Disability Research*, *51*(11): 866–74.

——— (2014). *Health Inequalities and People with Intellectual Disabilities*. Cambridge: Cambridge University Press.

Enabling Good Lives. (2021). *Principles*. Retrieved from https://www.enablinggoodlives.co.nz/about-egl/egl-approach/principles/

Evenhuis, H. M., Heermans, H., Hilgenkamp, T. I. M., Bastiaanse, L. P. & Echteld, M. A. (2012). Frailty and disability in older adults with intellectual disabilities: Results from the health ageing and intellectual disability study. *Journal of the American Geriatrics Society*, *60*: 934–8.

Gates, B. & Barr, O. (2009) (Eds.) *Oxford Handbook of Learning and Intellectual Disability Nursing*. Oxford, UK: Oxford University Press.

Gernand, A. D., Schulze, K. J., Stewart, C. P., West Jr, K. P. & Christian, P. (2016). Micronutrient deficiencies in pregnancy worldwide: health effects and prevention. *Nature Reviews Endocrinology*, *12*(5): 274–89.

Goldfarb, D. L. & Frankel, A. (2007). Intellectual disability etiologies and associated psychiatric disorders. *Mental Health Aspects of Developmental Disabilities*, *10*(1): 18–24.

Goodley, D. (2001). 'Learning difficulties', the social model of disability and impairment: Challenging epistemologies. *Disability & Society*, *16*(2): 207–31.

Health and Disability Commissioner Te Toihau Hauora Hauatanga. (1996). Code of Health and Disability Services Consumers' Rights. Retrieved from https://www.hdc.org.nz/your-rights/about-the-code/code-of-health-and-disability-services-consumers-rights/

Heard, E., Fitzgerald, L., Wigginton, B. & Mutch, A. (2020). Applying intersectionality theory in health promotion research and practice. *Health Promotion International*, *35*(4): 866–76.

Heslop, P., Turner, S., Read, S., Tucker, J., Seaton, S. & Evans, B. (2019). Implementing reasonable adjustments for disabled people in healthcare services. *Nursing Standard*, *34*(8): 29–34.

Janicki, M. P. (2009). The aging dilemma: Is increasing longevity among people with intellectual disabilities creating a new population challenge in the Asia-Pacific region? *Journal of Policy and Practice in Intellectual Disabilities*, *6*(2): 73–6.

King, T. L., Shields, M., Shakespeare, T., Milner, A. & Kavanagh, A. (2019). An intersectional approach to understandings of mental health inequalities among men with disability. *SSM – Population Health*, *9*: 100464.

Lott, I. T. & Head, E. (2019). Dementia in Down syndrome: Unique insights for Alzheimer disease research. *Nature Reviews Neurology*, *15*: 135–47.

Luckasson, R., Borthwick-Duffy, S., Buntinx, W. H. E., Coulter, D. L., Craig, E. M. (P.), Reeve, A., Schalock, R. L., Snell, M. E., Spitalnik, D. M., Spreat, S., Tassé, M. J. & The AAMR AD HOC Committee on Terminology and Classification. (2002). *Mental Retardation: Definition, classification, and systems of supports*, 10th edn. Silver Spring, MD: American Association on Mental Retardation.

Maulik, P. K., Mascarenhas, M. N., Mathers, C. D., Dua, T., & Saxena, S. (2011). Prevalence of intellectual disability: a meta-analysis of population-based studies. *Research in developmental disabilities, 32*(2): 419–36.

McCarron, M., Swinburne, J., Burke, E., McGlinchey, E., Mulryan, N., Andrews, V., Foran S. & McCallion, P. (2011). *Growing Older With an Intellectual Disability in Ireland 2011: First results from the intellectual disability supplement of the Irish longitudinal study on ageing.* Dublin: School of Nursing & Midwifery, Trinity College.

Ministry of Health (2011). *Health Indicators for New Zealanders with Intellectual Disability.* Wellington: Ministry of Health.

—— (2020). *Clinical Guidance for Responding to Patients with an Intellectual (Learning) Disability During COVID-19 in Aotearoa New Zealand.* Retrieved from https://www.health.govt.nz/ system/files/documents/pages/clinical-guidance-responding-patients-intellectual-learning-disability-during-covid-19-12may2020.pdf

Ministry of Social Development (MSD). (2016). *New Zealand Disability Strategy 2016–2026.* Wellington: Office for Disability Issues, Ministry of Social Development. Retrieved from https://www.odi.govt.nz/nz-disability-strategy/

Morris-Rosendahl, D. J. & Crocq, M.-A. (2020). Neurodevelopmental disorders: The history and future of a diagnostic concept. *Dialogues in Clinical Neuroscience, 22*(1): 65–72.

Nikfarid, L., Rassouli, M., Borimnejad, L. & Alavimajd, H. (2015). Chronic sorrow in mothers of children with cancer. *Journal of Pediatric Oncology Nursing, 32*(5): 314–19.

Nirje, B. (1969). The normalization principle and its human management implications. In R. Kugel, & W. Wolfensberger (eds), *Changing Patterns in Residential Services for the Mentally Retarded.* Washington, DC: President's Committee on Mental Retardation.

O'Brien, J. & Lyle, C. (1986). *Framework for Accomplishments.* Decatur, GA: Responsive Systems Associates.

Oliver, M. (2013). The social model of disability: Thirty years on. *Disability & Society, 28*(7): 1024–6.

Race, D., Boxall, K. & Carson, I. (2005). Towards a dialogue for practice: Reconciling social role valorisation and the social model of disability. *Disability & Society, 20*(5): 507–21.

Roth, E. A., Sarawgi, S. N. & Fodstad, J. C. (2019). History of intellectual disabilities. In J.L. Matson (ed.), *Handbook of Intellectual Disabilities: Integrating theory, research and practice* (pp. 3–16). New York: Springer.

Ruedrich, S. (2010). Disorders of the nervous system and neurodevelopment: Mental illness. In J. O'Hara, J. McCarthy & N. Bouras (eds), *Intellectual Disability and Ill Health* (pp. 165–77). Cambridge: Cambridge University Press.

Scior, K., Connolly, T. & Williams, J. (2013). The effects of symptom recognition and diagnostic labels on public health benefits, emotional reactions, and stigmas associated with intellectual disability. *American Journal of Intellectual and Developmental Disability, 118*(3): 211–23.

Shakespeare, T. & Watson, N. (2001). The social model of disability: An outdated ideology? In S. N. Barnartt & B. M. Altman (eds), *Exploring Theories and Expanding Methodologies: Where we are and where we need to go (Research in Social Science and Disability, Vol. 2)* (pp. 9–28). Bingley: Emerald Group Publishing Limited.

Sikabofori, T. & Iyer, A. (2012). Depressive disorders in people with intellectual disabilities. In R. Raghavan (ed.) *Anxiety and Depression in People with Intellectual Disabilities* (pp. 51–74). Pavilion Publishing and Media Ltd.

Stanton, L. R. & Coetzee, R. H. (2004). Down's syndrome and dementia. *Advances in Psychiatric Treatment, 10*(1): 50–8.

Statistics New Zealand. (2013). *Disability Survey: 2013.* Retrieved from https://www.stats.govt.nz/ informationreleases/disability-survey-2013

Taggart, L., Coates, V. & Truesdale-Kennedy, M. (2012). Management and quality indicators of diabetes mellitus in people with intellectual disabilities. *Journal of Intellectual Disability Research, 57*(2).

Tang, B., Byrne, C., Friedlander, R., McKibbin, D., Riley, M. & Thibeault, A. (2008). The other dual diagnosis: Developmental disability and mental health disorders. *British Columbia Medical Journal, 50*(6): 319–24.

Tonge, B. (2007). The psychopathology of children with intellectual disabilities. In N. Bouras & G. Holt (eds), *Psychiatric and Behavioral Disorders in Intellectual and Developmental Disabilities*, 2nd edn (pp. 92–112). Cambridge: Cambridge University Press.

Trip, H., Whitehead, L. & Crowe, M. (2020). Perceptions of ageing and future aspirations by people with intellectual disability: A grounded theory study using photo-elicitation. *Ageing and Society, 40*(5): 966–83.

Trip, H., Whitehead, L., Crowe, M., Mirfin-Veitch, B. & Daffue, C. (2019). Aging with intellectual disabilities in families: Navigating ever-changing seas – A theoretical model. *Qualitative Health Research, 29*(11): 1595–610.

Trollor, J., Srasuebkul, P., Xu, H. & Howlett, S. (2017). Cause of death and potentially avoidable deaths in Australian adults with intellectual disability using retrospective linked data. *BMJ Open, 7*(2): e013489.

United Nations. (2007). *Convention on the Rights of Persons with Disabilities*. Retrieved from https://www.refworld.org/docid/45f973632.html

Walker, E. R. & Shaw, S. C. K. (2018) Specific learning difficulties in healthcare education: The meaning in the nomenclature. *Nursing Education in Practice, 32*: 97–8.

Wehmeyer, M. L. (2013). Disability, disorder, and identity. *Intellectual and Developmental Disabilities, 51*(2): 122–6.

Whitehead, L. C., Trip, H. T., Hale, L. A., & Conder, J. (2016). Negotiated autonomy in diabetes self-management: the experiences of adults with intellectual disability and their support workers. *Journal of Intellectual Disability Research, 60*(4): 389–97.

Wolfensberger, W. (1972). *The Principle of Normalization in Human Services*. Toronto: National Institute on Mental Retardation.

——— (1983). Social role valorization: A proposed new term for the principle of normalization. *Mental Retardation, 21*(6): 234–9.

World Health Organization (WHO). (2001). *International Classification of Functioning, Disability and Health: ICF*. Geneva: WHO.

——— (2017). *Determinants of Health*. Retrieved from https://www.who.int/news-room/q-a-detail/determinants-of-health

Yim, S.-Y. (2015). Diagnostic approach for genetic causes of intellectual disability. *Journal of Genetic Medicine, 12*(1): 6–11.

Mental health of children and young people

Rhonda L. Wilson and Serena Riley

LEARNING OBJECTIVES

At the completion of this chapter, you should be able to:

1 Understand the importance of showing respect for and creating relationships with young people.
2 Consider the developmental needs of young people and how this influences their mental health.
3 Identify youth-friendly environments and contexts that enhance mental health care.
4 Identify enablers and barriers to developing therapeutic rapport with young people.
5 Recognise the importance of hopefulness and resilience in young people and how this influences their recovery experiences.
6 Identify some common mental health conditions experienced by young people.

Introduction

This chapter outlines a developmental orientation to understanding the mental health of children and young people. It examines the implications for mental health in children and young people in relation to the environment, the concept of nature and nurture, and brain development in the context of vulnerability, risk, resilience and protection. The chapter explores mental health promotion for young people, drawing from two real stories about bullying and altered eating patterns, including anorexia nervosa and bulimia, which include experiences of depression, anxiety and psychosis. Emphasis is given to prevention, awareness and early intervention for mental illness, including social media and e-mental health interventions for young people in relation to non-suicidal self-injury or suicide crisis, and popular public health initiatives to reduce suicide, such as R U OK? Day, headspace and other online services.

Respect for young people

Health professionals providing mental health care to children and young people should do so in a way that conveys respect and genuine concern. For children and young people, the first occurrence of a mental illness is likely to be a very confusing and perhaps frightening experience. An important priority is for healthcare professionals to develop a strong initial therapeutic rapport with the young people they are helping. Young people are unsure of what to anticipate in mental health care, especially if it is their first appointment, or their first experience of a mental illness (Watson, Rickwood & Vanags, 2013; Wilson, Cruickshank & Lea, 2012). Health professionals can do a great deal to allay the confusion, anxiety and apprehension that may accompany a first experience of mental health care, simply by creating a respectful and trusting relationship from the outset (Coughlan et al., 2013; Wilson et al., 2012).

Most mental health conditions are first encountered in the ages of 12–25 years, and approximately 20 per cent of the world's young people are affected (Wei et al., 2013). It is very important to promote mental health, provide accessible, youth-focused early intervention when it is needed, and to support the recovery care of young people. We know that the earlier mental health care is initiated, the more likely will be the success of recovery (Boyd et al., 2011; Coughlan et al., 2013; McAllister & Handley, 2008; Wilson, 2007; Wilson et al., 2012). Early commencement of mental health care reduces periods of disruption to the important developmental stages of growth, educational and vocational attainment, and social functioning (Coughlan et al., 2013; McAllister & Handley, 2008).

A shift towards a stronger focus on the mental health and well-being of young people is gaining international momentum (Coughlan et al., 2013). The objectives of *The International Declaration on Youth Mental Health* include:

youth-friendly – services, settings and health professionals in which authentic respect, care and congruence with the young person and their culture are conveyed

strength-based mental health care – acknowledges that positive attributes already present can be harnessed to enhance mental health recovery

- authentically involving young people and their families in meaningful youth mental health service development
- improving the understanding of youth mental health within communities
- improving accessibility of **youth-friendly** mental health services and supports
- the adoption of youth-focused, **strength-based mental health care**
- focusing on developing resilience, hope and recovery (Coughlan et al., 2013).

Developing a rapport with young people

Health professionals working with young people need to be aware of the dynamics of youth culture. It is important to understand the diverse language, social context, values and beliefs of young people so that a relevant and appropriate therapeutic relationship can be established (Wilson et al., 2012). In particular, it is important to ensure that the behaviours of the health professionals do not represent a barrier to young people engaging with mental healthcare providers (Wilson et al., 2012). An authentic and respectful relationship will need to be developed, to facilitate positive mental health care (Conradson, 2003; McAllister & Handley, 2008).

It can often be counterproductive for health professionals to adopt the behaviours or popular language of young people, as this can be taken as condescending and patronising to the young person. Additionally, obvious displays of shock or lack of awareness about the real-life experiences and cultures of young people can also have a negative effect on therapeutic rapport. Health professionals should maintain a fluid knowledge of the dynamics of young people's cultures, and should inform themselves about trends, spaces and places in which young people feel most comfortable (Conradson, 2003). In addition, practitioners should position themselves to find a point of congruence or agreement, operate with a positive regard for the person, and with warm empathy, so that a helping relationship can be developed and maintained (Rogers, 1980).

The following lists, while not exhaustive, represent some barriers and enablers to authentic engagement with young people, and practical assistance for students preparing for clinical placement or in transition to registration as a practitioner.

Barriers include:

- Clinical uniforms. To the young person, uniforms can present an overly pathological environmental context (Conradson, 2003).
- Formal clothes, outdated fashions and/or poor personal hygiene. These may repel young people, who may make subjective judgements about the trustworthiness of professionals and their emotional connections with them; these judgements may lack logic or reason, because the young people are still learning the social skills of extending respect and regard towards others (Conradson, 2003). Therefore, practitioners will need to take this developmental factor into consideration as part of their professional preparation for working with young people.
- Inauthentic use of the social language of young people. It is not considered 'cool' by young people for older people to use their language, or to assume intimate knowledge of their language, without having gained social permission and credibility to do so.
- Laughing at the cultures of young people or suggesting that 'they will grow out' of an undesirable stage.
- Sarcasm and lecturing about what is 'right' and 'wrong'. These approaches are unhelpful and demeaning to the person. Avoid taking an authoritarian approach.
- Long and drawn-out assessment appointments with multiple health professionals in attendance. Such practices can be daunting for young people, and are likely to be counterproductive to an accurate mental health assessment.
- Strict adherence to rules. Try to avoid demanding that young people adhere to rules.
- Alienating settings and attitudes within health services, such as treating adolescents like children rather than as emerging adults, labelling their experiences as 'typical teenager

issues' and admission to an adult facility. These practices can hinder recovery (Coughlan et al., 2011).

- A previous bad experience of mental health care and long waiting times or lists. Such experiences are detrimental to young people's engagement and recovery (Coughlan et al., 2011; McAllister & Handley, 2008; Wilson et al., 2012).
- Assumptions that social media is a 'bad thing'. For many young people, it is a good thing. Mocking them for their use or proficiency in their use of social media and their digital literacy can magnify dissonance between the healthcare professional and the client.

Enablers include:

- Introductions. Always introduce yourself and do so in a way that describes your role and availability to the young person. Introduce the young person to any other person who is involved in their care. It is appropriate to use first names in introductions because this represents contemporary culture, but it is equally important that the young person is informed about the delegations and roles of the people who are in helping positions.
- Dress code. Health professionals wearing contemporary and age-appropriate, smart casual, logo-free and modest clothing conveys respect and authenticity to young people. Young people are quick to identify 'fake' or imposter-like affiliation with their culture, and they have a low regard for it.
- Use of respectful plain language that is not laden with professional jargon or the casual lingo of young people. Keep yourself informed about the casual vocabulary of young people, because it is the role of health professionals to be able to interpret and understand the communication styles of the people they are trying to help (Wilson et al., 2012). It is appropriate to ask the young person for a definition of any term they use that you are unfamiliar with, because this conveys respect and interest in the person.
- Respect. Convey respect by responding appropriately to young people so that they feel they have been heard and that their experiences are regarded seriously (McAllister & Handley, 2008; Wilson et al., 2012).
- Sharing humour with young people (not laughing at them) and talking with (not at) the young person. Position yourself to journey with the young person towards recovery.
- Familiarity with young people's social and cultural connections. Build and maintain a general awareness of the popular music, TV, internet and social media preferences of young people. Perhaps engage in some of these activities (at least, occasionally) to gain some first-hand experience of these important social and cultural characteristics of young people's behaviour. This is of particular importance in regard to social media, because it has become a primary communication tool for young people, and on occasion can be a source of some discomfort as well (e.g. cyber-bullying) (Christensen, 2007; Christensen & Petrie, 2013a, 2013b; Department of Health and Ageing, 2012).
- Consultation. Check with young people about whether their basic needs have been met (e.g. when was the last time they ate, had a drink, a change of clothes and a safe place to sleep?). If the young person is hungry, then providing a simple sandwich and drink can convey care and will assist in establishing therapeutic rapport and trust.
- Time management. Provide opportunities for breaks in assessment sessions, so that engagement is optimised. Ensure that the young person has a support person present (preferably of their own choosing) if they would like that.
- Shared responsibility. Negotiate an agreement of shared responsibility, behaviours and actions that are achievable and safe for both the young person and the mental health

professional/s, and that these are based on the rights and responsibilities of both. Clarify what the consequences might be for breaking the agreement (e.g. mandatory reporting of abuse, invoking the Mental Health Act to promote and ensure safety etc.). Include young people and their families in the decision-making about mental healthcare interventions (Coughlan et al., 2011; McAllister & Handley, 2008).

- Reciprocal play and learning. Develop some basic skills in appropriate social activities; for example, playing electronic board games of interest to young people, sporting activities (e.g. shooting basketball hoops or pool/snooker, or ten pin bowling). There is no need to be proficient in any of these activities, but it is ideal to create an opportunity for young people to teach you how to develop skills in some of these types of activities. The reciprocal nature of learning and caring promotes horizontal rather than hierarchal relationships, which have helpful therapeutic qualities.

Developmental stages

There are several seminal theorists whose work explains the developmental stages of children and young people. A general knowledge of these developmental concepts will assist mental health practitioners to understand the related implications for mental health, recovery and well-being (McAllister & Handley, 2008). The psychological, intellectual and moral development of children and young people has been described across the lifespan, and with stages specifically relating to the need for successful schooling and cohesive social relationships (Erikson, 1968; Kolberg, 1963; Piaget, 1952; Vogel-Scibilia et al., 2009). Neurological developmental explanations are also relevant because the physiological development of the brain continues until about 22 years of age for humans, and thus cognitive abilities and capacities in young people are still forming at an early adult life stage (Blows, 2011; Geake, 2009).

It is equally important to consider the ecological systems that influence human development, and particularly any effects that magnify risk, vulnerability, strengths and resilience in regard to the mental health and well-being of young people (Bronfenbrenner, 1986, 2005). Young people need an environment in which they can be nurtured and in which their fundamental physical, social and psychological needs are met, in order to become robust individuals who are resilient and able to cope and thrive in all life domains (Candlin, 2008; Harms, 2010; Stein-Parbury, 2009).

Reducing risk and vulnerability

Mental health promotion is about reducing the risk factors and vulnerabilities that may predispose young people towards mental illness. A strengths-based focus is concerned with increasing opportunities to build psychological, physical and social strengths, because in doing so they offer protection and a buffer to various risks and vulnerabilities, and thus the effects of adverse conditions are minimised. Promoting sufficient support for families who care for children and young people is especially important in this regard, because healthy family contexts represent an ideal environment for children and young people to thrive (Lourey, Holland & Green, 2012).

There are many external factors that can arise outside of the control of the young person, or even their family unit. Within Australia and Aotearoa New Zealand, and across the world, natural disasters and adversities such as bushfires, floods, drought and pandemics have, historically and to this day, restricted access to support, intervention and treatment. The increased stress and anxiety experienced by family units during these challenging times often snowballs to young people, who may experience a decline in mental health as an indirect result. These natural adversities often unintentionally remove young people from their peer support groups by increasing the workload at home.

PERSONAL NARRATIVE

Serena – through the eyes of a paediatric RN, during a pandemic emergency

I had been working as a registered nurse in an eight-bed rural paediatric unit for four years. Over this time, I observed how unique this ward environment was compared to adult wards. Here, every ailment under the sun was admitted. There were no sub-categories or specialised units. Clinical, behavioural and mental health: all areas of paediatric nursing in one spot. This made it incredibly interesting, but also ridiculously challenging. With a premature infant needing nasogastric feeds in room 3, a teenager returning from surgery following the open repair of a broken arm in room 4a and a 5- year-old neutropenic patient admitted with a fever of unknown origin in isolation room 1, it was easy to occasionally forget about the 15-year-old girl in room 6b. She had been admitted with self-harm and suicidal ideation two days earlier and had spoken less than 10 words since then. Her habit of sending meals back to the kitchen untouched and avoiding drinking had been overlooked, but shortly after realising this the doctor assessed her, explained the implications of not eating or drinking and that the intervention of nasogastric feeding would be required if the behaviour continued. The girl began to eat, and drink, but not to speak. Over the following week the ward settled and I was able to spend more time with her. She began to speak, gradually. Board games became good icebreakers. A few more shifts passed, but the handovers were always the same: 'Reluctantly eating with +++ encouragement', 'Barely speaking and no expression', 'They're saying it's not eating disorder behaviour, more like self-punishment behaviour', 'She really just sits there all shift, it's impossible to engage with her'.

The girl never attempted to abscond. She self-harmed in hospital. She ate the minimum she was asked to. She didn't push the hospital's 'buttons' enough to be transferred to a higher facility. She 'behaved', and that saw her being overlooked.

Three weeks into her admission on the ward, at the end of a game of 'Rat–a–tat–cat' (a card game), she started to speak – *really* speak. I had asked about a photo of a newborn she kept on her bedside. She had said it was her little brother, who had passed away two years earlier. This led to a discussion about her 16-year-old brother, who had a young baby. She explained that her brother, his girlfriend and the baby had moved in to the family home 6 months earlier, due to the coronavirus outbreak. She said that not long after this she had also needed to start home-schooling as a result of the lockdown. Her brother had home-schooled her while caring for his baby, while her mother continued working. Her body language changed then, and her voice trembled. She alluded to a form of mistreatment, but she didn't disclose details. Later on that shift I made a mandatory report to Family and Community Service (FACS) regarding the alluded mistreatment. Over the following week the girl gradually shared her story and disclosed sexual abuse by her older brother prior to her admission, as well as two years earlier when he had last lived at the family home. She said, 'I hate COVID, it brought him [her older brother] back and took me away from my friends'.

This experience really stayed with me. I can't tell if it's the realisation of what the girl had endured and its potential for prolonged damage to her mental health. Or that it had seemed easier to keep treating the patients with fevers and broken bones than the teenager who refused to speak. I did learn though, that even a worldwide pandemic, experienced by all, is unique to each individual. It takes time, trust and rapport to learn the reality of another's experience, and it is often different to what we expect.

REFLECTIVE QUESTIONS

After reading about how unforeseen the effects of external disasters can be on a young person:

- How do you imagine you would respond to a teenage girl like this who was refusing to speak, eat or drink?
- What methods of communication do you think might help build rapport with her?
- Can you identify three other challenges young people may face due to natural disaster or adversity?

Drug and alcohol misuse

Alcohol abuse is highest among young people aged 16–24 years, with 11.1 per cent of the total Australian population of young people affected, which represents a significant vulnerability for the developing brains of people in this age group (Teesson et al., 2010). Cannabis use represents a further vulnerability for this age group, because it is the next most common drug used, with a first-use average age of 18 years, and it is associated with a risk of developing comorbid psychosis and/or anxiety and/or depression (Australian Institute of Health and Welfare (AIHW), 2011; Mental Health Council of Australia, 2006). More than one-third of people over 14 years of age use drugs in any given year in Australia, which is similar to other English-speaking countries (AIHW, 2011). This topic is further discussed in Chapter 12 of this book, and it is relevant to read that chapter in conjunction with this chapter, to further explore the drug and alcohol implications for young peoples' mental health.

Trauma and abuse

We know that it is far better that trauma or abuse should never occur, but if it has occurred, the younger the age at which it has occurred the more likely it is that the effects will be less overall than at older ages. This acknowledgement does not trivialise the experience of trauma or abuse at any life stage, but it does indicate that resilience and recovery is more strongly aligned with a younger exposure to adverse conditions (Harms, 2010).

Health practitioners are required by Australian law to mandatorily report any suspected or disclosed (direct or indirect) abuse, neglect or mistreatment to a child or young person, such as in Serena's narrative (Australian Institute of Family Studies (AIFS), 2020). The experience of **mandatory reporting**, alongside the confronting nature of what is often disclosed, can be difficult to process by the health professional. The opportunity to debrief within an

mandatory reporting – the legislative requirement for people in specific occupations to report suspected or confirmed child neglect or abuse to government authorities. It was first legally introduced in South Australia in 1969 to counteract the hidden nature of child neglect and physical abuse. Today, each Australian jurisdiction legislates which occupations are required to report and what types of abuse and neglect must be reported. Note that Australia wide, suspected or confirmed sexual abuse must always be reported, as must be the suspicion that future abuse or neglect is likely to occur.

appropriate and supportive environment has been expressed as exceptionally beneficial to the mental health of those involved.

In Aotearoa New Zealand, while the legislation does not require mandatory reporting of suspected case of child abuse and neglect, District Health Boards have within their child protection policies the requirement to report child protection concerns to police and or Oranga Tamariki/Ministry for Children (New Zealand Ministry of Health Manatū Hauora, 2021).

Trauma and abuse can take many forms (e.g. physical, emotional, sexual, refugee, war, neglect, family violence etc.) and bullying can be one such trauma for children and young people. The following exercise and real-life story can help to explore the mental health dynamics related to bullying in a school setting.

REFLECTIVE QUESTIONS

There is a schoolyard saying: 'Sticks and stones might break my bones, but words will never hurt me.'

- Why do you think reporting suspected or confirmed cases of child abuse and neglect is important?
- What are some of the challenges that health professionals might experience when lodging a child maltreatment notification?
- How can the health professional manage situations in which they are not sure whether a child maltreatment notification must be lodged?

Bullying – what it is like to be 12 years old and bullied

The following personal narrative is a real-life recount from Clare, who came to know a 12-year-old boy during her usual volunteering as a parent-helper at her local primary school. Some of the language in this story is very strong and unpleasant, but we have retained it because it is important that health practitioners who work in both general and mental health settings are aware of the challenges that young people face in their daily lives. It is relevant that health professionals should develop an appreciation of how uncomfortable some of their clients' circumstances of daily life can be. This is one such example.

PERSONAL NARRATIVE

Clare's story

He didn't have any hope that anything would change but said the pill would hopefully make him care less about it.

Jason is an extraordinary boy. I met him late last year when I was a parent-helper on a school excursion for Year 5 and 6 kids. Jason was in Year 6 in the combined Year 5/6 selective opportunity class for gifted children. He was and is an incredibly handsome kid: tall, olive skin and bright sparkly eyes. I immediately assumed he must be very popular because he was so well mannered and personable, along with being cute and clever. But it became clear that he was a loner.

I found Jason by himself a few times during the excursion and asked him why he wasn't off with the other boys. He told me they didn't like him and called him names, and it was easier for him to be by himself. I asked him what sort of names – he said 'queer, retard, gay, dancing queen, cock-sucker, faggot'. That's when I discovered that he had been dancing for several years (ballet, jazz, hip-hop). Jason said he really enjoyed dancing and that it kept him fit and flexible, and he seemed quite proud to show me his particularly muscular legs. But, clearly, some of the other boys at the school were merciless and relentless in their teasing. They didn't dare call him things when a teacher was around, but there were plenty of times when a teacher was not around. Jason told me that he was often shoved, had things thrown at him, was picked last and laughed at when he simply walked past those boys. He was sensitive to all the bullying behaviour.

I asked Jason if his mum and dad knew about it. He said they didn't know how bad it was, and just told him to ignore them. I told him he really needed to tell his teacher and his parents, and that I'd go with him to tell the teacher if he wanted that support. Jason said he didn't want to upset his mum more at that time. She was already crying a lot about his dad going overseas to work for 12 months. I urged him to tell his mum, ASAP! I also had a quiet word with his teacher.

Anyway, that was last year, and I didn't see Jason again until yesterday. He looked flat. There was no sparkle in his eye anymore. I asked him how he was finding high school and the selective gifted program there. That's when he told me about the five boys who have continued from primary school to the same high school as him, and how the teasing had worsened, and that he had been in a fight with one of them on Friday. He said one boy had hidden behind a pole and had kicked at him 'like a total coward'.

It was clear to me that Jason had initiated the fight, that he was just so angry and he really wanted to hurt that other boy. Jason said: 'He wouldn't even come out and fight like a man! And he calls me a sissy poofter!' I just thought that this poor, tortured kid, who is just a little boy on the inside, is alone and trying to prove his manhood. Jason said he was in trouble because of the fight, and on the weekend he had tried to kill himself. He had been in hospital all weekend, and was kept home on Monday and Tuesday, and then yesterday (Wednesday) was his first day back at school. Already that same boy Jason had tried to punch (the boy who had kicked out at him from behind the pole) had teased him again. Jason told me the name of the antidepressant he was on, the pill that he took with breakfast, how it was supposed to make him feel happier and how he would have to keep going back to see the psychologist for a while. He didn't have any hope that anything would change but said the pill would hopefully make him care less about it.

REFLECTIVE QUESTION

'Sticks and stones will break your bones, but words will never hurt you.'

- Have you heard that saying? Do you agree or disagree with the sentiment?
- What effects do you think unkind, unfair or disrespectful words have had on your own life?
- Have you developed some resilience to cope with unkind words when they are directed at you?
- What if hurtful words and actions occurred in your life on most days? How would you feel? What might you do? How do you think it might affect your mental health?

Mental health and schools

Increasingly, a focus on promoting inclusion and resilience within school student populations is seen as an important component of an holistic approach to promoting mental health and preventing mental illness in schools. There is a range of resources available to support mental health in schools. Be You (https://beyou.edu.au/) is an example of the model of integrated service delivery that supports schools in New South Wales, Australia. This model seeks to support schools to accumulate strengths and mitigate vulnerabilities to enhance the mental health and well-being of students, provide an opportunity for early help-seeking and early intervention and create a supportive environment for people who are in recovery with a mental health problem. Success in education and social successfulness are protective factors for mental health, learning and memory development are crucial for healthy neuro-development, and these further underpin mental health and well-being (Geake, 2009). Thus, collaboration of mental health professionals with schools and teachers has become an important strategy to support the holistic well-being of young people in general.

Mental health promotion, prevention and early intervention for young people

A focus on young people's mental health has gained some momentum in Australia in recent years, with a particular emphasis on the development of early intervention and youth-friendly services for people aged 15–24 years. The Australian government has sought to expand its *headspace* initiatives, which are considered by some to be flagship, integrated youth mental health services (Cohen et al., 2009; Hodges, O'Brien & McGorry, 2007; McGorry et al., 2007). However, the number of these centres is limited and there are many communities that lack these mental health services for young people, due to financial restraints. This significantly limits the availability and accessibility of youth-friendly services for young people, despite the aspirations and recognised need for appropriate mental health services for this age group (Boyd et al., 2011; Coughlan et al., 2011; Wilson et al., 2012). e-Mental health for young people is a concept that has the capacity to assist with some of the geographical limitations in service accessibility (Christensen & Petrie, 2013b; Griffiths, 2013; Smith, Skrbis & Western, 2012; Usher, 2010; Wilson et al., 2014; Wilson & Usher, 2015). See Chapter 11 for more about this topic.

What is it like to be a young person experiencing a mental illness?

Serena is a young woman who has been able to tell her story of experiencing a mental illness that was very disruptive in her life. She shares her experiences and, in doing so, illustrates some important aspects that helped her towards recovery.

PERSONAL NARRATIVE

Serena – a journey through darkness and a personal story of recovery: part one

For eight years I had struggled with anorexia nervosa and bulimia, never letting anyone know the secret that was killing me. From 13 to 20 years of age I was consumed by these undiagnosed mental illnesses. In December 2010 I realised that I needed help. For the first time in my life, I confided in a trusted adult and set about searching for treatment. A process that started with hope but ended in disappointment and despair as I searched without success for an eating disorder treatment facility in Australia.

On a morning in April 2011, I gave up. I could see no way out of the darkness I was in and no hope for a future. I felt so consumed and defeated that I attempted to end it all. After swallowing 40 paracetamol tablets, my 12-month journey through mental health hospitals began. My first encounter was the emergency department after my overdose. Laying on a stretcher, in a state of confusion, depression and physical shutdown, an empathetic nurse gently held my arm. She explained what was clinically happening to me, as my liver had begun to fail. More memorably though, she shared that she had been in my position 5 years earlier but was now better, and that planted a tiny flicker of hope for a future free from this darkness.

In contrast, the doctor on the ward that night treated me without respect or compassion. There was no understanding of mental illness, and I felt like a disgrace and shamed, wishing I was dead more than ever. One of the hardest things about that year was the shame of surviving. I experienced some nurses, doctors, family and friends who regarded me as simply an illness, a 'crazy', unstable, suicidal young girl, instead of a *person*. But inside I was *me*, scared, hopeless, *but still me*.

The months that followed, in ICU, low-security and high-security mental health wards, were like a bad dream. Even now, I wonder if it really happened. My body was failing and I was told that I could have a heart attack at any minute due to the eating disorders. In the hospitals there were nurses who understood, and those who didn't. One night in hospital, the negative self-talk playing on repeat in my head became incredibly intense and I resorted to self-harm to distract from those brutal thoughts. Afterwards I was helped by a compassionate nurse who thankfully showed me care and kindness. There was an understanding of my situation. An understanding that I was still just a girl, trapped in mental illness and feeling unable to escape from my own punishing thoughts.

As I was moved between psychiatrists, doctors, occupational therapists, dietitians, psychologists and nurses, I witnessed a range of treatment and care. Part of the treatment was the initiation of psychiatric medication. High doses of antidepressants, anti-psychotics, anti-convulsants and mood stabilisers employed with months of trial and error to find an effective combination. It was a horrible time. I had many adverse reactions (blurry vision, inability to void, facial and spinal muscular contortion and collapse) that even resulted in an emergency retrieval from the ward to the emergency department. For months I felt like a drugged-up zombie forced into a world of disturbed drowsiness by the medication.

Although the sedation seemed to dull my negative thoughts, it encouraged me to isolate and withdraw further.

One day in hospital, after fasting for 11 days due to the anorexia, I was made to eat. After the meal I couldn't cope. While vomiting in the bathroom a nurse pulled me out and dragged me by the back of my shirt through the ward to the isolation room, all the while telling me how disgusting and shameful I was. While I agree that the action of self-induced vomiting is disgusting and shameful, *I as a person am not*. But at that time, in that vulnerable state, *I believed I was*. The words of that nurse instilled in me more self-hatred and encouraged my decline into further depression. I found it particularly difficult that many staff members lacked understanding and knowledge about eating disorders and the intensity of the negative thoughts that are experienced. The contrast between healthcare practitioners who treated me as a person as opposed to a misunderstood illness was enormous. Their words had the ability to build hope or rip it away. The thing was, somewhere inside that broken, sick, depressed shell was me. *I was still there, not a word spoken or action taken toward me went unnoticed by my fragile inner self.*

When I spent some time out of hospital I was confronted with the stigma in the community about mental illness. Among many people the topic of my illness was avoided. Within my church, however, a project was commenced without my knowledge to create a quilt for me. While working on the project the members were freely discussing mental illness to educate themselves and break the stigma associated with it. This meant a lot to me as it removed some of the shame and judgement I had been feeling. [The perspective of the members was recorded in a nursing journal to assist and promote others to find innovative ways to support people in mental health recovery in their communities (Wilson, 2014).]

For the final three months of in-patient treatment, I was moved to an eating disorder-specific mental health hospital. It was a rough journey to break the cycle of illness that had developed over many years, but the staff were equipped to deal with the situations that arose. Understanding and knowledge allowed the nurses to treat their patients with dignity and informed care. There were still terribly hard times in which I thought I would break, but through therapy, support from loved ones, care from staff and a bucketful of determination, I was able to push through toward recovery.

REFLECTIVE QUESTION

Think about an occasion when you may have experienced feelings of shame or judgement in your life. Where there any actions by others that made you feel more or less comfortable?

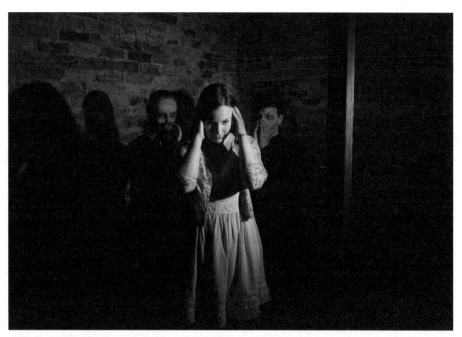

Figure 17.1   A representation of the experience of distress related to delusional thinking and auditory hallucinations, from *Immeasurable: The psychological experience of eating disorders*

Source: Elle Irvine (2015).

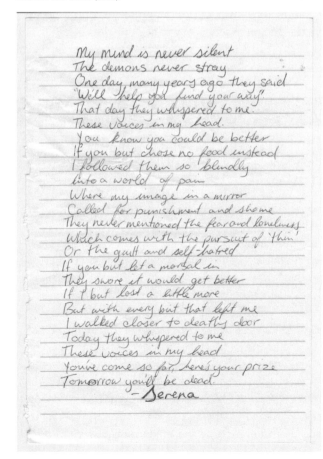

My mind is never silent
The demons never stray
One day many years ago they said
"We'll help you find your way".
That day they whispered to me.
These voices in my head.
You know you could be better
If you but chose no food instead
I followed them so blindly
Into a world of pain
Where my image in a mirror
Called for punishment and shame
They never mentioned the fear and loneliness
Which comes with the pursuit of 'thin'
Or the guilt and self-hatred
If you but let a mortal in
They swore it would get better
If I but lost a little more
But with every bit that left me
I walked closer to death's door
Today they whispered to me
These voices in my head
You've come so far, here's your prize
Tomorrow you'll be dead.
            — Serena

Figure 17.2   Poem written by Serena during a hospital admission

Source: Elle Irvine (2015).

Instilling hope

In Serena's story, she indicated that hope for the future was an important aspect in her recovery journey. Instilling hope for the future is a very important mental healthcare intervention, and one that all members of the interdisciplinary team are responsible for developing (Early Psychosis Writing Group, 2010; Kylma et al., 2006; Lourey et al., 2012). Serena described how some conversations and events developed in her a sense of hope for the future, and yet others diminished a sense of hopefulness while unhelpfully reinforcing stigma and feelings of shame and hopelessness. The following list provides some practical examples of ways in which health professionals can work towards fostering hope in the lives of other children and young people:

- Adopt a respectful and unhurried approach to listening.
- Sit next to the person. Physically and mentally position yourself to demonstrate care and interest in the person.
- Use words and language that are easily understood – avoid jargon. Explain what is happening and what will happen next so that there are no uncomfortable surprises.
- Ask about what the person is looking forward to in the future (today, next week, next year).
- Validate and reaffirm achievable, positive aspirations and goals for the future.
- Make sure basic immediate needs are met: safety (physical and psychological), enough good-quality food and drink, housing with a bed, appropriate clothing and privacy.
- Avoid flippant and judgemental comments – rather, reframe problems with a positive solution focus (Wand, 2010). Help the person to find a way to see the 'glass half-full, not half-empty'.

PERSONAL NARRATIVE

Serena – a journey through darkness and a personal story of recovery: part two

Since 2011, the year I spent in and out of hospitals receiving care from a multitude of health professionals, I have recovered … and relapsed … and recovered again. I learnt how intrinsic it is to recovery to have professionals and loved ones show understanding, patience, knowledge and empathy. Having professionals take the time and care to teach me about health, nutrition and how the body and brain work, in a non-judgemental manner, had a huge effect. Hope was planted the day I overdosed, in April of 2011, when a nurse held my arm and encouraged me with her empathetic words. I have had hard days since. I've had hard months since, but my hope for a healthy, happy future has slowly been restored and I am now living in the healthy reality of recovery.

The best part is that I have now developed therapeutic agency to encourage others and instil the sense of hope that was once instilled in me. I am now a paediatric-specialised registered nurse working with children and young people who are experiencing mental illnesses, including eating disorders, PTSD, self-harm, depression, suicidal ideation or attempts, and other related illnesses. I am humbled by them and reminded often how blessed I am to be here. How blessed I was to have had people instil irreplaceable hope during some of my darkest hours.

REFLECTIVE QUESTION

Think about the experiences of hope and empathy in Serena's story. In your own words, practise expressing hope and empathy for someone in similar circumstances as Serena. Try out your suggestions among your student peers. What feedback do they have for you to enhance your expressions of hope and empathy for others?

Common mental health conditions in young people

Suicide

According to *A Contributing Life: The 2012 national report card* (Lourey et al., 2012), 'more than 20 per cent of all deaths for young men and women in Australia are by suicide', making it a leading cause of death for young people (Lourey et al., 2012). While suicide is not an illness but a behaviour, the determinants of suicide are closely associated with mental illness. Suicide risk is accentuated by risk factors such as unemployment, social isolation, depression, recent bereavement, financial stress, disconnection from family and friends, and drug and alcohol misuse and abuse (Lourey et al., 2012). The greater the experience and accumulation of psychological stresses in a person's life, the greater the experience of suicidal thinking in that person's life (Lourey et al., 2012). Conversely, there are also protective factors that buffer individuals against suicide; for example, being connected with family and friends, being connected with culture, school and community, having another person care about their well-being, having a positive outlook on life, being creative with problem solving, experiencing sound financial stability, keeping physically fit and well, and being able to access mental health support when it is needed (Harms, 2010; Lourey et al., 2012).

Non-suicidal self-injury

Non-suicidal self-injury can be described as the deliberate destruction of bodily tissue without any suicidal intentions (Martin et al., 2010). It is considered a risk factor for suicide (Martin et al., 2010). All self-injury should be carefully considered on each occasion and should instigate a thorough mental health assessment. It is never appropriate to dismiss self-injury as a benign 'call for help'. It is a sign that the person's mental health is compromised, and that distress is occurring and is interfering with a healthy lifestyle. Such a person may benefit from mental health assessment and related interventions. Some examples of non-suicidal self-injury behaviours may include cutting, scratching, biting, burning or hitting (Martin et al., 2010). The motivation for non-suicidal self-injury includes emotional regulation and management, or self-punishment (Martin et al., 2010). Recalling Serena's story earlier in this chapter, health professionals can influence hope for the future with regard to non-suicidal self-injury, through their actions and words.

non-suicidal self-injury – the deliberate destruction of bodily tissue without any suicidal intentions

Psychosis

psychosis – a symptom
of mental illness that
affects a person's
thinking, behaviours
and emotions; in early
phases it is difficult to
pinpoint and can seem
as though 'something
is not quite right'. The
experiences of psychosis
are sometimes similar to
a normal developmental
phase of adolescence.
The problems become
acute when disorganised
thinking and/or
hallucinations, and/
or a deterioration in
maintaining social
relationships becomes
apparent and disrupts
daily life adversely.

Psychosis is most likely to be first experienced at around 18 years of age (Amos, 2012), and this age represents an important developmental stage in the life of young people as they transit between school and vocation or training, as young adults. This is sometimes a period of stress, important decision-making and participation in risk-taking behaviours that may include drug and alcohol misuse, and these activities may constitute risk factors for some people in regard to developing one or more episodes of psychosis (Early Psychosis Writing Group, 2010). Alcohol and cannabis consumption are both commonly noted in association with an onset of psychosis, and can be considered risk factors; however, it is not clear that a causal relationship is apparent (Early Psychosis Writing Group, 2010; Gregg, Barrowclough & Haddock, 2007; Henquet et al., 2006). Early intervention that addresses all life domains to support a young person with psychosis has been found to be highly successful and cost-effective (Amos, 2012; Yung, 2013).

Depression and anxiety

Depression and anxiety can affect young people, with the average onset of depression at about 25 years of age (that is, half of all people affected will have had their first experience of depression or anxiety as a young person) (Slade et al., 2009). Depression and anxiety problems affect people's emotions, thoughts, behaviours or motivation and physical health. A sustained lack of pleasure in life and a lack of hope for the future are some identifiable suicide risk factors. A range of psychological therapeutic actions can be administered by mental health practitioners to improve the mental health of people who experience depression and or anxiety (Ekers & Webster, 2012). A range of self-help and e-mental health resources, with a growing body of supporting evidence, is also useful (Christensen & Petrie, 2013a; Griffiths & Christensen, 2007).

REFLECTIVE QUESTIONS

You have read about the experiences of some young people, and some information about types of mental health difficulties that some young people may experience.

- Can you imagine what it must be like to be a young person who is experiencing a first episode of any type of mental illness?
- How do you think you would like to be helped, if this were you?
- What would be the most helpful things a mental health professional (e.g. a nurse) might do to assist you in getting help, and in recovering?

SUMMARY

This chapter has presented stories and information, supplemented with activities designed to deepen your understanding of:

- Seminal theorists whose work explains the developmental stages of children and young people. A general knowledge of these developmental concepts assists mental health practitioners to understand the related implications for mental health, recovery and well-being (McAllister & Handley, 2008). Young people need environments in which they can be nurtured and in which their fundamental physical, social and psychological needs are met, in order to become robust individuals who are resilient and able to cope and thrive in all life domains (Candlin, 2008; Harms, 2010; Stein-Parbury, 2009).
- The need for practitioners to ensure that youth-friendly services, environments and relationships exist between young people and health professionals and enhance timely engagement in mental health care by young people, when it is needed.
- Enablers and barriers to authentic engagement with young people. A respectful relationship will need to develop so that mental health care is achieved (Conradson, 2003; McAllister & Handley, 2008). In particular, it is important to ensure that the behaviours of the health professionals do not represent a barrier to young people engaging with mental healthcare providers (Wilson et al., 2012). For example, health professionals should not try to become like a young person by adopting the behaviours or popular language of young people; however, neither should they be shocked or unaware of the real-life experiences and culture of young people.
- Instilling hope for the future is a very important mental healthcare intervention, and one that all members of the interdisciplinary team are responsible for developing. There are several techniques that practitioners can adopt to instil hopefulness in young people.
- Common mental health conditions experienced by young people, including suicide ideation, non-suicidal self-injury, psychosis, depression and anxiety. It is important for practitioners to be aware of these conditions and to recognise that young people respond well to a range of mental healthcare interventions, and that best recovery and well-being are most likely where early interventions can be achieved.

CRITICAL THINKING/LEARNING ACTIVITIES

1   List some practical ways in which you could find a point of congruence or agreement with a young person. How could you find some common area of interest that allows you to demonstrate empathy and warmth towards a young person with a mental illness?
2   List some features of a youth-friendly environment in which to deliver mental health care.
3   List some ways in which a therapeutic rapport might be developed and maintained with young people.
4   In what ways does hope for the future (or lack of it) affect the recovery journey for a young person?
5   Visit some of the websites provided in this chapter. Which one appeals to you the most? Why?

LEARNING EXTENSION

Visit the website of Children of Parents with a Mental Illness (COPMI) at https://www.copmi .net.au, or the COPMI Facebook page at https://www.facebook.com/COPMIorg. These resources are designed to support and foster resilience while buffering vulnerability in children who are sometimes the carers of parents with mental illness. In addition, the siblings of children with disabilities often also share the burden of caring for them. An expert and carer group with representatives from Australia and Aotearoa New Zealand has developed a beginning discussion about this newly identified dynamic and an initial report advocates for support for vulnerable siblings (Royal Australian & New Zealand College of Psychiatrists, 2010).

Listen to this podcast from Radio National's *All In the Mind* program, which discusses the physical and mental health care of young people: https://www.abc.net.au/radionational/programs/allinthemind/newdocument/4689134

ACKNOWLEDGEMENT

We thank Sandy Butler for contributing some ideas in the development of this chapter.

Thanks to Dr Janene Carey for professional editorial assistance.

FURTHER READING

Coughlan, H., Cannon, M., Shiers, D., Power, P., Barry, C., Bates, T., Birchwood, M., Buckley, S., Chambers, D., Davidson, S., Duffy, M., Gavin, B., Healy, C., Healy, C., Keeley, H., Maher, M., Tanti, C. & McGorry, P. (2013). Towards a new paradigm of care: The International Declaration on Youth Mental Health. *Early Intervention in Psychiatry, 7*: 103–8.
The International Association for Youth Mental Health advocates for the mental health of young people worldwide. This article states the aims of the declaration and organisation.

Kids Helpline (Website). Retrieved from https://kidshelpline.com.au/
Kids Helpline is a resource to support the health and safety of children and young adults, including mental health and well-being.

Reachout (Website). Retrieved from https://au.reachout.com/
Online tools and online therapy for a range of mental illnesses suitable for children, young people and their parents and families.

REFERENCES

Amos, A. (2012). Assessing the cost of early intervention in psychosis: A systematic review. *Australian and New Zealand Journal of Psychiatry, 46*(8): 719–34.

Australian Institute of Family Studies (AIFS). (2020). *Mandatory Reporting of Child Abuse and Neglect*. Child Family Community Australia Resource Sheet. Retrieved from https://aifs.gov .au/cfca/sites/default/files/publication-documents/2006_mandatory_reporting_of_child_abuse_ and_neglect.pdf

Australian Institute of Health and Welfare (AIHW). (2011). 2010 *National Drug Strategy Household Survey Report*. Drug statistics series no. 25. Cat. no. PHE 145. Canberra: AIHW.

Blows, W. T. (2011). *The Biological Basis for Mental Health Nursing*, 2nd edn. New York: Routledge.

Boyd, C. P., Hayes, L., Nurse, S., Aisbett, D. L., Francis, K., Newnham, K. et al. (2011). Preferences and intention of rural adolescents toward seeking help for mental health problems. *Rural and Remote Health, 11*(1582): 1–13.

Bronfenbrenner, U. (1986). Ecology of the family as a context for human development: Research perspectives. *Developmental Psychology, 22*(6): 723–42.

——— (2005). Ecological systems theory. In U. Bronfenbrenner (ed.), *Making Human Beings Human: Bioecological perspectives on human development* (pp. 106–73). Thousand Oaks: Sage Publications.

Candlin, S. (2008). *Behaviour Change in Adolescence. Therapeutic communication: A lifespan approach.* Frenchs Forest, NSW: Pearson Education Australia.

Christensen, H. (2007). Internet-based Mental Health Interventions for Young Australians. Paper presented to the New South Wales Early Psychosis Forum, Westmead Hospital, Sydney.

Christensen, H. & Petrie, K. (2013a). Information technology as the key to accelerating advances in mental health care. *Australian and New Zealand Journal of Psychiatry, 47*(2): 114–16.

——— (2013b). State of the e-mental health field in Australia: Where are we now? *Australian and New Zealand Journal of Psychiatry, 47*(2): 117–20.

Cohen, A., Medlow, S., Kelk, N. & Hickie, I. B. (2009). Young people's experiences of mental health care. Implications for the headspace national youth mental health foundation. *Youth Studies Australia, 28*(1): 13–20.

Conradson, D. (2003). Spaces of care in the city: The place of a community drop-in centre. *Social and Cultural Geography, 4*(4): 507–25.

Coughlan, H., Cannon, H., Shiers, D., Power, P., Barry, C., Bates, T. et al. (2011). The Association of Child and Adolescent Mental Health Special Interest Group in Youth Mental Health in Ireland, 1–5. Retrieved from www.inspireireland.ie/wp-content/uploads/2011/10/YMH-Declaration_full-version_september-2011.-11.pdf

Coughlan, H., Cannon, M., Shiers, D., Power, P., Barry, C., Bates, T., Birchwood, M., Buckley, S., Chambers, D., Davidson, S., Duffy, M., Gavin, B., Healy, C., Healy, C., Keeley, H., Maher, M., Tanti, C. & McGorry, P. (2013). Towards a new paradigm of care: The International Declaration on Youth Mental Health. *Early Intervention in Psychiatry, 7*: 103–8.

Department of Health and Ageing. (2012). *E-Mental Health Strategy for Australia.* Canberra: Australian Government. Retrieved from www.health.gov.au/internet/main/publishing.nsf/Content/D67E137E77F0CE90CA257A2F0007736A/$File/emstrat.pdf

Early Psychosis Writing Group. (2010). *Australian Clinical Guidelines for Early Psychosis*, 2nd edn. Melbourne: Orygen Youth Health.

Ekers, D. & Webster, L. (2012). An overview of the effectiveness of psychological therapy for depression and stepped care service delivery models. *Journal of Research in Nursing, 18*(2): 171–84.

Erikson, E. (1968). *Identity, Youth and Crises.* New York: WW Norton.

Geake, J. G. (2009). *The Brain at School. Educational neuroscience in the classroom.* Berkshire: Open University Press.

Gregg, L., Barrowclough, C. & Haddock, G. (2007). Reasons for increased substance use in psychosis. *Clinical Psychology Review, 27*: 494–510.

Griffiths, K. M. (2013). A virtual mental health community: A future scenario. *Australian and New Zealand Journal of Psychiatry, 47*(2): 109–10.

Griffiths, K. M. & Christensen, H. (2007). Internet-based mental health programs: A powerful tool in the rural medical kit. *Australian Journal of Rural Health, 15*, 81–7.

Harms, L. (2010). *Coping with Stress. Understanding human development: A multidimensional approach.* South Melbourne: Oxford University Press.

Henquet, C., Krabbendam, L., Spauwen, J., Kaplan, C., Lieb, R., Wittchen, H. et al. (2006). Prospective cohort study of cannabis use, predisposition for psychosis, and psychotic symptoms in young people. *British Medical Journal, 330*(11): 1–5.

Hodges, C. A., O'Brien, M. S. & McGorry, P. D. (2007). headspace: National youth mental health foundation: Making headway with rural young people and their mental health. *Australian Journal Rural Health, 15*: 77–80.

Irvine, E. (2015). *Immeasurable: The psychological experience of eating disorders.* Brisbane: Elle Irvine.

Kolberg, L. (1963). The development of children's orientations toward moral order: Sequence in the development of moral thought. *Vita Humana, 6*(11): 33–173.

Kylma, J., Juvakka, T., Nikkonen, M., Korhonen, T. & Isohanni, M. (2006). Hope and schizophrenia: An integrative review. *Journal of Psychiatric and Mental Health Nursing, 13*: 651–64.

Lourey, C., Holland, C. & Green, R. (2012). *A Contributing Life: The 2012 national report card on mental health and suicide prevention.* Sydney: National Mental Health Commission. Retrieved from www.mentalhealthcommission.gov.au

Martin, G., Swannell, S., Harrison, J., Hazell, P. & Taylor, A. (2010). *The Australian National Epidemiological Study of Self-injury (ANESSI).* Brisbane: Centre for Suicide Prevention Studies.

McAllister, M. & Handley, C. (2008). Promoting mental health. In M. Barnes & J. Rowe (Eds), *Child, Youth and Family Health: Strengthening communities* (pp. 166–88). Marrickville, NSW: Elsevier.

McGorry, P. D., Tanti, C., Stokes, R., Hickie, I. B., Carnell, K., Littlefield, L. K. et al. (2007). headspace: Australia's national youth mental health foundation – where young minds come first. *Medical Journal of Australia*, *187*(7): S68–70.

Mental Health Council of Australia. (2006). *Where There's Smoke … Cannabis and mental health*. Melbourne: ORYGEN Youth Mental Health Service.

New Zealand Ministry of Health *Manatū Hauora*. (2021). Family Violence Questions and Answers (Webpage). Retrieved from https://www.health.govt.nz/our-work/preventative-health-wellness/family-violence/family-violence-questions-and-answers

Piaget, J. (1952). *The Origins of Intelligence in Children* (M. Cook, trans.). New York: International Universities Press.

Rogers, C. (1980). *A Way of Being*. Boston: Houghton Mifflin.

Royal Australian & New Zealand College of Psychiatrists. (2010). *Addressing the Needs of Siblings of Children with Chronic Conditions*. Melbourne: Royal Australian & New Zealand College of Psychiatrists. Retrieved from www.ranzcp.org/Files/ranzcp-attachments/Resources/siblings_report-pdf.aspx

Slade, T., Johnstone, A., Teesson, M., Whiteford, H., Burgess, P., Pirkis, J. et al. (2009). *The Mental Health of Australians 2: Report on the 2007 national survey of mental health and wellbeing*. Canberra: Department of Health and Ageing.

Smith, J., Skrbis, Z. & Western, M. (2012). Beneath the 'Digital Native' myth. *Journal of Sociology*, *49*(1): 97–118.

Stein-Parbury, J. (2009). *Challenging Interpersonal Encounters with Patients. Patient & person: Interpersonal skills in nursing*, 4th edn. Chatswood, NSW: Churchill Livingstone Elsevier.

Teesson, M., Hall, W., Slade, T., Mills, K., Grove, R., Mewton, L. et al. (2010). Prevalence and correlates of DSM-IV alcohol abuse and dependence in Australia: Findings of the 2007 National Survey of Mental Health and Wellbeing. *Addiction*, *105*(12): 2085–94.

Usher, W. (2010). Australian health professionals' social media (Web 2.0) adoption trends: Early 21st century health care delivery and practice promotion. *Australian Journal of Primary Health*, *18*: 31–41.

Vogel-Scibilia, S. E., McNulty, K. C., Baxter, B., Miller, S., Dine, M. & Frederick, J. F. (2009). The recovery process utilizing Erikson's stages of human development. *Community Mental Health Journal*, *45*: 405–14.

Wand, T. (2010). Mental health nursing from a solution focused perspective. *International Journal of Mental Health Nursing*, *19*: 210–19.

Watson, C., Rickwood, D. J. & Vanags, T. (2013). Exploring young people's expectations of a youth mental health care service. *Early Intervention in Psychiatry*, *7*: 131–7.

Wei, Y., Hayden, J. A., Kutcher, S., Zygmunt, A. & McGrath, P. (2013). The effectiveness of school mental health literacy programs to address knowledge, attitudes and help seeking among youth. *Early Intervention in Psychiatry*, *7*: 109–21.

Wilson, R. L. (2007). Out back and out-of-whack: Issues related to the experience of early psychosis in the New England region, New South Wales, Australia. *Rural and Remote Health*, *7*(715): 1–6.

——— (2014). Mental health recovery and quilting: Evaluation of a grass-roots community project in a small, rural Australian Christian church. *Issues in Mental Health Nursing*, *35*: 1–7.

Wilson, R. L., Cruickshank, M. & Lea, J. (2012). Experiences of families who help young rural men with emergent mental health problems in a rural community in New South Wales, Australia. *Contemporary Nurse*, *42*(2): 167–77.

Wilson, R. L., Ranse, J., Cashin, A. & McNamara, P. (2014). Nurses and Twitter: The good, the bad, and the reluctant. *Collegian*, *21*(2): 111–19.

Wilson, R. L. & Usher, K. (2015) Rural nurses: *A convenient co-location strategy for rural mental health care of young people. Journal of Clinical Nursing*, *24*: 2638–48.

Yung, A. (2013). Early intervention in psychosis: Evidence, evidence gaps, criticism and confusion. *Australian and New Zealand Journal of Psychiatry*, *46*(1): 7–9.

Mental health of older people

18

Helen P. Hamer, Debra Lampshire and Sue Thomson

LEARNING OBJECTIVES

At the completion of this chapter, you should be able to:

1 Understand the process of positive ageing and the life course of older people and their relationship to recovery focused care.
2 Consider the changing cultural norms of older people and the effects of ageism on older people and their loved ones.
3 Develop a deep awareness of the practice of human connectedness with older people.
4 Identify the skills in detecting and assessing the common mental health problems experienced by older people.
5 Describe the pharmacological and medico-legal aspects that relate to collaborative care planning with older people.
6 Understand and reflect on the future of care for older people and the application of an ethical framework to underpin practice.

Introduction

This chapter discusses the process of positive ageing, the life course and the changing cultural norms of older people within contemporary society. The chapter aims to assist nurses to consider and understand how **ageism** (Marques et al., 2020) and subsequent stigma and discrimination can affect the well-being of the older person and their family or loved ones. The multiple losses and associated mental health problems are presented. The specific approaches to nursing care required to support human connectedness with older people are also discussed. Common mental health problems, associated risk factors and considerations for treatment embedded within a recovery approach are explained. The chapter concludes with discussion of future issues for this area of specialty nursing practice.

ageism – an irrational prejudice based on a person's age

Background to the culture of older people

Many older people are ageing positively and continue to maintain their autonomy and well-being. Older people account for a considerable proportion of both Australia's and Aotearoa New Zealand's population. For example, Australia reports that in 2017, more than one in seven people was aged 65 and over (Australian Institute of Health and Welfare (AIHW), 2018). In Aotearoa New Zealand, census data from 2014 estimates that by 2036 around 1.2 million people, or 23 per cent of the total population, will be aged over 65 years (Ministry of Social Development, 2014).

Demographic projections of life expectancy suggest that New Zealanders over the age of 65 years will exceed 1 million by 2030. Further, ageing citizens will live longer; in the year 2010 the male population in the 80 years and older age group increased by 5.1 per cent (2900) to reach 60 200, while the female population increased by 2.8 per cent (2500) to 93 200 (Stats New Zealand, 2018). Likewise, the Australian government projects that the proportion of adults over 65 years will make up 25 per cent of the overall population by 2050 (AIHW, 2018).

Rather than being regarded as passive recipients of care, older people expect to continue to fulfil the same roles and responsibilities as others in society. Nurses, therefore, can expect to work alongside active, autonomous and informed older people who expect to participate in their care. Social cohesion, inclusion and belonging within their community also provide the vital protective factors for the older citizen's health and well-being, more so with the effects of the COVID-19 pandemic (Xie et al., 2020) and increased isolation.

Older people face many challenges, such as insecure housing and inaccessible health services and transport (Office for Seniors, 2017). Clearly, as this group continues to age, access to the latter resources that others in society take for granted is restricted because of the myths, stereotypes and stigma associated with ageing, and the resulting discrimination against older people.

The myths of ageing

Nurses must be mindful of the negative attitudes towards older people that proliferate within certain societies, including in Australia and Aotearoa New Zealand. According to Marques and colleagues (2020), ageism remains a widespread phenomenon and a significant threat to older people's well-being. For example, Bodner and colleagues (2018) report that ageism within health systems have led mental health professionals to rate older people as having poorer prognoses and as less appropriate for therapy than younger people with the same symptoms.

Older people and their families frequently experience prejudicial attitudes and discriminatory practices (Raymond, 2019; Werner & Segel-Karpas, 2020). Further, older people with mental illness carry a double burden of stigma and discrimination. Negative attitudes held by health professionals can prevent older people seeking help from services when needed, and this is compounded by the older person's fear that they will be coerced into involuntary treatment and rest homes, which further delays seeking treatment (Norvoll, Hem & Lindemann, 2018).

Of further concern is the risk of poly pharmacy (Fialová et al., 2018; Petrovic, Somers & Onder, 2016), due to multiple medications and the risk factors of memory problems, economic and social problems. Poly pharmacy thus requires highly individualised health care for both the older person and their family. Best practice tools, such as the Beers Criteria (American Geriatrics Society, 2015) and STOPP/START screening tool can support practitioners to prescribe safely (O'Mahony et al., 2014).

Practitioners who provide care and treatment for older people also experience courtesy stigma (Bachleda & El Menzhi, 2018), and are equally held in lower status by their professional peers. Stigma is associated with the degrading of a person and their loss of respect, due to some unique attribute or characteristic that is regarded as undesirable. Courtesy stigma is 'stigma by association', a term introduced by Erving Goffman (1963) in his book *Stigma: Notes on the management of spoiled identity*. Goffman describes courtesy stigma as when society also degrades or loses respect for a person because that person associates with someone who is stigmatised. Therefore, practitioners are required to reflect on their own attitudes and beliefs about older people and act as advocates to assist in the elimination of ageism and equity in the provision of health care (Adams & Collier, 2009).

REFLECTIVE QUESTIONS

- In pairs, write a list of some of the negative labels or words about older people that you have heard, in both your social and professional arenas.
- Briefly discuss how these labels and words are perpetuated by social media.
- What role do registered nurses have in changing these ageist assumptions?

Generativity and life tasks of older people

Villar (2012) suggests that successful ageing is related to good health and the ability to adapt to life changes through achievement in efficient functions of daily living and the sharing of life stories with others. Since older people may naturally reminisce and share their life stories, Cohen's (2001, 2009) seminal work proposes the process of **reminiscence therapy,** which benefits older people and is commonly practised (Cuevas et al., 2020; Elias, Neville & Scott, 2015).

Cohen (2009, 2001) proposes a theory about the life tasks in later life that could increase longevity, described as two phases in the final stages of the life cycle: these are *retirement/*

reminiscence therapy – the use of life stories – written, oral or both – to improve psychological well-being; video recordings are now increasingly popular in life story production

liberation and *summing up/swan song*. Cohen asserts that most people fare well, as retirement brings the liberating potential to explore new activities and relationships. Subsequently, the older person experiences renewed feelings of freedom, courage and self-confidence. The second life phase – *summing up/swan song* – relates to the inclination to appraise one's life work, ideas and discoveries, and to share them with family or society. The swan song, the final part of this phase, refers to a person's last act or final creative work before retirement or death.

Maintaining the narrative in practice is important when included in clinical notes and care planning, and this is equally as important as administering medication and other nursing tasks. Formally incorporating the narrative of the person's life story can strengthen the interpersonal alliance and preserve the dignity of the older person (Anderberg et al., 2007), and increase the human connectedness that many older people long for in their daily lives.

Recovery

recovery – 'a process, a way of life, and a way of approaching daily challenges of mental illness and to re-establish a new and valued sense of integrity and purpose … in a community in which one makes a significant contribution' (Deegan, 1988, p. 15)

The principles embedded within the **recovery** approach underpin mental health care within Australasia (Australian Government, 2012; Mental Health Commission, 2012); equally, having a life worth living is a core tenet of the recovery approach. As argued earlier, Fialová and colleagues (2018) suggest that ageist attitudes held by practitioners can influence the sense of hope that older people can live a life worth living, even in the face of multiple health problems. A stronger focus on what recovery means to older people has identified specific differences when compared to other younger age groups. Recovery for older people with mental distress can be described as 'continuing to be me' (NSW Ministry of Health, 2018), through an enduring sense of identity, and by drawing on a lifetime's experiences, coping strategies and resilience.

Copeland (2015) describes the six guiding principles of recovery: hope, education, self-advocacy, personal responsibility, support, and having meaning, purpose and direction. The complex combinations of mental health and addiction issues, disabilities, long-term conditions and/or dementia must not be a barrier to older people achieving the best quality of life. Recovery focused services are expected to deliver interventions and practices that promote recovery and reduce discrimination. Regaining and maintaining the major domains of one's life, namely housing, relationships, work and recreation, to live a satisfying, hopeful and contributing life are therefore essential for recovery (Deegan, 2005; Shanks et al., 2013).

ageing in place – when an older person continues to live in the facility of their choice for as long as they are able to do so, and have the necessary services and supports in place to accommodate changing needs and circumstances

However, older people face many challenges, such as having adequate resources, familiarity and stability; therefore, it is important for nurses to adapt their practice to bring the focus onto the broader social and economic needs of older people when planning care. As the population ages and older people continue to live in their own homes, **ageing-in-place** initiatives focus on supporting the three important aspects of home, home environment and the neighbourhood (Butcher & Breheny, 2016; van Hees et al., 2017). Adoption of a community focus will support a sense of human connectedness for the older person to their social structures and resources. Nurses will also be expected to ensure that older people feel safe and secure by offering a range of culturally appropriate services.

Debra's story

As a consumer academic and advisor, I have taught the recovery approach and the required competencies (Mental Health Commission, 2001) to many mental health professionals. It became apparent in these workshop discussions that many of the participants believed that the concept of recovery did not apply to older people with mental illness. These assumptions were based on the view that older people were unable to recover from dementia or other organic brain changes. I believe that the professionals were confusing 'cure' with recovery. Recovery, as a philosophy, equally applies to the older person. Older people have said to me: 'We are not robbed of the ability to recover as we age; we rob ourselves when others hold the belief that it is not possible'. Recovery is not limited by age. Moments of hope are precious to the older person and are to be celebrated. Any evidence of these moments tells us recovery is entirely possible. Experiences of distress, despair and confusion are not exclusive to the older person, and neither, thank goodness, is recovery. Recovery happens when nurses harness the enduring strengths of the person so they can continue to thrive, even when there are limited life years left. In sum, respect, love and being valued are universal imperatives required at any stage of the life span.

Culture of older people

Paying attention to the cultural aspects of nursing; that is, care that is congruent with the older person's cultural background and expectations (McBride, 2011; Zittoun & Baucal, 2021), will influence and cultivate the development of human connectedness within the nurse–older person alliance. For example, cultural differences can be ethnicity, or cultural or gender identity, such as being lesbian or gay. Specific tasks of developing the alliance with the older person involve **being-with** (Deegan, 2005; Russo & Rose, 2013). Being-with, rather than doing-to, in each encounter helps to foster human connectedness and a genuine interest, and conveys a sense of curiosity about the older person's narrative, in balance with the biomedical aspects of care.

> **being-with** – promotes the practitioner's deeper awareness of the meaning and dignity in human suffering

On a deeper level, it is important that nurses pay attention to the more existential aspects of being human (Bernstein, 2019), and recognise the barriers to exploring specific areas of the lives of the older person. Exploring aspects of the person's human experiences, such as sexual orientation, spirituality, experience of sexual abuse or trauma (see Chapters 2 and 15), substance abuse and suicidal ideation can be difficult for some nurses to discuss. We call these the '5 Ss'. For example, the connection between sexual orientation and well-being is important to explore with older people (Averett, Yoon & Jenkins, 2013), based on homophobia and prejudice extant in many health facilities.

Older people wish to continue to be sexually active and expect to talk about this with their health professionals (Bauer, Haesler & Fethersonhaugh, 2016; Malta et al., 2018). However, Bodley-Tickell and colleagues (2008) report that an increasing number of older people are contracting sexually transmissible infections due to unprotected sexual activity. This may be due to older people's perceptions of the use of condoms, for instance, as a contraceptive rather than as protection against infections. Therefore, sexual health programs, such as safe-sex messages aimed specifically at older people, can address any erroneous assumptions about sexual activity among older people.

REFLECTIVE QUESTIONS

- In pairs, choose one of the '5 S' topics above and discuss your own emotional and behavioural reactions when planning to address this aspect with an older person in your care.
- Discuss the types of appropriate questions that maintain the human connectedness with the older person when discussing this aspect of nursing assessment and care planning.

Human connectedness

To promote human connectedness in practice, nurses can undercut ageist assumptions and move beyond a primary focus on the biomedical understanding of people's distress, such as encouraging older people to explore other factors, such as grief and loss. Older people have diverse life experiences that bring a unique and individual set of beliefs and values accumulated over years of a life well-lived. Human connection is fostered by the respectful manner of the nurse. Taking the time to be-with the older person is also important.

Seminal work by Stebbins and colleagues (1999, 2002) reminds health professionals that giving people time to answer questions is important. Allowing time for the person to answer requires patience, respectful listening and deference. The notion of *presencing* (Benner, Tanner & Chesla, 2009; Candlin & Candlin, 2014) is the craft of being-with, rather than doing-to, and is equally important in the care of older people.

Human connectedness is also underpinned by the protection of the rights of older people and ensuring the provision of the range of services that promote their autonomy and well-being (Office for Seniors, 2017). Older people are entitled to excellent care from qualified specialist nurses, who can coordinate a range of options, such as psychosocial support, access to novel anti-psychotics and antidepressant medications, respite care, age-appropriate alcohol and other drugs treatment and, importantly, culturally appropriate services (Office for Seniors, 2017).

The dignity of risk

dignity of risk – the right to choose to take some risks in your daily life, based on making an informed choice and accepting the possibility of harm or failure

According to Lord (2011) and Gooding (2013), the term **dignity of risk** emerged from the disability sector and is increasingly being incorporated into the care of older people. However, mental health services have progressively become risk-averse environments (Higgins et al., 2016; Sawyer, 2005). Likewise, the care of older people with mental illness is equally dominated by risk management, often at the expense of the therapeutic relationship (Felton, Repper & Avis, 2018)

While assessment of risk is concerned primarily with avoiding or minimising harm to self or to others, the nurse needs to assess whether the older person is at risk from others. Rush and colleagues (2012) suggest that older people's understanding of risk is multifaceted and requires the balancing of risk-taking and risk avoidance, to support the autonomy and well-being of older people. The skill of safety and risk assessment develops as a nurse's practice advances and through experience in writing risk assessments that include the person's narrative in their treatment plans and clinical notes. The skill of assessing risk also requires that the nurse collaborates with the multidisciplinary team so that the nurse is not making such decisions alone.

Elder abuse

One of the most important aspects in the vulnerability of ageing is the risk of elder abuse. Fox (2012), and Lachs and Pillemer (2015) provide a comprehensive review of the mostly unreported, poorly defined and researched, yet growing problem of elder abuse and interpersonal violence within older people's own homes, by family members, in the wider society and by staff in residential care settings. Fox reports that five types of abuse are recognised: psychological, physical, sexual, financial and neglect (including self-neglect). Abuse of any kind is a violation of the person's human rights (World Health Organization, 2020), yet as one of the sensitive 'S' topics described earlier, nurses often do not feel confident in detecting, exploring and reporting elder abuse. The nurse must never feel alone with this disclosure as the degree of moral distress experienced by the nurse can be overwhelming; therefore, consulting a senior nurse to plan the next steps in care is recommended.

Medico-legal aspects

Nurses are both legally and ethically bound to ensure that older people are informed about their treatment and care options, or exercise their right to refuse treatment (Health and Disability Commission, n.d.; Nursing Council of New Zealand, 2012). Autonomous choices are voluntary and based on reasoning, and occur when people are adequately informed. If, because of dementia or other mental illness, a person cannot make autonomous choices, they are said to lack decision-making capacity (Sessums, Zembrzuska & Jackson, 2011).

Capacity and competency

The question of whether people have decision-making capacity or competence is frequently tested in the care of older people. Nurses need to be aware of the differences between decision-making capacity and competence. Decision-making capacity is when a clinician assesses a person's ability to make decisions about their health care, and is therefore a clinical assessment. To assess capacity, the clinician establishes whether the person can do the following: understand information relevant to the decision; retain the information, even if it is only for a short period of time; and can use or weigh the relevant information in the decision-making process. This includes the capacity to see both sides of the argument and the ability to communicate their decision by talking, using sign language or another form of communication understood by others (Braun et al., 2009; Pinsker et al., 2010).

Competence is a legal definition and is determined by the family court, based on whether the older person has the capacity to reason and makes decisions specific to the task, appreciates their circumstances and understands the information they are given. It is important to note that capacity can fluctuate over time, and lengthy and continuing medical procedures may need to repeat assessments of the person's capacity.

In Aotearoa New Zealand, if an older person no longer has capacity or competence to make these decision, then the person's rights are protected through the *Protection of Personal*

Property Rights Act 1988 (3PR Act). It is important for nurses to ascertain whether the older person has an identified enduring power of attorney (EPA) plan as part of the standard nursing assessment, because the person's decision-making ability can alter dramatically within a short period of time. The 3PR Act ensures that if the person has not nominated or appointed an EPA, and is now deemed to lack the capacity to do so, the family court will appoint both a property manager to protect and manage the person's property and financial matters, and a welfare guardian to protect future management of the person's health care and personal needs.

In Aotearoa New Zealand, the *Mental Health (Compulsory Assessment and Treatment) Act 1992* (Mental Health (CAT) Act) is invoked in situations where the person is assessed to have a high degree of risk, or their safety is compromised due to an associated serious mental illness, and where assessment and treatment without the older person's consent is required. However, an older person cannot be subject to the Mental Health (CAT) Act due to concerns about their competence alone.

Advance preferences and statements

Regardless of the impairments, a person is entitled to have their wishes respected; hence, the importance of planning in advance for one's preferences for care. There are continuing debates about the effects of health law on the care of older people, particularly competence, capacity and assessment of the value-laden concept of insight (Diesfeld & Sjöström, 2007; Hamilton & Roper, 2006). Such debates inform practitioners' decisions to use compulsory detention and treatment that suspend the rights and responsibilities of older citizens. To sustain their autonomy and preferences further, the nurse can support the older person to complete a written plan setting out information about what the person wishes to say to the treatment team, and to summarise the things that are important to the person.

These written plans are usually described as psychiatric advance directives (Lenagh-Glue et al., 2021; Ouliaris & Kealy-Bateman, 2017) or advance preferences statements (Lenagh-Glue et al., 2020). With older people, practitioners may need to also consider end-of-life advance care plans as people's physical health decline (Thomas, Lobo & Detering, 2017). Though nomenclatures vary, the emphasis of these plans is to support the practitioner to record and have a stronger recognition of the person's autonomy when they cannot account for themselves. However, there is no law that specifically protects a person's advance directive, which can be overridden if the person is subject to the Mental Health (CAT) Act.

So far, we have discussed the many sociopolitical, emotional and cognitive challenges that older people face as they age. The following section focuses on the factors that contribute to common mental health problems that bring older people to mental health services.

Common mental health problems

There are many challenges to growing older, such as increasing loneliness and isolation, developing medical conditions and cognitive decline. Stressful events or physical illness can increase anxiety and thus can reduce the older person's capacity to ward off trauma-related memories, images and feelings (Dinnen, Simiola & Cook, 2015; Hamilton & Atkinson, 2009). As well as risks of developing a depressive or anxiety illness, psychosis is one of the most common conditions in later life, with a lifetime risk of 23 per cent (Reinhardt & Cohen, 2015). However, manifestations of psychosis, such as hearing voices and talking to oneself can have an alternative explanation, as Margaret describes in her narrative.

PERSONAL NARRATIVE

Margaret's story

About 7 months after my husband died, I was out having lunch with my daughter. I came over all queer and demanded she take me home. I insisted she go home as I just needed to rest; I didn't want her there. I got out our photo albums and starting rummaging through them, taking out all the photos of my husband from different stages in our lives. You see, I had sat there with my daughter and I'd forgotten what my husband had looked like. I just couldn't bring his face to mind, and this terrified me. For 65 years he was my whole life, and suddenly I couldn't recall his face; I thought I'd really lost him then. I pasted his photos over everything – the cupboards, chairs, the toilet – everywhere I looked, so I wouldn't forget him. I started talking to him as if he was still around. I stopped going out. I just wanted to be with him and my memories. My kids thought I'd gone crazy. They came and took his photos down. I was furious and screamed at them to get out and never come into my house again. I had never in all their lives raised my voice to them; it must have been quite a shock when 'Mum blew her top'. Now they really thought I was going mad. They sent someone round to see me from the mental health services. I thought they were trying to put me in a home or the looney bin and forget about me, like they were trying to forget about their father. The nurse was very patient and kind, though, and finally I agreed to talk to her. She was a lovely woman, very easy to talk to. She said she didn't think I was crazy, which was a relief; she thought I was lonely and sad, and grieving for my husband. She was absolutely right, and she 'got' it. She helped me to cope with my loss and the enormity of it; she helped me link up with other widows and people with similar interests. She talked to my family and explained what was really going on for me. Everything is going well now. I have his photo by my bed and on the telly. His is the first face I see each morning and the last I see at night, just like it always was. I still talk to him about what's going on, but the nurse assured me that I am perfectly normal. So, I sit at night and tell him all about my day and what's happening on *Coronation Street*, and I feel content. You know, he's a much better listener since he died!

REFLECTIVE QUESTIONS

- On reading Margaret's narrative about her experiences, write down a summary of the important aspects of her story that need to be included in her clinical notes.
- Name three important elements of the communication style of the nurse in her interaction with Margaret.

This example highlights the importance of fostering human connectedness by undertaking a collaborative and shared formulation of the person's presentation, based on both the narrative and the biomedical understanding of the older person's current problems.

Cognitive decline, depression, delirium or dementia? Getting the diagnosis right

It is particularly difficult for health professionals to effectively recognise, identify and diagnose cognitive changes in older people. For example, the *Diagnostic and Statistical Manual of Mental Disorders* (DSM-5; American Psychiatric Association, 2013), provides criteria in a new category to determine the appropriate diagnoses of mild and major neurocognitive disorders. In this chapter, we focus on how nurses can develop a clear understanding of the different presentations, or the '4Ds' (Downing, Caprio & Lyness, 2013; Insel & Badger, 2002).

cognitive decline –
changes in one's thinking and remembering, and difficulty in retaining new information or juggling multiple mental tasks

Cognitive decline is part of the ageing process, and these changes are gradual; however, if the nurse notices a rapid decline, then the following diagnoses must be considered.

Depression

The prevalence rates for depression vary by age, peaking in older adulthood (above 7.5 per cent among females aged 55–74 years, and above 5.5 per cent among males) (World Health Organization, 2017). Unlike adults, depression in older people is often enduring in nature and associated with increased physical disability, cognitive impairment and mortality (Reinhardt & Cohen, 2015).

The similarity of symptoms between unresolved grief associated with multiple losses – for example, one's social status, employment or own home – and depression must also be considered and assessed. Pharmacological treatment of depression in older people places them at greater risk of injury because of adverse effects such as postural hypotension, leading to falls and fractures (Peron, Gray & Hanlon, 2011). Psychological interventions for depression, in an individual or group format, is often challenging because of age-related disabilities, in particular hearing loss and cognitive impairment. As discussed previously, nurses must work at a slower pace and be prepared to repeat conversations in all interactions with the older person (Lenze & Loebach Wetherell, 2011).

Delirium

Delirium or acute confusion and behavioural changes are evident in 10 to 40 per cent of people over 65 years of age admitted to hospital (Cerejeira & Mukaetova-Ladinska, 2011). Of those admissions, 25 to 60 per cent of people will develop delirium after discharge and, if left untreated, delirium effectively contributes to a mortality rate as high as 65 per cent of admissions. Of concern, Inouye (2018, 1990) asserts that poor reporting on episodes of delirium is not well recognised or recorded by nurses, hence her development of the tool titled Confusion Assessment Method (CAM), for the identification of delirium. The long-term consequences of less-than-optimal management of delirium results in falls, subsequent immobility and early admission to residential care (Fox et al., 2013). It is recommended that all nurses be alert to the complexity of such presentations and incorporate accurate diagnosis and treatment by using standardised assessment tools (National Institute for Health and Clinical Excellence, 2010).

Helen's story – the practitioner's role

As an advanced practice nurse working in the liaison psychiatry team within a general hospital, I received a referral from a registered nurse on a medical ward, requesting an assessment of Tom, a 75-year-old man with diabetes. Tom was assessed as being psychotic and deluded, and had refused to leave his bed for the past 24 hours. When I entered Tom's room, he immediately shouted at me to 'Get down, they will shoot you!' I crouched down close to his bed and at eye level with Tom. Maintaining a calm voice and gently probing Tom's reasons for his fear of harm to anyone who entered his room, I established that Tom was a war veteran who believed that he was back in the trenches and being shot at by snipers. The sudden onset of these beliefs, coupled with evidence of urinary incontinence and no prior history of mental health problems, led me to conclude that Tom was delirious. I subsequently read the clinical notes to identify the tell-tale signs and symptoms of delirium, such as spiking temperatures above 38°C, frequency and discomfort on micturition, fluctuating blood sugar levels, inadequate hydration noted on the fluid balance chart and reversal of his sleep–wake cycle. I explained to Tom about the cause of his fear and confusion, and contacted and explained this to his family, who had been very distressed about his out-of-character behaviour. I wrote a medical and nursing delirium treatment plan in his clinical notes and briefed the nursing team at their handover. Once the delirium plan was in place, Tom's confusion abated and he was able to start his activities of daily living again and was soon discharged.

Dementia

The numbers of people presenting in Aotearoa New Zealand and Australia with dementia is growing significantly. Age is the most significant risk factor for the development of dementia. Of the people over 65 years of age, 5 per cent will likely develop dementia, while in those aged 80 years or older, 20 per cent will develop dementia (Alzheimer's Disease International, 2011). However, Fox and colleagues (2013) report that the many clinical features that older adults present with lead them to conclude that there is no 'magic test' (p. 510) to diagnose dementia. These findings have implications for older people (Cook, 2008; Giezendanner et al., 2019), as Bradford and colleagues (2009) argue, at least two-thirds of this population attending primary and secondary healthcare providers will never receive the diagnosis of dementia and therefore will be ineligible for the available support services and pharmaceutical interventions. There are well-documented reasons for the sector's failure to diagnose dementia, including limited general practitioner time, lack of confidence in making the diagnosis and concern that making the diagnosis will have an adverse effect on the person and their family (Ahmad et al., 2010). For these reasons, there is clear evidence that the diagnosis and long-term management of dementia may be a role for advanced practice nurses (Boustani et al., 2007).

Offenders and dementia

Older offenders within the criminal justice system represent the most significant group to have considerable effect on both the aged residential care sector and the justice system (Baidawi et al., 2011; Kingston et al., 2011). Recent reports on child sexual abuse have led to survivors laying charges against their now elderly, former male caregivers, resulting in an increasing number of older persons ageing and dying in prisons (Australian Government, 2017; Christodoulou, 2012).

Further, most offenders will have comorbidities such as alcohol abuse, poor nutrition, traumatic brain injury and mental illness (Moore et al., 2016; Smith & Trimboli, 2010). Given the punitive prison environment, the offenders in this vulnerable population are ageing 10 to 15 years sooner than the general population, and the number of incarcerated offenders with dementia is growing significantly (Maschi et al., 2012; Skarupski et al., 2018).

PERSONAL NARRATIVE

Barbara's story

Barbara was a 77-year-old, gifted woman. She owned her own home and was incredibly house-proud. She was about to be discharged from mental health services, having been involved with the services for a number of years. Barbara had a history of childhood sexual abuse and later married an affluent but very violent man who had regularly assaulted her, leading to many admissions to the emergency department. After the birth of her third child, Barbara experienced a psychotic episode and was admitted to a psychiatric institution. Subsequently, her husband left her for another woman, she lost custody of her children and was denied visitation rights. She was discharged from hospital and was determined to gain control of her life and to see her children again. Barbara reconnected with her youngest son but her two older children were reluctant to have contact. She was thrilled with the relationship she had managed to develop with her son and was very careful not to burden him with discussion of the past. Two weeks prior to her discharge, Barbara went for an assessment at the memory clinic, as she had noticed a few memory lapses. More tests followed and Barbara was told that she had Alzheimer's dementia. The health professional told her that she probably had about 6 months before she would be significantly impaired, and advised her to immediately sell her home, give up her volunteer work and arrange to live with her son. Barbara went home in a state of shock; she locked herself in her home and wept. She wouldn't answer the door or the phone. She stopped seeing her friends, gave up her volunteer job and stopped eating. Everything that had brought her any pleasure had now ceased. She spoke to her son, and while he was sympathetic, he was concerned about the burden of caring for her as he was just beginning a new marriage with young children. Barbara then appeared to emerge from the state of shock; she put her house on the market, tidied everything up, packed her precious belongings away and made arrangements to go and visit her son. While a little thin, she seemed reasonably happy and content. Barbara died of heart failure 6 months after being given her diagnosis. Barbara had never had any heart problems prior to her diagnosis of Alzheimer's.

REFLECTIVE QUESTIONS

- How would you explain the diagnosis of Alzheimer's dementia to Barbara and her family?
- Do you think there is the connection between Barbara's heart failure and the diagnosis of Alzheimer's dementia? If so, discuss.

Older people and suicide

Depression is the most common cause of suicidal ideation in older people, with older men continuing to be at higher risk of completing suicide (Barak et al., 2020; Wand et al., 2018). In Australia, the highest rate of suicide in 2019 was observed in men aged 85 years and older. The highest rate in females was recorded in those aged 40–44 years (Australian Bureau of Statistics, 2019).

Wand and colleagues (2020) report that the adverse mental health effects of the COVID-19 pandemic on older adults need to be highlighted due risk of infection and isolation at home, thereby exacerbating already high suicide rates. As well as the physical health challenges, Barak and colleagues (2020) report that the high risk factors also include the psychosocial effects of loneliness, poverty and a move to residential care as the main reasons for the high suicide rates. These findings are consistent with the benefits of ageing-in-place and reduction in the effects of poly pharmacy in older people. Opportunistic screening, referral and appropriate treatment for depression and suicidal ideation in older people are required. The brief Ask Suicide-Screening Questions (National Institute of Mental Health, n.d.), has four brief questions and takes 20 seconds to administer; it is designed to give confidence to practitioners in detecting suicide ideation and prevention in older people.

An ethical framework to underpin practice

Hughes and colleagues' (2002) early work in the application of an ethical framework for dementia care reported that nurses working with older people lack confidence in the ethical aspects of their practice, specifically autonomy, consent, advance directives, truth-telling, research and end-of-life issues. Brannelly (2006), and Hughes and Common (2015), suggest that nurses can integrate ethical aspects of their care within the **ethic of care** framework (Tronto, 1999, p. 261).

The four elements of the ethic of care framework are:

1 *Caring about* – paying attention
2 *Taking care of* – taking responsibility for initiating caring activities
3 *Care giving* – attention to the person's specific care needs
4 *Care-receiving* – collaborating and ensuring the quality of the care process.

ethic of care – a framework concerned with the principles of ethics; not only avoiding wrong-doing but also reflection on and action towards affecting the conditions that make a good life possible

The adoption of an ethic of care framework by nurses to underpin their practice will strengthen the opportunity for increased autonomy, participation and inclusion of older citizens.

The future of older people's mental health care

We can expect that future health systems will need to prepare and adapt to provide more services for the current hidden population of younger adults (below 65 years) with chronic covid syndrome (CCS; Baig, 2020), neurological disorders, cognitive decline and/or dementia. The increasing problem and effects of poly pharmacy in older people, particularly in aged residential care settings, may be better served with an increase in the number of

deprescribing – the clinically supervised process of stopping or reducing the dose of an inappropriate medication that may cause harm or is no longer beneficial for the person (Royal Australian College of General Practitioners (RACGP), 2019)

nurse practitioner prescribers (Prasad, et al., 2014), and the specialist skills of **deprescribing** (Linsky et al., 2019). As the ageing population increases worldwide, recruiting and retaining experienced nurses within the aged-care sector are also challenges for the future. Recruitment and retention initiatives are underway in Australia to increase this specialist workforce (Commonwealth of Australia, 2020).

The family and loved ones of older people

Observing the decline of a loved one, described as a 'social death' (Brannelly, 2011; Spicker, 2000), and loss of their personhood, begins the journey of grief for the carer. The carer may experience a range of emotions, and their resilience may be tested. It is important therefore that nurses maintain the human connectedness with the family and loved ones of consumers, to support and offer appropriate interventions that assist the carer to maintain their own physical and mental health (Watson, Tatangelo & McCabe, 2018). Supporting the psychosocial needs of family members caring for people with dementia is vital (Hopwood et al., 2018). Taking regular breaks, through arranging respite and home support for carers, is also important (Mast, 2013). Further, Rosness and colleagues (2011) report that the risk of depression and anxiety in those who are caring for family members with dementia can be reduced by regular home visits by professionals.

INTERPROFESSIONAL PERSPECTIVES

Sue's story

As a nurse, I am the care partner for Olivia, a 65-year-old Māori woman with a long history of bipolar affective disorder (BPAD). Olivia has been discharged from the acute in-patient unit and has a history of managing her illness really well with the support of her partner and her children. Olivia's partner died six months ago and all her children now live in Australia. In the past four weeks, Olivia has felt increasingly sad and alone, and has quickly become unwell. Once in hospital, with 24-hour care Olivia stabilised quickly once she began taking her regular medication and with support from the staff. She began eating and exercising regularly, and regained social contact with her extended *whānau* (family), who came from out of town to support her.

I reviewed Olivia's care at my multidisciplinary team meeting and advised the team of my plans for Olivia's discharge into her community. I collaborated with the social worker to arrange meals-on-wheels to support her nutritional requirements, as well as visits from a support person to visit Olivia twice a week to take her to the supermarket, undertake the heavier housework and provide some regular social contact and monitoring of Olivia's well-being. After gaining Olivia's consent, a cultural support worker from Māori services visited her twice weekly. The cultural worker invited Olivia to join the **kāumātua** and **kuia** weekly support group so that Olivia could meet and converse in *te reo* Māori, with her peers. This support is vital for Olivia to nurture her spiritual needs and assist with grieving for her partner.

kāumātua – Māori term for a respected male elder

kuia – Māori term for a respected female elder

I also rang her local pharmacy and arranged for Olivia's medication to be dispensed in a blister-pack to support her regular medication regimen. Given that Olivia now lives alone, I contacted the St John's Ambulance service and arranged for Olivia to receive a monitored alarm bracelet so that she can feel safe in knowing that she can summon help in the event of a fall or an intruder in her home. Overall, reconnecting Olivia to the variety of support structures is paramount so that she can continue to use her own resources and resilience, and continue living as independently as possible within her community.

SUMMARY

This chapter has presented stories and information, supplemented by activities designed to deepen your understanding of:

- The care of older people. Older people can thrive and have lives worth living, even in the face of adversity related to biopsychosocial and cultural issues, and cognitive decline.
- The role of the mental health practitioner in supporting the recovery process and acting as a change agent to challenge and reduce the effects of ageism and stigma in society towards this age group within the medical and social arenas.
- What health practitioners can learn from older people; their life experiences have prepared most for adversity, and by offering deference and human connectedness to older people, this specialist area of practice can be rewarding.
- The ability of practitioners working within the specialist area to offer the advanced specialist practice to deliver interventions for the complicated nature of the mental health and neurological challenges, consideration of the legal and ethical aspects, and to advocate and model best practice care to other professions.
- The uncertainty of the potential effects of COVID-19 on the future health and well-being of those who live through the pandemic. As an international community of health practitioners, working with older people and their families the future will require us to work in partnership with the broader health agencies.
- The importance of partnership with older people and their families as they too will have the answers that practitioners seek to rise to this global challenge.

CRITICAL THINKING/LEARNING ACTIVITIES

1   What are some of the important priorities that you would need to consider in your plan of nursing care for a person experiencing cognitive decline?
2   What should be at the forefront of a nurse's mind when considering admitting an older person into an acute mental health unit?
3   An older person in your care tells you that they feel frightened when at home with their partner, who gets inebriated, becomes 'aggro' and starts yelling and shouting at them. On one occasion the older person sustained a broken rib. You are concerned for their safety; what is your next step?

4 Unresolved grief is often not detected or may manifest as a depressive illness. It can have a profound effect on the older person. What are the contributing factors to unresolved grief?

5 The notion of recovery has been regarded as not having a place in the care of the older person with dementia. How would you instil hope for an older person with dementia and their loved ones?

LEARNING EXTENSION

In pairs, discuss and write a short paragraph on the following:

- Is an offender entitled to be nursed within an appropriate dementia unit in the community setting? What are some of the risk factors to both the offender and the residents if the person is to be nursed in the dementia unit?
- Go to the Ask Suicide-Screening Questions (ASQ) Toolkit and practise asking the questions. Formulate the responses you would give to the older person: https://www.nimh.nih.gov/research/research-conducted-at-nimh/asq-toolkit-materials/index.shtml
- How would you coach a primary care clinician (nurse or GP) to increase their confidence and ability to provide appropriate responses in the use of this tool in their practice setting with older people?
- How would you start a conversation with an older person? View the short video *Depression in Older People* from Choose Psychiatry, designed by Dr Sophia Bennett, National Health England and available on YouTube: https://www.youtube.com/watch?v=mrqgaLnQ5zQ. Depression in older people is not inevitable, it is preventable, and it can be treated. The content supports nurses to start a conversation with older people by asking two simple questions to assess or diagnose depression. The content will be relevant to new mental health nurses working with older people and is also suitable to show older people and/or their loved ones. The key message to all practitioners is to see the person, not their age.

FURTHER READING

Read the following articles and consider the advantages and disadvantages in the use of this technology in the care of older people. How might this new technology help older people and their loved ones?

Bradwell, H. L., Edwards, K. J., Winnington, R., Thill, S. & Jones, R. B. (2019). Companion robots for older people: Importance of user-centred design demonstrated through observations and focus groups comparing preferences of older people and roboticists in south west England. *BMJ Open*, *9*(9): e032468.

Hopwood, J., Walker, N., McDonagh, L., Rait, G., Walters, K., Iliffe, S., Ross, J. & Davies, N. (2018). Internet-based interventions aimed at supporting family caregivers of people with dementia: Systematic review. *Journal of Medical Internet Research*, *20*(6): e216.

Jecker, N. S. (2020). You've got a friend in me: Sociable robots for older adults in an age of global pandemics. *Ethics and Information Technology*. Retrieved from https://doi.org/10.1007/s10676-020-09546-y

Te Pou o Te Whakaaro Nui. (2010). *Talking therapies for older adults: Best and promising practice guide for mental health and addiction services*. Auckland: Mental Health Programmes

Limited. Retrieved from https://www.tepou.co.nz/resources/talking-therapies-for-older-adults

Though medication remains important for older people with depression or anxiety disorders, increasingly older people are also referred to receive talking therapy. This resource provides a summary of the best and promising practices when using talking therapies with older people.

REFERENCES

Adams, T. & Collier, E. (2009). Services for older people with mental health conditions. In P. Barker (ed.), *Psychiatric and Mental Health Nursing: The craft of caring*, 2nd edn (pp. 486–92). London: Hodder Arnold.

Ahmad, S., Orrell, M., Iliffe, S. & Gracie, A. (2010). GPs' attitudes, awareness, and practice regarding early diagnosis of dementia. *British Journal of General Practice*, *60*(578): 360–5.

Alzhiemer's Disease International. (2011). *World Alzheimer's Report 2011: The benefits of early diagnosis and intervention. Executive summary*. Retrieved from http://www.alz.co.uk/research/WorldAlzheimerReport2011ExecutiveSummary.pdf

American Geriatrics Society. (2015). Beers criteria update expert panel 2015: Updated Beers criteria for potentially inappropriate medication use in older adults. *Journal of the American Geriatrics Society*, *63*(11): 2227–46.

American Psychiatric Association (APA). (2013). *Diagnostic and Statistical Manual of Mental Disorders: DSM-V*, 5th edn. Washington, DC: APA.

Anderberg, P., Lepp, M., Berglund, A.-L. & Segesten, K. (2007). Preserving dignity in caring for older adults: A concept analysis. *Journal of Advanced Nursing*, *59*(6): 635–43.

Australian Bureau of Statistics. (2019). *Intentional self-harm by age and sex: Age-specific death rates*. Retrieved from https://www.abs.gov.au/statistics/health/causes-death/causes-death-australia/latest-release#intentional-self-harm-suicides-key-characteristics

Australian Government. (2012). *Ten year road map for national mental health reform*. Retrieved from http://www.coag.gov.au/sites/default/files/The%20Roadmap%20for%20National%20Mental%20Health%20Reform%202012-2022.pdf.pdf

—— (2017). *Royal commission into institutional responses to child sexual abuse*. Retrieved from https://www.childabuseroyalcommission.gov.au

Australian Institute of Health and Welfare (AIHW). (2018). *Older Australia at a Glance*. Retrieved from https://www.aihw.gov.au/reports/older-people/older-australia-at-a-glance/contents/summary

Averett, P., Yoon, I. & Jenkins, C. L. (2013). Older lesbian experiences of homophobia and ageism. *Journal of Social Service Research*, *39*(1): 3–15.

Bachleda, C. L. & El Menzhi, L. (2018). Reducing susceptibility to courtesy stigma. *Health Communication*, *33*(6): 771–81.

Baidawi, S., Turner, S., Trotter, C., Browning, C., Collier, P., O'Connor, D., & Sheehan, R. (2011). Older prisoners: A challenge for Australian corrections. *Trends and Issues in Crime and Criminal Justice Series*, (426): 1–8.

Baig, A. M. (2020). Deleterious outcomes in long-hauler covid-19: The effects of Sars-Cov-2 on the CNS in chronic covid syndrome. *ACS Chemical Neuroscience*, *11*(24): 4017–20.

Barak, Y., Cheung, G., Fortune, S. & Glue, P. (2020). No country for older men: Ageing male suicide in New Zealand. *Australasian Psychiatry*, *28*(4): 383–5.

Bauer, M., Haesler, E. & Fetherstonhaugh, D. (2016). Let's talk about sex: Older people's views on the recognition of sexuality and sexual health in the health-care setting. *Health Expectations*, *19*(6): 1237–50.

Benner, P. E., Tanner, C. A. & Chesla, C. A. (2009). *Expertise in Nursing Practice: Caring, clinical judgment and ethics*, 2nd edn. New York: Springer.

Bernstein, S. (2019). Being present: Mindfulness and nursing practice. *Nursing*, *49*(6): 14–17.

Bodley-Tickell, A. T., Olowokure, B., Bhaduri, S., White, D. J., Ward, D., Ross, J. D. C., Smith, G., Duggal, H. V. & Goold, P. (2008). Trends in sexually transmitted infections (other than HIV) in older people: Analysis of data from an enhanced surveillance system. *Sexually Transmitted Infections, 84*, 312–7.

Bodner, E., Palgi, Y. & Wyman, M. F. (2018). Ageism in mental health assessment and treatment of older adults. In L. Ayalon & C. Tesch-Römer (eds.), *Contemporary Perspectives on Ageism* (pp. 241–62). New York: Springer Open.

Boustani, M., Schubert, C. & Sennour, Y. (2007). The challenge of supporting care for dementia in primary care. *Clinical Interventions in Aging, 2*(4): 631–6.

Bradford, A., Kunik, M. E., Schulz, P., Williams, S. P. & Singh, H. (2009). Missed and delayed diagnosis of dementia in primary care: Prevalence and contributing factors. *Alzheimer Disease and Associated Disorders, 23*(4): 306–14.

Brannelly, T. (2006). Negotiating ethics in dementia care: An analysis of an ethic of care in practice. *Dementia, 5*(2): 197–212.

———— (2011). Sustaining citizenship: People with dementia and the phenomenon of social death. *Nursing Ethics, 18*(5): 662–71.

Braun, M., Gurrera, R., Karel, M., Armesto, J. & Moye, J. (2009). Are clinicians ever biased in their judgments of the capacity of older adults to make medical decisions? *Generations, 33*(1): 78–91.

Butcher, E. & Breheny, M. (2016). Dependence on place: A source of autonomy in later life for older Māori. *Journal of Aging Studies, 37*: 48–58.

Candlin, S. & Candlin, C. N. (2014). Presencing in the context of enhancing patient well-being in nursing care, In H. Hamilton & W.-Y. S. Chou (eds.), *The Routledge Handbook of Language and Health Communication* (pp. 259–78). London and New York: Routledge.

Cerejeira, J. & Mukaetova-Ladinska, E. B. (2011). A clinical update on delirium: From early recognition to effective management. *Nursing Research and Practice, 2011*: Art. 875196.

Christodoulou, M. (2012). Locked up and at risk of dementia. *The Lancet Neurology, 11*(9): 750–1.

Cohen, G. D. (2001). The course of unfulfilled dreams and unfinished business with aging. *American Journal of Geriatric Psychiatry, 9*(1): 1–5.

———— (2009). New theories and research findings on the positive influence of music and art on health with ageing. *Arts & Health, 1*(1): 48–62.

Commonwealth of Australia. (2020). *Aged Care Workforce Retention Bonus Payment for Residential and Home Care Workers*. Retrieved from https://www.health.gov.au/initiatives-and-programs/aged-care-workforce-retention-bonus-payment-for-residential-and-home-care-workers

Cook, A. (2008). *Dementia and Wellbeing*. Dunedin: Dunedin Academic Press.

Copeland, M. E. (2015). *Wrap: Wellness recovery action plan*. West Dummerston, VT: Peach Press.

Cuevas, P. E. G., Davidson, P. M., Mejilla, J. L., & Rodney, T. W. (2020). Reminiscence therapy for older adults with Alzheimer's disease: A literature review. *International Journal of Mental Health Nursing, 29*(3): 364–71.

Deegan, P. E. (1988). Recovery: The lived experience of rehabilitation. *Psychosocial Rehabilitation Journal, 4*(11): 11–19.

———— (2005). *Recovery as a Journey of the Heart*. Boston, MA: Center for Psychiatric Rehabilitation: Boston University.

Diesfeld, K. & Sjöström, S. (2007). Interpretive flexibility: Why doesn't insight incite controversy in mental health law? *Behavioral Sciences and the Law, 25*(1): 85–101.

Dinnen, S., Simiola, V. & Cook, J. M. (2015). Post-traumatic stress disorder in older adults: A systematic review of the psychotherapy treatment literature. *Aging & Mental Health, 19*(2): 144–50.

Downing, L. J., Caprio, T. V. & Lyness, J. M. (2013). Geriatric psychiatry review: Differential diagnosis and treatment of the 3 d's – delirium, dementia, and depression. *Current Psychiatry Reports, 15*(6): 365.

Elias, S. M. S., Neville, C. & Scott, T. (2015). The effectiveness of group reminiscence therapy for loneliness, anxiety and depression in older adults in long-term care: A systematic review. *Geriatric Nursing, 36*(5): 372–80.

Felton, A., Repper, J. & Avis, M. (2018). Therapeutic relationships, risk, and mental health practice. *International Journal of Mental Health Nursing, 27*(3): 1137–48.

Fialová, D., Kummer, I., Držaić, M. & Leppee, M. (2018). Ageism in medication use in older patients. In L. Ayalon & C. Tesch-Römer (eds), *Contemporary Perspectives on Ageism* (pp. 213–40). New York: Springer Open.

Fox, A. W. (2012). Elder abuse. *Medical Science and Law, 52*: 128–36.

Fox, C., Lafortune, L., Boustani, M. & Brayne, C. (2013). The pros and cons of early diagnosis in dementia. *British Journal of General Practice, 63*(612): e510–e512.

Giezendanner, S., Monsch, A. U., Kressig, R. W., Mueller, Y., Streit, S., Essig, S., Zeller, A. & Bally, K. (2019). General practitioners' attitudes towards early diagnosis of dementia: A cross-sectional survey. *BMC Family Practice, 20*(1): 65.

Goffman, E. (1963). *Stigma: Notes on the management of spoiled identity.* New York: Simon & Schuster.

Gooding, P. (2013). Supported decision-making: A rights-based disability concept and its implications for mental health law. *Psychiatry, Psychology and Law, 20*(3): 431–51.

Hamilton, B. & Roper, C. (2006). Troubling 'insight': Power and possibilities in mental health care. *Journal of Psychiatric and Mental Health Nursing, 13*(4): 416–22.

Hamilton, C. & Atkinson, D. (2009). 'A story to tell': Learning from the life-stories of older people with intellectual disabilities in Ireland. *British Journal of Learning Disabilities, 37*(4): 316–22.

Health and Disability Commission. (n.d.). *The HDC Code of Health and Disability Services Consumers' Rights Regulation.* Retrieved from http://www.legislation.govt.nz/regulation/public/1996/0078/latest/DLM209080.html

Higgins, A., Doyle, L., Downes, C., Morrissey, J., Costello, P., Brennan, M. & Nash, M. (2016). There is more to risk and safety planning than dramatic risks: Mental health nurses' risk assessment and safety-management practice. *International Journal of Mental Health Nursing, 25*(2): 159–70.

Hopwood, J., Walker, N., McDonagh, L., Rait, G., Walters, K., Iliffe, S., Ross, J., & Davies, N. (2018). Internet-based interventions aimed at supporting family caregivers of people with dementia: Systematic review. *Journal of Medical Internet Research, 20*(6): e216.

Hughes, J. C. & Common, J. (2015). Ethical issues in caring for patients with dementia. *Nursing Standard, 29*(49): 42–7.

Hughes, J. C., Hope, T., Savulescu, J. & Ziebland, S. (2002). Carers, ethics and dementia: A survey of the review of the literature. *International Journal of Geriatric Psychiatry, 17*(1): 35–40.

Inouye, S. K. (2018). Delirium: A framework to improve acute care for older persons. *Journal of the American Geriatrics Society, 66*(3): 446–51.

Inouye, S. K., Van Dyck, C. H., Alessi, C. A., Balkin, S., Siegal, A. P. & Horwitz, R. I. (1990). Clarifying confusion: The confusion assessment method. A new method for detecting delirium. *Annals of Internal Medicine, 113*(12): 941–8.

Insel, K. C. & Badger, T. A. (2002). Deciphering the 4 D's: Cognitive decline, delirium, depression and dementia – a review. *Journal of Advanced Nursing, 38*(4): 360–8.

Kingston, P., Le Mesurier, N., Yorston, G., Wardle, S. & Heath, L. (2011). Psychiatric morbidity in older prisoners: Unrecognized and undertreated. *International Psychogeriatrics, 23*(8): 1354–60.

Lachs, M. S. & Pillemer, K. A. (2015). Elder abuse. *New England Journal of Medicine, 373*: 1947–56.

Lenagh-Glue, J., Potiki, J., O'Brien, A., Dawson, J., Thom K., Casey, H. & Glue, P. (2021). Help and hindrances to completion of psychiatric advance directives. *Psychiatric Services, 72*(2): 216–18.

Lenagh-Glue, J., Potiki, J., O'Brien, A., Dawson, J., Thom K., Casey, H., Glue, P., Thom, K., O'Brien, A., Potiki, J., Casey, H., Dawson, J. & Glue, P. (2020). The content of mental health advance preference statements (MAPS): An assessment of completed advance directives in one New Zealand Health Board. *International Journal of Law and Psychiatry, 68*: 101537.

Lenze, E. J. & Loebach Wetherell, J. (2011). State of the art: A lifespan view of anxiety disorders. *Dialogues in Clinical Neuroscience, 13*(4): 381–99.

Linsky, A., Gellad, W. F., Linder, J. A. & Friedberg, M. W. (2019). Advancing the science of deprescribing: A novel comprehensive conceptual framework. *Journal of the American Geriatrics Society, 67*(10): 2018–22.

Lord, J. (2011). *Ageism is a Human Rights Issue: Equality reform law project.* Human Rights Law Centre. Retrieved from http://www.humanrightsactionplan.org.au/nhrap-blogs/ageism-is-a-human-rights-issue

Malta, S., Hocking, J., Lyne, J., McGavin, D., Hunter, J., Bickerstaffe, A. & Temple-Smith, M. (2018). Do you talk to your older patients about sexual health. *Australian Journal for General Practitioners, 47*: 807–11.

Marques, S., Mariano, J., Mendonça, J., De Tavernier, W., Hess, M., Naegele, L., Peixeiro, F. & Martins, D. (2020). Determinants of ageism against older adults: A systematic review. *International Journal of Environmental Research and Public Health, 17*(7): 2560.

Maschi, T., Kwak, J., Ko, E. & Morrissey, M. B. (2012). Forget me not: Dementia in prison. *Gerontologist, 52*(4): 441–51.

Mast, M. E. (2013). To use or not to use. A literature review of factors that influence family caregivers' use of support services. *Journal of Gerontological Nursing, 39*(1): 20–8.

McBride, M. (2011). *Ethnogeriatrics and Cultural Competence for Nursing Practice.* New York: Hartford Institute of Geriatric Nursing. Retrieved from https://nursing.nyu.edu/innovation/hartford-institute-geriatric-nursing

Mental Health (Compulsory Assessment and Treatment) Act 1992, 46 Stat. N.Z. (1992). Retrieved from http://www.health.govt.nz/publication/guidelines-mental-health-compulsory-assessment-and-treatment-act-1992

Mental Health Commission. (2001). *Recovery Competencies for New Zealand Mental Health Workers.* Retrieved from https://files.eric.ed.gov/fulltext/ED457512.pdf

——— (2012). *Blueprint II: Improving mental health and wellbeing for all New Zealanders: How things need to be.* Retrieved from http://www.hdc.org.nz/media/20764kk2/blueprint%20ii%20how%20things%20need%20to%20be.pdf

Ministry of Social Development. (2014). *Annual Report 2013/2014.* Retrieved from https://www.msd.govt.nz/documents/about-msd-and-our-work/publications-resources/corporate/annual-report/2014/annual-report-2013-2014.pdf

Moore, E., Sunjic, S., Kaye, S., Archer, V. & Indig, D. (2016). Adult ADHD among NSW prisoners: Prevalence and psychiatric comorbidity. *Journal of Attention Disorders, 20*(11): 958–67.

National Institute for Health and Clinical Excellence. (2010). *Delirium: Diagnosis, Prevention and Management.* Retrieved from http://www.nice.org.uk/guidance/CG103/PublicInfo

National Institute of Mental Health. (n.d.). The Ask Suicide Screening Questions (ASQ) Toolkit. Retrieved from https://www.nimh.nih.gov/research/research-conducted-at-nimh/asq-toolkit-materials/index.shtml

Norvoll, R., Hem, M. H. & Lindemann, H. (2018). Family members' existential and moral dilemmas with coercion in mental healthcare. *Qualitative Health Research, 28*(6): 900–15.

NSW Ministry of Health. (2018). *NSW Older People's Mental Health Recovery-oriented Practice Improvement Project: Statewide project report.* Retrieved from https://www.health.nsw.gov.au/mentalhealth/resources/Publications/opmh-recovery-project-report.pdf

Nursing Council of New Zealand. (2012). *Code of Conduct for Nurses.* Retrieved from http://www.nursingcouncil.org.nz/download/283/coc-printsept12.pdf

Office for Seniors. (2017). *Briefing for Incoming Minister.* Retrieved from https://www.msd.govt.nz/documents/about-msd-and-our-work/publications-resources/corporate/bims/2017/seniors-bim-2017.pdf

O'Mahony, D., O'Sullivan, D., Byrne, S., O'Connor, M. N., Ryan, C. & Gallagher, P. (2014). STOPP/START criteria for potentially inappropriate prescribing in older people: Version 2. *Age and Ageing, 44*(2): 213–18.

Ouliaris, C. & Kealy-Bateman, W. (2017). Psychiatric advance directives in Australian mental-health legislation. *Australasian Psychiatry, 25*(6): 574–7.

Peron, E. P., Gray, S. L. & Hanlon, J. T. (2011). Medication use and functional status decline in older adults: A narrative review. *The American Journal of Geriatric Pharmacotherapy, 9*(6): 378–91.

Petrovic, M., Somers, A. & Onder, G. (2016). Optimization of geriatric pharmacotherapy: Role of multifaceted cooperation in the hospital setting. *Drugs & Aging, 33*(3): 179–88.

Pinsker, D. M., Pachana, N. A., Wilson, J., Tilse, C. & Byrne, G. J. (2010). Financial capacity in older adults: A review of clinical assessment approaches and considerations. *Clinical Gerontologist*, *33*(4): 332–46.

Prasad, S., Dunn, W., Hillier, L. M., McAiney, C. A., Warren, R. & Rutherford, P. (2014). Rural geriatric glue: A nurse practitioner–led model of care for enhancing primary care for frail older adults within an ecosystem approach. *Journal of the American Geriatrics Society*, *62*(9): 1772–80.

Raymond, É. (2019). The challenge of inclusion for older people with impairments: Insights from a stigma-based analysis. *Journal of Aging Studies*, *49*: 9–15.

Reinhardt, M. M. & Cohen, C. I. (2015). Late-life psychosis: Diagnosis and treatment. *Current Psychiatry Reports*, *17*(2): 1.

Rosness, T. A., Mjørud, M. & Engedal, K. (2011). Quality of life and depression in carers of patients with early onset dementia. *Aging & Mental Health*, *15*(3): 299–306.

Royal Australian College of General Practitioners (RACGP). (2019). Deprescribing. Retrieved from https://www.racgp.org.au/clinical-resources/clinical-guidelines/key-racgp-guidelines/view-all-racgp-guidelines/silver-book/part-a/deprescribing

Rush, K. L., Murphy, M. A. & Kozak, J. F. (2012). A photovoice study of older adults' conceptualizations of risk. *Journal of Aging Studies*, *26*(4): 448–58.

Russo, J. & Rose, D. (2013). 'But what if nobody's going to sit down and have a real conversation with you?' Service user/survivor perspectives on human rights. *Journal of Public Mental Health*, *12*(4): 184–92.

Sawyer, A.-M. (2005). From therapy to administration: Deinstitutionalisation and the ascendancy of psychiatric 'risk-thinking'. *Health Sociology Review*, *14*(3): 283–96.

Sessums, L. L., Zembrzuska, H. & Jackson, J. L. (2011). Does this patient have medical decision-making capacity? *JAMA*, *306*(4): 420–7.

Shanks, V., Williams, J., Leamy, M., Bird, V. J., Boutillier, C. L. & Slade, M. (2013). Measures of personal recovery: A systematic review. *Psychiatric Services*, *64*(10): 974–80.

Skarupski, K. A., Gross, A., Schrack, J. A., Deal, J. A. & Eber, G. B. (2018). The health of America's aging prison population. *Epidemiologic Reviews*, *40*(1): 157–65.

Smith, N. E. & Trimboli, L. (2010). Comorbid substance and non-substance mental health disorders and re-offending among NSW prisoners. *BOCSAR NSW Crime and Justice Bulletins*, 16.

Spicker, P. (2000). Dementia and social death. *Self Agency and Society*, *2*: 88–104.

Stats New Zealand. (2018). Population. Retrieved from https://www.stats.govt.nz/topics/population

Stebbins, G. T., Carrillo, M. C., Dorfman, J., Dirksen, C., Desmond, J. E., Turner, D. A., Bennett, D. A., Wilson, R. S., Glover, G. & Gabrieli, J. D. E. (2002). Aging effects on memory encoding in the frontal lobes. *Psychology and Aging*, *17*: 44–55.

Stebbins, G. T., Gabrieli, J. D. E., Masciari, F., Monti, L. & Geotz, C. G. (1999). Delayed recognition memory in parkinson's disease: A role for working memory? *Neuropsychologia*, *37*(4): 503–10.

Thomas, K., Lobo, B. & Detering, K. (2017). *Advance Care Planning in End of Life Care*. Oxford: Oxford University Press.

Tronto, J. C. (1999). Age-segregated housing as a moral problem: An exercise in re-thinking ethics. In M. Urban Walker (ed.), *Mother Time: Women, aging, and ethics* (pp. 261–77). Lanham, MD: Rowman & Littlefield Publishers.

van Hees, S., Horstman, K., Jansen, M. & Ruwaard, D. (2017). Photovoicing the neighbourhood: Understanding the situated meaning of intangible places for ageing-in-place. *Health & Place*, *48*: 11–19.

Villar, F. (2012). Successful ageing and development: The contribution of generativity in older age. *Ageing & Society*, *32*(7): 1087–105.

Wand, A. P. F., Peisah, C., Draper, B. & Brodaty, H. (2018). Why do the very old self-harm? A qualitative study. *The American Journal of Geriatric Psychiatry*, *26*(8): 862–71.

Wand, A. P. F., Zhong, B.-L., Chiu, H. F. K., Draper, B. & De Leo, D. (2020). Covid-19: The implications for suicide in older adults. *International Psychogeriatrics*, *32*(10): 1225–30.

Watson, B., Tatangelo, G. & McCabe, M. (2018). Depression and anxiety among partner and offspring carers of people with dementia: A systematic review. *The Gerontologist*, *59*(5): e597–e610.

Werner, P. & Segel-Karpas, D. (2020). Depression-related stigma: Comparing laypersons' stigmatic attributions towards younger and older persons. *Aging & Mental Health*, *24*(7): 1149–52.

World Health Organization. (2017). *Depression and Other Common Mental Disorders Global Health Estimates*. Retrieved from https://apps.who.int/iris/bitstream/handle/10665/254610/WHO-MSD-MER-2017.2-eng.pdf?sequence=1

———— (2020). *Elder Abuse*. Retrieved from https://www.who.int/news-room/fact-sheets/detail/elder-abuse

Xie, B., Charness, N., Fingerman, K., Kaye, J., Kim, M. T. & Khurshid, A. (2020). When going digital becomes a necessity: Ensuring older adults' needs for information, services, and social inclusion during Covid-19. *Journal of Aging & Social Policy*, *32*(4–5): 460–70.

Zittoun, T. & Baucal, A. (2021). The relevance of a sociocultural perspective for understanding learning and development in older age. *Learning, Culture and Social Interaction*, *28*: 100453.

Rural and regional mental health

Rhonda L. Wilson

19

LEARNING OBJECTIVES

At the completion of this chapter, you should be able to:

1 Describe the mental health needs of rural people.
2 Identify and discuss rural vulnerability and resilience with regard to mental health.
3 Understand the implications of travel, distance and access to mental health services for rural people.
4 Recognise lifestyle practicalities of mental health care in a rural community, and how these relate to recovery.
5 Identify forms of mental health care delivery for people in rural communities.

Introduction

This chapter begins with an overview of the clinical context in rural and regional areas, and explores the connections that rural mental health practitioners have within rural communities. Models of mental health promotion and service delivery are discussed. The nature of life in rural settings and the ways in which climate and geographical location affect the mental health of people are also considered in the context of mental health resilience and vulnerability. Attention is given to the effects of natural disasters, agribusiness, mining, the itinerant rural workforce and under-employment, and their associated mental health consequences. This chapter discusses some rural community benefits with regard to mental health promotion, such as a deeply felt sense of closeness in social proximity despite significant geographical distances between rural people. The chapter encourages readers to reflect upon, and critically think about, the ways in which mental health promotion, well-being and recovery can be enhanced in rural populations.

What is *rural*?

rural – a multi-dimensional concept that includes aspects of a person's culture, place, identity and geography, and the extent to which these align with standardised measures of rurality and remoteness

Rural is a multi-dimensional concept, which includes aspects of a person's culture, place, identity and geography, and the extent to which these align with standardised measures of rurality and remoteness (Wilson, Wilson & Usher, 2015). A range of perceptions and factors needs to be considered when understanding what it is to *be* a rural person. People who live in rural communities often identify closely with a deep sense of 'place', which includes psychological, emotional, socio-economic and geographical factors (Campbell, Manoff & Caffery, 2006; Wilson & Waqanaviti, 2021). In Australia, approximately one-third of the population lives in rural and regional areas (Australian Bureau of Statistics (ABS), 2019). People in rural and regional communities may refer to themselves as being 'from the bush', or as a 'country person', or as 'rural', and all of these descriptions convey a sense of identity. People from within a similar geographical region usually share a connection that includes an inherent sense of mutual support for each other, which can also be thought of as 'mateship' (Wilson, 2014). It is important that mental health professionals incorporate uncontrived respect for this culture into their professional practice and therapeutic interactions (Wilson et al., 2015).

In terms of mental health care, the rural person and the rural community are central to the concept of recovery. The cultural aspects underpinning what it is to be a rural person, and the places, people and interconnectedness that make up the rural lifestyle, are critical to understanding the whole picture of rural recovery processes (Wilson et al., 2015). Attention to these aspects will assist in developing mental health care plans that are realistic, achievable and person-centred (Wilson, 2014). If we confine our thinking to a health service-focused perspective, we will discover that there are perpetual service shortcomings that we cannot hope to address sufficiently within the bounds of usual resources. However, if we consider the strengths that are inherent within rural communities and cultures, we will discover creative ways in which the mental health of rural people can be improved (Lourey, Holland & Green, 2012; Wilson, 2014; Wilson & Waqanaviti, 2021).

Government departments need to utilise pragmatic measures to define rurality, so that they can plan to distribute resources and services equitably. Rurality has been defined in

Australia by an equation that accounts for both the population size and the distance required to travel to services by road transport. The Accessibility Remoteness Index of Australia (ARIA+) describes the relative ease or difficulty for rural people to access services by road (Hugo Centre for Population and Housing, 2020). The ARIA+ scale rates from 0 (high accessibility) to 15 (high remoteness), with five bands of remoteness identified in Australia (see Figure 19.1).

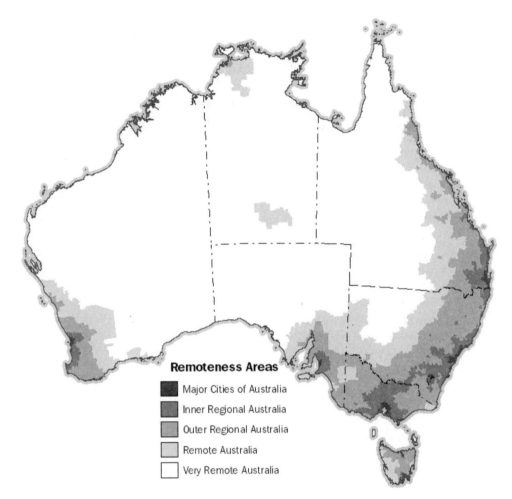

Figure 19.1   Map of the 2016 remoteness areas in Australia
Source: ABS (2016).

Thus, rurality is not a straightforward concept, and care needs to be taken in both urban and rural clinical settings to ensure that when planning for recovery in collaboration with people residing in rural communities, therapy is conducted with a positive regard to rural cultures and circumstances.

Waltzing Matilda

Perhaps nothing epitomises rural mental health, and rural context, in Australia as much as the Banjo Patterson poem that has become the unofficial national song: Waltzing Matilda.

The song is about a rural itinerant worker, a man who travels alone in search of work, and with his possessions carried in his backpack (swag). He has no transport and so he walks (waltzes). He could be considered impoverished, and perhaps homeless and lonely. He comes to the attention of the police because he has stolen a sheep (jumbuck) for food. He feels that his circumstances are hopeless, and that his only option is to die by suicide, which he does by drowning himself in an oxbow dam (billabong). Perhaps he experiences a litany of mental health risk factors and vulnerabilities that continue to describe the hardship and struggles that many rural people face, too frequently with the same outcome. It seems that Australian people – and cultures – find it easier to sing about the hardships and make light of the difficulties in life than to find ways to prevent the overwhelming burden of mental health conditions.

REFLECTIVE QUESTION

Have you ever thought about the story behind this popular Australian song? Read the lyrics below and consider the effects this song, and perhaps the meaning of the lyrics, has in relation to Australian culture, and how this aligns with mental health disadvantages today.

Once a jolly swagman camped by a billabong
Under the shade of a coolibah tree,
And he sang as he watched and waited till his billy boiled:
'Who'll come a Waltzing Matilda with me?'

…

Down came a jumbuck to drink at that billabong.
Up jumped the swagman and grabbed him with glee.
And he sang as he shoved that jumbuck in his tucker bag:
'You'll come a Waltzing Matilda with me.'

…

Up rode the squatter, mounted on his thoroughbred.
Down came the troopers, one, two and three.
'Whose is that jolly jumbuck you've got in your tucker bag?
You'll come a Waltzing Matilda with me.'
Up jumped the swagman and sprang into the billabong.
'You'll never catch me alive!' said he.
And his ghost may be heard as you pass by that billabong:
'Who'll come a Waltzing Matilda with me?'

Overview of the rural and regional clinical contexts

Rural and regional communities vary in size, environment and public amenity. Geographical distance is often a factor in the isolation of people from a wide range of health and other services. The distribution of mental health nurses, representing the largest proportion of the mental health workforce in Australia, decreases as remoteness increases, with 46 per cent of local government areas having no full-time equivalent mental health nurses (Sutarsa et al., 2021). The economic base is another significant factor that, for rural and regional communities, influences the social determinants of health (World Health Organization (WHO), 2013). There are benefits and limitations in residing in a rural community, and these influence the health outcomes of people in those communities (Wilson et al., 2015). The challenges for rural and regional communities include promoting healthy conditions, opportunities and environments, and to provide people with sufficient resources to access mental health care that is equitably distributed, as compared to that of their urban counterparts (WHO, 2013; Wilson et al., 2015; Perkins et al., 2019).

In rural and regional communities, access to health services is problematic and is frequently raised as a matter of concern by rural citizens, health service managers and policy planners. Public opinion and political lobbying frequently demand a response by governments in providing improved access for rural citizens, with a view that more services will provide better mental health care for rural populations (Wilson & Usher, 2015). A tension remains because there is disproportionate access to mental health services between urban and rural or regional populations, and this circumstance perpetuates inequities in mental health and well-being for rural people (Young & McGrath, 2011; Wilson & Waqanaviti, 2021). People with longer-term mental health conditions are more likely to find mental health service provision in rural and regional areas, while younger people with emerging mental health conditions are less likely to experience successful access to appropriate care (Wilson, Cruickshank & Lea, 2012).

Additionally, studies have demonstrated that in rural communities and in age groups in which mental health problems are more prevalent, an increased physical comorbidity usually exists (Morgan et al., 2011). For example, increases in emergency department presentations, chronic pain, asthma, cardiac conditions, headache, diabetes and stroke have been shown to be higher among people with mental health conditions, and these problems are further exacerbated by rurality (Morgan et al., 2011).

Governments, which fund public mental health services, have traditionally taken the view that **community participation** should be promoted as both an appropriate approach and an intervention to buffer rural health disadvantages (Preston et al., 2010; COAG, 2012). Community participation is defined as the involvement of local people in assessing their own needs and planning their own strategies to address those needs. Despite widespread adoption of community participation models, there is scant evidence to support such an approach (Preston et al., 2010). Only a few studies have attempted to evaluate the effectiveness of this approach, and more research about effective models of rural healthcare delivery are needed to advance rural and regional health care into the future (Wilson & Usher, 2015).

community participation – the involvement of local people in assessing their own needs and planning strategies to address those needs

A possible benefit of living in rural and regional settings is that strong community participation models contribute to the helpfulness and effectiveness of social and health or well-being capacities within the community (Wilson et al., 2015). In small communities, health service practitioners represent a unique element of that social helpfulness, and they are able to develop informal linkages and intrinsically prompt well-being capacity because of their embedded, close social proximity and shared social experiences with the rural people in their community (Boyd et al., 2008; Wilson & Usher, 2015).

Health professionals, simultaneously, hold dual roles as resident community members and health services providers, and both roles are thought to be important because community linkages are enhanced between health systems and the communities if they are served by health professionals (Kilpatrick, 2009). This circumstance places practitioners in challenging situations at times as they seek to manage their personal and professional relationships within rural and regional communities. It is inevitable in small communities that practitioners will be required to provide health care for people with whom they have a personal relationship (Endacott et al., 2006). Thus, mental health professionals in rural communities are adding value to the communities in which they live and work, across two domains, professional and personal, and these domains are interconnected to some extent (Wilson & Usher, 2015). Therefore, maintaining ethical standards of care and confidentiality in such circumstances is of high importance for all health professionals (Australian Nursing and Midwifery Council, Royal College of Nursing Australia & Australian Nursing Federation, 2008).

REFLECTIVE QUESTION

How difficult would you find separating the professional and personal aspects of your relationships in a clinical setting if you were a practitioner in a small rural health service? Think about some of the challenges you might encounter. List some of the people, or organisations, you could consult with to assist you to maintain ethical standards as a health care professional.

PERSONAL NARRATIVE

Edwina – a new graduate

Edwina is a new graduate who recently gained employment as a registered nurse in a small rural hospital. Filled with enthusiasm for her new role, in the first couple of weeks Edwina met some people with mental health conditions and discovered that helping these people in the rural context was particularly challenging. This is Edwina's story about two people she helped and how it made her feel.

A 48-year-old woman and a 25-year-old man were admitted to the ward on the same day; both of them had overdosed. The woman had taken an overdose of benzodiazepines and paracetamol the previous night, with the intention of repeating her actions the next morning if she woke up. Luckily, her husband found her in the early morning and called the ambulance. The young man had overdosed on escitalopram, an antidepressant, and he had sent a text message to his wife, who was in Brisbane, telling her about what he was doing, and she rang the police. The man's wife and two children had recently moved from Brisbane, but not long afterwards his wife left him and took the two children back to Brisbane.

The woman was initially in the high dependency unit (HDU), and after she was moved onto the ward it was decided that she would be sent to the nearest mental health facility, about 1.5 hours away by road.

The man remained in hospital so his health could be monitored – his pupils were dilated to 9 millimetres! 'The biggest pupils I have *ever* seen'. An appointment was made with the mental health team, but these appointments are so scarce, and the waiting list is never-ending. An appointment was made for 2.5 weeks' time, and the man was sent home.

I couldn't believe this! I expressed my concern to the nurse-in-charge, and she said that mental health appointments are so scarce and far away in this region that most people re-present to the emergency department before attending the appointment.

I had a lot of time for this young man. He was only a few years older than me, and I wanted to help him as much as I could, even if it was just getting him a bundle of magazines from the waiting room, because he had no belongings with him and the TVs weren't working. He needed something to take his mind off things!

As predicted, the young man did re-present to the emergency department. This time he had taken a chainsaw to his leg. Apparently, his injuries weren't too severe but, as I was off duty at that time, from what I heard his injuries were treated and he was sent home … *again*! After that, I heard he got involved with the police (he had anger-management issues) and then, only then, was he sent to the nearest mental health facility.

To me, this was wrong, and I think more needs to be done about mental health in rural areas – it took *three* emergency admissions for this man to get the attention that he needed. That's *three* times this man was crying out for help. If this man had had an infection in his body with the potential to kill him, he would undoubtedly have been kept in hospital until it was cleared up, not sent home to simply hope for the best, and that he would be okay.

I remember being in university nursing classes and learning about how mental health was underfunded and that awareness of mental health needed to be improved in rural and regional areas. It is not until now, though, that I truly understand how essential it really is!

People can be so flippant and/or sceptical about mental health, and it frustrates me … My mental health clinical placement last year opened my eyes to the reality of mental health needs and how prevalent it really is, as did these experiences.

REFLECTIVE QUESTIONS

Edwina found her first experiences in caring for people with mental health conditions in the hospital setting rather confronting.

- What strategies can you use to manage your own feelings about challenging situations you might experience in a rural setting?
- How can you participate positively in the wider health are team to facilitate timely and respectful help for people in general health settings who have mental health conditions?

Prevalence of mental health problems in rural and regional communities

Self-reports by people in rural communities indicate that they experience mental health conditions and behavioural problems at a rate of 16 per cent higher than their urban counterparts (ABS, 2011). Idyllic notions about achieving a healthier lifestyle and greater well-being in rural communities may be based more on optimistic hopes than on facts. Unemployment and under-employment are higher in rural areas than in urban areas, and there are generally fewer senior positions available in most sectors, which limits career progression at an early stage and at lower remuneration for many people. Careers in rural communities are sometimes more vulnerable to the 'boom and bust' dynamics of the agricultural sector, and to related environmental changes such as drought, poor crop yields, loss of stock, and the fluctuations of livestock sale prices and markets. These dynamics place stresses on the mental health and well-being of rural people, such as family pressures to 'stay on the land' or fears of 'losing the farm', despite a widely held view that rural people are stoic and resilient (Austin et al., 2018; Wilson et al., 2015; Lawrence-Bourne et al., 2020). Sometimes, the stoic expectation of rural people to endure hardship is a barrier to rural people seeking assistance for mental health conditions and related services, and rural men are particularly vulnerable in this regard. By contrast, rural women are more likely to seek help for mental health conditions when they need it, and especially for problems such as depression and anxiety (Buikstra, Fallon & Eley, 2007).

Suicide rates in rural and remote areas are higher than in capital cities. In 2016, the rate of suicide in all of Australia's greater capital cities combined was 10.0 per 100 000, while the rate of suicide for the combined areas outside the greater capital cities was over 50 per cent higher at 15.3 per 100 000 (Hazell et al., 2017). Suicide rates among rural males, and especially young men aged 15–29 years, have been increasing over the past 20 years (Department of Health and Ageing, 2013) and at rates twice as high as young men who live in urban communities (ABS, 2011). Rural older men aged 85 years and over have been reported as having the highest rate of death by suicide, at 40 deaths per 100 000 men, and this is thought to be influenced by increased financial insecurity and agricultural stresses sometimes brought about by the experience of environmental events such as floods, droughts and bush fires (ABS, 2011). It has been suggested that people in rural communities often have access to more lethal means when they intend to harm themselves (ABS, 2011). Edwina's story demonstrates this to some extent, a situation that could have had a much worse outcome. In addition, loneliness and difficulty accessing mental health care are factors related to suicide (ABS, 2011). It may also be that a novel taxonomy for rural of depression among males is necessary and rural-specific treatments for the condition are yet to be adequately developed and tested (Sharpley, Bitsika & Agnew, 2021).

Some risk factors in combination with rural residency have been noted as having an association with the prevalence of mental health conditions, including:

- poverty
- unemployment
- female gender
- LGBTIQ identification
- being unmarried
- low socio-economic circumstances
- alcohol and/or substance abuse
- history of childhood sexual abuse
- poor social networks
- small size of primary support groups (Campbell, Manoff & Caffery, 2006).

Rural mental health promotion and prevention

Rural and regional mental health services vary in type and service mix across communities. Access to specialist mental health services, and specialist practitioners, is usually restricted to larger regional centres. Occasionally, however, these services send visiting teams to outlying rural communities and regional centres on semi-regular and ad hoc bases (Wilson et al., 2015) using a **'hub and spoke' model** of service. The hub represents the centralisation or home base of services and the spokes the outreach to specific communities or community events (see Table 19.1). In most cases, people seeking assistance for mental health conditions attend centre-based or bed-based mental health services, and usually in larger regional or metropolitan centres. Sometimes, major rural events such as agricultural field days are targeted for health promotion activities because they attract large concentrations of rural people, and this makes it convenient and cost-effective for health services to provide mental health education and information to larger groups. e-Mental health and telehealth are becoming more available to rural and regional communities, with the COVID-19 pandemic triggering a telehealth services pivot to incorporating digital health and telehealth services more generally.

'hub and spoke' model – of service, whereby the hub represents the centralisation or home base of services and the spokes the outreach to specific communities or community events

Table 19.1   Interprofessional rural mental health services

Type of health service	Descriptions and examples
Public, rural, multi-purpose centres or rural hospitals and primary health networks	• Multidisciplinary, clinic-based services that require people seeking help to attend either a scheduled individual appointment or a group session • Some bed-based services – mostly aged-care related; some acute-care beds and first-response emergency services; these centres vary in size (e.g. 12–40 beds) • Visiting mental health services may be available on a regular or ad hoc basis, and the range of practitioners who attend includes several (e.g. 1–4) mental health nurses, psychiatrists, psychologists, social workers, occupational therapists and counsellors • Other non-mental health services co-located in a service such as this might include child and family nurses, community nurses, aged care assistants, podiatrists, dietitians, sexual health and women's health nurses, drug and alcohol counsellors and general practitioners • For more information about this service see: http://www.health.nsw.gov.au/rural/rhhsp/Pages/default.aspx • An example of a rural hospital: https://www.health.qld.gov.au/darlingdowns
Telehealth and e-mental health	• Videoconferencing, telephone-conferencing or internet-based services. Frequently, the practitioners providing the mental health service are located in major metropolitan areas and the recipients of this care are situated in rural communities. Telehealth services help to reduce the barrier of poor access to specialist mental health services for rural people; however, they do rely on quality internet and telephone or data connectivity. An additional challenge for this type of service delivery is establishing trust and rapport at a distance, and with a fundamental difference in lifestyle and experiences • A useful resource: Jakowenko (2014)

(cont.)

Table 19.1   (cont.)

Type of health service	Descriptions and examples
Community health services	• Services available to ambulatory clients who are able to attend a community health centre for regular health appointments, or clients who are able to remain at home with the support of a visiting practitioner to provide in-home care • An example of services provided by a community health service: https://www.dhhs.tas.gov.au/mentalhealth/mhs_tas/gvt_mhs/adult_community_mental_health_services
Case management	• Occurs at large regional centres, and some smaller centres, but requires a team for optimum functionality • Sometimes, outreach versions of case management apply to outlying rural communities
Indigenous emotional and social well-being or mental health services	• Indigenous people have a significantly higher propensity for mental health conditions. This video describes how one community was able to positively address some of the mental health conditions encountered in their Bathurst Island community and to focus further on promoting mental well-being: https://www.youtube.com/watch?v=jQWqBWy8HRE • Primary Health Networks are involved in developing care connections and facilitating mental health and social health and well-being support for Aboriginal and Torres Strait Islander peoples in Australia. An example of this service type is found at HealthWISE (http://www.healthwisenenw.com.au/) • A further example of mental health care in remote Aboriginal communities can be found in Purdie, Dudgeon & Walker (2010)

TRANSLATION TO PRACTICE

Rural partnerships

Partnerships between mental health services and other sectors contribute to building rural mental health and well-being capacity in innovative ways, such as in the example of a partnership between the Rural Adversity Mental Health Program and a national rural newspaper, *The Land* (2016; 'Glove box guide to mental health'). This was a useful strategy because it conveniently placed mental health information where many rural people would access it, with potential to trigger further research on the topic by people who could benefit from the information. However, a limitation of these types of programs is that they are often short-term in nature and are difficult to sustain beyond pilot stages, as funds are frequently not available for replication or for more sustainable and long-term ventures.

Rural early intervention mental health services

Early intervention services are needed, especially for young people, because most mental health conditions are known to first develop in late adolescence and during early adulthood (Wilson & Usher, 2015). Specialist early intervention programs are very important, especially for the treatment of early psychosis; research suggests that early and continuing interventions for up to 5 years are critical, and cost effective, in the reduction of the long-term effects of untreated psychosis (Yung, 2013). However, rural communities are often limited in the diversity of mental health services available. Generic mental health services are saturated with practitioner caseloads predominated by people with long-term, and somewhat consolidated, mental health conditions. Access to mental health services for young people is especially challenging because few face-to-face local services are available in rural communities. It can be extremely difficult for the general public, and non-mental health professionals, to determine whether the odd behaviours and 'not quite right' interactions that sometimes accompany emergent mental health conditions such as early psychosis and bipolar disorder are because a mental health condition is developing (Callaly et al., 2010; Rodd & Stewart, 2009; Wilson & Usher, 2015). Rural young women are more likely than young men to access, or attempt to access, mental health services, especially for conditions such as depression. However, they sometimes have difficulty finding appropriate help because of the lack of services in their communities and long waiting periods (Black, Roberts & Li-Leng, 2012). National mental health plans have recognised that more needs to be done to better address young people's mental health needs in rural communities (COAG, 2012). One aspect that is showing promise is the inclusion of social models to promote conversations and support about mental health and inclusion more generally. For example, Men's Sheds are a resource in many rural communities that can reduce the barriers to accessing early mental health care for rural men (Wilson et al., 2019).

The *headspace* (https://headspace.org.au) model of care has been the Australian government's most determined recent initiative to address the mental health needs of young people. There are more than 100 centres nationally in which face-to-face services may be accessed, but most of these are located in urban or large regional centres. Rural communities remain under-serviced, and there is an expectation that young people, and their families, should travel to major centres to address their mental healthcare needs. Headspace is advancing its e-mental health approach, because this is seen by the Australian government as a more inclusive and equitable approach for young people's mental health programs (Department of Health and Ageing, 2012).

An alternative is to engage in telehealth and/or e-mental health linkages to specialist services based in metropolitan centres (e.g. early psychosis services). It has been argued that small communities are unlikely to have sufficient quantities of people with early mental health problems to sustain the establishment of specialist face-to-face services (Early Psychosis Writing Group, 2016), and this highlights the compromises that are often required in the struggle for cost-efficiency and equity of service distribution, which rural communities continue to battle. Early mental health interventionists have noted that telehealth and e-mental health services should not be seen as a substitute for face-to-face, early intervention services, and some suggest that visiting services may be the next best alternative for rural communities (Early Psychosis Writing Group, 2016).

Community mental health and primary health services

Community mental health services are available in many rural communities, and in some cases, these are delivered in an outreach mode. A **case management** model is often used to manage the services delivered by a multidisciplinary team, some of which will 'fly in/ fly out' on a monthly rotation, with combinations of mental health practitioners, psychologists, social workers, occupational therapists, counsellors and psychiatrists. Case management models have a variety of subtypes, but they have in common the goals that mental health services should be provided in a coordinated way (Purtell, Dowling & Fossey, 2008). There are four key phases to coordinated care: planning, implementation, monitoring and review (Purtell et al., 2008). In general, practical terms, teams of practitioners work together and meet regularly to consult about complex care planning for the people they help. Each team member is allocated a few people because mental health services are increasingly striving towards person-centred approaches; however, the vocabulary used to describe service activities needs to be modified, and 'case management' is becoming outdated, although a proposed alternative description is yet to emerge. It is no longer acceptable to refer to people who require mental health care as 'cases to be managed'. Case-manager roles should bear a title that is person-centred, reflecting activities that are recovery-focused, such as enablers and facilitators of well-being and functioning (Purtell et al., 2008). There is a call for reform, so that people are encouraged to make informed decisions about their own recovery, rather than expected to comply passively with health professionals' advice. Thus, it is appropriate that service delivery should incorporate person-centred recovery models of care that reflect evidenced-based practice (Keen & Lakeman, 2009).

Bed-based mental health services

Bed-based units for mental health care in rural communities are extremely limited. Most bed-based units are both involuntary (following administration of a Mental Health Act), and voluntary units within regional or metropolitan hospital services. Bed-based units care for people who are experiencing acute mental health symptoms and who are unable to cope at home or with the assistance of community mental health services alone. It is preferable that people are helped towards recovery prior to this acute stage, but this is not always possible. Bed-based units require staffing levels that may not be possible to achieve in communities other than larger centres, because there may not be sufficient mental health practitioners to resource a bed-based unit. Traditionally, health services have experienced difficulty in recruiting mental health professionals to rural communities.

In regional communities, bed-based units are likely to service a wider-reaching rural community. It is important for these units to work closely with the mental health practitioners of their clients' home communities. Discharge poses multiple challenges, and careful consideration of medication, suicide risk, travel arrangements and future appointments need to be planned so there is efficient continuation of care. In addition, it is fundamental to collaborate with the person receiving mental health care and any carers or family. The successful continuation of care, and the transition to home following discharge, is extremely important so that relapse can be minimised and prevented.

Telehealth

Over the past 15 years, telehealth has emerged as a cost-effective strategy to improve mental health service delivery in rural and regional communities. An example of how a telehealth service operates is described in a Queensland Health video: *Extending the Reach of Clinical Health Services Throughout Queensland* (Statewide Telehealth Services, 2013). Telehealth clinical consultations are usually conducted in a videoconferencing format, whereby parties communicate in real time, using a computer, video or TV screen (Christensen et al., 2020). More recently, interactions have begun to develop within the Web 2.0 social media forum, especially regarding mental health promotion, awareness and information delivery. Examples are social media channels such as Facebook, Instagram and Twitter, where progressive health services work with interest groups in social media settings to improve navigation, help-seeking and psychosocial education for early invitation to assessment and treatment pathways. This demonstrates the potential for integration of social media into a more comprehensive and far-reaching e-mental health framework (Cronin, Hungerford & Wilson, 2020). Similar to telehealth, e-mental health services can be delivered in digital, electronic or telephone-based formats, and can take effect in synchronous or asynchronous episodes. e-Mental health is an evolving area of practice that is likely to see significant development in the future (Rickwood, 2012). It will be impossible for Australia, or Aotearoa New Zealand, to develop adequate and equitable mental health plans for rural communities without also adopting e-mental health interventions, because the cost of placing specialist, face-to-face mental health services in all rural and regional communities would be cost prohibitive (Early Psychosis Writing Group, 2016; Rickwood, 2012; Smith, Skrbis & Western, 2012). There are many examples of internet-based, or mobile device-supported, mental health interventions that might be applied to the rural context – see Chapter 11 for more information.

Recovery and rehabilitation

Recovery planning commences at first consultation wherever, and whenever, it takes place. A recovery focus promotes well-being and engages people purposefully in their own decision-making about their future health, including the lifestyle changes they decide to make (Caldwell et al., 2010), enabling people to lead meaningful and contributing lives (Lourey et al., 2012). Some people living with complex long-term illnesses find coping with daily life extremely challenging, and they must work hard to maintain a sufficient life balance in order to manage their own activities and to maximise their wellness. Community based recovery and rehabilitation centres and groups can be very helpful for these people (Cruwys et al., 2020). In rural communities, recovery services such as these are likely to be delivered by non-government organisations (NGOs) such as in the example provided in this chapter.

Billabong Clubhouse

Billabong Clubhouse, located in regional Tamworth, New South Wales, is a member of an international clubhouse movement (clubhouse-intl.org). In Australia and Aotearoa New Zealand, it operates as an NGO. There are several other clubhouses in Australia and Aotearoa New Zealand, but what is most interesting about Billabong Clubhouse is that it is a community participation response to address the needs of people with long-term mental health conditions in their own community. The Tamworth community recognised that the needs of people with long-term mental health conditions in their midst were not being met. In the face of insufficient public health resources, community members formed an organisation to address the matter. Billabong Clubhouse has been operational for about 20 years, which is an outcome that many rural programs have been unable to achieve. The members of the Clubhouse are equally responsible for the management and day-to-day operations of the Clubhouse. Members gather daily to give support and encouragement to each other, to care for each other in practical ways, to socialise, develop a routine, share or cook meals together, and to undertake work or vocational activities. The structure of the Clubhouse model fosters wellness, and many members report that it 'keeps them out of hospital', which is a very important personal outcome. Initiatives such as this may be useful in other rural and regional communities that have similar populations and conditions as Tamworth.

INTERPROFESSIONAL PERSPECTIVES

Collaborative mental health care has the potential to improve quality of care for under-resourced and geographically isolated communities. Health professionals usually have limited support, resources and supervision when working in rural areas. However, initiatives aimed at providing mental healthcare training for community professionals have shown promising results in rural communities in Canada. A 20-week training course on evidence-based mental health intervention was delivered to different professionals (e.g. nurses, social workers, physician, pharmacists, ambulance attendants, community development workers) working closely with people. Participants indicated that the training created new opportunities for 'interprofessional and intersectoral partnerships in providing mental health care that had the potential to benefit clients and the community' (Heath et al., 2015, p. 200). For more details, see the original paper published by Heath and collaborators (Heath et al., 2015). Similar initiatives in Australia and Aotearoa New Zealand need to be tested and implemented.

Travel implications for rural people with mental healthcare needs

A challenge for people seeking mental health care – and their practitioners alike – is that, often, rural people need to travel many hours to attend mental health appointments, and this means that other personal, vocational and educational activities are disrupted (Wilson et al., 2015). Significant personal expenses may also be incurred, adding an additional financial burden to people who are experiencing mental health conditions. Managing these travel requirements can be very difficult for people and their carers, because frequently they also experience symptoms that affect their logical thinking, motivation and planning. There is not an abundance of public transport systems for rural communities, and if people do not have access to a personal vehicle, or are not able to drive, they are further isolated and have to rely on the goodwill of others for transport. Thus, any therapy that is dependent upon significant personal resources for rural people is a factor for consideration by practitioners when planning short and long-term recovery goals.

Natural disasters and the implications for rural communities

Australia and Aotearoa New Zealand are prone to natural disasters. The climate and environment in rural Australia make rural communities especially vulnerable to the effects of bush fires, heatwaves, storms or cyclones, floods and droughts, while Aotearoa New Zealand has experienced devastating earthquakes. Research has demonstrated that an important contribution to the disaster response phase is the inclusion of immediate psychosocial support (Ranse et al., 2014). There have been investments in Australia to improve preparation and early warning systems to assist rural people to cope with these adverse conditions (Jones, 2013). For example, sending population-wide emergency alert text messages to warn people of impending natural disasters in their area; rural residents have been informed about developing self-plans to improve their survival of storms and bush fires; and water storage and timing of releases have been improved. All these improvements are of great importance to rural communities.

The mental health effects of disasters for rural people are also significant (Ranse et al., 2014), affecting poorer rural people, farmers and rural men, in particular (Saniotis & Irvine, 2010; Austin et al., 2018). The immediate crisis that accompanies a natural disaster can be traumatic, and this requires monitoring and intervention of individuals and, sometimes, the entire population. However, the longer-term effects of disaster-related trauma can include serious and/or longer-term consequences, which become the focus of targeted mental health assessment and intervention in those communities (Hayward, 2020). The prevalence of mental health conditions following natural and other disasters is not well known, and this is a field in which more research is needed (Ranse et al., 2015; Hayward, 2020). The robust nature of rural communities and the close social connections within them are thought to be protective for mental health, and so there is capacity to strengthen resilience (Boyd et al., 2008) through mental health promotion and awareness before, during and after these events.

Assisting communities during natural disasters

A story broadcast on Australian national radio recounted the experiences of nurses in the rural town of Moree, New South Wales, in which their response to flood conditions provided an example of the roles of health professionals in times of natural disaster (Fuller, 2012).

Another example of health professionals taking the initiative to protect their rural community in challenging times is the small town of Bellingen on the Mid North Coast of New South Wales (Keers, 2020). As the COVID-19 pandemic began to take hold nationally in March 2020, local GPs banded together and used their own resources to set up a drive-through testing clinic, because they were concerned that a COVID-positive case entering their premises would cause a two-week shutdown of services. This clinic, the first in the region, diagnosed its first case a week later. See Keers (2020) for more information.

TRANSLATION TO PRACTICE

REFLECTIVE QUESTIONS

Can you imagine what it would be like to experience first-hand flood, bushfire or earthquake conditions? (Or perhaps you have done so in your own life?)

- Imagine (or recall) the feelings and emotions of uncertainty, anxiety, worry, fear, loss and the pressure of having to make a quick decision to evacuate your home.
- What could others do to help you cope with these types of challenges?
- As a health worker, list some of the ways you think you may be able to help others to cope with the emotional and practical difficulties people may face in this situation.

Agriculture, mining and itinerant workforces

Rural communities are shaped by some unique vocational groups: the agricultural workforce, the itinerant and seasonal rural workforces (e.g. in fruit harvesting) and the mining workforce. The uncertainty and seasonality of these industries have population-wide effects that, in turn, influence the mental health of these groups, and the wider rural community. The mining industry has developed significantly in recent times in rural Australia, and this has implications for community health and well-being for both new mining residents and long-term residents in rural communities. The mining workforce has to contend with shift work and fly-in, fly-out (FIFO) conditions, both of which affect families and the personal connections people have with places and people in their lives. These circumstances may predispose vulnerable individuals towards mental health conditions on occasion, and this is emerging as an area of concern to health services in these communities (Wilson et al., 2015). Relative shifts in population sizes, and especially sudden increases in populations, place additional demands on current health services and other rural amenities, such as housing and employment. An example is in Mt Isa, Queensland, where local people and services have noticed an increased need for mental health services as the mining industry has expanded.

SUMMARY

This chapter has presented stories and information, supplemented with activities designed to deepen your understanding of:

- The diverse and unique mental health needs of rural people. Respect should be afforded to rural culture in promoting mental health recovery. There are many mental health vulnerabilities and risk factors that can be identified in rural communities. However, resilience can be fostered and mental health and well-being nurtured by the close social connections rural people have with each other.
- Recovery in rural communities, entailing understanding the unique rural culture, geography and opportunities. e-Mental health is showing promise in helping to overcome some of the practical barriers to accessing specialist services and to minimise the burden of travel for some people.

- The delivery of mental health services using a variety of service models. The service dynamics between communities often differ; however, some similarities are noted, such as the use of outreach services, community services and bed-based services. Models of service continue to be adapted to provide equitable mental health care for all people.

CRITICAL THINKING/LEARNING ACTIVITIES

1   Describe some benefits and some vulnerabilities of mental health that may be experienced by rural people.
2   How can rural people and communities participate in rural mental health promotion?
3   What are some of the strengths and limitations of e-mental health strategies?
4   Describe how a person-centred recovery could be achieved in a rural community.

LEARNING EXTENSION

Activity one

1   Watch the news report about the experiences of young people in Mt Isa and their need for mental health support: https://www.youtube.com/watch?v=MsjYhKjBlX4 ('Rural mining town battles mental health issues', ABC News (Australia)).
2   Think about the following question. What types of mental health care might be suitable for use with rural young people to help reduce the burden of mental health conditions and suicide in rural communities?

Activity two

Review some examples of rural mental health promotion and information using social media, including these Facebook open groups and Twitter streams and handles:

- Rural Mental Health Australia: https://www.facebook.com/RuralMH/info and #RuralMH
- Rural Mental Health: http://anzmh.asn.au/rrmh/ and #anzmh

ACKNOWLEDGEMENT

Thanks to Edwina Casey RN BN, who shared her story and contributed to this chapter to provide a perspective from a recent graduate nurse.

FURTHER READING

ABC News. (2011). Mental health clients feel stigmatised. *7:30 Report*. Retrieved from
     https://www.youtube.com/watch?v=xqlQS3IANdQ
This news report discusses the stigma attached to mental health conditions, particularly with regard to health professionals. Are health professionals guilty of this discrimination?

Fairfax Agricultural Media. (2012). Mental health resources for the bush. *The Land*, 1 November. Retrieved from https://www.theland.com.au/story/3599288/mental-health-resources-for-the-bush/

The Land is an agricultural news outlet based in New South Wales.

The Land. (2016). *Glove box guide to mental health*, Volume 8. Retrieved from
https://specialpubs.austcommunitymedia.com.au/e-mags/2019/TL5/1003_01/

The eighth volume of this publication is a partnership between *The Land* and the Rural Adversity
in Mental Health Program. It aims to start conversations about mental health.

Lourey, C., Holland, C. & Green, R. (2012). *A Contributing Life: The 2012 national report card
on mental health and suicide prevention.* Sydney: National Mental Health Commission.
Retrieved from http://www.mentalhealthcommission.gov.au/media/39273/nmhc_
reportcard_lo-res.pdf

This report assesses the mental health of Australians and the services that aid recovery. The
report also makes recommendations for improvements to services across a variety of sectors.

REFERENCES

Austin, E. K., Handley, T., Kiem, A. S., Rich, J. L., Lewin, T. J., Askland, H. H., Askarimarnani, S. S.,
Perkins, D. A. & Kelly, B. J. (2018). Drought-related stress among farmers: findings from the
Australian Rural Mental Health Study. *The Medical Journal of Australia, 209*(4): 159–65.

Australian Bureau of Statistics. (ABS). (2011). *Australian Social Trends, March 2011. Health outside
major cities.* Canberra: ABS.

————— (2016). *Australian Statistical Geography Standard (ASGS): Volume 5 – Remoteness Structure,
July 2016.* (Cat. no. 1270. 0.55.005). Retrieved from https://www.abs.gov.au/ausstats/abs@
.nsf/Latestproducts/1270.0.55.005Main%20Features5July%202016

————— (2019). *Rural and Remote Health.* Retrieved from https://www.aihw.gov.au/reports/australias-
health/rural-and-remote-health

Australian Nursing and Midwifery Council, Royal College of Nursing Australia & Australian Nursing
Federation. (2008). *Code of Ethics for Nurses in Australia.* Dickson, ACT: Australian Nursing
and Midwifery Council.

Black, C., Roberts, R. M. & Li-Leng, T. (2012). Depression in rural adolescents: Relationships with
gender and availability of mental health services. *Rural and Remote Health, 12*(2092): 1–11.

Boyd, C. P., Hayes, L., Sewell, J., Caldwell, K., Kemp, E., Harvie, L. ... Nurse, S. (2008). Mental health
problems in rural contexts: A broader perspective. *Australian Psychologist, 43*(1): 2–6.

Boyd, C. P., Hayes, L., Wilson, R. L. & Bearsley-Smith, C. (2008). Harnessing the social capital of rural
communities for youth mental health: An asset-based community development framework.
Australian Journal of Rural Health, 16: 189–93.

Buikstra, E., Fallon, A. B. & Eley, R. (2007). Psychological services in five south-west Queensland
communities – supply and demand. *Rural and Remote Health, 7*(543): 1–11.

Caldwell, B. A., Sclafani, M., Swarbrick, M. & Piren, K. (2010). Psychiatric nursing practice and the
recovery model of care. *Journal of Psychosocial Nursing, 48*(7): 42–8.

Callaly, T., Ackerly, C. A., Hyland, M. E., Dodd, S., O'Shea, M. & Berk, M. (2010). A qualitative
evaluation of a regional early psychosis service 3 years after its commencement. *Australian
Health Review, 34*: 382–5.

Campbell, A., Manoff, T. & Caffery, J. (2006). Rurality and mental health: An Australian primary care
study. *Rural and Remote Health (online), 6*(595).

Christensen, L. F., Wilson, R., Hansen, J. P., Nielsen, C. T. & Gildberg, F. A. (2020). A qualitative study
of patients' and providers' experiences with the use of videoconferences by older adults with
depression. *International Journal of Mental Health Nursing, 30*(2): 427–39.

Council of Australian Governments (COAG). (2012). *Roadmap for National Mental Health Reform
2012– 2022.* Retrieved from www.coag.gov.au/node/482

Cronin, C., Hungerford, C. & Wilson, R. L. (2020). Using digital health technologies to manage the
psychosocial symptoms of menopause in the workplace: A narrative literature review. *Issues
in Mental Health Nursing, 42*(6): 541–8.

Cruwys, T., Stewart, B., Buckley, L., Gumley, J. & Scholz, B. (2020). The recovery model in chronic mental health: A community-based investigation of social identity processes. *Psychiatry Research, 291*: 113241.

Department of Health and Ageing. (2012). *e-Mental Health Strategy for Australia*. Canberra: Australian Government. Retrieved from www.health.gov.au/internet/main/publishing.nsf/Content/D67E137E77F0CE90CA257A2F0007736A/$File/emstrat.pdf

——— (2013). *Better Access to Psychiatrists, Psychologists and General Practitioners through the MBS (Better Access) initiative*. Retrieved from www.health.gov.au/internet/main/publishing.nsf/content/mental-ba

Early Psychosis Guidelines Writing Group and EPPIC National Support Program. (2016). *Australian Clinical Guidelines for Early Psychosis*, 2nd edn. Melbourne: Orygen, The National Centre of Excellence in Youth Mental Health.

Endacott, R., Wood, A., Judd, F., Hulbert, C., Thomas, B. & Grigg, M. (2006). Impact and management of dual relationships in metropolitan, regional and rural mental health practice. *Australian and New Zealand College of Psychiatry, 40*: 987–94.

Fuller, K. (2012). Beyond the call of duty. *ABC Local*, 10 February. Retrieved from https://www.abc.net.au/local/stories/2012/02/10/3428111.htm

Glove Box Guide to Mental Health & The Land Publishers. (2016). *The Land, 5*. Retrieved from http://specialpubs.fairfaxregional.com.au/theland/magazines/mental-health/2016/

Hayward, B. A. (2020). Mental health nursing in bushfire-affected communities: An autoethnographic insight. *International Journal of Mental Health Nursing, 29*(6): 1262–71.

Hazell, T., Dalton, H., Caton, T. & Perkins, D. (2017). Rural Suicide and its Prevention: A CRRMH position paper. Centre for Rural and Remote Mental Health, University of Newcastle.

Heath, O., Church, E., Curran, V., Hollett, A., Cornish, P., Callanan, T., Bethune, C. & Younghusband, L. (2015). Interprofessional mental health training in rural primary care: findings from a mixed methods study. *Journal of Interprofessional Care, 29*(3): 195–201.

Hugo Centre for Population and Housing. (2020). ARIA (Accessibility/Remoteness Index of Australia). Retrieved from https://www.adelaide.edu.au/hugo-centre/services/aria

Jakowenko, J. (2014). *Implementation guidelines for video consultations in general practice: A telehealth initiative*, 3rd edn. East Melbourne: Royal Australian College of General Practitioners.

Jones, R. (2013). In search of the 'prepared community': The way ahead for Australia? *Australian Journal of Emergency Management, 28*(1): 15–18.

Keen, T. & Lakeman, R. (2009). Collaboration with patients and families. In P. Barker (ed.), *Psychiatric and Mental Health Nursing. The craft of caring*, 2nd edn. (pp. 149–61). London: Hodder Education.

Keers, J. (2020). COVID-19 testing clinic opens for Bellingen Shire. *The Macleay Argus*, 24 March. Retrieved from https://www.bellingencourier.com.au/story/6693684/covid-19-testing-clinic-opens-for-bellingen-shire/

Kilpatrick, S. (2009). Multi-level rural community engagement in health. *Rural and Remote Health, 17*: 39–44.

Lawrence-Bourne, J., Dalton, H., Perkins, D., Farmer, J., Luscombe, G., Oelke, N. & Bagheri N. (2020). What is rural adversity, how does it affect wellbeing and what are the implications for action? *International Journal of Environmental Research and Public Health, 17*(19): 7205.

Lourey, C., Holland, C. & Green, R. (2012). *A Contributing Life: The 2012 national report card on mental health and suicide prevention*. Sydney: National Mental Health Commission. Retrieved from www.mentalhealthcommission.gov.au.

Morgan, V. A., Waterreus, A., Jablensky, A., Mackinnon, A., Mcgrath, J. J., Carr, V. J. ... Saw, S., (2011). *People Living with Psychotic Illness 2010. Report on the second Australian national survey*. Canberra: Department of Health and Ageing.

Perkins, D., Farmer, J., Salvador-Carulla, L., Dalton, H. & Luscombe, G. (2019). The Orange Declaration on rural and remote mental health. *Australian Journal of Rural Health, 27*: 374–9.

Preston, R., Waugh, H., Larkins, S. & Taylor, J. (2010). Community participation in rural primary health care: Intervention or approach? *Australian Journal of Primary Health, 16*: 4–16.

Purdie, N., Dudgeon, P. & Walker, R. (eds). (2010). *Working Together: Aboriginal and Torres Strait Islander mental health and wellbeing principles and practice*. Canberra: Commonwealth of Australia.

Purtell, C., Dowling, R.-M. & Fossey, E. (2008). Case management models: Similarities and differences. In G. Meadows, B. Singh & M. Grigg (eds), *Mental Health in Australia: Collaborative practice*, 2nd edn. (pp. 343–5). Melbourne: Oxford University Press.

Ranse, J., Hutton, A., Jeeawody, B. & Wilson, R. (2014). What are the research needs for the field of disaster nursing? An international Delphi study. *Prehospital and Disaster Medicine, 29*: 448–54.

Ranse, J., Hutton, A., Wilson, R. & Usher, K. (2015). Leadership opportunities for mental health nurses in the field of disaster preparation, response, and recovery. *Issues in Mental Health Nursing, 36*(5): 391–4.

Rickwood, D. J. (2012). Entering the e-spectrum: An examination of new interventions for youth mental health. *Youth Studies Australia, 31*(4): 18–27.

Rodd, H. & Stewart, H. (2009). The glue that holds our work together. The role and nature of relationships in youth work. *Youth Studies Australia, 28*(4): 4–10.

Saniotis, A. & Irvine, R. (2010). Climate change and the possible health effects on older Australians. *Australian Journal of Primary Health, 16*: 217–20.

Sharpley, C. F., Bitsika, V. & Agnew, L. L. (2021). Does 'male' depression exist in rural Australian men? *The Journal of Men's Studies, 29*(1): 73–85.

Smith, J., Skrbis, Z. & Western, M. (2012). Beneath the 'digital native' myth. *Journal of Sociology, 49*(1): 97–118.

Statewide Telehealth Services. (2013). *Extending the Reach of Clinical Health Services Throughout Queensland.* Retrieved from www.youtube.com/watch?v=Hfl3iPk6t2o

Sutarsa, N., Banfield, M., Passioura, J., Konings, P. & Moore, M. (2021). Spatial inequities of mental health nurses in rural and remote Australia. *International Journal of Mental Health Nursing, 30*(1): 167–76.

Wilson, N. J., Cordier, R., Parsons, R., Vaz, S. & Ciccarelli, M. (2019). An examination of health promotion and social inclusion activities: A cross-sectional survey of Australian community Men's Sheds. *Health Promotion Journal of Australia, 30*(3): 371–80.

Wilson, R. L. (2014). Mental health recovery and quilting: Evaluation of a grass-roots project in a small, rural, Australian christian church. *Issues in Mental Health Nursing, 35*(4): 292–8.

Wilson, R. L., Cruickshank, M. & Lea, J. (2012). Experiences of families who help young rural men with emergent mental health problems in a rural community in New South Wales, Australia. *Contemporary Nurse, 42*(2): 167–77.

Wilson, R. L. & Usher, K. (2015). Rural nurses: A convenient co-location strategy for the rural mental health care of young people. *Journal of Clinical Nursing, 24*: 2638–48.

Wilson, R. L. & Waqanaviti, K. (2021). Emotional and social well-being for First Nations people in the mental health context. In O. Best & B. Fredericks (eds). *Yatdjuljin: Aboriginal and Torres Strait Islander Nursing and Midwifery Care*, 3rd edn. Port Melbourne: Cambridge University Press.

Wilson, R. L., Wilson, G. G. & Usher, K. (2015). Rural mental health ecology: A framework for engaging with mental health social capital in rural communities. *EcoHealth, 12*: 412–20.

World Health Organization (WHO). (2013). *Social Determinants of Health.* Retrieved from www.who.int/social_determinants/en

Young, J. & McGrath, R. (2011). Exploring discourses of equity, social justice and social determinants in Australian health care policy and planning documents. *Australian Journal of Primary Health, 17*: 369–77.

Yung, A. (2013). Early intervention in psychosis: Evidence, evidence gaps, criticism and confusion. *Australian and New Zealand Journal of Psychiatry, 46*(1): 7–9.

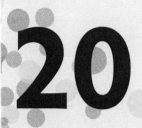

Learning through human connectedness on clinical placement

Translation to practice

Denise McGarry and Kerry Mawson

LEARNING OBJECTIVES

At the completion of this chapter, you should be able to:

1 Develop strategies to prioritise and personalise your learning objectives when undertaking mental health study as an undergraduate student or beginning in mental health practice.
2 Recognise opportunities and your responsibility to develop your learning to meet the needs of the clinical practice environment.
3 Develop strategies to work within a trauma-informed care and practice framework, with awareness of vicarious and secondary trauma and plans to sustain your personal resilience.
4 Describe ways to support the recovery model through alliance with people experiencing mental ill-health and their carers to achieve goals developed collaboratively.
5 Develop self-reflective, emotional competence to support therapeutic interactional skills that are applicable across a range of mental health and non-mental health practice settings.
6 Practise with skill in the environment of health services, utilising evidence-based approaches.

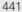

Introduction

This chapter explores a range of challenges arising for students as they learn to apply interpersonal skills within the mental health practicum placement and other non-mental health settings. The chapter begins with an exploration of the student's own attitudes, expectations and positive engagement within practice. This is followed by discussion of power relations that characterise the therapeutic relationship, including the development of emotional competence. The chapter outlines reflective practice as a critical thinking process, and clinical supervision for the beginning nursing student within mental health nursing. It explores the importance of developing skills to work within a trauma-informed care and practice framework that is mindful of potential **vicarious trauma** or **secondary trauma** at the personal level. How to go about developing objectives for practice, and the process of self-assessment and personal problem-solving are discussed in the context of various clinical settings. Self-care planning is emphasised. Reflection, self in-action and post-placement are also explored as they relate to learning in mental health. Throughout this chapter, critical examination of the ethical and political influences on care that extend beyond individual engagement with the person experiencing mental ill-health are highlighted. The chapter also considers non-traditional opportunities to learn, and the experience of **transition programs** into mental health nursing.

vicarious trauma – the effect on health professionals who work with people who have experienced trauma; it frequently has a cumulative, disruptive effect on the helper's own spiritual well-being, meaning or sense of hope

secondary trauma – the response to stress that results from exposure to the first-hand trauma of another person; it can resemble post-traumatic stress disorder

transition program – a formalised, often competitive, program designed to orientate and support newly graduated nurses into clinical practice. These programs may also be offered to experienced RNs transitioning to specialist practice, or to RNs returning following a break from practice.

Mental health education: An overview

Curricula in mental health education conform broadly with those elsewhere in health: a combination of theoretical instruction and clinical application. The implementation of curricula varies across different education programs, but increasingly the preparation of undergraduate nurses and other health professionals shares fundamental minimal characteristics. This is partially because national regulatory authorities have standardised requirements for every beginning practitioner. In nursing, theoretical study must include mental health. There is no requirement for a clinical placement in mental health (Australian Nursing & Midwifery Accreditation Council (ANMAC), 2019). Aotearoa New Zealand requires nursing students to undertake mental health placement (Nursing Council of New Zealand, 2012).

There are increasing pressures in Australia for the provision of the clinical placement component. Competition between different health disciplines for placement and a reduction in suitable placements have both intensified. This has resulted in clinical placements being provided across a broad range of services that are now involved in the provision of care for people experiencing mental ill-health. Thus, the public in-patient mental health service is no longer the dominant setting for clinical placement in preregistration education. Forensic, community, non-government and general health services are increasingly being used as clinical placement settings for mental health students.

Alternatives have been developed in a small number of instances. An example of this is a mental health service specifically developed by the University of Wollongong, in New South Wales, to provide health professional students with clinical placement opportunities in recreational services provided in community settings for people diagnosed with enduring mental ill-health. The Recovery Camp (http://recoverycamp.com.au/) presents challenges to the ordinary learning styles of health professional programs, but has been developed to align with the requisite standards of accreditation bodies (Cowley et al., 2016; Patterson et al., 2017).

Not all theoretical curricula for mental health are designed exclusively for work in this field. Many skills in specialist fields of health, especially at the beginning health-practitioner level are shared. Communication skills is a good case in point, as are infection control principles. Therefore, not all theoretical preparation for mental health practice is labelled as such. At times, the relevance and contribution of these fields of study to a beginning practice in mental health can be challenging to recall and recognise.

This may contribute to an often-reported phenomenon: the self-perceived lack of preparation for clinical placement in mental health reported by nursing students. In turn, this can contribute to the fear reported by many nurses prior to their first placement in a mental health service. This fear is often described as arising from three major concerns:

1   the assumed unpredictable nature of behaviour associated with mental health problems
2   expectations of high levels of violence associated with mental ill-health
3   concern that a failure to speak or respond in a 'correct' manner may cause harm to a consumer (Kameg et al., 2014; Stuhlmiller & Tolchard, 2019).

It is important, first, to acknowledge that some of these ideas and beliefs are remnants of unexamined **stigma** and **stereotyping**. The role of the media should also be acknowledged in this context (Maiorano et al., 2017). Health practitioners ordinarily have a range of socially determined beliefs about the nature of mental health problems (Carrara et al., 2019). Even direct instruction or education may not alter these, as this teaching is filtered through the lens of prior beliefs and is constantly reinforced by many prominent social institutions, such as the media (Thornicroft et al., 2016).

The **therapeutic use of self** has become a commonly used expression in mental health services, yet definitions can differ and the concept remains ambiguous (Currid & Pennington, 2010). However, the establishment of the therapeutic relationship requires the therapeutic use of self and reflective practice. For the clinician, this means developing an understanding of self-knowledge, self-awareness, empathy, ethical practice, boundaries and the limits within the professional role. The therapeutic use of self requires the use of communication techniques such as active listening, ability to sit with silence, reflection, focusing, validating, open-ended questions, paraphrasing, clarifying and summarising (Jones, 2012). This highlights the extensive skills and the importance of reflecting on self and connecting with others through the encounter (Jones, 2012).

The nature of therapeutic interventions in mental health can be in stark contrast to the procedural delivery model applicable elsewhere in health care. Therapeutic use of self has prominence that can be unsettling (Wyder et al., 2017). It is, however, what those experiencing mental ill-health most value, but are not always accorded by health practitioners (Browne, Hurley & Lakeman, 2014; McAllister et al., 2019).

Therapeutic use of self can be unsettling as there is an often-unspoken requirement that clinicians should be self-aware and understand their own thoughts, emotions and the effects of their behaviour on others, which means they must examine their own personal issues. The self-awareness of transference and counter-transference, power dynamics, assumptions, prejudices, involuntary admissions and use of coercion are examples in which therapeutic use of self becomes challenging. Being open to examination of practice can be confronting; however, this scrutiny can bring an awareness of self not previously

stigma – a form of prejudice against people diagnosed with mental ill-health that involves inaccurate and hurtful representations of them; in some instances, those representations might be as violent, comical or incompetent. This form of stigma is dehumanising and makes people with mental health problems the object of fear or ridicule.

stereotype – a taken-for-granted assumption about a person, based on the presumed qualities of the group to which they belong; stereotypes can lead to inaccurate assessments of people's personal qualities and characteristics

therapeutic use of self – 'nurses employing their emotions and perceptions to understand clients' health needs and their knowledge and skills to facilitate the healing process' (Williams & Davis, 2005, ch. 1)

acknowledged (Currid & Pennington, 2010). Therapeutic use of self is not an instant transformation in a professional sense, but rather a gradual unfolding of one's practice with time and experience (Jones, 2012).

INTERPROFESSIONAL PERSPECTIVES

Character of the mental health workforce

Clinical placements in mental health services can differ from those in other areas of health care because of the range of disciplines encountered and the nature of the relationships between these professionals. The distinct delineation of respective scopes of practice between professions in mental health services is less distinct than elsewhere. This can be confusing for people experiencing mental health problems and their families or carers, and the same can be true for students. Indeed, the formation of professional identity can be challenging, and this is witnessed by definitional difficulties seen in mental health nursing (Happell, 2014; Hercelinskyj et al., 2014; Hurley & Lakeman, 2011; Lakeman & Hurley, 2021).

An environment characterised by a dynamic interprofessional workforce can have many strengths. The consultative characteristics can bring to bear a wide range of perspectives and skill sets. Ideally, this meets the person and their family and loved-ones' needs more comprehensively.

A key aspect of the interprofessional workforce in mental health services is the centrality of the person who has the lived experience of mental health problems and their families. Although not fully realised across all service jurisdictions, it is clearly the policy direction of mental health services (Stewart, Crozier & Wheeler, 2016). This establishes the person seeking help for their mental health problems as the expert in devising their care. Person-centred care becomes person-led care (Fraher & Brandt, 2019).

An additional feature in mental health services is the increasing profile of the peer workforce, which is the employment of people with lived experience of mental health problems across all areas of mental health services, including in clinical roles.

TRANSLATION TO PRACTICE

Interprofessional practice in mental health

The complexity of professions and disciplinary roles is a known point of confusion across all health care. Nurses have employed a range of means to support orientation into these roles and identities, for both the person seeking help and their families. List several of these aids that you may have observed across health services. Consider their positive features and those aspects that remain challenging. Which of these approaches could be used in provision of mental health services, and which are less successfully adopted by mental health services? Consider a range of mental health service settings, including in-patient and community settings, and the emergency department. In your answer, look at the roles of peer workers and of mental health liaison services. You may also include in your answer how these aids could also be used by students on clinical placement, or by staff new to the team.

Shane's story – what was helpful

Experiencing severe psychological distress can be an isolating, frightening and even traumatic experience. As someone who has a lived experience of this, including being hospitalised on a few occasions, I can attest to the importance of genuine person-centred care in supporting people toward recovery. Unfortunately, this was not always what I experienced in the health system. At its worst, I experienced moments of feeling unheard and was treated as though I was 'just another person' in the system. Interactions with those caring for me were few-and-far between, often limited to brief consultations with a treating psychiatrist or to receiving medication from nursing staff. There were, however, key people and moments that were central to the beginning of my recovery process. I can vividly recall one nurse who showed genuine care and concern for my well-being. Amid their busy schedule, they made the time to sit with me, to listen and hold the space with both compassion and hope. This nurse was able to see, despite the situation I was in, the strengths and potential I had to recover and flourish once again. They were able to genuinely connect with me and acknowledge how I was feeling in the moment. The time spent in conversation with this nurse left me feeling a little less distressed and, instead, a little lighter and more hopeful. This was, likewise, the case with one particular treating psychiatrist. As opposed to simply being diagnosed and pathologised, this psychiatrist encouraged and held out hope for me when I was unable to see it for myself. I felt genuinely heard when I expressed the thoughts and feelings that I was experiencing. I was more than a cluster of symptoms: I was, and am, a human being with hopes, dreams and fears. Being treated as such made all the difference. It was these people and qualities, I believe, that had a tangible and positive effect on me and my recovery journey.

REFLECTIVE QUESTIONS

- List the helpful and less helpful actions identified by Shane that influenced their recovery journey.
- How do these relate to recovery-orientated and trauma-informed practice?

Attitudes, expectations and positive engagement within practice

The ability to engage in a positive manner within mental health draws on the therapeutic use of 'self'. The aim of this type of practice is to establish a therapeutic alliance with the person experiencing mental ill-health to help in achieving their desired recovery goals. It is part of the central tradition of caring in nursing but has some different features and emphases in the domain of mental health nursing. The strength of the therapeutic alliance has been shown to be associated with lower symptoms early in therapy (Flückiger et al., 2020).

The therapeutic relationship is the foundational component of mental health nursing care, which facilitates any other interventions or therapies. Its ascendancy in mental health nursing is often attributed to the work of Peplau (1952, 1997), especially in the United States. However, the details of how to use the therapeutic relationship in mental health nursing are complex and are sometimes contested (Hurley & Rankin, 2008; Hutchinson & Hurley, 2013; Lakeman & Molloy, 2018).

Empathy, collaboration, alliance and presence have been suggested as critical elements of the therapeutic relationship (Geller & Greenberg, 2012; Lindquist, Tracy & Snyder, 2018; Miller et al., 2014; Norcross, Beutler & Levant, 2006), and these are explored more closely in this chapter. However, the claims for the importance of the therapeutic relationship must be judged by the effect it has on recovery for people experiencing mental health problems. Norcross and colleagues (2006) have suggested that, although much of the variation in therapeutic outcomes is related to the severity of mental ill-health and the characteristics of those experiencing them, the remaining unexplained variance is understood to be attributable not to a particular intervention, but to the therapeutic relationship itself (Norcross et al., 2006). Flückiger and colleagues (2020), in a meta-analysis of the relationship between the therapeutic alliance and early treatment symptoms, suggest a reciprocity that underlines the importance of the therapeutic relationship for recovery outcomes.

Empathy

There are many definitions, descriptions and features of empathy. In caring for a person, it has been described as arising 'out of a natural desire to care about others' (Hojat, 2007, p. 79). In the context of person-centred care, empathy is a tool that contributes to understanding the person's experiences, concerns and perspectives (Hojat, 2007; Hojat et al., 2015). This construct comprises two aspects: a cognitive and an affective component. It is sometimes characterised as feeling 'with' rather than 'for' the person experiencing mental ill-health. This rough characterisation attempts to emphasise the importance of understanding the other person's situation and their feelings. This is often contrasted with the emotion of sympathy, which is concerned with a personal response to the consumer's situation. It is perhaps helpful to conceptualise empathy and sympathy as differing on the dimensions of understanding and emotion. Empathy incorporates a cognitive element of understanding the other's experience, whereas sympathy involves a greater emotional component of sharing the other's feelings. The two concepts overlap in what might be understood as compassion (Hojat, 2007, pp. 8–11).

Collaboration

Collaboration refers to a mutual endeavour by the health practitioner and consumer: the engagement of both in the (therapeutic) relationship. Mutual goals can be established for the relationship when agreement is reached about the problems of the person experiencing mental ill-health. Collaboration requires the practitioner to follow the lead of the consumer regarding their goals for recovery. This is an empowering element of the therapeutic relationship.

Therapeutic alliance and presence

therapeutic presence
– a way of being open, receptive and ever-emerging in our states of being as we connect with others and with our inner world

Essentially, the therapeutic alliance refers to the strength of goal-directed activity between healthcare practitioners and consumers. If a person-centred negotiation of goals is undertaken, the therapeutic alliance is reinforced (Horvath & Bedi, 2002; Sharp, McAllister & Broadbent, 2016). However, the therapeutic alliance will not be reinforced if a therapeutic presence is not part of the groundwork. **Therapeutic presence** is the clinician's ability to be present and completely in the moment. It is a state of being relationally present with the consumer. 'Therapeutic presence involves contact with one's integrated and healthy self, while being open and receptive' to what is happening in that moment with consumers (Geller & Greenberg, 2012, p. 7).

Mindfulness is a practice that has been used interchangeably with presence and has contributed to confusion in terminology. Mindfulness is a technique that can have a profound influence on the present moment by enhancing and contributing to our way of being with a consumer. Mindfulness is one technique, whereas therapeutic presence is a stance that can be supported and developed, both personally and professionally, by the practice of mindfulness.

To fully prepare to be present with others we need to learn to be present and connect with ourselves. This is inclusive of the self-care practised in one's personal life. Preparing for presence professionally can be harder due to the practitioner not understanding the importance of self-care in a professional sense. Techniques in the work place include the following: preparing the physical space prior to seeing a consumer; 'clearing a space by putting aside personal concerns, needs and experiences from one's daily life' (Geller & Greenberg, 2012, pp. 75–7); and not meeting the consumer as a category of illness, but as a whole being.

Therapeutic presence creates and supports a strong therapeutic alliance (Geller, Greenberg, & Watson, 2010; Oghene, Pos & Geller, 2010). Therapeutic presence 'promote[s] agency and responsibility; reconnect[s] to pain and attune[s] to opportunities to transform pain and allow[s] for the development of a safe therapeutic relationship that is growth promoting' (Geller & Greenberg, 2012, p. 62). However, difficulties in clinicians' professional and personal lives, such as stress, unresolved personal issues, lack of self-care and fatigue, can be obstacles to developing presence (Geller & Greenberg, 2012). Illness-related distress contributes to people feeling disconnected, though at the same time increases a person's drive for connectedness. There is a healing effect when people experience connectedness (Hojat, 2007). Presence supports the requirements of safety and the relational connection that is a part of the foundation of the therapeutic relationship.

Professional boundaries

Counter-transference is a phenomenon that may occur in any field of health care. Defined as an unconscious response to a consumer's **transference**, it may be a significant factor requiring explicit monitoring. It may be a support to the therapeutic relationship, or it may affect it detrimentally, but it risks being a factor in transgression of **professional boundaries**.

The engagement in therapeutic alliances with people experiencing mental health problems exposes workers to risks of both vicarious trauma and secondary trauma. Vicarious trauma is common among those working in many fields of human services, and is associated with witnessing the trauma experienced by others. In some health fields, this can be developed by exposure to injuries suffered by others – for example, motor-vehicle accidents attended by first responders such as paramedics, emergency department staff and law enforcement services.

In the field of mental health services, even as students, you may witness people experiencing high levels of distress. This may be expressed in aggressive or even violent ways and witnessing this can be disturbing. Interventions employed in such circumstances may involve coercive techniques, such as the use of physical restraint, seclusion and administration of non-consensual medication. Witnessing or participating in these interventions presents

mindfulness – being aware of the present moment or experience, with intention and purpose, without grasping onto judgements (Siegel, 2012)

counter-transference – the response that is elicited in the recipient (therapist) by the other's (client's) unconscious transference

transference – the phenomenon whereby we unconsciously transfer feelings and attitudes from a person or situation in the past onto a person or situation in the present; the process is at least partly inappropriate to the present

professional boundaries – limits that protect the space between the professional's power and the consumer's vulnerability; the borders between a professional, therapeutic relationship and a non-professional or personal relationship of a nurse and a person in their care

staff with profound ethical challenges, especially to their common self-characterisation as a 'caring' profession. Vicarious trauma may result (Rossi et al., 2012).

Vicarious trauma is not necessarily only the result of extreme scenarios. There is emerging evidence that it can be cumulative due to exposure over time to lesser traumatic events. This can include witnessing the effects of involuntary detention, separation from home and family, or the loss of autonomy and self-determination experienced by many people within (mental) health services (Bywood & McMillan, 2019; Louth et al., 2019).

Secondary trauma shares many of the features of vicarious trauma in people working in the mental health field. It can be differentiated by attributing it to exposure to the experiences of people having had prior traumas. Listening to or reading about the past traumatic experiences of others can cause a secondary traumatic effect in the person exposed to these accounts. Again, this may be cumulative as the worker learns of many people's traumatic pasts – especially as people experiencing mental health problems are known to have experienced higher rates of trauma than the general population (Shevlin et al., 2008; Varese et al., 2012).

In addition, many health workers themselves may have experienced personal trauma. Working with other people who are experiencing trauma or who have a significant history of trauma may 're-activate' your own distress.

The key to maintaining professional boundaries and avoiding the potential for harm to consumers and oneself is the development of self-awareness by mental health clinicians. This helps to highlight counter-transference and other factors that may affect the maintenance of a therapeutic relationship that incorporates empathy, alliance, presence and collaboration. Developing an understanding of how a consumer's behaviour affects you, and why, can help to ensure that interactions remain focused on the consumer's needs and goals. This can be achieved by reflective practice, most usefully by clinical supervision or personal therapy. As a student, this may be difficult to achieve, yet it is perhaps a time when it can be most critical. The preceptor, mentor and **clinical facilitator** and **clinical supervisor** can be excellent sources for this support. **Debriefing** discussion, either alone with the facilitator or with a group of fellow students, can serve as a proxy.

Power relations and the therapeutic relationship

Power is a pervasive and multifaceted aspect of mental health services that affects the therapeutic relationship. It has origins in many of the contextual elements of the delivery of care, including the physical environment, knowledge, interprofessional teams, the law and models of holistic care. Its effects may be both limiting and strengthening within the therapeutic relationship, where judicious use may support a consumer in regaining resilience in recovery (Hixson, 2016; Johnstone et al., 2018; Salzmann-Erikson & Eriksson, 2012).

Knowledge – both having and lacking knowledge – contributes to the power differential in the therapeutic relationship. A healthcare practitioner has knowledge of all manner of things that may be mysterious, confusing and not self-evident to consumers. Some questions that may arise for the consumer include: *What is wrong with me? What will happen to me? Who are the people in the treatment team and how significant are they?* A healthcare practitioner may have knowledge of such matters, whereas consumers may not. The knowledge in question may be quite prosaic: *What is the layout of the venue? What is the timetable of events (meals, visits, appointments)?* However, the imbalance undercuts an

---

clinical facilitator – a registered nurse employed on a sessional basis by a school of nursing to work with a group of students allocated to a designated health facility while on their clinical placement; the clinical facilitator, who performs many linking roles between the school of nursing and the clinical facility, works with the facility's staff to ensure clinical learning opportunities for students and to assess their attainment of learning objectives for the placement

clinical supervisor – usually an experienced clinicians who acts as a teacher, coach, mentor, role model, advisor or a combination of these. Their exact role depends on the context, their supervisees' clinical experience and many other factors (Clinical Supervision Guidelines, 2013).

debriefing – a process frequently employed in nursing as a means by which to provide support and ensure learning possibilities are realised from clinical (real or simulated) experiences; it is often facilitated by teaching staff and encourages critical reflection and contribution from nursing students in a shared space removed but adjacent in time and place to the clinical experience

otherwise equal relationship, as the consumer is dependent upon the healthcare practitioner to provide information about such matters.

The therapeutic relationship between a person with mental ill-health and the healthcare practitioner occurs in limited contexts. These contexts are frequently those characterised by greatest need or distress and, in certain organisational arrangements such as administration of medication and assessment interviews. The healthcare practitioner rarely knows the person presenting with mental distress beyond them being the recipient of care. The healthcare practitioner constructs the therapeutic relationship within its limits, which is when mental health need is highest. Acknowledging the person beyond the diagnostic label, respecting each person as an individual and holding hope are essential to service users when presenting to services (Cleary et al., 2012; Horgan et al., 2020).

Due to a wide range of environments in which mental health care occurs and its engagement in both primary and secondary preventative activities, positioning the therapeutic relationship in terms of mental health problems being experienced is problematic. Development of strengths-based models of care, with its emphasis on resilience, continues to regard the consumer in a traditional, objectifying manner, through the lens of medicalisation and psychiatric diagnosis (Horgan et al., 2020).

Maintaining professional boundaries also serves to establish power differentials between the clinician and consumer. Mutual sharing of confidences, personal thoughts and information is not regarded as being therapeutic and is potentially detrimental, by removing the focus of the relationship from the needs of the consumer. Maintaining professional boundaries also helps to avoid the potential for misuse of power arising from the power differential between the clinician and the consumer and their family.

Consumers cannot be seen to have a legitimate right to insist on the disclosure of the clinician's personal world in the same manner that a nurse may ask of the consumer. Indeed, failure to 'play the patient game' and comply with the expectation of self-disclosure may have the undesired consequence of **pathologising** the behaviour (Foucault, 1986). What is accepted in ordinary social discourse may be regarded as evidence of problems in the context of a mental health service. A person who refuses to divulge intimate information or who demands that the clinician reveals personal information is poorly regarded. Yet, these behaviours may be defining characteristics of egalitarian relationships. The clinician, further, is involved in reinterpreting the consumer's experience, an exercise of power that effectively invalidates the consumer's personal experience (Horgan et al., 2020).

Application of interpersonal skills

Learning to use interpersonal skills is a daunting challenge for all health practitioners. Often, students feel confounded by how to achieve an opportunity to rehearse and acquire these elusive skills, which take on a mysterious and reified nature that contributes to these difficulties.

In the main, an attitude of courteous curiosity may be a sound manner in which to start exploring how to use interpersonal skills in your mental health practice. Observe the styles and methods of your colleagues. What do you admire about the ways in which they communicate? What do you feel falls short of skilful interpersonal communication? Take note of these observations – how can you ensure that you do not replicate the communication and interpersonal skills that you find wanting? If you are able to analyse

power – a complex and multifaceted construct that in health care and other social environments centres on the ability to influence people's behaviour; closely associated with constructs such as coercion, authority and influence

pathologising – the interpretation of beliefs and behaviours as evidence of an underlying disease or disorder. In mental health settings, the use of the term can indicate feelings, thoughts and behaviours not considered normal (GoodTherapy, 2021).

those aspects of interpersonal communication that are less helpful, can you understand why they are sometimes used? If you gain this insight, perhaps you may be able to devise alternate strategies to replace the less-helpful interpersonal skills that you have observed.

Encountering a nurse with admirable interpersonal skills – a role model – offers a great opportunity for learning (Cleary, Horsfall & Jackson, 2013; Jack, Hamshire & Chambers, 2017). Approach this person and request a chance to discuss your observations. They may be able to give you an in-depth understanding of how to develop skilful interpersonal abilities. Discuss these observations with your peers, preceptor, mentor, clinical facilitator or clinical supervisor.

Finally, request feedback about your interpersonal skills. This may be difficult and confronting, but these observations can highlight your strengths and weaknesses in ways that are difficult to discern on your own. Remember that you are a student: this is an acceptable time to make mistakes and try different approaches. Take advantage of this.

Legal framework of practice

Establishing a therapeutic relationship in a context in which treatment is legally determined, whether as an involuntary in-patient or under involuntary provisions in a community setting, clearly skews power relationships from the initial encounter (Light et al., 2014). The existence of a legal framework of compulsion for treatment within which the therapeutic relationship is engaged is problematic (Courtney & Moulding, 2014). A subtext, frequently unacknowledged, is that the failure to comply with the construction of the relationship may incur a legal consequence. The consumer who has engaged voluntarily in treatment may lose their voluntary status, and someone being treated in a community setting may have this freedom curtailed. Clearly, the law vests significant power in nurses in this regard, either formally, for example, as accredited persons under a Mental Health Act, or informally, as a discipline whose professional assessment has weight in determining a consumer's treatment.

Wyder and colleagues (2015), in their study of involuntary treatment, concluded that there was growing evidence that involuntary hospital admission can erode the therapeutic relationship (Wyder et al., 2015). The coercive nature of involuntary treatment is widely recognised as corrosive for the viability of a therapeutic alliance critical for attaining recovery goals (Corring et al., 2018; Goulet et al., 2020; Lagarde & Msellati, 2017; Stensrud et al., 2016).

REFLECTIVE QUESTION

How might the clinician maintain a therapeutic alliance in these circumstances?

Ethical and political influences on care

Mental health services have been the focus of a reform agenda since the early 1990s in Australia. The ways in which mental health services have changed, from predominantly separate, in-hospital services to services delivered primarily in community settings and 'mainstream' health settings. These services now employ a broader range of providers, including non-government organisations (Happell, 2010).

The most important, and in some ways revolutionary, change to mental health workforces has been the development of peer workers positions (see Chapter 8).

Some political factors have had some unforeseen and unfortunate consequences for consumers. It has been common for people with mental ill-health to find it difficult to get adequate living arrangements. Homelessness and involvement in the criminal and justice systems have seen significant rises following these political decisions about health care. These changed circumstances represent challenges to mental health nursing, not only in the provision of services but in ethical dimensions as well. Mental health nurses may feel that their professional practice is compromised by some of the circumstances of care delivery. Their delivery of care may be constrained by limitations in resources, especially when working with some of the most vulnerable groups, such as homeless people and asylum seekers.

REFLECTIVE QUESTIONS

- How can the role of advocacy be undertaken in an ethical manner?
- What consent should be obtained? Where might mental health nurses undertake advocacy?
- What conflicts might arise in adopting this role?

Development of emotional competence

Emotional intelligence (EI) is an idea with resonance in working within mental health services. It is important for both the effectiveness of the care offered and the interprofessional nature of this work, and also for the self-care that is important in mental health and health care more generally (Freshwater & Stickley, 2004; Montes-Berges & Augusto, 2007; Riley & Weiss, 2016).

Some of the seminal work in this field is associated with Peter Salovey and John Mayer (1990) and Daniel Goleman (1996). These authors challenged traditional views that emotions were a countervailing force to intelligence, and required firm control to ensure rational behaviour. According to Salovey and Mayer (1990, p. 189) emotional intelligence is:

> ... the ability to monitor one's own and others' feelings and emotions, to discriminate amongst them and to use this information to guide one's thinking and actions.

Emotional competence therefore refers to the ability to recognise, interpret and respond constructively to emotions in oneself and in others (Beaumont, 2005; Mayer, Caruso & Salovey, 2016). This can be recognised in empathetic responses to other's emotional reactions in health care, which is dependent upon an ability to recognise feelings and appreciate their nature.

How to achieve this ability is challenging, but it is proposed that it is a skill that can be developed with practice or increase over time (Foster et al., 2017; Hurley & Rankin, 2008; Judge, Opsahl & Robinson, 2018; Louth et al., 2019). Successful leadership within health contexts, particularly in nursing, is recognised as built on emotional intelligence (Abraham & Scaria, 2017).

Well-being in the workplace

Well-being is essential to having highly skilled and confident mental health clinicians. Well-being in the workplace has been shown to have a positive correlation with self-care activities. Clinicians' well-being and the quality of care given have been shown to be interdependent (Adams et al., 2020; Mills, Wand & Fraser, 2018). Viewing well-being from the professional and personal perspective demonstrates the importance of how domains overlap and inform each other. Domains identified by Cleary and colleagues (2020) include physical, psychological, emotional, spiritual, relational, recreational and other interests. Other domains include workload, time management and the professional role. The inclusion of peer support, protected time, debriefing with trusted colleagues and clinical supervision are important to ongoing well-being (Cleary et al., 2020).

To truly care for others, mental health clinicians need to learn to care for themselves. A positive correlation when participating in self-care activities and an enhancement in well-being are evident in the literature (Mills et al., 2018). This aspect of well-being is mostly left unspoken in the workplace; however, it holds a very important place in achieving reduced levels of stress and burnout.

Mental health professionals need to embody self-care and become role models of the practice of self-care through health promotion. Caring for the self is not selfish, but instead shows the importance of well-being in the workplace. Leadership that values and incorporates emotional safety for all is vital in achieving well-being in the workplace.

Reflective practice as a critical thinking process

The way in which one might approach the work of mental health nursing can be unclear. What is it that mental health nurses 'do'? How do they set priorities?

Mental health nursing shares with all fields of nursing certain habits of mind and ways of thinking, albeit with some aspects being at different levels of importance. The familiar cycle of clinical reasoning in nursing (also known as the nursing process) is applicable to mental health nursing (Levett-Jones et al., 2011; Levett-Jones et al., 2009). This six-step process, developed from the work of Ida Jean Orlando, progresses through the following predictable phases: assessment, problem identification, outcome of problem identification, planning, implementing and assessment (Funnell, Koutoukidis & Lawrence, 2009). In this context, a nurse undertakes a predictable series of activities when determining a course of action in clinical practice. Ordinarily, this starts with consideration of the consumer's mental health condition and experiences, in collaboration with the consumer and the collection of cues and information relevant to the consumer. This information requires processing to understand the relevant factors for the consumer and through the synthesis of these to establish the definitive problem for support or resolution. The outcome or goal of resolving the problem requires clarification prior to taking action, by selecting between alternatives. Following this action – perhaps an intervention – an evaluation is made of the outcomes achieved. The final component of the nursing process is reflection directed at the process undertaken and to discern the possible learning achieved.

A component of this clinical reasoning cycle of the nursing process is the utilisation and development of a habit of critical thinking (Heaslip, 2008). Kanbay and Okanli (2017) have suggested that nursing requires a questioning disposition and a reflective capacity, to ensure that safety and high standards are achieved. Critical thinking contributes to this by supporting an ability to think in a systematic and logical manner that is non-judgemental. It acts as the guide to establishing beliefs and courses of skilful action.

Critical thinking can be understood to be part of a reflective process, in which both actions and emotions are considered. Reflection examines assumptions, particularly those underlying opinion, actions and beliefs. Its aim is to deepen the understanding of the clinical situation and of the self (Rosser et al., 2019; Rubenfeld & Scheffer, 2006; Scheffer & Rubenfeld, 2000; Stewart, 2017).

Support frameworks for working in mental health services

Clinical supervision is an important component of professional practice in mental health. It is a concept that can be confusing and is at times spoken of interchangeably with the practices of preceptorship and mentorship. It does differ from those practices, and it is helpful to understand the distinction between these three supportive practices (Mills, Francis & Bonner, 2005).

Preceptorship

A preceptorship may be distinguished as a relationship that occurs within the bounds of the work environment. Ordinarily, a particular skill or set of skills forms the focus of the relationship. The **preceptor** is appointed to support the novice in attaining proficiency in these skills or procedures. The duration of the relationship is usually limited to the period that it takes to achieve this expertise.

The term 'preceptorship' is commonly used to describe the staff member assigned to support the student's learning while on clinical placement or as part of the new graduate year. At times this takes the form of 'buddying', or the student working entirely with this staff member. At other times, working arrangements cannot support such a consistent and exclusive relationship over the period of clinical placement. In such instances, the preceptor may be responsible for negotiating the learning opportunities for the student in their absence. It is common for a preceptor also to have a role in the assessment of skills (Billay & Myrick, 2008; Trede, Sutton & Bernoth, 2016).

Mentorship

This is a broad-based relationship with with a more expert nurse (Harding & Mawson, 2017). It is usually a relationship initiated by the novice, with a view to seeking support for their personal and career development through qualities in the expert nurse's practice that the novice may seek to emulate. The relationship is negotiated between the two parties and can occur in the workplace, but will ordinarily occur outside of working hours. It may be a long-term relationship in which the novice seeks advice from the mentor on a range of practice matters over extended periods of time. The frequency of these consultations may reflect the needs of the novice or may be more formally convened at regular intervals. Sometimes these **mentor** relationships may last for the nurse's entire career!

The mentoring relationship differs from the admiration one may hold for an esteemed expert nurse and their practice. It is an exclusive relationship that acknowledges the role

clinical supervision – 'a process within which the clinician brings their practice under scrutiny in order to more fully appreciate the meaning of their experience, to develop their abilities, to maintain standards of practice and to provide a more therapeutic service to the client' (Consedine, 2001)

preceptor – 'a clinical staff member – as opposed to a faculty member – who provides supervision and clinical instruction to new practitioners, undergraduate or newly registered, or new to a specific clinical environment' (Mills, Francis & Bonner, 2005)

mentor – 'a teaching–learning process acquired through personal experience within a one-to-one, reciprocal, career-development relationship between two individuals diverse in age, personality, life cycle, professional status and/or credentials' (Stewart & Krueger, 1996) of the expert nurse in the provision of advice to the novice. Although the management of the relationship may in many ways be the responsibility of the novice, there is mutuality in the concern and commitment to the development of the novice nurse (Hoover et al., 2020).

Clinical supervision

The term 'clinical supervision' has often been criticised as being prone to misunderstanding. Supervision has a managerial connotation that is the antithesis of the relationship of clinical supervision. In fact, the frank and confidential nature of the clinical supervision role precludes the conflict of interest inherent in any attempt to develop such a relationship with one's direct or line manager.

Clinical supervision is a supportive relationship that is focused on the development of improved clinical practice. It may occur under the guidance of a supervisor with specific expertise (who also engages in their own clinical supervision to maintain a good standard in the supervisory role), or between peers. It may occur on an individual basis between a single supervisee and clinical supervisor, or as part of a group.

The frequency of meetings varies, but research has established that it is most effective when occurring at no less than monthly intervals (White & Winstanley, 2011). It is usually acknowledged that the duration of the meetings should be 60 minutes. There is increasing use of innovative means to access clinical supervision, especially by nurses who practice in rural, isolated or remote environments. Videoconferencing and other media and information technologies are used to facilitate participation.

The form of clinical supervision that has been most frequently adopted in nursing contexts over the past 25 years has been that developed by Bridget Proctor (Proctor, 1986, 2008; White & Winstanley, 2011). This model conceptualises clinical supervision as having three functions: the so-called normative, formative and restorative domains. Normative functions are those that aid in developing and maintaining standards for clinical practice and clinical review. Developing knowledge and skills are those represented by the formative domain. Personal well-being of participants is the restorative function. There is some evidence that these domains become effective at differing rates (White & Winstanley, 2010). Changes are first seen in normative and restorative domains. It is later that the formative domain shows change, suggesting that improvements for consumers may become possible when organisational culture responds to the benefits of the normative and restorative domains in practitioners (White & Winstanley, 2010).

There is emerging evidence that clinical supervision contributes to both improved consumer outcomes by facilitating improvements in clinical skills as well as improved wellness and therapeutic orientation of nurses involved with clinical supervision (Cutcliffe, Sloan & Bashaw, 2018; Gonge & Buus, 2015; White & Winstanley, 2014).

Overall rates of clinical supervision in mental health nursing have been low in Australia and Aotearoa New Zealand, despite support from health authorities and professional associations. This presents a challenge for novice nurses who wish to access this form of structured professional support and development. As a newcomer to the workforce, the novice nurse may find it difficult to persevere to secure access to clinical supervision in the absence of overt and explicit managerial support (Cutcliffe et al., 2018).

REFLECTIVE QUESTIONS

- By what means could clinical supervision be secured by a novice mental health nurse?
- How might student nurses utilise clinical supervision?
- What reasons would you suggest to explain the low clinical supervision participation rates in mental health nursing in Australia and Aotearoa New Zealand?

Preparing for clinical placement

Clinical placements may not occur in a designated mental health service for every student in an undergraduate health program. Nevertheless, it is clear that both knowledge and skills for supportive practice with people experiencing mental distress are essential for all, due to the prevalence of mental health issues throughout society. You, as the student, can equip yourself to attain some level of mental healthcare proficiency, even if this engages in non-traditional settings. Initial independent knowledge can be gained by undertaking a first-aid focused program, such as that offered by Mental Health First Aid Australia (https://mhfa.com.au/) and the Mental Health Foundation of New Zealand (https://www.mentalhealth.org.nz/).

Developing objectives for clinical placements

It is helpful to set yourself objectives prior to clinical placement, which offers an opportunity to deepen your mental health skills and knowledge,. This will help ensure that you maximise opportunities that become available, whether placed in a non-traditional environment such as the Recovery Camp program, or in tertiary health services such as emergency departments. Indeed, if you do not encounter mental health placement until after graduation – during a transition program, for example – setting objectives for your learning will be valuable.

Setting learning objectives for clinical placement is dependent upon three factors:

1   Knowledge of the learning objectives of the unit of study associated with the placement
2   Knowledge of the opportunities available within the clinical placement setting at that point in time
3   Knowledge of one's own learning needs based on the objectives to be accomplished in the formal unit of study and personal objectives arising from reflection on one's areas of weakness or challenge in this area of nursing practice.

Achieving alignment of these three factors may be difficult. However, it offers an opportunity to rehearse negotiating skills as you attempt to achieve these objectives. Negotiation with clinical staff of the placement setting may help to determine the objectives that may be supported during the placement, and negotiation with the university's clinical facilitator is required to achieve this. Additionally, the self-scrutiny of what you do well, what you might improve upon and what you may not as yet be able to perform can help you to develop the habit of critical questioning and prioritising of your own learning objectives.

Sometimes, clinical placements may appear to be restricted in what they offer for learning. This may be a first impression and based on a misunderstanding of the nature and experience of people with mental distress and/or ill-health, mental health nursing or mental health services associated with the placement. Learning may need to be considered in a different manner than in other domains of health. If you have concentrated on achieving skills in clinical procedures, the relatively low profile of these skills in mental health nursing may be unsettling. Although such aspects of nursing practice form part of mental health nursing, pursuit of these as learning opportunities may be misplaced. Utilisation of such clinical skills may, however, prove a valuable way to engage in the more central activities of mental health nursing.

Another aspect of mental health nursing that is arguably in contrast with other fields of nursing is a further feature of the relationship between mental health nurse and consumer. Nurses work *with* consumers to achieve the recovery goals established by the consumer. This may be contrasted with other fields of nursing, where the work is about doing *for* or *to* the recipients of nursing care. Procedures provide a clear example of this contrast. In medical and surgical fields of nursing, procedures have a high profile in mediating the relationship between the nurse and the consumer of the services.

The time in clinical placement serves to help rehearse and deepen communication skills. These skills will be valuable across the entire range of nursing practice and are also helpful in one's personal life. They may include developing an ability to tolerate uncertainty and ambiguity in communication, and improving your ability to recall the content and features of communication for documentation at a later time. Rehearsing communication skills that enhance your ability to respond in a therapeutic manner, and tolerating silence, are important learning opportunities. All these communication skills are useful to learn.

It is sometimes tempting to listen to accounts from peers and assume that their placements offer superior learning opportunities. While there are certainly occasions when this might be an accurate assessment, changing placement location frequently in pursuit of a 'better' learning opportunity can be counter-productive. The experiences may be elusive and may only offer themselves by dint of your own effort and growing familiarity with the environment in which you are placed.

The therapeutic relationship is central to working in mental health nursing. Time can be a very helpful factor in establishing such a relationship. Clinical placement that allows for your presence on a continuing basis and an opportunity to persevere in this regard is valuable. Take it!

Pragmatic strategies for learning

Several approaches are available to help you make the best of your clinical placements in mental health services. These can be summarised as preparation, communication and self-care. The following sections give some direction and suggestions.

Preparation

- Find out about the service prior to the commencement of your placement. To whom does it offer help? Who runs the service? How big is the service – does it offer a range of services? There may be a website that provides this type of overview, or your university may supply some information. It is probably not advisable to ring the service as it may provide a great many clinical placements, making repeated provision of this type of information a burden on staff. However, it is often true that a show of interest and initiative on the part of students is very well regarded.

- Be clear about meeting venues and times for your first day. It may be advisable to visit the service prior to your placement, to ensure you are clear as to the location of the mental health service and the meeting venue.
- Clarify dress codes. Some mental health services discourage the wearing of uniforms because of their potential to stigmatise people with mental ill-health, especially in rehabilitation and community services. In other services, uniforms are seen as helpful to identify your role to staff and consumers.
- Make sure that your requisite vaccinations, police-check and student identification documentation are in order prior to commencing your placement.
- Wear comfortable and safe footwear.
- Review the theory subject that has prepared you for this placement. Clarify the learning objectives expected from the placement and your university's specific requirements.

Communication

- Identify your facilitator or preceptor and their contact details. Ensure you keep the relevant staff of the health facility and university apprised of any variation in your attendance.
- Introduce yourself to staff and consumers in a friendly and courteous manner.
- Make an effort to get to know the members of the team and the consumers of the service.
- Request feedback on your performance. This is a valuable learning opportunity, and as a student you are allowed to make mistakes.
- Avoid gossip.
- Spend your time engaged with the consumers of the service as much as you can. The service exists to help these people, and you are there to learn how to make your contribution. Meetings, case notes and university assignments can be completed in many other venues – time spent with people who are experiencing mental ill-health will be invaluable to your learning.
- Anticipate that some services may not be structured for your needs as a student, but rather to meet the needs of consumers as a priority. Additionally, consumers may not wish to interact with you because of their experiences of mental health disorders. Be patient, be present. Do not seek to 'sight-see' by requesting to visit other services if you are 'feeling bored', as this approach is both superficial and disrespectful. Perseverance can bring unexpected insight and opportunities.
- Maintain professional boundaries. Do not keep confidences for consumers and do not divulge personal details such as your phone number or address. Do not arrange to meet socially with consumers you meet on your clinical placement.
- Ensure that your use of social media does not breach policy and guidelines.

Looking after yourself

- Ask questions and seek clarification about the things you observe on clinical placement.
- Actively engage in tutorials or meetings arranged by your clinical facilitator or preceptor. It can be helpful to make a note of the topics you wish to talk about.
- If you experience difficulties or feel emotionally affected by your experiences, make sure that you report this to your clinical facilitator and ward staff. Actively prepare a plan of action to re-establish your equilibrium.
- Exercise, eat and sleep well. This advice may seem clichéd, but it does help.

- Avoid excessive consumption of caffeine or alcohol.
- Have fun, get involved, enjoy your experience – this is your education.

Self-assessment and personal problem-solving

Understanding one's learning needs and devising ways to address these can be a challenging task. *What do I know? How do I ensure my understanding is accurate and comprehensive? How do I respond to gaps I am aware of?*

Utilising a personal learning plan is a useful device. This log of learning objectives and possible courses of action may take a variety of forms that is best suited to your own style. All nurses are now required to keep a log of their professional development; commencing this process by utilising a learning plan and/or a journal on clinical placement will start habits that will be valuable later in your career.

TRANSLATION TO PRACTICE

Reflection, self-in-action and post-placement

Your conceptualisation of the experience and your learning from mental health clinical placement will develop over time. As you consider your experiences, both within the clinical placement and through theoretical preparation, fresh understandings will develop. Reflection about your prior attitudes and understandings of mental health, and how these may have changed as a result of these experiences, will deepen and expand your capacity to provide therapeutic care.

Many students report greater appreciation of the prevalence of distress and mental ill-health among people throughout healthcare services following their education in mental health, along with a deeper understanding of holistic and person-centred care.

REFLECTIVE QUESTION

How might you incorporate mental health care in nursing practice in other clinical domains?

SUMMARY

This chapter has presented information and a lived-experience perspective, supplemented by activities designed to deepen your understanding of:

- Why active development of personal learning objectives enhances the benefits for a student in clinical placement. A range of techniques was suggested to help ensure that formal learning objectives required by the students' educational body are met and also that students are able to recognise their own personal learning needs.

- The range of slightly different learning opportunities offered by each clinical placement, as no two environments are identical. Indeed, the same clinical placement may offer different opportunities over time. Students are encouraged to actively engage with opportunities while ensuring that they prioritise engagement with the consumers of services.
- The high prevalence of trauma in the backgrounds of people seeking mental health services. Students are alerted that this exposes them in a mental health setting (as in very many health settings) to potential personal and vicarious trauma, due to working in or being present on clinical placement. Strategies for maintaining personal wellness are suggested so students can remain resilient, avoid personal harm and continue to contribute to health care.
- The requirement in the policy environment for collaborative development of healthcare objectives in mental health services. The challenge of possible disparate views between health practitioners and health service consumers of what constitutes desirable outcomes can be challenging. It requires development of critical reflective skills to understand the potential contribution of transference and counter-transference.
- The contribution of emotional intelligence in the capacity to interact in a therapeutic manner.
- The personal attributes, interpersonal skills and professional skills that are necessary for success, not only in your clinical placements but also in your future practice. With this knowledge, you should be able to work skilfully in the health service environment.

CRITICAL THINKING/LEARNING ACTIVITIES

1 How do the standards for mental health nursing attempt to reconcile the inherent conflict between mental health service's dual roles of control and care?
2 What constraints affect learning on clinical placement in mental health?
3 Many factors interfere with self-care. List factors in your daily life that stop you meeting ideal standards of self-care. What other issues might arise when you begin your health career? What methods can be used to ensure that you employ self-care strategies throughout your career?
4 Trauma-informed care and practice challenge health professionals to ensure that their practices do not inflict trauma or re-traumatise recipients of their care. However, the emotional labour in mental health work may open these health professionals to experiencing secondary or vicarious trauma. Consider those feelings and behaviours that may indicate that this is developing. What strategies could be employed to redress this? How could secondary or vicarious traumatisation be prevented?
5 Recovery principles of mental health practice are based on notions of collaborative, person-led care. Discuss the challenges for health professionals to meet this practice standard in a responsive and individualised manner. What skills are required?

LEARNING EXTENSION

When you complete your education, you will be required to undertake continuing professional development to maintain your registration as a health practitioner.

Prepare a learning portfolio in which you set your learning objectives for your mental health placement, record evidence of meeting these objectives and keep a record that will meet the requirements of registration.

FURTHER READING

Australian College of Mental Health Nursing Inc (ACMHN). (2018). *National Framework for Mental Health Content in Pre-registration Nursing Programs 2018: Survey summary data and results.* Canberra: ACMHN.

This report itemises features of mental health nursing preparation in Australia and sets an agenda for the future characteristics of preparation.

Cleary, M., Horsfall, J., Happell, B. & Hunt, G. E. (2013). Reflective components in undergraduate mental health nursing curricula: Some issues for consideration. *Issues in Mental Health Nursing, 34*(2): 69–74.

This article draws the reader's attention to the variety of possible reflective exercises available for pre-registration nursing students from their mental health clinical placement. It incorporates discussion from the perspective of both educators and students and raises relative ethical concerns that are involved.

Flückiger, C., Rubel, J., Del Re, A. O., Horvath, A., Wampold, B. E., Crits-Christoph, P., Atzil-Slonim, D., Compare, A., Falkenström, F., Ekeblad, A., Errázuriz, P., Fisher, H., Hoffart, A., Huppert, J. & Kivity, Y. (2020). The reciprocal relationship between alliance and early treatment symptoms: A two-stage individual participant data meta-analysis. *Journal of Consulting and Clinical Psychology, 88*(9): 829–49.

This research article explores the therapeutic alliance and the reduction of symptoms, suggesting that the first stage of the alliance is critical for this effect.

Health Education and Training Institute. (2016). *Student Training and Rights of Patients. Policy Directives.* NSW Department of Health. Retrieved from http://www1.health.nsw.gov.au/PDS/pages/doc.aspx?dn=PD2005_548

This NSW Health policy directive aims to cover the principles for appropriate conduct standards in relation student clinical placement. This is representative of the concerns of health services providers in many jurisdictions as they seek to balance patients' rights and the responsibilities to support education of student health professionals.

REFERENCES

Abraham, J. & Scaria, J. (2017). Emotional intelligence: The context for successful nursing leadership: a literature review. *Nursing & Care Open Access Journal, 2*(6): 160–4.

Adams, M., Chase, J., Doyle, C. & Mills, J. (2020). Self-care planning supports clinical care: Putting total care into practice. *Progress in Palliative Care, 28*(5): 305–7.

Australian Nursing & Midwifery Accreditation Council (ANMAC). (2019). *Registered Nurse Accreditation Standards 2019.* Canberra ACT: ANMAC.

Beaumont, L. R. (2005). *Emotional Competency.* Retrieved from http://www.emotionalcompetency.com/

Billay, D. & Myrick, F. (2008). Preceptorship: An integrative review of the literature. *Nurse Education in Practice, 8*(4): 258–66.

Browne, G., Hurley, J. & Lakeman, R. (2014). Mental health nursing: What difference does it make? *Journal of Psychiatric and Mental Health Nursing, 21*(6): 558–63.

Bywood, P. & McMillan, J. (2019). *Cumulative Exposure to Trauma at Work: Phase 2: Prevention and intervention strategies.* Melbourne: Worksafe Australia and Monash University.

Carrara, B. S., Ventura, C. A. A., Bobbili, S. J., Jacobina, O. M. P., Khenti, A. & Mendes, I. A. C. (2019). Stigma in health professionals towards people with mental illness: an integrative review. *Archives of Psychiatric Nursing, 33*(4): 311–8.

Cleary, M., Horsfall, J. & Jackson, D. (2013). Role models in mental health nursing: The good, the bad, and the possible. *Issues in Mental Health Nursing*, 34(8): 635–6.

Cleary, M., Hunt, G. E., Horsfall, J. & Deacon, M. (2012). Nurse–patient interaction in acute adult inpatient mental health units: A review and synthesis of qualitative studies. *Issues in Mental Health Nursing, 33*(2): 66–79.

Cleary, M., Schafer, C., McLean, L. & Visentin, D. C. (2020). Mental health and well-being in the health workplace. *Issues in Mental Health Nursing, 41*(2): 172–5.

Clinical Supervision Guidelines. (2013). *Definition and Purpose*. Retrieved from: http://www.clinicalsupervisionguidelines.com.au/definition-and-purpose

Consedine, M. (2001). Using role theory in clinical supervision. *Australian and New Zealand Psychodrama Association Journal, 10*: 37–49.

Corring, D., O'Reilly, R., Sommerdyk, C. & Russell, E. (2018). What families have to say about community treatment orders (CTOs). *Canadian Journal of Community Mental Health, 37*(2): 1–12.

Courtney, M. & Moulding, N. T. (2014). Beyond balancing competing needs: Embedding involuntary treatment within a recovery approach to mental health social work. *Australian Social Work, 67*(2): 214–26.

Cowley, T., Sumskis, S., Moxham, L., Taylor, E., Brighton, R., Patterson, C. & Halcomb, E. (2016). Evaluation of undergraduate nursing students' clinical confidence following a mental health recovery camp. *International Journal of Mental Health Nursing, 25*(1): 33–41.

Cutcliffe, J. R., Sloan, G. & Bashaw, M. (2018). A systematic review of clinical supervision evaluation studies in nursing. *International Journal of Mental Health Nursing, 27*(5): 1344–63.

Currid, T. & Pennington, J. (2010). Continuing professional development: Therapeutic use of self. *British Journal of Wellbeing, 1*(3): 35–42.

Flückiger, C., Rubel, J., Del Re, A. O. Horvath, A., Wampold, B. E., Crits-Christoph, P., Atzil-Slonim, D., Compare, A., Falkenström, F., Ekeblad, A., Errázuriz, P., Fisher, H., Hoffart, A., Huppert, J. & Kivity, Y. (2020). The reciprocal relationship between alliance and early treatment symptoms: A two-stage individual participant data meta-analysis. *Journal of Consulting and Clinical Psychology, 88*(9): 829–49.

Foster, K., Fethney, J., McKenzie, H., Fisher, M., Harkness, E. & Kozlowski, D. (2017). Emotional intelligence increases over time: A longitudinal study of Australian pre-registration nursing students. *Nurse Education Today, 55*: 65-70.

Foucault, M. (1986). Afterword: The subject and power. In H. L. Dreyfus & P. Rabinow (eds), *Beyond Structuralism and Hermeneutics* (pp. 208–27). Brighton, UK: Harvester.

Fraher, E. & Brandt, B. (2019). Toward a system where workforce planning and interprofessional practice and education are designed around patients and populations not professions. *Journal of Interprofessional Care, 33*(4): 389–97.

Freshwater, D. & Stickley, T. (2004). The heart of the art: Emotional intelligence in nurse education. *Nursing Inquiry, 11*(2): 91–8.

Funnell, R., Koutoukidis, G. & Lawrence, K. (2009). *Tabbner's Nursing Care*, 5th edn. Port Melbourne: Elsevier.

Geller, S. M. & Greenberg, L. S. (2012). *Therapeutic Presence: A mindful approach to effective therapy*. Washington, DC: American Psychological Association.

Geller, S. M., Greenberg, L. S. & Watson, J. C. (2010). Therapist and client perceptions of therapeutic presence: The development of a measure. *Psychotherapy Research, 20*(5): 599–610.

Goleman, D. (1996). *Emotional Intelligence: Why it can matter more than IQ*. New York: Bantam Books.

Gonge, H. & Buus, N. (2015). Is it possible to strengthen psychiatric nursing staff's clinical supervision? RCT of a meta-supervision intervention. *Journal of Advanced Nursing, 71*(4): 909–21.

GoodTherapy. (2021). *Pathologizing*. Retrieved from https://www.goodtherapy.org/blog/psychpedia/pathologizing

Goulet, M.-H., Pariseau-Legault, P., Côté, C., Klein, A. & Crocker, A. G. (2020). Multiple stakeholders' perspectives of involuntary treatment orders: a meta-synthesis of the qualitative evidence toward an exploratory model. *International Journal of Forensic Mental Health, 19*(1): 18–32.

Happell, B. (2010). Moving in circles: A brief history of reports and inquiries relating to mental health content in undergraduate nursing curricula. *Nurse Education Today, 30*(7): 643–8.

———— (2014). Let the buyer beware! Loss of professional identity in mental health nursing. *International Journal of Mental Health Nursing*, *23*(2): 99–100.

Harding, T. & Mawson, K. (2017). Richness and reciprocity: Undergraduate student nurse mentoring in mental health. *SAGE Open Nursing*, *3*: 2377960817706040.

Heaslip, P. (2008). *Critical Thinking: To think like a nurse*. Kamloops, BC: Thompson Rivers University.

Hercelinskyj, G., Cruickshank, M., Brown, P. & Phillips, B. (2014). Perceptions from the front line: Professional identity in mental health nursing. *International Journal of Mental Health Nursing*, *23*(1): 24–32.

Hixson, K. A. (2016). *Understanding Power in the Therapeutic Relationship*. Oregon: Oregon State University.

Hojat, M. (2007). *Empathy in Patient Care: Antecedents, development, measurement and outcomes*. New York: Springer Science+Business Media.

Hojat, M., Bianco, J. A., Mann, D., Massello, D. & Calabrese, L. H. (2015). Overlap between empathy, teamwork and integrative approach to patient care. *Medical Teacher*, *37*(8): 755–8.

Hoover, J., Koon, A. D., Rosser, E. N. & Rao, K. D. (2020). Mentoring the working nurse: A scoping review. *Human Resources for Health*, *18*(1): 52.

Horgan, A. O., Donovan, M., Manning, F., Doody, R., Savage, E., Dorrity, C., O'Sullivan, H., Goodwin, J., Greaney, S., Biering, P., Bjornsson, E., Bocking, J., Russell, S., Griffin, M., MacGabhann, L., van der Vaart, K.J., Allon, J., Granerud, A., Hals, E., Pulli, J., Vatula, A., Ellilä, H., Lahti, M. & Happell, B. (2020). 'Meet Me Where I Am': Mental health service users' perspectives on the desirable qualities of a mental health nurse. *International Journal of Mental Health Nursing*, 30(1).

Horvath, A. O. & Bedi, R. P. (2002). The alliance. In J. C. Norcross (ed.), *Psychotherapy Relationships That Work: Therapist contributions and responsiveness to patients* (pp. 37–70). New York: Oxford University Press.

Hurley, J. & Lakeman, R. (2011). Becoming a psychiatric/mental health nurse in the UK: A qualitative study exploring processes of identity formation. *Issues in Mental Health Nursing*, *32*(12): 745–51.

Hurley, J. & Rankin, R. (2008). As mental health nursing roles expand, is education expanding mental health nurses? An emotionally intelligent view towards preparation for psychological therapies and relatedness. *Nursing Inquiry*, *15*(3): 199–205.

Hutchinson, M. & Hurley, J. (2013). Exploring leadership capability and emotional intelligence as moderators of workplace bullying. *Journal of Nursing Management*, *21*(3): 553–62.

Jack, K., Hamshire, C. & Chambers, A. (2017). The influence of role models in undergraduate nurse education. *Journal of Clinical Nursing*, *26*(23–24): 4707–15.

Johnstone, L., Boyle, M., with Cromby, J., Dillon, J., Harper, D., Kinderman, P., Longden, E., Pilgrim, D. & Read, J. (2018). The Power Threat Meaning Framework: Towards the identification of patterns in emotional distress, unusual experiences and troubled or troubling behaviour, as an alternative to functional psychiatric diagnosis. Leicester: British Psychological Society. Retrieved from www.bps.org.uk/PTM-Main

Jones, K. A. (2012). Developing the therapeutic use of self in the health care professional through autoethnography: Working with the borderline personality disorder population. *The International Journal of Qualitative Methods*, *11*(5): 573–84

Judge, D. S., Opsahl, A. & Robinson, D. (2018). Collaboration between two schools of nursing: Emotional intelligence education for prelicensure students. *Teaching and Learning in Nursing*, *13*(4): 244–6.

Kameg, K. M., Szpak, J. L., Cline, T. W. & McDermott, D. S. (2014). Utilization of standardized patients to decrease nursing student anxiety. *Clinical Simulation in Nursing*, *10*(11): 567–73.

Kanbay, Y. & Okanli, A. (2017). The effect of critical thinking education on nursing students' problem-solving skills. *Contemporary Nurse*, *53*(3): 313–21.

Lagarde, V. & Msellati, A. (2017). The effects of the care program on the therapeutic process. *L'information Psychiatrique*, *93*(5): 381–6.

Lakeman, R. & Hurley, J. (2021). What mental health nurses have to say about themselves: A discourse analysis. *International Journal of Mental Health Nursing*, *30*: 126–35.

Lakeman, R. & Molloy, L. (2018) Rise of the zombie institution, the failure of mental health nursing leadership, and mental health nursing as a zombie category. *International Journal of Mental Health Nursing*, *27*(3): 1009–14.

Levett-Jones, T., Gersbach, J., Arthur, C. & Roche, J. (2011). Implementing a clinical competency assessment model that promotes critical reflection and ensures nursing graduates' readiness for professional practice. *Nurse Education in Practice*, *11*(1): 64–9.

Levett-Jones, T., Hoffman, K., Dempsey, Y., Jeong, S. Y.-S., Noble, D., Norton, C. A., Roche, J. & Hickey, N. (2009). The 'five rights' of clinical reasoning: an educational model to enhance nursing students' ability to identify and manage clinically 'at risk' patients. *Nurse Education Today*, *30*(6): 515–20.

Light, E. M., Robertson, M. D., Boyce, P., Carney, T., Rosen, A., Cleary, M., Hunt, G. E., O'Connor, N., Ryan, C. & Kerridge, I. H. (2014). The lived experience of involuntary community treatment: a qualitative study of mental health consumers and carers. *Australasian Psychiatry*, *22*(4): 345–51.

Lindquist, R., Tracy, M. F. & Snyder, M. (2018). *Complementary and Alternative Therapies in Nursing*. Springer Publishing Company.

Louth, J., Mackay, T., Karpetis, G. & Goodwin-Smith, I. (2019). Understanding vicarious trauma. Exploring cumulative stress, fatigue and trauma in a frontline community services setting. Adelaide: The Australian Alliance for Social Enterprise, University of South Australia. Retrieved from https://centacare.org.au/wp-content/uploads/corporate/VicariousTraumaReport.pdf

Maiorano, A., Lasalvia, A., Sampogna, G., Pocai, B., Ruggeri, M. & Henderson, C. (2017). Reducing stigma in media professionals: Is there room for improvement? Results from a systematic review. *The Canadian Journal of Psychiatry*, *62*(10): 702–15.

Mayer, J. D., Caruso, D. R. & Salovey, P. (2016). The ability model of emotional intelligence: Principles and updates. *Emotion Review*, *8*(4): 290–300.

McAllister, S., Robert, G., Tsianakas, V. & McCrae, N. (2019). Conceptualising nurse-patient therapeutic engagement on acute mental health wards: An integrative review. *International Journal of Nursing Studies*, *93*: 106–18.

Miller, S. D., Hubble, M. A., Seidel, J. A., Chow, D. & Bargmann, S. (2014). Focus on clinical practice: Feedback informed treatment (FIT) – Achieving clinical excellence one person at a time. *Bulletin of Psychologists in Independent Practice*, Summer: 78–82.

Mills, J., Wand, T. & Fraser, J. A. (2018). Exploring the meaning and practice of self-care among palliative care nurses and doctors: A qualitative study. *BMC Palliative Care*, *17*(1): 63.

Mills, J. E., Francis, K. L. & Bonner, A. (2005). Mentoring, clinical supervision and preceptoring: Clarifying the conceptual definitions for Australian rural nurses. A review of the literature. *Rural and Remote Health*, *5*(3): 70.

Montes-Berges, B. & Augusto, J. M. (2007). Exploring the relationship between perceived emotional intelligence, coping, social support and mental health in nursing students. *Journal of Psychiatric and Mental Health Nursing*, *14*(2): 163–71.

Norcross, J. C., Beutler, L. E. & Levant, R. F. (2006). *Evidence-based Practices in Mental Health: Debate and dialogue on the fundamental questions*. Washington, DC: American Psychological Association.

Nursing Council of New Zealand. (2012). *Competencies for Registered Nurses*. Retrieved from www.nursingcouncil.org.nz

Oghene, J., Pos, A. & Geller, S. (2010). Therapist presence, empathy and the alliance in experiential treatment for depression. Unpublished honors thesis, York University, Toronto, Canada.

Patterson, C., Cregan, A., Moxham, L., Perlman, D., Taylor, E. K., Brighton, R., Molloy, L., Cutler, N. & Picton, C. (2017). Recovery camp: An innovative, positive education. *Australian Nursing and Midwifery Journal*, *25*(2): 42.

Peplau, H. E. (1952). Interpersonal relations in nursing. *American Journal of Nursing*, *52*(6): 765.

——— (1997). Peplau's theory of interpersonal relations. *Nursing Science Quarterly*, *14*(2): 162–7.

Proctor, B. (1986). Supervision: A cooperative exercise in accountability. In M. Marken & M. Payne (eds), *Enabling and Ensuring: Supervision in practice* (pp. 21–34). Leicester, UK: National Youth Bureau and Council for Education and Training in Youth and Community Work.

——— (2008). *Group Supervision: A Guide to creative practice*, 2nd edn. Thousand Oaks, CA: Sage Publications Ltd.

Riley, R. & Weiss, M. C. (2016). A qualitative thematic review: Emotional labour in healthcare settings. *Journal of Advanced Nursing*, *72*(1): 6–17.

Rosser, E. A., Scammell, J., Heaslip, V., White, S., Phillips, J., Cooper, K., Donaldson, I. & Hemingway, A. (2019). Caring values in undergraduate nurse students: A qualitative longitudinal study. *Nurse Education Today*, *77*: 65–70.

Rossi, A., Cetrano, G., Pertile, R., Rabbi, L., Donisi, V., Grigoletti, L. ... Amaddeo, F. (2012). Burnout, compassion fatigue, and compassion satisfaction among staff in community-based mental health services. *Psychiatry Research, 200*(2): 933–8.

Rubenfeld, M. & Scheffer, B. (2006). *Critical Thinking Tactics For Nurses*. Boston: Jones and Bartlett.

Salovey, P. & Mayer, J. D. (1990). Emotional intelligence. *Imagination, Cognition and Personality, 9*(3): 185–211.

Salzmann-Erikson, M. & Eriksson, H. (2012). Panoptic power and mental health nursing – Space and surveillance in relation to staff, patients, and neutral places. *Issues in Mental Health Nursing, 33*(8): 500–4.

Scheffer, B. & Rubenfeld, M. (2000). A consensus statement on critical thinking in nursing. *Journal of Nursing Education, 39*: 352–9.

Siegel, D. J. (2012). *The Norton series on interpersonal neurobiology. Pocket guide to interpersonal neurobiology: An integrative handbook of the mind*. New York: W W Norton & Co.

Sharp, S., McAllister, M. & Broadbent, M. (2016). The vital blend of clinical competence and compassion: How patients experience person-centred care. *Contemporary Nurse, 52*(2–3): 300–12.

Shevlin, M., Houston, J. E., Dorahy, M. J. & Adamson, G. (2008). Cumulative traumas and psychosis: an analysis of the national comorbidity survey and the British Psychiatric Morbidity Survey. *Schizophrenia Bulletin, 34*(1): 193–9.

Stensrud, B., Høyer, G., Beston, G., Granerud, A. & Landheim, A. S. (2016). 'Care or control?': A qualitative study of staff experiences with outpatient commitment orders. *Social Psychiatry and Psychiatric Epidemiology, 51*(5): 747–55.

Stewart, A. (2017). *Critical Thinking in Nursing: A critical discourse analysis of a perpetual paradox*. Auckland: Auckland University of Technology.

Stewart, B. M. & Krueger, L. E. (1996). An evolutionary concept analysis of mentoring in nursing. *Journal of Professional Nursing, 12*: 311–321.

Stewart, V., Crozier, M. & Wheeler, A. (2016). Interprofessional learning issues in postgraduate mental health education. *Journal of Social Inclusion, 7*(1).

Stuhlmiller, C. & Tolchard, B. (2019). Understanding the impact of mental health placements on student nurses' attitudes towards mental illness. *Nurse Education in Practice, 34*: 25–30.

Thornicroft, G., Mehta, N., Clement, S., Evans-Lacko, S., Doherty, M., Rose, D., Koschorke, M., Shidhaye, R., O'Reilly, C. & Henderson, C. (2016). Evidence for effective interventions to reduce mental-health-related stigma and discrimination. *The Lancet, 387*(10023): 1123–32.

Trede, F., Sutton, K. & Bernoth, M. (2016). Conceptualisations and perceptions of the nurse preceptor's role: A scoping review. *Nurse Education Today, 36*: 268–74.

Varese, F., Smeets, F., Drukker, M., Lieverse, R., Lataster, T., Viechtbauer, W. ... Bentall, R. P. (2012). Childhood adversities increase the risk of psychosis: A meta-analysis of patient-control, prospective-and cross-sectional cohort studies. *Schizophrenia Bulletin, 38*(4): 661–71.

White, E. & Winstanley, J. (2010). A randomised controlled trial of clinical supervision: Selected findings from a novel Australian attempt to establish the evidence base for causal relationships with quality of care and patient outcomes, as an informed contribution to mental health nursing practice development. *Journal of Research in Nursing, 15*(2): 151–67.

—— (2011). Clinical supervision for mental health professionals: The evidence base. *Social Work and Social Sciences Review, 14*(3): 77–94.

—— (2014). *Clinical Supervision: Predicting best outcomes. Research monograph*. Sydney: Osman Consulting Pty Ltd.

Williams, C. L. & Davis, C. M. (2005). *Therapeutic Interaction in Nursing*. Ontario: Jones and Bartlett Publishers.

Wyder, M., Bland, R., Blythe, A., Matarasso, B. & Crompton, D. (2015). Therapeutic relationships and involuntary treatment orders: service users' interactions with health-care professionals on the ward. *International Journal of Mental Health Nursing, 24*(2): 181–9.

Wyder, M., Ehrlich, C., Crompton, D., McArthur, L., Delaforce, C., Dziopa, F. ... Powell, E. (2017). Nurses experiences of delivering care in acute inpatient mental health settings: A narrative synthesis of the literature. *International Journal of Mental Health Nursing, 26*(6): 527–40.

Conclusions

Leadership and mentoring for person-centred mental health practice

Nicholas Procter, Mark Loughhead and Davi Macedo

21

Introduction

By now, readers of this book will have been thinking quite deeply about how to collaborate with and support people with a mental illness and their families and carers. The preceding chapters have given considerable emphasis to a narrative approach. This final chapter is orientated towards a discussion of leadership – particularly for new entrants into mental health settings.

Effective clinical care is person-centred and family centred. It seeks to understand and involve consumers, carers and families in rich discussions about their needs, preferences and values. This understanding and involvement is also combined with evidence-based practice to support consumers in their treatment and recovery goals.

At the heart of the decision to take this approach in this book has been a fundamental belief in human connectedness. By working through each of the chapters, readers will have been challenged to think about how and when to move in new ways when working with resilient and vulnerable people, which might be helpful across a range of practice settings when seeking to make a difference in the lives of people experiencing a mental illness. And while this is important in providing a theoretical and practical basis for care, it is at the point of care that effective leadership is required.

A message of leadership

What we say, do, think and feel as health professionals can be an expression of leadership. This approach speaks directly to the process of making sense of what people around us are doing together and how best to understand, engage and be committed to support each other (Holm & Severinsson, 2010). Why is this important? Because there have been and continue to be reports of people with mental illness not accessing mental health care. Many in the sector advocate that change is urgently needed, and that to continue with the current inadequate rate of reform, to utilise the same governance structures and fail to invest in innovation, is to condemn many of the most disadvantaged to many more years of poor mental and physical health (Procter, 2003). This points towards the importance of shared leadership and systems change.

Trust and compassion in leadership

Recent discussions among consumers, carers, practitioners and policymakers have centred upon finding new ways to express leadership in mental health practice (Mental Health and Substance Use Research Group (MHSURG), 2016). Compassion – the ability to provide genuine understanding, kindness and care – is a key attribute needed by everyone across the continuum of care. The emerging idea of *compassionate leadership* in mental health service delivery means that staff at all levels should demonstrate active empathy as a therapeutic means of making an emotional connection with people in mental distress.

Such activity is also central to building trust in mental health care. In *trust leadership*, carers and practitioners are poised to create a guiding partnership towards consumer recovery processes that have value and meaning, primarily for the consumer.

Trust is what brings people together in mental health care; it has the potential to do much more than help people achieve the same health outcomes or objectives. In the context of clinical leadership, trust is embedded in the everyday professionalism of practitioners: the ways in which they seek to provide interventions marked by quality and safety across care episodes; in what they say, do, think and feel; in documentation; in telephone conversations; and during face-to-face contact. In *trust leadership*, therapeutic processes are not limited by professional disciplinary boundaries. Trust also runs two ways. Recovery requires clinicians to trust the priorities of the consumer, to recognise opportunities and look beyond a focus on risk. Trust requires clinicians to support the perspectives of consumers and to recognise and actively work to reduce power differentials in the relationship, and across organisations.

Lived experience leadership

Lived experience leadership is the activity of consumers and carers who lead change in mental health. There are many areas of activity where people with lived experience have acted to assist others, to shape local services and to shape national policy. This leadership operates in teaching environments, in advocacy, service-level governance, research and in peer support work (Stewart et al., 2019). *Lived experience leadership* is playing a stronger role in the commissioning and co-production of services in Australia, including the emergence of peer-run organisations and services.

Lived experience leaders, particularly consumer leaders, play a critical role in the reform of Australian mental health care. Experienced consumer advocates, as well as peer support leaders, work to apply their lived experience with a clear purpose. This involves communicating on common topics in mental health care, from the collective perspective of consumers. This might reflect common experiences of help-seeking, acute care or emergency department experience, or being under an order of a Mental Health Act. A consumer 'lens' is likely to include insights about discrimination, stigma and trauma due to mental health service use, or experience of other services, as well as preferred helping roles. Leaders seek change from the perspectives of social justice, human rights and citizenship, with some advocating for a radical reshaping of the sector, while others seek reform within the current psychosocial, clinically led models of care (Daya, Hamilton & Roya, 2019). The skill set of leaders is to articulate a vision for change, raise awareness of other decision makers and lead a culture of inclusion (Stewart et al., 2019).

The recognition and valuing of *lived experience leadership* is vital for emerging health practitioners. This should occur on all levels including in the recovery or clinical relationship, within local organisations and in the ways in which state, territory and national services are produced. Health practitioners, including nurses, can play an important role by being allies in supporting the changes that lived experience recommends. This includes recognising the role of peer support, values of acceptance, inclusion and justice, and people's preferred language for describing distress and trauma. Being an ally or supporter of lived experience encourages health practitioners to see that services can be disempowering, and limiting, and to recognise the privilege that professionals have in decision-making and providing access to resources. Using this privilege, allies can support the principles of *lived experience leadership* and co-production, and can work to create spaces for the voices of those with lived experience. This is in contrast to the common professional role of speaking for consumer and carer experience and interests (Happell & Scholz, 2018). The saying 'nothing about us, without us' has been an enduring anthem of the lived-experience movement in Australia, and in contemporary terms, demands that health practitioners share agenda-setting, knowledge production and decision-making, acknowledging that lived expertise sits alongside professional, learned expertise. This acknowledgement of the need for co-production means there are times when health practitioners should take the back seat as listeners and learners, and engage with the ideas, considerations and leadership of lived experience. This stance enables emerging lived-experience leaders to access increased opportunities for development of skills and knowledge in leading groups, chairing meetings, shaping deliberation and activating networks. A further role in supporting lived-experience leadership is to encourage emerging leaders to find pathways for peer-based learning, supervision, mentoring and connection.

The need to self-question

Leadership in mental health is across all levels of practice, education and service delivery (Sayers et al., 2015). Embracing a leadership role at all levels is fundamental in clinical practice, in order to influence consumer-centred care (Sayers et al., 2015). There will be, among many things, the need to self-question (Rozuel & Ketola, 2012). Clinical leaders at all levels can begin by reflecting upon what it is they do and to what extent it is in the best interest of consumers, their families and clinical colleagues (Procter, 2003). Is the person primarily a leader or a manager? Do they make long-term decisions about their development, or does the employer? Does the leader have the opportunity or right to challenge those decisions? Do they have the obligation to challenge what is happening within the practice setting (adapted from Goldsmith, 2003)?

What then might be the best way to influence and lead? Perhaps the answer begins with communicating respect and warmth, because 'Warmth is the conduit to influence: It facilitates trust and the communication and absorption of ideas. Prioritising warmth helps you connect immediately with those around you, demonstrating that you hear them, understand them, and can be trusted by them' (Cuddy, Kohut & Neffinger, 2013, p. 56).

Also important are positive working relationships, healthy resolution of conflict, debriefing, support and discussion. This involves focusing on what practitioners say, do, think and feel, for leadership growth and capacity-building. Empowerment for new and emerging leaders is, in this sense, more than 'being able to simply voice an opinion (although clearly that is important too); it gives a broad range of people the authority to make decisions and express points of view that matter' (Kets de Vries, 2001, p. 272).

Empowerment also contributes to the positive workplace culture required in an interdisciplinary world marked by potential collaborative failures across nursing and allied healthcare disciplines (see Freshwater, Cahill & Essen, 2014). The cultivation of positive workplace cultures can also be a platform for delivery of evidence-based practices and can foster a collaborative and supportive work environment (Clearly et al., 2011). Extending this stance, clinical leaders also need to shape workplace cultures to be inclusive, supportive and acknowledging of lived-experience workforces. Positive culture, here, often entails continuing self-reflection on power and privilege, working with resistance, and supporting the recovery and citizenship paradigm.

Clinical mentoring and empowerment

Clinical leadership and mentoring opportunities for beginning practitioners in mental health can also be seen as a reciprocal process whereby people learn from each other to recognise areas for personal and professional growth and further development (Blegen & Severinsson 2011). Leadership and management in the context of person-centered care are human activities that imply strong values of respect, embedded in mutual relationships. The idea is that personal and professional leadership development can be inclusive of personal and professional goal-setting and feedback to help identify best practices and how to grow and move in new ways. Central to this learning is information about consumer experience and recovery outcomes, both from the practitioner's own practice and their team. Here, professional development is informed by positive or negative feedback from consumer, carer and peer-worker perspectives, as well as other recovery and safety data.

When workplace mentoring and support are done well, they can be greatly empowering, facilitating self-discovery and the creation of new learning about emotional well-being (Kets de Vries, 2013; Phoenix 2013). Mentoring in clinical practice is marked by a supportive learning relationship. Having a trusted advisor (for example) to facilitate practice-based mentoring can be an effective way to encourage and develop emerging leaders, with particular emphasis upon their creativity and imagination (Sayers et al., 2015). This, in turn, enables those working in mental health to learn about how self-motivation and drive can assist in abandoning ineffective practices, attitudes and beliefs (Procter, 2003). Moreover, effective mentoring becomes a crucial means through which to help maintain a sense of purpose, commitment and ethical comportment in practice.

Expressed in this way, leadership in mental health draws upon formal and informal relationships and supports, which are mutually beneficial and incentive-building. In meeting these challenges, some enabling objectives include:

- Entering into a productive relationship with consumers and carers, as well as with clinical colleagues, clinical mentors and lived-experience leaders, for continuous self-reflection and personal and professional development.
- Facilitating personal and professional development initiatives that target areas for future growth and the advancement of recovery with dignity for consumers and their families; seeking out opportunities for information exchange and support in the workplace.
- Demonstrating cultural and emotional intelligence (see Hurley, 2013). Emerging leaders know how to manage their own emotions, read the emotions of others and communicate effectively.
- Creating a dedicated time for confidential debriefing with managers and/or mentors in a variety of settings about the nature and scope of your involvement with consumers and other mental health professionals.

Viewed in this way, your journey as an emerging leader is marked by personal and professional growth. At the outset of this process, mentors and other trusted guides are central to discussion of professional and personal goals. These initial discussions – to be incorporated into a personalised professional development plan – are intended to discuss the range of perceived needs *before* planning any specific learning objectives. There should also be scope and freedom to receive feedback from others and, consequently, to review goals (Procter, 2003). The main intention is to create learning opportunities within a cohesive, dynamic team in which people feel valued and involved. Mentoring and career support in mental health settings are, therefore, ways to identify personal characteristics, enhance inherent skills and improve individual development (Jenkins, 2012).

REFERENCES

Blegen, N. E. & Severinsson, E. (2011). Leadership and management in mental health nursing. *Journal of Nursing Management*, *19*(4): 487–97.

Clearly, M., Horsfall, J., Deacon, M. & Jackson, D. (2011). Leadership and mental health nursing. *Issues in Mental Health Nursing*, *32*: 632–9.

Cuddy, A. J. C., Kohut, M. & Neffinger, J. (2013). Connect, then lead. *Harvard Business Review* (July–August): 55–61.

Daya, I., Hamilton, B. & Roper, C. (2019). Authentic engagement: A conceptual model for welcoming diverse and challenging consumer and survivor views in mental health research, policy, and practice. *International Journal of Mental Health Nursing*, *29*(2): 299–311.

Freshwater, D., Cahill, J. & Essen, C. (2014). Discourses of collaborative failure: Identity, role and discourse in an interdisciplinary world. *Nursing Inquiry*, *21*(1): 59–68.

Goldsmith, M. (2003). The changing role of leadership. In L. Segil, M. Goldsmith & J. Belasco (eds), *Partnering: The new face of leadership*. New York: American Management Association.

Happell, B. & Scholz, B. (2018). Doing what we can, but knowing our place: Being an ally to promote consumer leadership in mental health. *International Journal of Mental Health Nursing*, *27*(1): 440–7.

Holm, A. L. & Severinsson, E. (2010). The role of mental health nursing leadership. *Journal of Nursing Management*, *18*: 463–71.

Hurley, J. (2013). Perceptual shifts of priority: A qualitative study bringing emotional intelligence to the foreground for nurses in talk-based therapy roles. *Journal of Psychiatric & Mental Health Nursing*, *20*(2): 97–104.

Jenkins, D. M. (2012). Exploring signature pedagogies in undergraduate leadership education. *Journal of Leadership Education*, *11*: 1–27.

Kets de Vries, M. (2001). *The Leadership Mystique: A user's manual for the human enterprise*. London: Prentice Hall.

——— (2013). Coaching's 'good hour': Creating tipping points. *Coaching: An International Journal of Theory, Research and Practice*, *6*(2): 152–75.

Mental Health and Substance Use Research Group (MHSURG). (2016) *Shared Learning in Clinical Practice: Mental Health Practice Development Newsletter*. September: 11. Retrieved from http://www.unisa.edu.au/PageFiles/152570/SLICP%20Newsletter%20Issue%2011%20 September%202016.pdf

Phoenix, B. J. (2013). Developing a culture of mentoring in psychiatric mental health nursing. *Journal of the American Psychiatric Nurses Association*, *19*(4): 215–16.

Procter, N. G. (2003). Leadership and mentoring for mental health service reform (Editorial). *Contemporary Nurse*, *14*: 223–6.

Rozuel, C. & Ketola, T. (2012). A view from within: Exploring the psychology of responsible leadership. Guest editorial. *Journal of Management Development*, *31*: 444–8.

Sayers, J., Lopez, V., Howard, P. B., Escott, P. & Cleary, M. (2015). The leadership role of nurse educators in mental health nursing. *Issues in Mental Health Nursing*, *36*(9): 718–24.

Stewart, S., Scholz, B., Gordon, S. & Happell, B. (2019). 'It depends what you mean by leadership': An analysis of stakeholder perspectives on consumer leadership. *International Journal of Mental Health Nursing*, *28*(1): 339–50.

Index